An Algorithm Approach to

PEDIATRIC DIAGNOSIS

An Algorithm Approach to
PEDIATRIC DIAGNOSIS

Editor-in-Chief

GV Basavaraja
MBBS MD DNB
Professor of Pediatrics and Head of PICU
Department of Pediatrics
Indira Gandhi Institute of Child Health
Bengaluru, Karnataka, India
National President, 2024

Managing Editors

Vasant M Khalatkar
MD FIAP PG Dip Inf Dis (UNSW)
Director
Khalatkar Hospital for Mother and Child
Nagpur, Maharashtra, India
President Elect 2024

Yogesh N Parikh
MD (Pediatrics)
Professor, Department of Pediatrics
Government Medical College, Surat
Former Professor and Head
Department of Pediatrics
PDU Government Medical
College and KT Children Hospital
Rajkot, Gujarat, India
Secretary General
Indian Academy of Pediatrics (2024–2025)

Atanu Bhadra
DCH FIAP
Superintendent
ESI Hospital
Asansol, West Bengal, India
National Treasurer
Indian Academy of Pediatrics (2024–2025)

Academic Editors

Gnanamurthy Narasimha
FIAP FAAP DCH
Private Practitioner
Mother and Child Care Centre
Bengaluru, Karnataka, India

Sumitha Nayak
MD DNB FIAP Adv Certificate in Vaccinology
(IVI KOREA & CMC Vellore)
Consultant Pediatrician
Shishu—The Children's Clinic
Bengaluru, Karnataka, India

Executive Editors

Janani Shankar
DNB PhD
Medical Director and Senior Consultant
Department of Pediatric Medicine
Kanchi Kamakoti CHILDS Trust Hospital
Chennai, Tamil Nadu, India

B Rajsekhar
MD (Pediatrics)
Associate Medical Director and
Senior Consultant Pediatrician
Department of Pediatrics
Giggles by Omni Hospital
Visakhapatnam, Andhra Pradesh, India

Kripasindhu Chatterjee
MD DCH FIAP
Professor and Head
Department of Pediatrics
Gouri Devi Institute of Medical Sciences and Hospital
Rajbandh, West Bengal, India

Nehal Patel
MBBS MD (Pediatrics) IBCLC
Professor and Head
Department of Pediatrics
GMERS Medical College and Hospital
Ahmedabad, Gujarat, India

Rupesh Masand
MD (Pediatrics)
Professor
Department of Pediatrics
National Institute of Medical Sciences and Research
Jaipur, Rajasthan, India

Foreword
GV Basavaraja

JAYPEE
JAYPEE BROTHERS MEDICAL PUBLISHERS
The Health Sciences Publisher
New Delhi | London

Jaypee Brothers Medical Publishers (P) Ltd

Headquarters
Jaypee Brothers Medical Publishers (P) Ltd
EMCA House, 23/23-B
Ansari Road, Daryaganj
New Delhi 110 002, India
Landline: +91-11-23272143, +91-11-23272703
+91-11-23282021, +91-11-23245672
Email: jaypee@jaypeebrothers.com

Corporate Office
Jaypee Brothers Medical Publishers (P) Ltd
4838/24, Ansari Road, Daryaganj
New Delhi 110 002, India
Phone: +91-11-43574357
Fax: +91-11-43574314
Email: jaypee@jaypeebrothers.com

Overseas Office
JP Medical Ltd.
83, Victoria Street, London
SW1H 0HW (UK)
Phone: +44 20 3170 8910
Fax: +44 (0)20 3008 6180
Email: info@jpmedpub.com

Website: www.jaypeebrothers.com
Website: www.jaypeedigital.com

Inquiries for bulk sales may be solicited at: jaypee@jaypeebrothers.com

An Algorithm Approach to Pediatric Diagnosis

First Edition: **2025**

ISBN: 978-93-6616-434-2

Printed at: Samrat Offset Pvt. Ltd.

Dedicated to

All the children and adolescents who have helped to hone our skills and who will continue to challenge our knowledge and skills in the future.

Contributors

Aaradhana Singh MD (Pediatrics)
Professor
Department of Pediatrics
University College of Medical Sciences
and Guru Teg Bahadur Hospital
New Delhi, India

Abhay Shivpuri DNB (Pediatrics) IAP
Fellowship Pediatric Rheumatology RCPCH
Fellowship Pediatric Rheumatology, GOSH UK,
EULAR Cert Pediatric Rheumatology and MSK
Ultrasound
Consultant
Department of Pediatric Rheumatology
Neo Clinic Children's Hospital
Jaipur, Rajasthan, India

Aditi MD DM
Assistant Professor
Department of Pediatrics
All India Institute of Medical Sciences
Bhubaneswar, Odisha, India

Ajeitha Loganathan
MD (Pediatrics) Post Doctoral Fellowship
in Ped Hemato– Oncology
Consultant
Department of Oncology
G Kuppuswamy Naidu Memorial
Hospital
Coimbatore, Tamil Nadu, India

Akash Bang MD DNB MNAMS PGDMLS
IDPCCM
Additional Professor
Department of Pediatrics
All India Institute of Medical Sciences
Nagpur, Maharashtra, India

Akshay BK
MS (ENT & Head & Neck Surgery)
Associate Consultant
Department of ENT
Trustwell Hospitals Pvt Ltd
Bengaluru, Karnataka, India

Amulya K MBBS MD
Clinical Associate
Department of Pediatrics
Rainbow Children Hospital
Hyderabad, Telangana, India

Ananda Kesavan TM MD MNAMS FIAP
FIAMS PGDDN FRCP (Edin)
Professor
Department of Pediatrics
Government Medical College
Thrissur, Kerala, India

Anita Sharma MD DM (Child Neurology)
Senior Consultant, Former Senior
Professor and In-charge
(Child Neurology)
Department of Pediatrics
Centre for Epilepsy and Child Neurology
Arcus Health Services
New Delhi, India

Antony Robert Charles MCh DNBE MS
MRCS (Edin)
Senior Consultant
Department of Pediatric Surgery and
Pediatric Urology
Rainbow Children's Hospital
Bengaluru, Karnataka, India

Anurag Bajpai MD (Ped) FRACP
Pediatric Endocrinology, RCH, Melbourne SCE
(Endocrinology)
Pediatric and Adolescent
Endocrinologist
Department of Pediatric Endocrinology
Regency Centre for Diabetes,
Endocrinology and Research
Kanpur, Uttar Pradesh, India

Arathi Srinivasan DNB Post-Doctoral
Fellowship in Pediatric Hemato-oncology
Head and Senior Consultant
Pediatric Hemato-oncology
Kanchi Kamakoti CHILDS Trust Hospital
Chennai, Tamil Nadu, India

Arijit Chattopadhyay DCH MD MRCP
FRCPCH CCST (Pediatric Neurology, UK)
Senior Consultant
Department of Pediatric Neurology
Apollo Multispecialty Hospital
Kolkata, West Bengal, India

Arti Pawaria MD (Ped) PDCC (Ped
Gastroenterology) DM (Ped Hepatology and
Transplant)
Clinical Lead, Senior Consultant and
Assistant Professor
Department of Pediatric
Gastroenterology, Hepatology and Liver
Transplantation
Amrita Institute of Medical Sciences
Faridabad, Haryana, India

Arun YB MBBS MD DNB Fellowship in
Pediatric Neurology
Assistant Professor
Department of Pediatrics
Indira Gandhi Institute of Child Health
Bengaluru, Karnataka, India

AS Kireeti MD
Professor
Department of Pediatrics
SVRR Government General Hospital
Tirupati, Andhra Pradesh, India

Ashim Kumar Ghosh DCH PGDAP
Senior Practicing Pediatrician and
Adolescent Pediatrician
Department of Pediatrics
Practising Pediatrician Chamber...
Pratiksha
Asansol, West Bengal, India

Ashish Mehta MD (Ped) DCH (Sydney Uni)
Fellow in Neonatology, College of Pediatric,
Australia
Director and Consultant Neonatologist
Arpan Newborn Care Center Pvt Ltd
Ahmedabad, Gujarat, India

Contributors

Ashka Prajapati MD (Pediatrics)
Fellowship in Clinical Genetics
Consultant Clinical Geneticist
Department of Inherited Genomic Medicine
Genetic Care Clinic, Neuberg Centre for Genomic Medicine
Ahmedabad, Gujarat, India

Asok Kumar Datta MD FIAP
Professor
Department of Pediatrics
Santiniketan Medical College
Bolpur, West Bengal, India

Atanu Bhadra DCH FIAP
Superintendent
ESI Hospital
Asansol, West Bengal, India

Aathira Ravindranath MD DM
Superintendent
ESI Hospital
Asansol, West Bengal, India
National Treasurer
Indian Academy of Pediatrics
(2024–2025)

B Rajsekhar MD (Pediatrics)
Associate Medical Director and Senior Consultant Pediatrician
Department of Pediatrics
Giggles by Omni Hospital
Visakhapatnam, Andhra Pradesh, India

Balachandra BV MBBS MD (Pediatrics)
Consultant Pediatrician and Allergy Asthma Specialist
MedTrain, Allergy Central, Aadya Health Sciences Pvt Ltd
Manipal Hospital
Bengaluru, Karnataka, India

Bela Verma MD DCH
Professor and Head
Department of Pediatrics
Grant Govt Medical College and Sir JJ hospital
Mumbai, Maharashtra, India

Bhadra Trivedi MD (Pediatrics) Fellowship in Pediatric Cardiology
Consultant Pediatric Cardiologist and Professor of Pediatrics
Department of Pediatrics and Pediatric Cardiology
Parul Sevashram Hospital
Vadodara, Gujarat, India

Bhaskar Shenoy MD (Ped) FRCPCH
Fellowship in Pediatric ID, Dip in Infectious Diseases
Head (Pediatrics)
Chief, Division of Pediatric Infectious Diseases
Manipal Hospital
Bengaluru, Karnataka, India

Bhavi S Barchha MD (Ped) FPC (Pediatric Cardiology)
Consultant
Department of Pediatric Cardiology
Plexus Med Care
Rajkot, Gujarat, India

Bhavya Verma MD (Pediatrics)
Assistant Professor
Department of Pediatrics
Vyas Medical College
Jodhpur, Rajasthan, India

Biraj Thakker DNB (Pediatric) FIAP (Neonatology)
Consultant Neonatologist and In-charge NICU
Department of Neonatal Intensive Care
Akanksha Hospital and Research Institute
Anand, Gujarat, India

C Vijayabhaskar MD (Dermatology)
Professor
Department of DVL
Government Stanley Medical College
Chennai, Tamil Nadu, India

Chidananda NK MBBS DNB (Pediatrics)
Consultant
Department of Pediatrics
Chiguru Child Care Centre
Bengaluru, Karnataka, India

Chiranjeet Narayan Dev MD (Pediatrics) Fellowship Pediatric Pulmonology
Clinical Fellow, Pediatric Pulmonology and Sleep Medicine
Department of Pediatrics
National University Hospital
Singapore

Chirantap Oza MBBS MD (Pediatrics)
Fellowship in Pediatric Endocrinology
Visiting Pediatric Endocrinologist
Department of Pediatrics
BJ Medical College and Civil Hospital, Ahmedabad
Consultant Pediatric Endocrinologist
EndoGrow Clinic
Ahmedabad, Gujarat, India

Chitra Sankar DCH MRCP PGDDN
Consultant (Developmental Pediatrics)
Manipal Hospital
Department of Pediatrics
Bengaluru, Karnataka, India

Debaditya Das DNB (Ped) DM (Endo)
Senior Resident
Department of Pediatrics
IPGMER and SSKM Hospital
Kolkata, West Bengal, India

Debasis Panigrahi MD (Pediatrics) PDF Pediatric Neurology
Consultant Pediatric Neurologist
Department of Pediatrics
Jagannath Hospital
Bhubaneswar, Odisha, India

Deepak V Haldipur MS (ENT & Head & Neck Surgery)
Director
Department of ENT
Trustwell Hospitals Pvt Ltd
Bengaluru, Karnataka, India

Dhiraj Mohan Gupta DCH DPAA
Consultant Pediatrician and Allergologist
Department of Pediatrics
Pankhuri Hospital Pvt Ltd
Varanasi, Uttar Pradesh, India

Dipti Pujari MD (Pediatrics) DNB DCH MRCPCH (UK) EAACI FACI
Consultant Pediatrician
Department of Pediatrics
Deenanath Mangeshkar Hospital and Research Centre
Pune, Maharashtra, India

Eshita Bhowmik MD (Pediatrics) PDCC (Pediatric Endocrinology) ESPE Fellow
Consultant Pediatrician and Pediatric Endocrinology
Department of Pediatrics
Aster Aadhar Hospital
Kolhapur, Maharashtra, India

Fagun Shah MD (Pediatrics) Fellowship in Pediatric Nephrology
Pediatric Nephrologist
Department of Pediatric Nephrology
Child's Kidney Care Center
Surat, Gujarat, India

G Sudhakar MD (Ped) DCH AASC (Allergy Asthma Specialist Course) FAAP (Fellowship Allergy Asthma Procedures) DPSM (Diploma Pediatric Sleep Medicine)
Former Professor
Department of Pediatrics
KIMS Hospital
Kurnool, Andhra Pradesh, India

Ganesh Jevalikar MD DNB (Ped) PDCC (Ped Endocrinology)
Principal Consultant
Department of Endocrinology and Diabetes
Max Healthcare
New Delhi, India

Ganesh Kulkarni DCH DNB
Director and CEO
Department of Pediatrics
Sanjeevani Children's Hospital
Aurangabad, Maharashtra, India

Gnanamurthy Narasimha FIAP FAAP DCH
Private Practitioner
Mother and Child Care Centre
Bengaluru, Karnataka, India

Gowri Somayaji MD
Consultant
Department of Pediatrics
Aruna Clinic
Bengaluru, Karnataka, India

GV Basavaraja MBBS MD DNB
Professor of Pediatrics and Head of PICU
Department of Pediatrics
Indira Gandhi Institute of Child Health
Bengaluru, Karnataka, India
National President, 2024

H Ravi Ramamurthy MD (Ped) FNB (Ped Cardiology)
Professor
Department of Pediatric Cardiology
Armed Forces Medical College
Army Institute of Cardiothoracic Sciences
Pune, Maharashtra, India

Hamsa V MBBS MD DM (Ped Nephro)
Assistant Professor
Department of Pediatrics
Ramaiah Medical College Hospital
Bengaluru, Karnataka, India

Hania Qamar Khan MBBS MD DVL FRGUHS Paediatric Dermatology, RCPUK SCE Dermatology
Specialty Doctor Dermatology
Department of Dermatology
Mersey and West Lancashire Teaching Hospitals NHS Trust
England, UK

Harshini T Reddy MBBS DNB (Paediatrics)
Fellow
Department of Pediatric Infectious Diseases
Manipal Hospital
Bengaluru, Karnataka, India

Hema Gupta Mittal MD (Pediatrics) European Diploma in Pediatric Respiratory Medicine (ERS) DPAA
Professor (Pediatrics) and In-charge
Division of Pediatric Pulmonology
Atal Bihari Vajpayee Institute of Medical Sciences and Dr Ram Manohar Lohia Hospital
New Delhi, India

Hriday De MD (Ped) Fellowship in Pediatric and Adolescent Endocrinology
Assistant Professor
Department of Pediatrics
Institute of Child Health
Kolkata, West Bengal, India

HS Arora MD (Pediatrics) FNB (Pediatric Cardiology)
Professor and Consultant
Department of Pediatric Cardiology
Army Hospital (Research and Referral)
Dehradun, Uttarakhand, India

Hunsi Giri MD (Ped)
Faculty DCh Course
Department of Pediatrics
Ganesh Das Government MCH Hospital
Shillong, Meghalaya, India

Jagdish Prasad Goyal MD (Pediatrics)
Professor
Department of Pediatrics
All India Institute of Medical Sciences
Jodhpur, Rajasthan, India

Janani Shankar DNB PhD
Medical Director and Senior Consultant
Department of Pediatric Medicine
Kanchi Kamakoti CHILDS Trust Hospital
Chennai, Tamil Nadu, India

Jasodhara Chaudhuri MD (Pediatric Medicine) MRCPCH (UK) FRCPCH UK DM (Neurology)
Assistant Professor
Department of Pediatrics
NRS Medical College and Hospital
Kolkata, West Bengal, India

Javeed Iqbal Bhat MD (Pediatrics)
Additional Professor
Department of Pediatrics
Sher-i-Kashmir Institute of Medical Sciences
Srinagar, Jammu and Kashmir, India

Jay T Dhirwani MBBS MD (Pediatrics)
Consultant Pediatrician
Department of Pediatrics
Amrutaa Hospital and Samanvay Hospital
Rajkot, Gujarat, India

Jaydeb Ray MD (Paed) DCH DNB (Paed) MD (Com Med) FIAP FNNF FIAMS
Principal and Professor
Department of Pediatrics
Institute of Child Health
Kolkata, West Bengal, India

Jeevan Silwal MD DNB FIPN
Director
Department of Pediatric Neurologist
Athena Child Neuro Clinic
Siliguri, West Bengal, India
Member of AOCN, IAN, ICNA, IES

Joyance James Mammen MS (Orthopedics)
Senior Fellow Pediatric Orthopedics
Department of Pediatric Orthopedics
Ortho Kids Clinic
Ahmedabad, Gujarat, India

Joydeep Das MD
Professor and Head
Department of Pediatrics
Jagannath Gupta Institute of Medical Sciences College and Hospital
Kolkata, West Bengal, India

K Radhakrishna MD DCH
Chief Consultant
Department of Pediatrics
Giggles by Omni RK Hospital
Visakhapatnam, Andhra Pradesh, India

Kakoli Roy MD Fellowship in Paediatric and Adolescent Endocrinology
Assistant Professor
Department of Pediatrics
Nil Ratan Sircar Medical College and Hospital
Kolkata, West Bengal, India

Kalpana Datta Chatterjee MD FIAP
Professor and Head
Department of Pediatrics
Government Medical College
Kolkata, West Bengal, India

Kalpana Panda MBBS MD (Pediatrics) DNB DM
Associate Professor
Department of Pediatrics
Institute of Medical Sciences and SUM Hospital
Bhubaneswar, Odisha, India

Kana Ram Jat MD (Pediatrics)
Additional Professor
Department of Pediatrics
All India Institute of Medical Sciences
New Delhi, India

Kaustav Nayek MD
Director of Medical Education and Ex-Officio Secretary to the Government of West Bengal
Department of Health
Government of West Bengal

Keyur Mahajan MBBS DNB DPID (Oxford, UK)
Consultant
Department of Pediatric Infectious Diseases
Deenanath Mangeshkar Hospital and Research Centre
Pune, Maharashtra, India

Kinnari Vala Fellow in Pediatric Nephrology MD (Ped)
Head and In-charge
Department of Pediatric Nephrology
Smt. GR Doshi and KM Mehta Institute of Kidney Disease and Research Center
Ahmedabad, Gujarat, India

Kripasindhu Chatterjee MD DCH FIAP
Professor and Head
Department of Pediatrics
Gouri Devi Institute of Medical Sciences and Hospital
Rajbandh, West Bengal, India

Krishna Mohan DNB MNAMS DAA
Consultant Pediatrician
Kerala Government Health Services
Kozhikode, Kerala, India

Kunal P Ahya MD (Peds) Fellow in Neonatology
Director and Consultant
Department of Neonatology
MAAHI Newborn Care Centre
Rajkot, Gujarat, India

Lalit Bharadia MD DNB PDCC Fellowship Ped Gastro
Consultant
Department of Pediatric Gastroenterology
Neo Clinic Children Hospital
Jaipur, Rajasthan, India

Lalitha Wadhwa MD (Pediatrics)
Professor and Head
Department of Pediatrics
GITAM Institute of Medical Sciences and Research
Visakhapatnam, Andhra Pradesh, India

Madhu S Pujar MD (Ped)
Professor of Pediatrics and In-charge PICU
Bapuji Child Health Institute and Research Centre
Davanagere, Karnataka, India

Mahima Mittal MD
Professor and Head
Department of Pediatrics
All India Institute of Medical Sciences
Gorakhpur, Uttar Pradesh, India

Mandira Roy DNB (Pediatrics) PGDDN (Kerala)
Assistant Professor
Department of Pediatrics
Santiniketan Medical College and Hospital
Bolpur, West Bengal, India

Manikumar S DCH DNB (Pediatrics) DM (Neonatology)
Assistant Professor of Neonatology
Department of Neonatology
Government Chengalpattu Medical College
Chennai, Tamil Nadu, India

Manini Moudgal MBBS Diploma American Board of Pediatrics
Consultant Pediatrician
Kid Care Clinic
Mysuru, Karnataka, India

Manjusha K MBBS MD DCH DNB MNAMS MRCPCH MBA (HHSM) PGDMLE
Associate Professor
Department of Pediatrics
Sree Narayana Institute of Medical Sciences
Ernakulam, Kerala, India

Maulin Shah MS (Orthopedics) DNB (Orthopedics) Fellowship Pediatric Orthopedics
Chief
Department of Pediatric Orthopedics
Ortho Kids Clinic
Ahmedabad, Gujarat, India

Meena Sivasankaran DNB (Ped) FAIP (Ped Hemato-oncology) FNB (Ped Hemato-oncology)
Senior Consultant
Department of Pediatric Hemato-Oncology and BMT
Kanchi Kamakoti CHILDS Trust Hospital
Chennai, Tamil Nadu, India

Minal Ambade MD Fellowship Developmental and Behavioral Pediatrics
Assistant Professor
Department of Pediatrics
Datta Meghe Medical College
Nagpur, Maharashtra, India

MM Zameer MBBS MS (Gen Surg) MCh (Ped Surgery, PGIMER) MRCS (Edinburgh)
Senior Consultant
Department of Pediatric Surgery
Narayana Health
Bengaluru, Karnataka, India

Mohammad Asif MD (Pediatrics) DPAA
Professor and Head
Department of Pediatrics
RNT Medical College
Udaipur, Rajasthan, India

Mounika B DNB
Resident
Department of Pediatric Medicine
Kanchi Kamakoti CHILDS Trust Hospital
Chennai, Tamil Nadu, India

Mrutunjay Dash MD (Pediatrics)
Professor
Department of Pediatrics
Institute of Medical Sciences and SUM Hospital
Bhubaneswar, Odisha, India

M S Viswanathan MBBS MD (Paed) MRCPCH FRCPCH CCT (UK)
Senior Consultant
Department of Pediatric Gastroenterology
Apollo Children's Hospital
Chennai, Tamil Nadu, India

Munesh Tomar MD FNB (Pediatric Cardiology) FACC
Director and Head
Department of Pediatric Cardiology
Max Superspecialty Hospital
New Delhi, India

Nagalatha Chidananda MBBS DNB IBCLC
Pediatrician and Lactation Consultant
Department of Pediatrics
Rangadore Memorial Hospital
Bengaluru, Karnataka, India

Nagendra Kumar VR MD (Pediatrics) PDCC DM (Ped Gastroenterology)
Consultant
Department of Pediatric Gastroenterology and Hepatology
Rainbow Children Hospital and Indira Gandhi Institute of Child Health
Bengaluru, Karnataka, India

Nagesh A MBBS DCH DNB
Senior Pediatrician
Kidcare Clinic
Banashankari III Stage
Bengaluru, Karnataka, India

Naveen Parkash Gupta MD (Pediatrics) DNB (Neonatology) Fellowship in Neonatology (BC Children's Hospital, Vancouver, Canada)
Senior Consultant
Department of Neonatology
Madhukar Rainbow Children's Hospital
New Delhi, India
Secretary, NNF-Delhi (2024)

Neeraj Aggarwal MD (Pediatrics) Fellowship Ped Cardiology
Director Pediatric Cardiology
Department of Pediatric Cardiac Sciences
Sir Gangaram Hospital
New Delhi, India

Neha Agarwal MD PDCC (Ped Endocrinology)
Consultant Pediatric Endocrinologist
Department of Pediatrics
Regency Health Care
Lucknow, Uttar Pradesh, India

Nehal Patel
MBBS MD (Pediatrics) IBCLC
Professor and Head
Department of Pediatrics
GMERS Medical College and Hospital
Ahmedabad, Gujarat, India

Neminathan MD (Pediatrics) DCH
Consultant Pediatrician
Department of Pediatrics
Coimbatore Child Trust Hospital
Coimbatore, Tamil Nadu, India

Nihaz Naha MD Fellowship IAP
Senior Consultant
Department of Neonatology
Crescent Pediatrics and Neonatology
Aspire Children's Speciality Centre
Kozhikode, Kerala, India

Nitin Rao MD DNB (Paed) DM DNB (Cardio)
Chief
Department of Pediatric Cardiology
Star Hospital
Hyderabad, Telangana, India

Nivedita Kamath MBBS MD FPN DM (Ped Nephro)
Associate Professor
Department of Pediatric Nephrology
St John's Medical College Hospital
Bengaluru, Karnataka, India

Nuthan Kumar MK MD Post Doctoral Fellowship in PHO
Associate Professor
Department of Pediatric Oncology
Kidwai Memorial Institute of Oncology
Bengaluru, Karnataka, India

P Anil Kumar DCH DNB FIAMS (Paed Nephro) FIAMS (Paed) FIAP Fellow in Pediatric Nephrology
Professor
Department of Pediatrics
Siddhartha Medical College
Vijayawada, Andhra Pradesh, India

Palash Das MD (Pediatrics) PDF Pediatric Hemato–oncology
Associate Professor
Department of Pediatrics
KIMS-KIIT University
Bhubaneswar, Odisha, India

Partha Pratim Borah DCH DPSM
Consultant Pediatrician
Department of Pediatrics
Pratiksha Hospital
Guwahati, Assam, India

Pavithra Nagaraj MBBS MD Fellowship in Pediatric and Adolescent Endocrinology
Consultant
Department of Pediatric Endocrinology
Mazumdar Shaw Medical Centre, Narayana Health City
Bengaluru, Karnataka, India

Pawan Kalyan Pinnamaneni MD (Pediatrics) FACI FIAP Fellow in Pediatric Pulmonary & Sleep Medicine
Consultant Pediatrician
Department of Pediatrics
Dr Pinnamaneni Siddhartha Institute of Medical Sciences and Research Foundation
Vijayawada, Andhra Pradesh, India

Payal Mittal DNB (Pediatrics) MNAMS
Associate Professor
Department of Pediatrics
FH Medical College
Agra, Uttar Pradesh, India

Piyali Bhattacharya MD (Pediatrics) DCH FRCP FIAP
Consultant Pediatrician
General Hospital Institute, SGPGIMS
Lucknow, Uttar Pradesh, India

Pooja Gujjal Chebbi MD (Ped) DM (Ped Oncology)
Associate Professor of Pediatrics and Pediatric Hemato-oncologist
Department of Pediatric Medicine
Indira Gandhi Institute of Child Health
Bengaluru, Karnataka, India

Poornima RN DNB FAPE
Assistant Professor
Department of Pediatrics
St John's Medical College and Hospital
Bengaluru, Karnataka, India

Pradip Paria DPM MD (Pediatrics) DM (Pediatric Neurology)
Assistant Professor
Department of Pediatrics
Government Medical College
Raiganj, West Bengal, India

Prarthana Karumbaiah K MD (Pediatrics) FDBP (Developmental and Behavioral Pediatrics (IAP)
Associate Professor and Consultant Pediatrician
Department of Pediatrics
Ramaiah Medical College and Hospitals
Bengaluru, Karnataka, India

Prasad BS
MBBS DCH DNB (Pediatrics) PDCC (Pediatric Gastroenterology, SGPGI, Lucknow)
Consultant
Department of Pediatric Gastroenterologist
AJ Hospital and Research Centre
Mangaluru, Karnataka, India

Prasant Kumar Saboth MD
Professor
Department of Pediatrics
Institute of Medical Sciences and SUM Hospital
Bhubaneswar, Odisha, India

Prashanth SN MD DNB FIAP
Professor and Head
Department of Pediatrics
JSS Medical College
Mysuru, Karnataka, India

Prathik Bandiya MD DM (Neonatology)
Associate Professor
Department of Neonatology
Indira Gandhi Institute of Child Health
Bengaluru, Karnataka, India

Preeti M Galagali MD PGDAP FIAP
Director and Consultant Adolescent Health Specialist
Department of Pediatrics and Adolescent Medicine
Radha Ortho and Paediatric Centre
Bengaluru, Karnataka, India

Prem Kumar P MS (ENT)
Associate Professor and Head
Department of ENT
Indira Gandhi Institute of Child Health
Bengaluru, Karnataka, India

Priya Shivalli DCH DNB Fellowship in Neonatology (IAP)
Senior Consultant Neonatologist and Pediatrician
Narayana Superspeciality Hospitals
Bengaluru, Karnataka, India

Puneetha B MBBS DVD FRGUHS
Consultant
Department of Pediatric Dermatology
Rajiv Gandhi University of Health Sciences
Kangaroo Care Women and Children Hospitals
Mysuru, Karnataka, India

R Venkateswari DCH DNB (Pediatrics)
Senior Consultant Pediatrician
Department of Pediatrics
Kanchi Kamakoti CHILDS Trust Hospital
Chennai, Tamil Nadu, India

Raja Rajeswari DCH DNB (Pediatrics) MRCPCH
Fellow in Pediatric Oncology
Department of Pediatric Oncology
The Royal Marsden Hospital
Sutton, UK

Rajni Sharma MD
Additional Professor
Department of Pediatrics
All India Institute of Medical Sciences
New Delhi, India

Rajyashree Chamaria MBBS DCH MRCPCH (UK) PGDAP (Kerala)
Consultant Pediatrician and Adolescent Health Specialist
Caring Hands Clinic
Siliguri, West Bengal, India

Rakesh Mishra MD (Pediatrics)
Professor
Department of Pediatrics
Miracles Hospital, Chirayu Medical College
Bhopal, Madhya Pradesh, India

Ramesh Santhana Krishnan MBBS MS DNB MCh
Professor and Former Head
Department of Pediatric Surgery
Indira Gandhi Institute of Child Health
Bengaluru, Karnataka, India

Rashmi Agarwal MD DNB FRGUHS
Consultant
Department of Dermatology
Rainbow Children's Hospital
Bengaluru, Karnataka, India

Rashmi Ranjan Das MD (Pediatrics) FRCPCH
Professor
Department of Pediatrics
All India Institute of Medical Sciences
Bhubaneswar, Odisha, India

Ravi Bhatia DNB (Pediatrics)
Professor
Department of Pediatrics
Pacific Medical College
Udaipur, Rajasthan, India

Ravi Hiremagalur MD
Assistant Professor
Department of Dermatology
University of Alabama
Birmingham

Ravishankara Marpalli MBBS DCH DNB FIAP
Head
Department of Pediatrics
SS Sparsh Hospital
Bengaluru, Karnataka, India

Ritesh Sukharamwala MBBS MD (Pediatrics) Fellowship in Pediatric Cardiology
Consultant Pediatric Cardiologist
Department of Pediatric Cardiology
Shri BD Mehta Mahavir Heart Institute
Surat, Gujarat, India

Rupesh Masand MD (Pediatrics)
Professor
Department of Pediatrics
National Institute of Medical Sciences and Research
Jaipur, Rajasthan, India

Sahana Devadas MD (Pediatrics) FIPM
Professor and Head
Department of Pediatrics
Bengaluru Medical College and Research Institute
Bengaluru, Karnataka, India

Sahana M Srinivas MBBS DNB DDVL FRGUHS (Pediatric Dermatology)
Consultant
Department of Pediatric Dermatology
Indira Gandhi Institute of Child Health
Bengaluru, Karnataka, India

Saloni A Thakur MBBS
Jr Resident
Department of Pediatrics
Ramaiah Medical College
Bengaluru, Karnataka, India

Sandeep PS DNB (Pediatrics) MRCPCH
Senior Resident
Department of Pediatrics
All India Institute of Medical Sciences
New Delhi, India

Sanjay KS MD FIAP
Director, Professor and Unit Chief
Department of Pediatrics
Indira Gandhi Institute of Child Health
Bengaluru, Karnataka, India

Santanu Deb MD FIAP
Senior Consultant and Head
Department of Pediatrics
Nazareth Hospital
Shillong, Meghalaya, India

Sathya Srivatsav MD (Pediatrics) DM (Pediatric Pulmonology)
Senior Resident
Department of Pediatrics
All India Institute of Medical Sciences
Jodhpur, Rajasthan, India

Saumil Gaur MD Advanced Paediatric Nephrology Fellowship
Senior Consultant
Department of Pediatric Nephrology
Rainbow Children's Hospital
Bengaluru, Karnataka, India

Sayan Banerjee MD (Ped) Fellowship in Pediatric Endocrinology CDER Kanpur DM (Ped Endo), PGIMER Chandigarh
Senior Resident
Department of Pediatrics, Diabetes and Pediatric Endocrinology Unit
Postgraduate Institute of Medical Education and Research
Chandigarh, India

Sayoni Roy Chowdhury MD DM (Pediatric Neurology)
Assistant Professor
Department of Pediatrics
Lady Hardinge Medical College and Associated
Kalawati Saran Children's Hospital
New Delhi, India

Shaad Abqari MD (Pediatrics) FNB (Pediatric Cardiology)
Professor and In-charge
Division of Pediatric Cardiology
Department of Pediatrics
Jawaharlal Nehru Medical College
Aligarh Muslim University
Aligarh, Uttar Pradesh, India

Shalini Sharma MD MRCPCH Fellowship (IAP) and PG Diploma (University of Oxford) in Pediatric Infectious Diseases
Consultant Pediatrician and Pediatric ID Specialist
Department of Pediatrics
Manipal Hospital Hebbal
Bengaluru, Karnataka, India

Shama Sowdagar MBBS DNB (Pediatrics) PDF Rheumatology
Consultant Rheumatologist
Department of Rheumatology and Clinical Immunology
Medigo Multispecialty Hospital
Tirupati, Andhra Pradesh, India

Shamik Ghosh DCH (AFMC, Pune) DNB (Paediatrics) MRCP (Edinburgh) MRCPCH (London)
Senior Consultant Pediatrician
Manipal Hospital
Kolkata, West Bengal, India

Shashikiran KB MD DNB DM DrNB
Associate Professor and Head
Department of Nephrology
Institute of Nephro-urology
Mysuru, Karnataka, India

Sheetal Sajjan MBBS MD
Registrar
Department of Pediatrics
Sagar Hospital
Bengaluru, Karnataka, India

Sheffali Gulati MD FRCPCH (UK) FAMS FIAP FIMSA FNASc FIANS
Faculty In-Charge
Centre of Excellence and Advanced Research for Childhood Neurodevelopmental Disorders
Department of Pediatrics
All India Institute of Medical Sciences
New Delhi, India

Shikha Garg MBBS DCH DNB Diploma in Developmental Neurology
Developmental Behavioral Pediatrician
Babylon's Newton Institute of Child and Adolescent Development
Jaipur, Rajasthan, India

Shilpi Siddhanta Talukdar DNB (Ped) MRCPCH (UK) DCH (UK)
Divisional Medical Officer, ER
Department of Pediatrics
BR Singh Hospital
Kolkata, West Bengal, India

Showkat Hussain Tali MD (Pediatrics) DrNB (Neonatology)
Associate Professor and Head
Department of Pediatrics
Government Medical College
Anantnag, Jammu & Kashmir, India

Shreekrishna GN DCH DNB
Professor
Department of Pediatrics
AJ Institute and Research Center
Mangaluru, Karnataka, India

Shreepal Jain MD FNB FPICS
Consultant
Department of Cardiology
Bai Jerbai Wadia Hospital for Children
Mumbai, Maharashtra, India

Shrikiran Aroor Hebbar MBBS MD (Pediatrics)
Professor
Department of Pediatrics
Kasturba Medical College
Manipal, Karnataka, India

Siddhant Chavan MBBS MD FPGHN (Pediatric Gastroenterology)
Associate Consultant Pediatric Gastroenterologist
Department of Liver Sciences
Ruby Hall Clinic
Pune, Maharashtra, India

Sinchana Bhat MBBS DCH DNB DAA
SNCU Pediatrician
Department of Pediatrics
Government Wenlock Hospital
Mangaluru, Karnataka, India

Sumalatha Soppa MBBS MRCPCH AASC FAAP (Fellowship in Allergy and Asthma Procedures)
Pediatrician and Allergy Asthma Specialist
Chirayu Multispeciality Clinic
Bengaluru, Karnataka, India

Somashekar AR DCH DNB FIAP
Professor
Department of Pediatrics
Ramaiah Memorial Hospital
Bengaluru, Karnataka, India

Somu Sivabalan MD (Pediatrics) DNB (Pediatrics) FCCP FIAP FAPSR FRCP (Edin)
Consultant Pediatrician and Pulmonologist
Department of Pediatrics
Rainbow Children's Hospital
Chennai, Tamil Nadu, India

Sonia Bhatt MD (Pediatrics) DAA PGCAP
Professor and Head
Department of Pediatrics
FH Medical College
Agra, Uttar Pradesh, India

Soundharya S MBBS MS MCh (Pediatric Surgery)
Assistant Professor
Department of Pediatric Surgery
Indira Gandhi Institute of Child Health
Bengaluru, Karnataka, India

Sowmya A Nagarajan MBBS DCH Fellowship in Paediatric Allergy and Asthma, Diploma in Allergy and Asthma, Certificate of Excellence in Allergy (EAACI)
Consultant Pediatrician
Sanjeevini Specialist Clinic
Kangaroo Care Hospitals and Motherhood Hospitals
Bengaluru, Karnataka, India

Srikrishna RSV MBBS DNB (Pediatrics)
Associate Professor
Department of Pediatrics
Dr VRK Women's Medical College
Kaloji Narayana Rao University of Health Sciences
Hyderabad, Telangana, India
Treasurer, Indian Academy of Pediatrics Twin Cities Branch
Secretary, IAP-IYCF Telangana State

Srinivasa Murthy D MBBS MD (Ped) MRCPCh (UK) Fellowship in Neonatal Medicine (McMaster Univ Canada)
Professor of Pediatrics
Department of Pediatrics
JSS Medical College
Mysuru, Karnataka, India

Srujan Reddy Salukati MBBS DCH DNB (Peds) DrNB (Pediatric Cardiology)
Senior Resident
Department of Pediatric Cardiology
Star Hospitals
Hyderabad, Telangana, India

Subhasish Bhattacharyya DCH MD (Del) DNB MNAMS
Professor and Head
Department of Pediatrics
CSS College of Obstetrics, Gynecology, and Child Health
Kolkata, West Bengal, India

Suchitra Pusapati MBBS MRCPCH (UK) DCH (UK)
Associate Professor
Department of Pediatrics
GITAM Institute of Medical Sciences and Research
Visakhapatnam, Andhra Pradesh, India

Sukanta Chatterjee MD FIAP
Former Professor and Head
Department of Pediatrics
Government Medical College
Kolkata, West Bengal, India

Sumana Kundagrami MD (Ped) MRCPH (UK) Fellowship in Pediatric Endocrinology (Grow Society)
Associate Professor and Pediatric Endocrinologist
Department of Pediatrics
KPC Medical College and Hospital
Kolkata, West Bengal, India

Sumitha Nayak
MD DNB FIAP Adv Certificate in Vaccinology (IVI KOREA & CMC Vellore)
Consultant Pediatrician
Shishu—The Children's Clinic
Bengaluru, Karnataka, India

Supratim Datta MBBS DCH MD (Ped)
Professor of Pediatrics
Department of Pediatrics
KPC Medical College
Kolkata, West Bengal, India

Suprita Kalra MD DNB (Pediatrics)
Fellowship in Pediatric Nephrology
Professor
Department of Pediatrics
Command Hospital
Pune, Maharashtra, India

Suraj S Shetty MD
Postgraduate
Department of Pediatrics
AJ Institute of Medical Sciences
Mangalore, Karnataka, India

Susrut Das DNB APGPN
Practicing Pediatrician
Department of Pediatrics
Balyashree Clinic
Bhubaneswar, Odisha, India
Founder Director
SAMBHAV–Early Childhood
Development Center

Swapan Kumar Ray MBBS DCH DNB (Ped) MNAMS FIAP
Professor
Department of Pediatrics
MGM Medical College
Kishanganj, Bihar, India

Sweta Mandal MD (Ped) DM (Endo) DrNB (Endo)
Senior Resident
Department of Pediatrics
Murshidabad Medical College
Berhampore, West Bengal, India

Taraknath Ghosh MBBS MD
Professor
Department of Pediatrics
Burdwan Medical College and Hospital
Burdwan, West Bengal, India

Uday A Pai MD DCH FIAP
Consultant Pediatrician
Aangan Clinic
Mumbai, Maharashtra, India

Urvi Sanghvi MD (Ped) DrNB (Neonatology)
Neonatal Intensivist
Department of Neonatology
Anmol Newborn Care
Mumbai, Maharashtra, India

V Spandana DNB (Pediatrics)
Assistant Professor
Department of Pediatrics
SV Medical College
Tirupati, Andhra Pradesh, India

Vaibhav Shah MD (Ped) FPGHN (India)
Consultant
Department of Pediatric
Gastroenterology and Hepatology
Gujarat Superspeciality Clinic
Ahmedabad, Gujarat, India

Vani HN MD (Ped) Fellowship in Paediatric and Adolescent Endocrinology
Associate Professor and Pediatric
Endocrinologist
Department of Pediatrics
Indira Gandhi Institute of Child Health
Bengaluru, Karnataka, India

Vasundhara Chugh MD (Ped) Fellowship in Pediatric and Adolescent Endocrinology
Consultant
Department of Pediatric Endocrinology
Neoclinic Children Hospital and Aermed
Super Specialty Clinic
Jaipur, Rajasthan, India

Veeraraja Basavanthappa Sathenahalli MBBS MD DNB (Paediatrics)
Associate Professor
Department of Pediatrics
Indira Gandhi Institute of Child Health
Bengaluru, Karnataka, India

Vikram Sakaleshpur Kumar MD
Professor
Department of Pediatrics
Subbaiah Institute of Medical Sciences
Shivamogga, Karnataka, India

Vishal Gohil MD (Pediatrics) Fellowship in Neonatology at RCPCH NNF Fellowship in Neonatology
Consultant Neonatologist
Department of NICU
Arpan Newborn Care Centre
Ahmedabad, Gujarat, India

Vishnu D Biradar
MBBS MD PDCC (Ped Gastro)
Consultant Pediatric Gastroenterologist
Department of Liver Sciences
Ruby Hall Clinic and Kamal
Endoscopy Centre
Pune, Maharashtra, India

Vishnu Mohan PT MBBS MD Fellowship in Neonatology PGDMLS
Senior Consultant
Department of Neonatology
Aster MIMS Hospital
Kozhikode, Kerala, India

Yogesh Chintaman Sathe MD (Pediatrics) FNB (Pediatric Cardiology)
Senior Consultant and Head
Department of Pediatric Cardiology
Sri Sathya Sai Sanjeevani Hospital
Nava Raipur, Chhattisgarh, India

Foreword

"Knowledge is the understanding we gain through learning, while skill is knowing what action to take next."

It gives me great pleasure to write the foreword for this significant book, *An Algorithm Approach to Pediatric Diagnosis*. Despite the vast knowledge we accumulate over years of learning and practice, there are often moments in clinical settings when we find ourselves uncertain about the next step. Managing challenging symptoms in a busy outpatient department can sometimes be overwhelming, leaving us questioning whether to treat, refer, or further investigate.

This exceptional book offers a clear and structured approach to these dilemmas, providing pediatricians with practical, easy-to-follow guidance for navigating such situations. With detailed coverage of 140 different symptoms, the book walks readers through history-taking, clinical features, and a systematic approach to diagnosis. The inclusion of differential diagnoses, recommended investigations, and critical "red flag" signs ensures that every patient receives the appropriate care and attention.

Not only does this book enhance the reader's diagnostic skills, but it also empowers them to make informed decisions that will lead to better outcomes for their young patients.

I extend my heartfelt congratulations to the authors for the tremendous effort invested in creating this valuable resource.

With Warm Regards

GV Basavaraja
National President, 2024

Message

Dear Colleagues, Friends, and Esteemed Guests,

As the President 2025 of the Indian Academy of Pediatrics (IAP), it is my privilege to introduce *An Algorithm Approach to Pediatric Diagnosis (AAAPD)* book, a valuable resource that promises to enhance the clinical practice of pediatric healthcare providers across the nation. In an era where the demands of patient care often compete with the need for accurate and timely diagnosis, this book stands as a beacon of support for practitioners navigating the complexities of pediatric symptoms.

The symptom-based approach presented in this book is especially commendable. By focusing on 140 common symptoms, the authors have created an accessible guide that aligns seamlessly with the fast-paced environment of outpatient departments (OPDs). This practicality is vital, as healthcare professionals are increasingly required to make quick and informed decisions in their clinical practice.

Moreover, the inclusion of relevant differentials and investigations adds significant value to the text. It encourages a comprehensive evaluation process, ensuring that practitioners consider all possible avenues in their diagnostic approach. The algorithm guiding clinicians to the most probable diagnosis further streamlines decision-making, allowing for swift and effective patient management.

As we move towards a future that emphasizes both efficiency and accuracy in pediatric care, resources like the AAAPD book are essential. They empower practitioners with the knowledge and tools necessary to provide the best possible care for our children.

I extend my heartfelt congratulations to the authors and contributors for their dedication to this project. I am confident that this book will be an invaluable addition to the libraries of pediatric practitioners, enhancing their ability to provide high-quality care.

Wishing you all the success with this publication.

Warm regards

Vasant M Khalatkar
MD FIAP PG Dip Inf Dis (UNSW)
Director
Khalatkar Hospital for Mother and Child
Nagpur, Maharashtra, India
President Elect 2024

Message

In the dynamic and demanding field of Pediatrics, the ability to swiftly and accurately diagnose common symptoms is crucial as well as paramount. *An Algorithm Approach in Pediatric Diagnosis (AAAPD)* book is a remarkable resource that addresses this need with a comprehensive, symptom-based approach that is both practical and insightful.

This book meticulously covers 140 common symptoms, providing an easy-to-use guide, an invaluable resource for practitioners navigating the complexities of a busy outpatient department (OPD). Its format allows healthcare professionals to quickly access relevant differentials and investigations, streamlining the diagnostic process.

One of the standout features of this book is its well-structured algorithms, which guide practitioners towards the most probable diagnosis with precision and clarity. This systematic approach not only enhances diagnostic accuracy but also improves patient outcomes by facilitating timely and appropriate interventions.

The "AAAPD" book is more than just a guide; it is a trusted companion for pediatricians, offering support and confidence in their clinical decisions. It embodies the commitment to excellence and the dedication to patient care that define our profession.

As the Secretary General of the Indian Academy of Pediatrics for 2024–2025, I am proud to endorse this book. It is a reflection of our collective efforts to advance pediatric care and education. I am confident that this book will become an indispensable tool for practitioners, postgraduate students enriching their practice and ultimately benefiting the children we serve.

Yogesh N Parikh
MD (Pediatrics)
Professor
Department of Pediatrics
Government Medical College
Surat, Gujarat, India
Former Professor and Head
Department of Pediatrics
PDU Government Medical College and
KT Children Hospital, Rajkot, Gujarat
Secretary General
Indian Academy of Pediatrics (2024–2025)

Message

It is my pleasure to write a message for this important book titled *An Algorithm Approach to Pediatric Diagnosis (AAAPD)*.

This book is designed to serve as a practical guide, offering clear, step-by-step algorithms that can be applied in clinical settings. These algorithms are based on the latest evidence and best practices, ensuring that clinicians have a reliable resource at their fingertips when faced with the complex task of diagnosing pediatric conditions.

The salient features of this book include a symptom-based approach of 140 common symptoms. It is an easy guide for practitioners in a busy OPD and includes relevant differentials and investigations. Finally, the algorithm in every chapter guides the readers to the most probable diagnosis.

I am confident that this book will serve as a valuable educational resource and invaluable asset for practitioners, teachers, students and all who are managing children in their clinical practice. They will find the structured approach helpful in mastering the complexities of pediatric diagnosis, ultimately supporting you in providing the best possible care to your young patients, helping them to lead healthy lives and achieving full potential.

I am grateful to all the children and adolescents for their inspiration, leading to desired output in due course of time.

With warm regards,

Atanu Bhadra
DCH FIAP
Superintendent
ESI Hospital
Asansol, West Bengal, India
National Treasurer
Indian Academy of Pediatrics (2024–2025)

Preface

The field of pediatrics is vast, with a unique set of challenges and intricacies that demand a precise, nuanced approach to diagnosis. Children are not simply small adults; their developmental stages, physiological differences, and the ways they manifest symptoms require specialized attention. Accurate diagnosis in pediatric medicine is crucial, as early detection and appropriate intervention can significantly alter the trajectory of a child's health and development.

An Algorithm Approach to Pediatric Diagnosis was conceived out of a desire to streamline the diagnostic process for pediatric healthcare professionals. The book serves as a practical guide, offering clear, step-by-step algorithms that can be applied in clinical settings. These algorithms are based on the latest evidence and best practices, ensuring that clinicians have a reliable resource at their fingertips when faced with the complex task of diagnosing pediatric conditions.

The book is organized by symptomatology, covering 140 common symptoms in childhood. Each chapter is structured to guide the readers through a logical sequence including differential diagnosis, relevant investigations and red flag signs. The readers are kept aware of what are danger signals that require immediate and urgent attention and care.

We have taken great care to ensure that this book is both accessible and authoritative. The algorithms are designed to be user-friendly, allowing for quick reference during patient encounters in a busy outpatient setting.

In addition to its utility as a clinical tool, we hope this book will also serve as a valuable educational resource. Medical students, residents, and fellows will find the structured approach helpful in mastering the complexities of pediatric diagnosis, while experienced clinicians may discover new insights and strategies to enhance their practice.

The journey of creating this book has been one of collaboration, learning, and reflection. It would not have been possible without the contributions of many experts in the field of pediatrics, who generously shared their knowledge and experience. We are also deeply grateful to the children and families who inspire our work and remind us daily of the profound impact that accurate diagnosis and compassionate care can have.

As you navigate through the pages of this book, we hope that you find the algorithms clear, the guidance practical, and the approach empowering. Our ultimate goal is to support you in providing the best possible care for your young patients, helping them to lead healthy, fulfilling lives.

Gnanamurthy Narasimha
Sumitha Nayak
Academic Editors

Contents

Anxiety

1

***Section Editor:* Sumitha Nayak**
***Section Co-Editor:* Priya Shivalli**
***Author:* Aaradhana Singh**

Introduction

Anxiety is defined as fear or apprehension and is a normal human emotion involving cognitive-behavior component (worry, fear) and physiologic component mediated by the autonomic nervous system (pallor, tachycardia, tremors). Often, anxiety is normal and adaptive response among children and adolescents, especially during specific development periods, for example, stranger anxiety among infants, school and performance anxiety among school-going kids, and fear of peer rejection among adolescents. In the presence of red flag signs, it is pathological and is referred to as anxiety disorder and is the most common psychiatric disorder among children with a prevalence of 5–18%.

Etiology of Anxiety in Children

- Normal adaptive response
- Known or unrecognized medical conditions
- Substance abuse
- Anxiety disorders

Red Flag Signs and Categories of Anxiety Disorder

ANXIETY DISORDER	SOURCE OF THREAT	RED FLAG SIGNS
Separation anxiety disorder	Excessive worries about separation from home and caregivers	Refusal to go to school, to sleep without caregiver, nightmares of being alone
Social anxiety disorder (social phobia)	Excessive anxiety in social settings	Avoidance of speaking in class, attending social gatherings, poor school performance, and decreased quality of life
Panic disorder (PD)	Recurrent episodes of excessive fear along with psychological and physical symptoms	Fear of death, impending doom, fear of having future episodes, palpitation, sweating, shortness of breath, and nausea
Generalized anxiety disorder (GAD)	Marked fear and anxiety in various situations like using public transportation, being in open or enclosed spaces, standing in line or in crowds, and concerns about performance in school and athletics	Sleep disturbance, restlessness, irritability, fatigue, muscle tension, and poor concentration
Obsessive compulsive disorders (OCD)	Recurrent thoughts and repetitive behaviors over which the patient has little control and which cause distress, consume time, and interfere with social or occupational functioning	Thoughts of harming loved ones or oneself, washing and cleaning compulsions, and checking
Post-traumatic stress disorder (PTSD)	Behavioral and physiological sequelae of trauma	Recurrent distressing memories, dreams of traumatic event

Risk Factors of Anxiety Disorder in Children

- Anxiety disorders in parents
- Behavioral inhibition in early childhood
- Early childhood adversity
- Exposure to physical and sexual abuse early in life

Approach

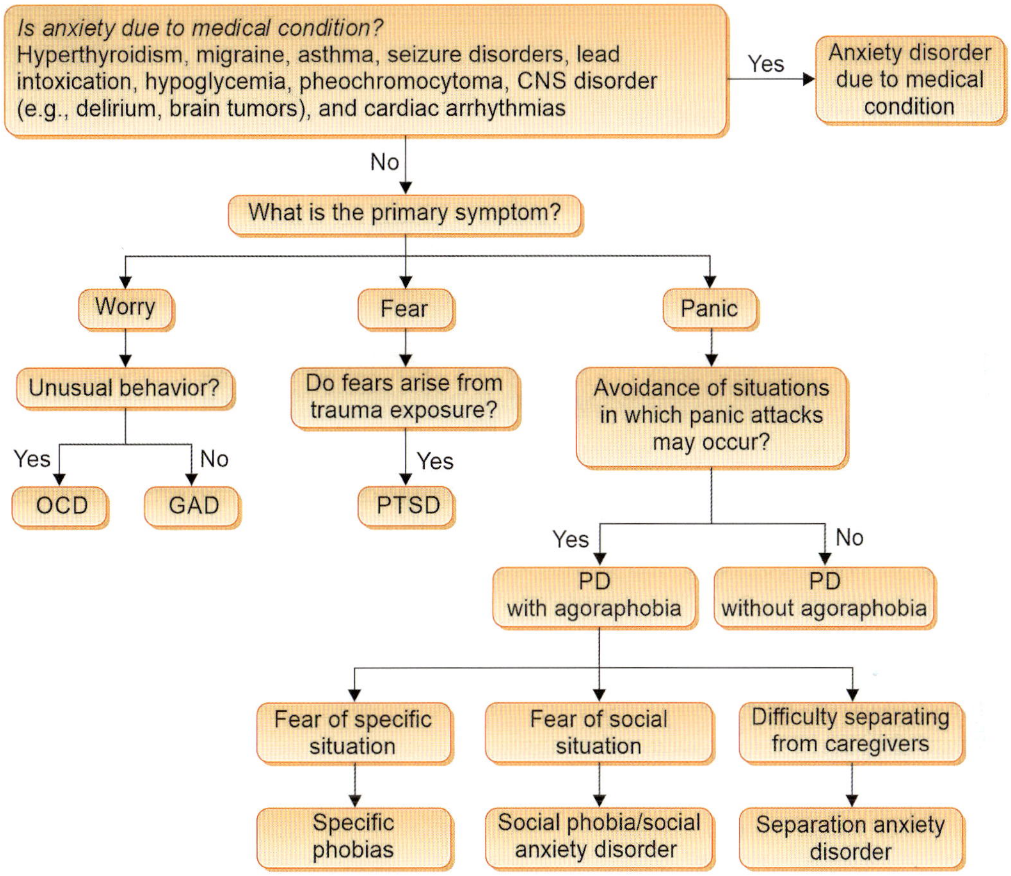

Treatment: Behavioral therapy or/and medications like selective serotonin uptake inhibitors

Suggested Reading

- Connolly SD, Bernstein GA; Work Group on Quality Issues. Practice parameter for the assessment and treatment of children and adolescents with anxiety disorders. J Am Acad Child Adolesc Psychiatry. 2007;46(2):267-83.
- Freidl EK, Stroeh OM, Elkins RM, Steinberg E, Albano AM, Rynn M. Assessment and Treatment of Anxiety Among Children and Adolescents. Focus (Am Psychiatr Publ). 2017;15(2):144-56.
- Kliegman RM, St. Geme III JW. Nelson Textbook of Pediatrics, 21st edition. Amsterdam: Elsevier; 2019.

Learning Disability

2

Section Editor: **Sumitha Nayak**
Section Co-Editor: **Priya Shivalli**
Author: **Manini Moudgal**

Introduction

Learning disability (LD) is a **group of neurodevelopmental disorders** wherein a child has difficulty acquiring, retrieving, and using information, especially with reading, writing, and/or mathematics. LD usually manifests in preschool years and is unrelated to neurological or motor disorders, intellectual disability, and socioeconomic and environmental disadvantages. Based on the child's overall intelligence, academic achievement is lower than expected.

The prevalence of LD in India is 1.6–15%. Under Rights of Persons with Disability Act, India, 2016, people with LD have a right to free education till 18 years. They also have 5% reservation for higher education in government institutes and 1% for government jobs.

Etiology

- *Heredity (accounts for 50% of LD):* Chromosomal abnormalities; single gene, imprinting and mitochondrial disorders
- *Prenatal, birth, and postnatal factors:* Congenital infections (rubella, CMV, toxoplasmosis), birth asphyxia, teratogens (alcohol, anticonvulsants), prematurity
- *Environment:* Lead poisoning
- *Inborn errors of metabolism:* Wilson's disease

Common Types

- *Dyslexia:* Difficulty in reading
- *Dysgraphia:* Difficulty in visual spatial perception and handwriting
- *Dyscalculia:* Difficulty with understanding how numbers work
- *Nonverbal LD:* Difficulty reading facial cues, body language, social appropriateness, and coordination

All these may exist alone or in varying degrees in the same person.

Comorbidities

- Attention-deficit hyperactivity disorder (ADHD)
- Autism spectrum disorders (ASD)
- *Dyspraxia:* Difficulty with movement and coordination, speech and language
- Anxiety
- Depression

Red Flag Signs

Symptoms in each column are cumulative with the next.

Concerns in two or more of these areas warrant further investigation.

PRESCHOOL	PRIMARY SCHOOL	MIDDLE AND HIGH SCHOOL
Late speech development with unclear speech	Poor memory for poems, tasks, facts, and numbers	Trouble understanding abstract concepts and reading comprehension
Difficulty recognizing simple letters, words, and numbers	Errors connecting letters to sounds and differentiating similar or rhyming words	Confusion with complex arithmetic, signs, and word problems
Clumsy, fidgety, and easily distracted	Slow learner compared to kids of own age	Difficulty with friendships
Difficulty following directions	Poor fine motor skills and organizational ability	Hates school because of constant poor academic performance, bullying
	Odd pencil grip, jumbled handwriting, and writing avoidance	

Approach

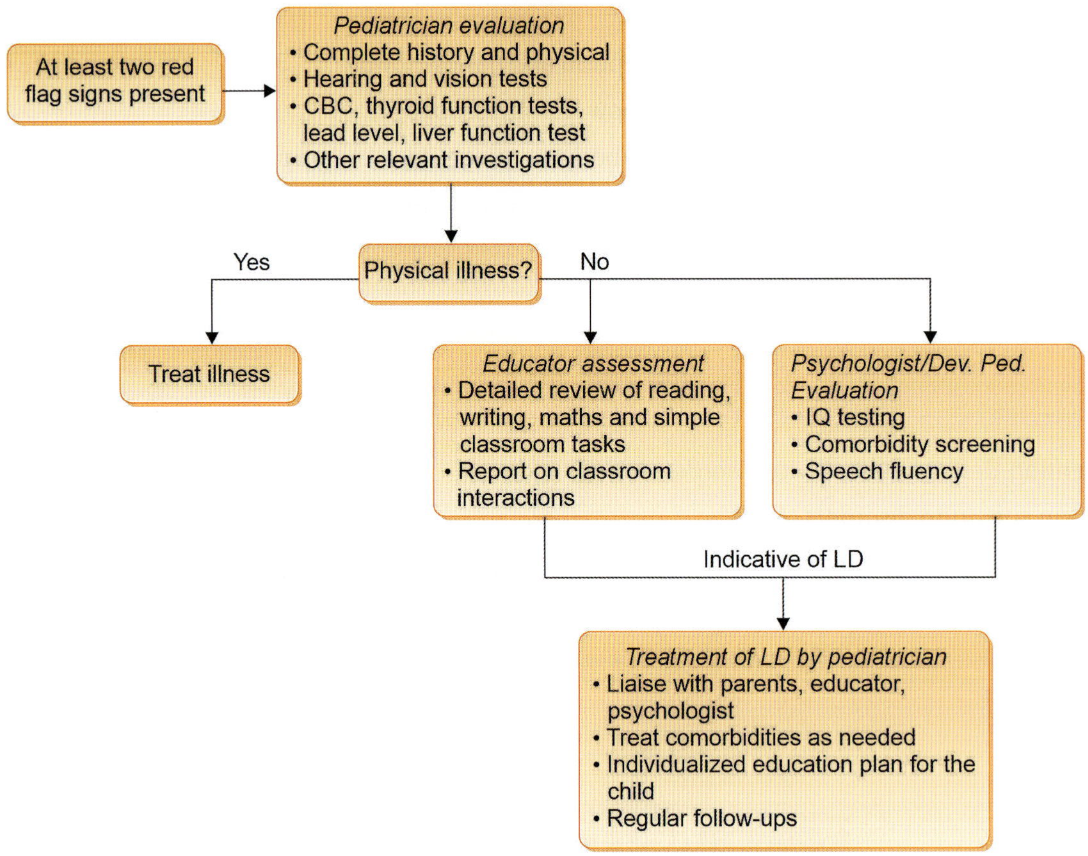

Suggested Reading

- American Psychiatric Association Diagnostic and Statistical Manual of Psychiatric Disorders (DSM V). Washington, DC: American Psychiatric Association; 2013.
- Foster A, Titheradge H, Morton J. Genetics of learning disability. Paediatr Child Health. 2015;25(10):450-7.
- Indian Academy of Pediatrics. D'Souza N, Somasundaram A, Vinchurkar S. (2022). Standard Treatment Guidelines 2022. [online] Available from https://iapindia.org/pdf/Ch-081-Specific-Learning-Disorders.pdf [Last accessed December, 2023].
- Ministry of Social justice and Empowerment. Rights of Persons with Disability Act 2016 (RPWD Act 2016). Government of India.

Fever with Rash in Children

3

Section Editor: **B Rajsekhar**
Section Co-Editor: **Suchitra Pusapati**
Authors: **K Radhakrishna, Amulya K**

Introduction

- Fever with rash is one of the leading complaints among children.
- Most causes are viral in origin and benign in nature.
- A few life-threatening cause of rashes needs to be recognized.

Life-threatening Causes of Fever with Rash

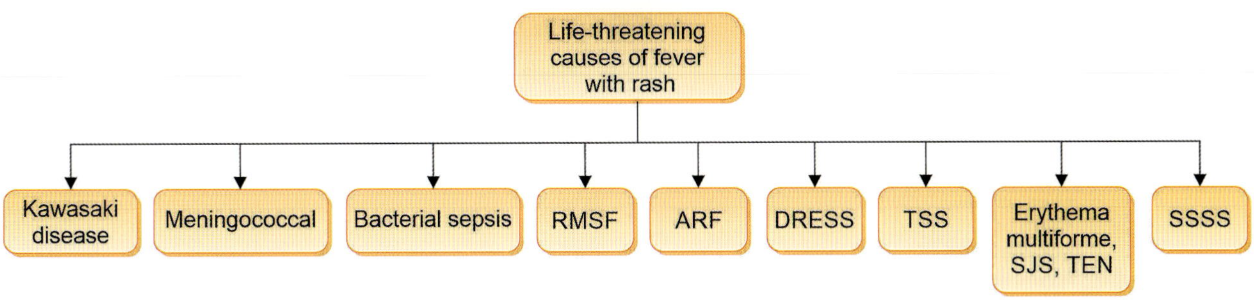

(ARF: acute rheumatic fever; DRESS: drug reaction with eosinophilia and systemic symptoms; RMSF: Rocky mountain spotted fever; SJS: Steven–Johnson syndrome; SSSS: staphylococcal scalded skin syndrome; TEN: toxic epidermal necrolysis; TSS: toxic shock syndrome)

Red Flag Signs

- Petechial/purpuric rash specially < 2 years of age
- With meningeal signs
- Associated with weight loss, anorexia
- Associated with unstable vitals
- Toxic appearance

Approach Based on Associated Clinical Features

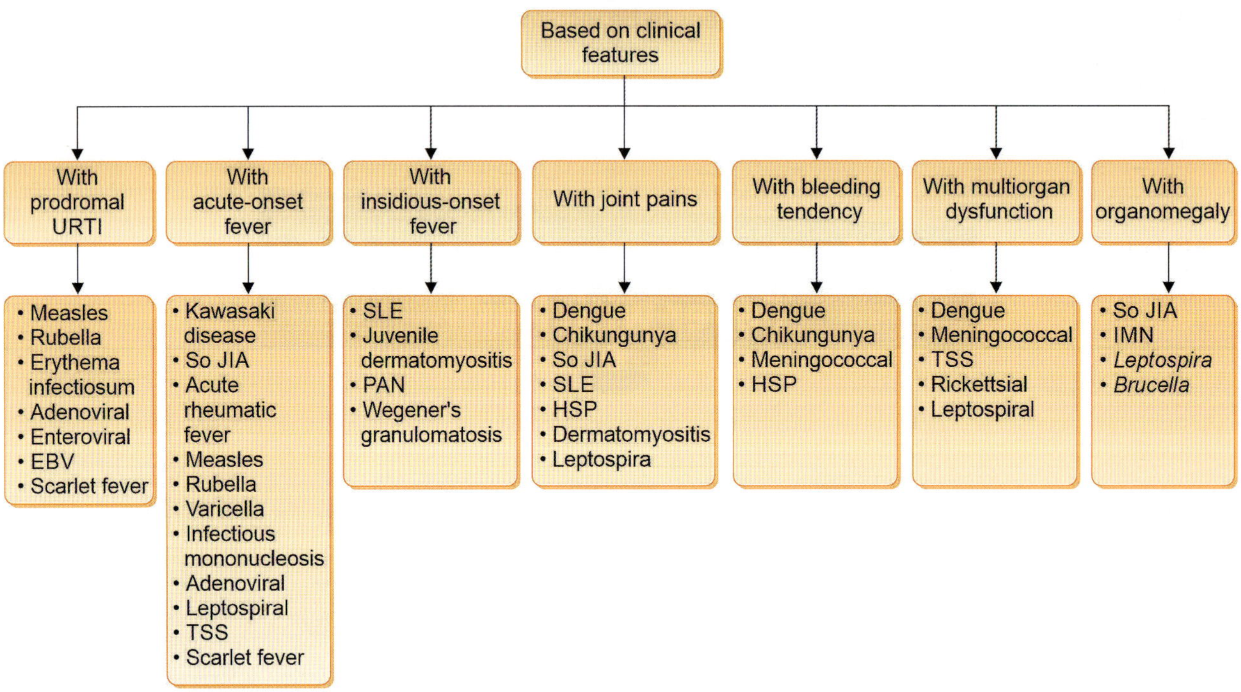

(EBV: Epstein–Barr virus; So JIA: systemic onset juvenile idiopathic arthritis; HSP: Henoch–Schonlein purpura; SLE: systemic lupus erythematosus; PAN: polyarteritis nodosa; IMN: infectious mononucleosis)

Approach Based on Rash Morphology

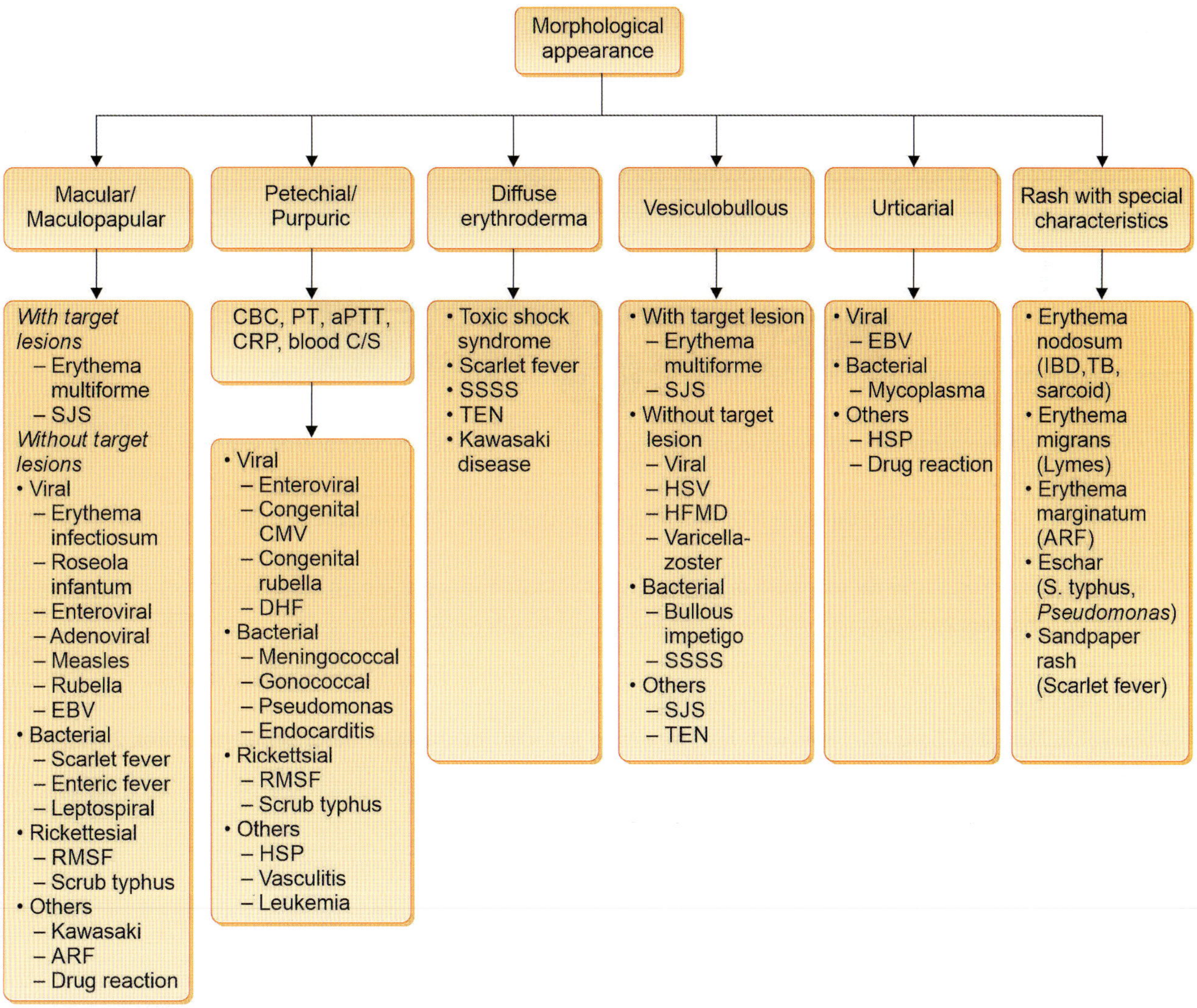

(CBC: complete blood test; CMV: cytomegalovirus; CRP: C-reactive protein; DHF: dengue hemorrhagic fever; HFMD: hand foot mouth disease; HSV: herpes simplex virus; PT: prothrombin time; TB: tuberculosis; TEN: toxic epidermal necrolysis; IBD: inflammatory bowel disease)

Drug Rash

- Commonly maculopapular eruptions
- Appear within 7–14 days of start of the treatment
- The commonly implicated drugs are beta lactams, sulfonamides, nonsteroidal anti-inflammatory drugs (NSAIDs), and anticonvulsants.
- Diagnosed by absence of prodromal symptoms, presence of severe itching, absence of high-grade fevers commonly, temporal relation to drug intake, confluence of rash on dependent areas
- Reappearance of rash on drug provocation confirms diagnosis.

Suggested Reading

- Doshi BR, Manjunathswamy BS. Maculopapular drug eruption versus maculopapular viral exanthem. Indian J Drugs Dermatol. 2017;3:45-7.
- Khandpur S, Ahuja R. Drug-Induced vs. Viral Maculopapular Exanthem-Resolving the Dilemma. Dermatopathology (Basel). 2022;9(2):164-71.
- Kliegman RM, St. Geme III JW. Part XVI: Infectious disease. Nelson Textbook of Pediatrics, 21st Edition. Amsterdam: Elsevier. [Chapters 201–204]
- Pomeranz AJ Sabnis S Busey SL Kliegman R. Pediatric Decision-Making Strategies, 2nd edition. Philadelphia: Elsevier/Saunders; 2016. pp. 223-25 [Chapter 59].
- Sarkar R, Mishra K, Garg VK. Fever with rash in a child in India. Indian J Dermatol Venereol Leprol. 2012;78(3): 251-62.

4

School Refusal and Absenteeism

***Section Editor:* Sumitha Nayak**
***Section Co-Editor:* Priya Shivalli**
***Author:* Prarthana Karumbaiah K**

Introduction

- In India, school refusal accounts to 1–8% of school attendance problems.
- Refusal is mainly seen in 10–13 years age group.
- This is mainly due to transition years when less play-oriented and more task-oriented curriculum occurs, along with homework load and sudden increase in school hours.

Berg's definition of operational criteria includes:

- School attendance <80% in the classroom during the prior 2 weeks
- Parents aware of their child's whereabouts
- Associated anxiety disorder
- Absence of conduct disorder problems

Etiology

- *Temperament:* Difficult personality, maladaptive coping skills
- *Home environment:* Dependency toward parents, shifting residence, socioeconomic status, help in house job, neighborhood crime, screen time (television, mobile, ipad)
- *School environment:* Lack of interest in any academic activities, irregular classes, school far from home
- *Family stressors:* Parental divorce, dysfunctional family environments, poor familial cohesion, poor communication, lack of financial support
- *Interpersonal/peer problems:* Victimization, social isolation

Red Flags

- Reluctance/frequent refusal to go to school
- Seeking comfort and security of home and parent figures during school hours
- Display of the following just before school time/the previous evening/at school before certain classes
  - Physical or psychosomatic forms (e.g., nausea, pain abdomen, severe headaches, back pain, pain in limbs, fainting spells)
  - Behavioral forms (upset, distressed, anxious)
  - Cognitive forms (panic attack)
  - Problems with emotional regulation, sleep

Consequences

- *Short-term:* Social isolation, poor academic performance, suicidal ideation
- *Long-term:* Increased susceptibility to adjustment problems, attendance, school dropout rates, major depression, adult income, health

Management Algorithm

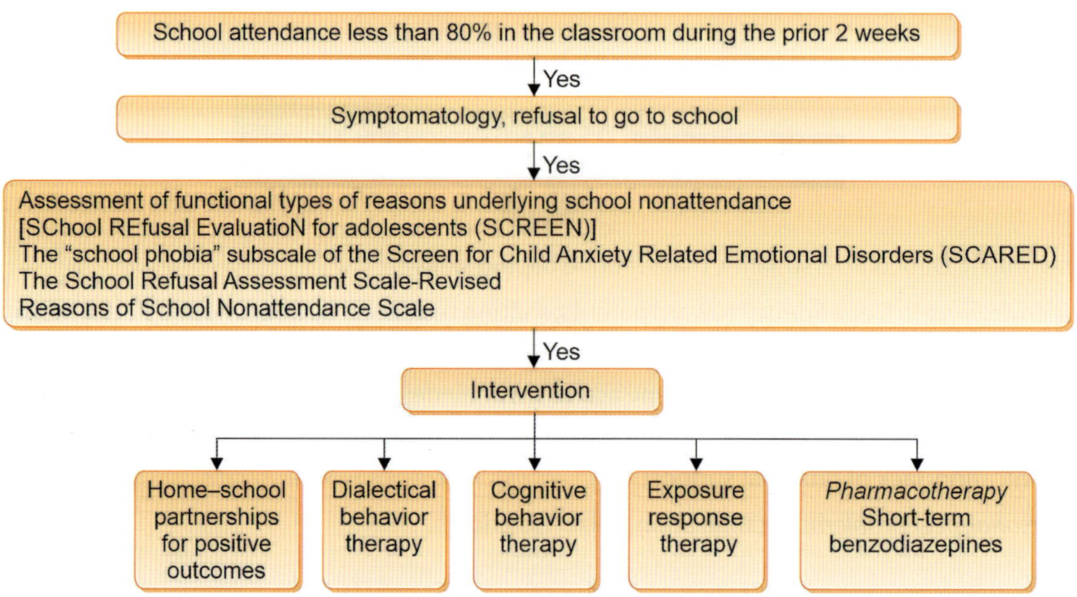

Suggested Reading

- Berg I. School avoidance, school phobia and truancy. In: Lewis M (Ed). Child and Adolescent Psychiatry: A Comprehensive Textbook. London: Williams & Wilkins; 1996. pp. 1104-10.
- Berg I. School avoidance, school phobia, and truancy. In: Lewis M (Ed). Child and Adolescent Psychiatry: A Comprehensive Textbook. Sydney: Lippincott Williams & Wilkins; 2002. pp. 1260-6.
- Biswas H, Sahoo MK. A study on psychiatric conditions in children with school refusal—A clinic based study. J Family Med Prim Care. 2023;12(1):160-4.
- Henderson T, Hill C, Norton K. (2014). The connection between missing school and health: a review of chronic absenteeism and student health in Oregon. Upstream Public Health. [online] Available from https://www.attendanceworks.org/wp-content/uploads/2017/08/Chronic-Absence-and-Health-Review-10.8.14-FINAL-REVISED.pdf [Last accessed December, 2023].
- Heyne D, King NJ, Tonge BJ, Cooper H. School refusal: Epidemiology and management. Paediatr Drugs. 2001;3: 719-32.
- Kearney CA. Forms and functions of school refusal behavior in youth: An empirical analysis of absenteeism severity. J Child Psychol Psychiatry. 2007;48:53-61.
- King NJ, Bernstein GA. School refusal in children and adolescents: A review of the past 10 years. J Am Acad Child Adolesc Psychiatry. 2001;40:197-206.
- Leduc K, Tougas AM, Robert V, Boulanger C. School Refusal in Youth: A Systematic Review of Ecological Factors. Child Psychiatry Hum Develop. 2022;1-19.
- Nayak A, Sangoi B, Nachane H. School refusal behavior in Indian children: Analysis of clinical profile, psychopathology and development of a best-fit risk assessment model. Indian J Pediatr. 2018;85:1073-8.
- U.S. Department of Education. (2016). Chronic absenteeism in the nation's schools: an unprecedented look at a hidden educational crisis. [online] Available from https://www2.ed.gov/datastory/chronicabsenteeism.html [Last accessed December, 2023].

Precocious Puberty

5

Section Editor: **Kripasindhu Chatterjee**
Section Co-Editors: **Ashim Kumar Ghosh, Atanu Bhadra**
Authors: **Kakali Roy, Rajni Sharma**

Definition

- Precocious puberty (PP) is defined as onset of secondary sexual characteristics before the age of 8 years in girls (thelarche) and 9 years in boys (testicular enlargement ≥4 mL/penile growth).
- It is usually associated with height spurt (due to sex steroids) and bone age advancement.

Classification

- *Central:* Due to activation of the hypothalamic pituitary gonadal (HPG) axis/gonadotropin dependent
- *Peripheral:* Without hypothalamic pituitary activation/gonadotropin-independent

Peripheral precocity →
- Isosexual (features are commensurate with sex of the child)
- Heterosexual (features are not commensurate with the sex of the child)

- Variations in pubertal development/absence of other features
  - *Premature (isolated) thelarche:* No growth spurt/bone age advancement
  - *Premature pubarche:* Development of pubic hair
  - Isolated menarche

Etiology

Central precocious puberty (CPP)

- Idiopathic
- Hypothalamic hamartoma
- Brain tumor (germinoma, astrocytoma, pineal tumor)
- Head trauma
- Hydrocephalus

Peripheral precocious puberty

GIRLS

Isosexual:

- Functioning ovarian cyst
- Ovarian tumor (granulosa-theca cell tumor)
- Adrenal tumor (feminizing adrenocortical tumor)
- McCune–Albright syndrome
- Exogenous estrogens

Heterosexual (virilization in girls):

- Congenital adrenal hyperplasia, adrenal tumors
- Exogenous androgens

BOYS

Isosexual:

- Congenital adrenal hyperplasia
- Adrenocortical tumors
- *Testicular tumor:* Leydig cell tumor
- hCG-secreting tumors (teratoma)
- Exogenous androgens

Heterosexual (feminization in boys):

- Feminizing adrenocortical tumor
- Exogenous estrogens

Premature pubarche: Premature adrenarche
Isolated menarche: Local gynecological causes like vulvovaginitis, trauma, abuse, UTI, foreign body

(hCG: human chorionic gonadotropin; UTI: urinary tract infection)

Approach

Examination

- Height, weight, BMI, head circumference
- *Tanner staging:* Axillary/pubic hair, genital examination
- *General physical exam:* Café-au-lait spots/bony deformities (MAS)
- Features of hypothyroidism
- CNS examination (CNS lesion)

Investigations

- Basal sex hormones (testosterone/estradiol)
- Basal and gonadotropin hormone-releasing hormone (GnRH-stimulated gonadotropin levels [luteinizing hormone (LH), follicle-stimulating hormone (FSH)]
- *GnRH agonist stimulation test:* Leuprolide 20 μg/kg subcutaneus (SC) or triptorelin 100 μg/m^2 SC followed by LH and FSH after 4 hours and sex steroids (estradiol/testosterone) after 24 hours
- *Bone age:* Left hand and wrist AP
- Ultrasound pelvis (girls)
- *MRI brain:* For all boys with CPP; girls <6 years with CPP
- *Other investigations when needed:*
  - *Hypothyroidism*: Thyroxine (T3), triiodothyronine (T4), thyroid stimulating hormone (TSH)
  - *Congenital adrenal hyperplasia (CAH):* Serum 17-hydroxyprogesterone (17-OHP)
  - *MAS:* Skeletal survey for fibrous dysplasia, bone scan

Red Flags

- Short stature/delayed bone age and ovarian cysts
- Recurrent ovarian cysts
- Very high serum estradiol (>75 pg/mL)
- History of headaches, visual disturbance, or vomiting
- Isolated pubarche in boys and girls or peripheral precocity in boys
- Unilateral enlargement of testes in boys

Diagnostic Approach

Features of PP

- Gonadal hormone levels are increased to pubertal range (serum estradiol >10 pg/mL/37 pmol/L in girls: Testosterone >30 ng/dL in boys)
- Advanced bone age
- In girls, ovarian volume >1 cm^3 and uterine length >3.5 cm, endometrial thickness >2 mm

Distinguishing Central and Peripheral PP

- In boys with peripheral precocity, testicular volume is prepubertal (<4 mL) or small for genital stage
- Increased baseline serum LH levels >0.2–0.3 IU/L by ECLIA method
  - LH > 3.5–5 IU/L and LH:FSH ratio >1.0 after GnRH stimulation test suggests CPP. FSH response is highly exaggerated in isolated thelarche.
  - Baseline serum LH levels are prepubertal (<0.2 IU/L) with no response to GnRH stimulation test in peripheral PP.
- *USG abdomen and pelvis:* Look for gonadal or extragonadal tumors.

Approach to Precocious Puberty in Boys

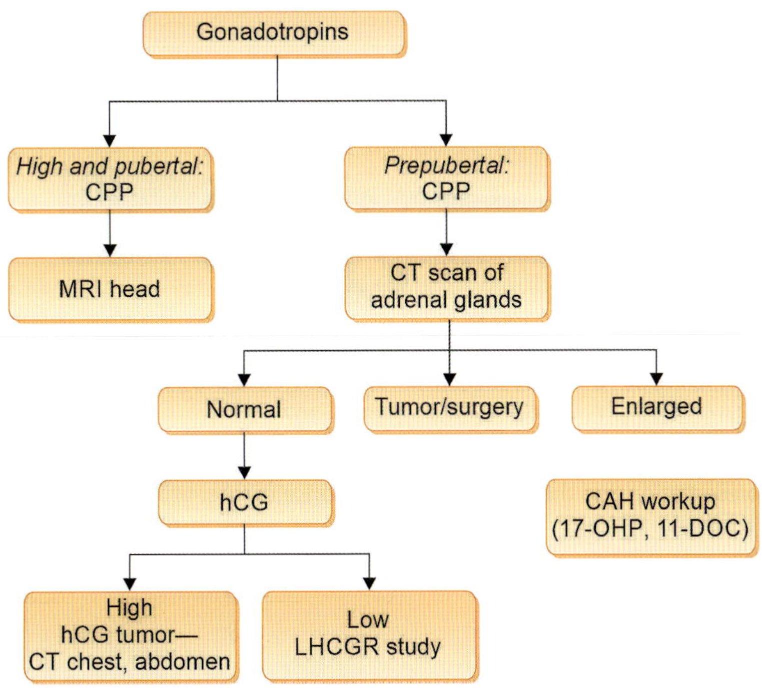

(11-DOC: 11-desoxycortisol; LHCGR: luteinizing hormone/choriogonadotropin receptor)

Approach to Precocious Puberty in Girls

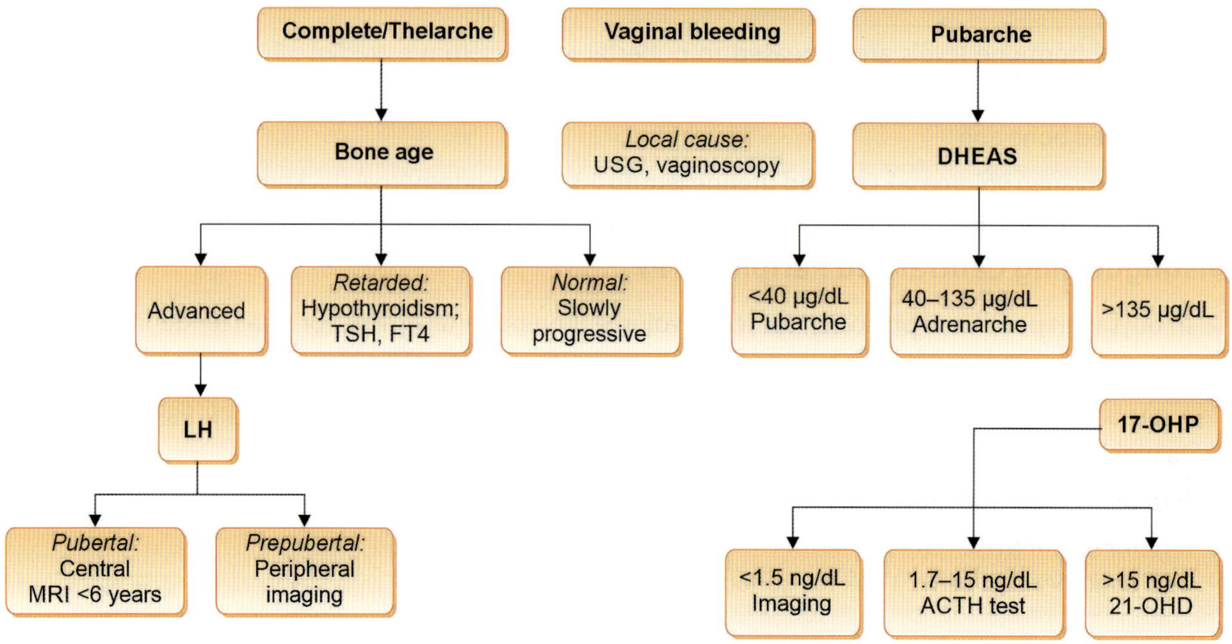

Suggested Reading

- Alghamdi A. Precocious Puberty: Types, Pathogenesis and Updated Management. Cureus. 2023;15(10):e47485.
- Cheuiche AV, da Silveira LG, de Paula LCP, Lucena IRS, Silveiro SP. Diagnosis and management of precocious sexual maturation: an updated review. Eur J Pediatr. 2021;180(10):3073-7.
- Pescovitz OH, Hench KD, Barnes KM, Loriaux DL, Cutler GB Jr. Premature thelarche and CPP: the relationship between clinical presentation and the gonadotropin response to luteinizing hormone-releasing hormone. J Clin Endocrinol Metab. 1988;67(3):474-9.

Tall Stature

6

Section Editor: **Kripasindhu Chatterjee**
Section Co-Editors: **Ashim Kumar Ghosh, Atanu Bhadra**
Authors: **Sumana Kundagrami, Neha Agarwal**

Introduction

- Tall stature is a relatively uncommon presenting complaint in children.
- It is rare and usually physiological.
- It is important to differentiate the physiological causes from pathological and diagnose the rare causes and treat them accordingly.

Definition

- Height standard deviation score (SDS) >2.
- Height velocity >90th centile.

Etiology

- Several causes could result in tall stature.
- Most are due to physiological reasons.
- Genetic and endocrine factors are sometimes responsible:
  - *Constitutional:* Normal at birth, peak from 4 years ending in tall stature/advanced bone age
  - *Familial:* Early onset, increased adult height
  - *Childhood obesity:* Increased free insulin-like growth factor-1 (IGF-1) levels due to inhibition of IGF binding protein (BP) production by hyperinsulinism, increased estradiol levels causing increased growth but chondrocyte apoptosis causing premature fusion and hence normal adult height.

Pathological

- *Endocrine:* GH excess—rare
  - Thyrotoxicosis
  - Precocious puberty
  - Delayed puberty—delayed epiphyseal fusion leads to increased final height
- *Overgrowth syndromes:* Paracrine dysregulation
  - Beckwith–Wiedemann syndrome
  - Simpson–Golabi–Behmel syndrome
  - Sotos syndrome
- *Syndromes:* Klinefelter (XXY)
  - Marfan syndrome
  - Homocystinuria

Red Flag Signs

- Gynecomastia
- Lens dislocation
- Hypoglycemia
- Mental retardation

Specific Diagnostic Pointers

- *Large for gestational age:* Beckwith–Wiedemann syndrome, Simpson, Sotos
- *Café-au-lait spots:* McCune–Albright syndrome
- *Gynecomastia:* Klinefelter, aromatase excess
- *Lens dislocation:* Marfan, homocystinuria
- *Macrocephaly:* Sotos, growth hormone (GH) excess
- *Mental retardation:* Sotos, Simpson

Investigations

- *Blood:* Thyroid profile, IGF-1
- Genetic studies (karyotype in Klinefelter syndrome)
- *Bone age:* X-ray left hand and wrist
- GH axis assessment to be done after excluding physiological and syndromic causes.
- IGF-1 levels above +2 SDS for age and gender indicate GH excess.
- This is to be confirmed by GH suppression tests (GH >1 ng/mL after 2 hours of 1.75 g/kg oral glucose).
- Pituitary MRI, cortisol levels, etc., may be done as indicated.

Approach to Tall Stature

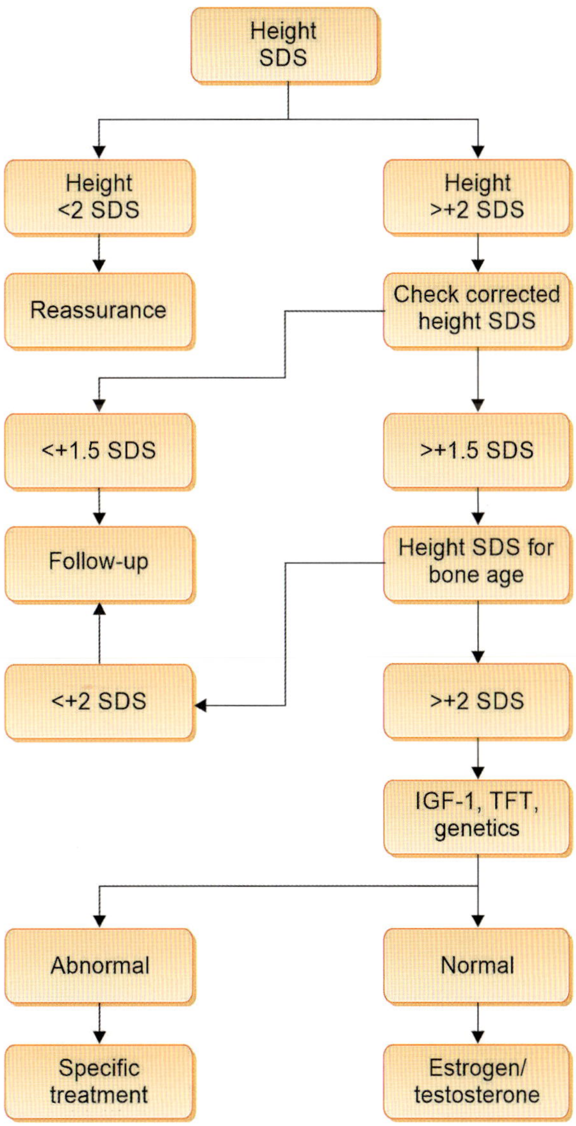

Suggested Reading

- Bajpai A, Patel R. Tall stature. Advanced Pediatric Endocrinology, Volume I, 1st edition. MedEClasses Publications: Kanpur; 2021. pp. 175-82.
- Cooke DW, Divali SA, Redovick S. Normal and aberrant growth in children. In: Melmed S, Auchus RJ, Goldfine AB, Koenig RJ, Rosen CJ (Eds). Williams Textbook of Endocrinology, 14th edition. Philadelphia: Elsevier; 2020. p. 941.
- Kaiser U, Ho K. Pituitary physiology and diagnostic evaluation. In: Melmed S, Auchus R, Goldfine A, Koenig R, Rosen C (Eds). Williams Textbook of Endocrinology, 14th edition. Gurugram : Elsevier ; 2019. pp. 184-235.
- Khadilkar V, Kondpalle S. Normal growth. In: Khadilkar V, Bajpai A, Prasad HK (Eds). IAP Textbook on Pediatric Endocrinology. New Delhi: Jaypee Brothers Medical Publishers; 2019. p. 37.
- Murray PG, Clayton PE. Disorders of growth. In: Dattani M, Brook CG (Ed). Brook's Clinical Pediatric Endocrinology, 7th edition. Oxford: Willey; 2020. p. 201.

Depression

7

Section Editor: **Sumitha Nayak**
Section Co-Editor: **Priya Shivalli**
Authors: **Akash Bang, Minal Ambade**

Depression in Pediatric Population in Office Practice

- Pediatric depression is complex and difficult to diagnose.
- The highest prevalence is reported in adolescents.
- It presents as social exclusion, discrimination, poor academic performance, risk-taking behaviors, physical ill-health, self-harm/suicidality, etc.

Etiology

- Physical and comorbid illnesses predispose to depression.
- *Other associations:* Autism, attention deficit hyperactivity disorder (ADHD), gender discrimination, child abuse and trafficking, failure in examinations, school dropouts, poverty, failed relationships, unemployment, bullying and cyberbullying, substance use, bereavement, environmental disasters, foster care/adoption, etc.

Red Flag Signs

These signs warrant immediate care:

- *Nonsuicidal self-injury (NSSI) behavior:* Deliberate destruction or alteration of body tissue without suicidal intent. It is commonly noted in adolescents as a coping mechanism for mental distress/secure attention and as a form of self-punishment.
- High risk of suicide using the mnemonic "IS PATH WARM" as below:

I—Ideation (talking or writing or posting online about death, threatening to hurt or kill self, and giving away prized possessions)
S—Substance use
P—Purposelessness (having no reason to live)
A—Anxiety
T—Trapped
H—Hopelessness
W—Withdrawal
A—Anger (uncontrolled)
R—Recklessness
M—Mood changes

Investigations

- Complete evaluation including current symptoms (externalizing and internalizing)
- Personal history, especially psychological development, response to life transitions, and major life events
- Diagnostic tests to rule out systemic effects of depression/associated chronic disorders

DSM-5 Criteria for Diagnosis of Depression (five or more of criteria during the same 2-week period and at least one of either A1 or A2)

A1	Depressed mood—by subjective report/observation by others (in children and adolescents, can be irritable mood)
A2	Loss of interest or pleasure in almost all activities—by subjective report/observation by others
A3	Significant (>5% in a month) unintentional weight loss/gain/decrease/increase in appetite (failure to make expected weight gains).
A4	*Sleep disturbance:* Insomnia/hypersomnia
A5	*Noticeable psychomotor changes:* Agitation or retardation
A6	Tiredness, fatigue, low energy, decreased efficiency for completion of routine tasks
A7	Sense of worthlessness, excessive, inappropriate, or delusional guilt
A8	Impaired ability to think, concentrate, or make decisions by subjective report or observation by others
A9	Recurrent thoughts of death, suicidal ideation, suicide attempts

- All adolescents above 12 years of age should be screened annually using the HEEADSSS Tool—Home environment, Education and Employment, Eating, peer-related Activities, Drugs, Sexuality, Suicide/depression and Safety psychosocial screening (HEEADSSS)
- *Other screening questionnaires:* Children's Depression Rating Scale, Patient Health Questionniare-9-A, Beck Depression Inventory, Hamilton Depression Rating Scale, Screening for Childhood Anxiety Related Emotional Disorders (SCARED), etc.
- *Teen Screening Questionnaire: Mental Health (TSQ-M):* A validated tool

Quick Tools for a Busy OPD

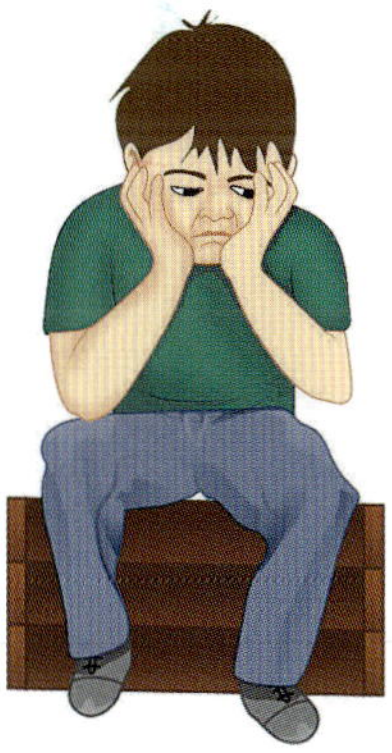

Pictorial Instrument for Children and Adolescents (PICA-R): For 6–16-year-old children.

- Ask, "How much you are like him/her?, "Do you get like him? How much? Do you feel sad the way he does? Do people tell you that you look sad? How much? What about crying? How much does it happen to you?"
- Then provide a *five-point rated visual analog scale*, which quantifies things, i.e., showing with hands how much they mean.

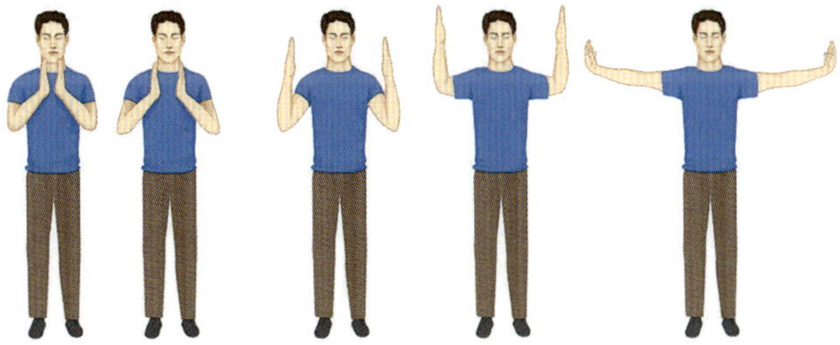

- *Ask* short nonjudgmental questions to assess intent or thoughts/plan for suicide.
- Disclosure of suicidality information with a trustworthy caregiver is pivotal.

Approach

According to the Diagnostic Statistical Manual of Mental Disorders, 5th edition (DSM-5) criteria for diagnosis of adolescent depression:
These symptoms should be present for at least 2 weeks, on most of the days

Causes and risk factors present
HEEADSSS screening, clinical history, examination, mental state examination, past and family history of psychiatric issues, screening for comorbid psychiatric disorders, assessment of caregivers

- Differentiate from mood changes secondary to organic problems (e.g., anemia, hypothyroidism, Wilson's disease) by doing a detailed clinical assessment and relevant investigations
- Assess severity and level of dysfunction

Psychometric tests in office practice: Patient Health Questionnaire-2 (PHQ-2), PHQ-9 modified for adolescents (PHQ-A), and Teen Screening Questionnaire-Mental Health (TSQ-M)

Mild depression: Positive lifestyle changes, mood diary, journal, counseling and psychotherapy—cognitive behavior therapy (CBT) or rational emotive behavioral therapy (REBT)

Moderate and severe depression: Pharmacotherapy—selective serotonin reuptake inhibitors (SSRIs)—continued for a period of 6–12 months and slowly tapered off over 4–6 weeks

- A team approach
- Anticipatory guidance and imparting psychoeducation regarding pubertal changes, communication, conflict management, peer affiliation, parental expectation, drugs and sexuality
- Healthy balanced eating plan, sleep, screen time, physical activity, mindfulness
- Create a safety plan—emergency numbers, helpline 1098

Suggested Reading

- American Psychiatric Association. Depressive disorders. The Diagnostic and Statistical Manual of Mental Disorders, 5th edition (DSM-5) TR.
- Croke L. Depression in Adolescents: AAP Updates Guidelines on Diagnosis and Treatment. American Family Physician. 2018;98(7):462-3.
- Grover S, Avasthi A. Clinical Practice Guidelines for the management of depression in children and adolescents. Indian J Psychiatry. 2019;61(Suppl 2):226-40.
- Nair MKC. Adolescent anxiety and depression. Indian J Pract Pediatr. 2015;17(2):122-6.
- Nair MKC. Anticipatory Guidance in Adolescents. Standard Treatment Guidelines. 2022.
- Patra S. Assessment and management of Pediatric Depression. Indian J Psychiatry. 2019;61(3):300-6.

Developmental Delay

8

Section Editor: **Sumitha Nayak**
Section Co-Editor: **Priya Shivalli**
Author: **Chitra Sankar**

Introduction

Developmental delay refers to a failure to achieve the expected milestones in one or more domains within the expected age range or time frame. There is a normal age range for every milestone in the developmental domains—gross motor, fine motor, communication, cognition, and personal–social domains. Delay may be specific to one or more domains of development. If present in two or more domains, it is called global developmental delay.

Etiology

The etiology of developmental delay is given in **Table 1**.

TABLE 1: Genetic and nongenetic etiology of developmental delay.

Genetic	*Nongenetic*
Chromosomal abnormalities (e.g., trisomy 21 and Klinefelter syndrome)	Prenatal infections (TORCH, Zika, chickenpox), brain malformations, and congenital hypothyroidism
Single-gene disorders [e.g., fragile X syndrome, Rett syndrome, tuberous sclerosis, PKU, and inborn errors of metabolism (small molecule and lysosomal storage disorders)]	Perinatal factors (severe birth asphyxia, infections, prematurity, PVL, LBW, IUGR, hypoglycemia, and bilirubin encephalopathy)
Defects of genomic imprinting (Prader–Willi syndrome and Angelman syndrome)	Environmental factors (traumatic brain injury, abuse, neglect, poverty, malnutrition, micronutrient deficiency—iron, folate, vitamin D, and calcium)
Mutations (Duchenne muscular dystrophy and spinal muscular atrophy)	Sequalae of childhood illnesses (meningitis, encephalitis, and seizure disorders)
Deletion syndromes (Williams syndrome and DiGeorge syndrome)	Teratogens/toxins (smoking, fetal alcohol syndrome, lead, other toxins, maternal antiseizure medications, and cytotoxic drugs)
Undetermined (familial)	Undetermined (nonfamilial)

[PKU: phenylketonuria; PVL: periventricular leukomalacia; LBW: low birth weight; IUGR: intrauterine growth restriction; TORCH: toxoplasmosis, others (syphilis, hepatitis B), rubella, cytomegalovirus, herpes simplex]

Absolute Indications for Further Workup

- No social smile, poor visual behavior, and response to sounds by 2 months
- No head control by 5–6 months and no bilateral transfer by 8 months
- No independent sitting by 9 months and no pincer grasp by 12 months
- No independent walking by 16 months and no running by 24 months
- No babbling, index-finger pointing, and gestures by 12 months
- No single words by 16 months, nonecholalic two-word sentences by 24 months, and three-word sentences by 3 years
- Regression or loss of skills at any age

Red Flag Signs

- Dysmorphic features
- Clenched hands/dystonic posture/hand preference before 1 year of age
- Microcephaly or macrocephaly
- Tone abnormalities—hypertonia and hypotonia
- Muscle weakness
- Tongue fasciculations
- Hepatosplenomegaly
- Poor eye contact and strabismus
- Hyperactivity

Relevant Investigations and Referrals

A comprehensive history, physical and neurological examination, and use of developmental screening tools are essential for further evaluations.

Early intervention services including physical, occupational, and speech therapy are required for further management.

Do not refer directly for therapy without an appropriate workup.

Do not take a "wait and watch" approach without screening and basic investigations.

Basic screening and investigations include:

- Hearing and vision check. In preterm, retinopathy of prematurity (ROP) screening is compulsory.
- Complete blood count, serum calcium, phosphorus, alkaline phosphatase, vitamin D, liver function tests, and glucose
- *Developmental delay with dysmorphic features:* Karyotyping, chromosomal microarray
- *Motor delay with high tone:* Neuroimaging, preferably magnetic resonance imaging (MRI) of the brain
- *Motor delay with normal/low tone:* Check thyroid functions and creatine phosphokinase (CPK).
- *Developmental delay with microcephaly:* Neuroimaging—MRI brain, TORCH [toxoplasmosis, others (syphilis, hepatitis B), rubella, cytomegalovirus, herpes simplex] screening, and retinal examination
- *Developmental delay with the following signs suggestive of neurometabolic conditions:* Unexplained delay in development with or without family history and worsening with illness/high-protein diet/fasting
  - Hypoglycemia
  - Hepatosplenomegaly
  - Coarse facial features
  - Neurological regression
  - Seizures
  - Dysmorphism
  - Unexplained ataxia/spasticity
  - Abnormal urinary or body odors, hair abnormalities, ocular abnormalities like cataracts, and increased/decreased pigmentation
- *Isolated speech delay:* Check hearing status, screen with MCHAT (modified checklist for autism in toddlers).
- *Global developmental delay:* Investigate as above and refer for further management.
- *Screening tools:* Trivandrum Developmental Screening Tool (TDSC) or Denver Developmental Screening Tool (DDST) is to be used.

Approach

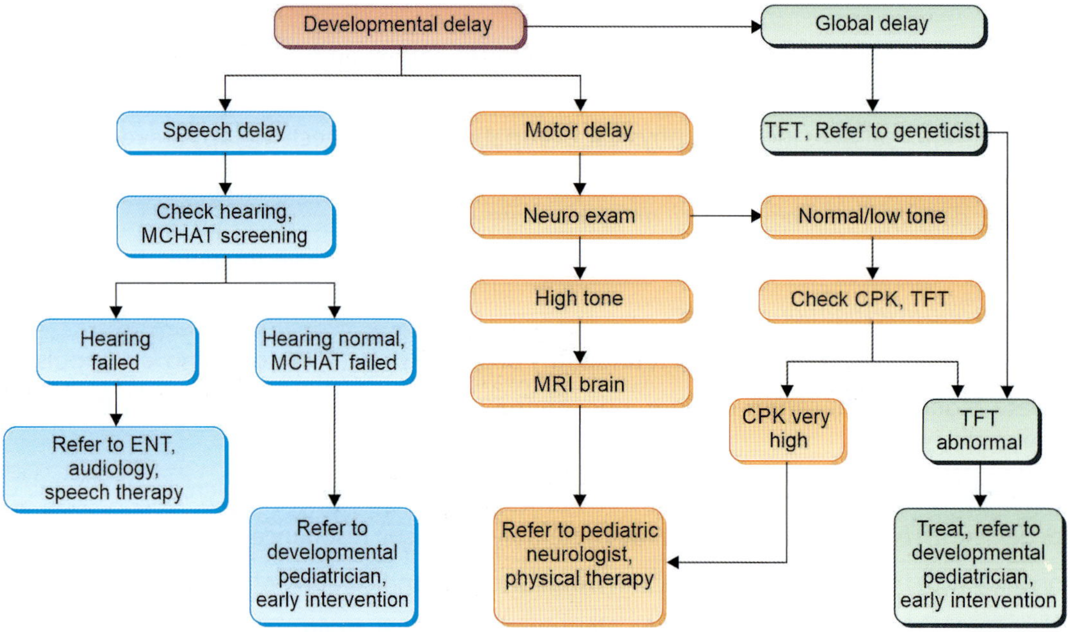

(CPK: creatine phosphokinase; ENT: ear, nose, and throat; MCHAT: modified checklist for autism in toddlers; MRI: magnetic resonance imaging; TFT: thyroid function tests)

Suggested Reading

- AlMutiri R, Malta M, Shevell MI, Srour M. Evaluation of individuals with non-syndromic global developmental delay and intellectual disability. Children (Basel). 2023;10(3):414.
- Cleary MA, Green A. Developmental delay: When to suspect and how to investigate for an inborn error of metabolism. Arch Dis Child. 2005;90:1128-32.
- Jullien S. Screening for language and speech delay in children under five years. BMC Pediatr. 2021;21(Suppl 1):362.
- Juneja M, Gupta A, Sairam S, Jain R, Sharma M, Thadani A, et al. Diagnosis and management of global development delay: Consensus guidelines of growth, development and behavioral pediatrics chapter, neurology chapter and neurodevelopment pediatrics chapter of the Indian Academy of Pediatrics. Indian Pediatr. 2022;59(5):401-15.
- Khan I, Leventhal BL. Developmental Delay. In: StatPearls [Internet]. Treasure Island (FL): StatPearls Publishing; 2023. [online] Available from https://www.ncbi.nlm.nih.gov/books/NBK562231/ [Last accessed January, 2024].
- Sharma AR, Siddiqui MS, Magar S, Kale A, Nelanuthala M, Singh SP. The etiological profile of global developmental delay at a tertiary care hospital in India: An observational study. Cureus. 2023;15(6):e41066.

Phimosis

9

Section Editor: **Gnanamurthy Narasimha**
Section Co-Editor: **Nagalatha Chidananda**
Author: **Antony Robert Charles**

Introduction

- Phimosis is one of the most commonly diagnosed conditions in young boys. Up to the age of 5 years, it is physiological to have the prepuce not opening and does not require treatment unless symptomatic or in special urological conditions.
- Pathological phimosis is present only in about 10% of all boys with phimosis.

Etiology

When it is pathological, the etiology is usually inflammatory with a nonretractile, scarred prepuce. This does not respond to standard medical therapy. In majority of boys, it is a physiological phenomenon.

Red Flags

- Recurrent urinary tract infections in a boy
- Red, edematous prepuce
- Scarred prepuce with whitish discoloration
- Balanitis xerotica obliterans (BXO)/lichen sclerosus seen in 10–15% of older children
- Paraphimosis, a condition where a retracted prepuce does not come back and cause extreme edema

Approach to Management

Common Symptoms

- Ballooning of prepuce while passing urine
- Itching/constantly holding the penis
- After passing urine, a few droplets of urine falling in underwear
- Complaints of painful micturition and frequency
- Skin color changes and pain while retracting
- Inability to retract, even after the age of 5 years
- Small swellings under the prepuce—innocuous epithelial pearls

Algorithm for the approach to management of phimosis.

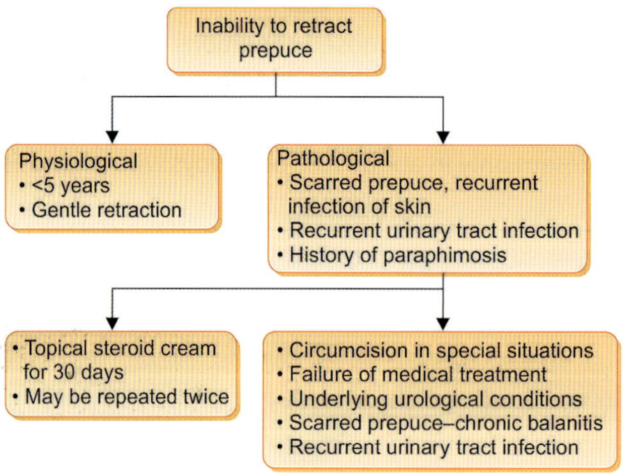

Suggested Reading

- Babu R, Harrison SK, Hutton KA. Ballooning of the foreskin and physiological phimosis: Is there any objective evidence of obstructed voiding? BJU Int. 2004;94(3):384-7.
- Yang SS, Tsai YC, Wu CC, Liu SP, Wang CC. Highly potent and moderately potent topical steroids are effective in treating phimosis: A prospective randomized study. J Urol. 2005;173(4):1361-3.

Hematuria

10

Section Editor: **Gnanamurthy Narasimha**
Section Co-Editor: **Nagalatha Chidananda**
Author: **Shashikiran KB**

Introduction

Evaluation of hematuria proceeds as follows:

- Confirmation of the presence of hematuria and differentiating it from other causes of red/brown urine
- Identifying the potential site of bleeding (glomerular vs. nonglomerular)
- Algorithmic approach based on symptomatology

Definition

Hematuria is defined as the presence of an increased number of red blood cells (RBCs) in the urine.

Classification:

- *Gross hematuria:* Visible to the naked eye
- *Microscopic hematuria:* Apparent only upon urinalysis
  It refers to the presence of >5 RBCs per high-power field (latest guidelines say >3 RBCs/high-power field).
- *Persistent hematuria:* Presence of hematuria on two to three occasions for a period beyond 4 weeks
- *Transient microscopic hematuria:* It is caused by exercise, fever, trauma to urinary tract, and urinary tract infection.

Urinary Dipstick Test

Centrifuge 10 mL of a fresh urine sample at 2,000 rpm for 5 minutes.

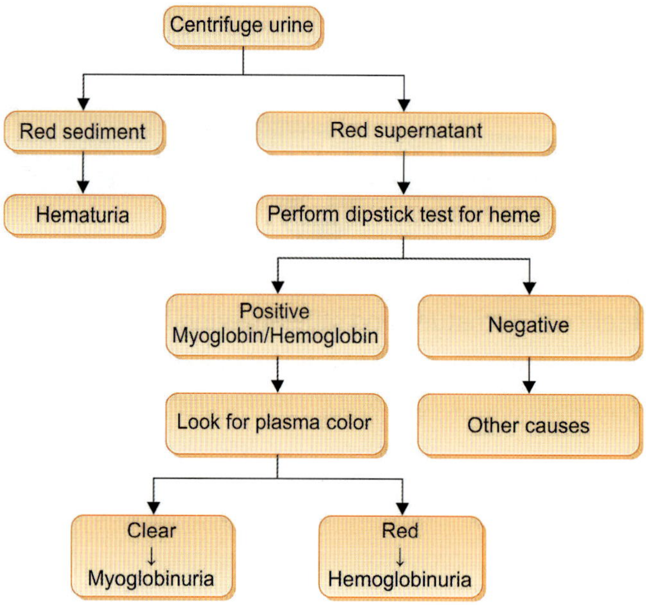

Other causes of dipstick-negative red/brown urine:

- *Medications:* Rifampin, doxorubicin, chloroquine, deferoxamine, ibuprofen, iron sorbitol, nitrofurantoin, and phenolphthalein
- *Food dyes:* Beets and food coloring agents
- *Metabolites:* Bile pigments, homogentisic acid, methemoglobin, porphyrin, and tyrosinosis

Microscopic Urine Examination

It is the gold standard for the detection of microscopic hematuria.

Glomerular hematuria:

- Presence of RBC casts
- Presence of >20% dysmorphic RBCs or >5% acanthocytes is highly suggestive.
- Associated with significant proteinuria

Pointers to Etiology

ETIOLOGY	DIAGNOSIS
Unilateral flank pain that radiates to the groin	Ureteric calculi
Dysuria, frequency, urgency, new-onset enuresis	Urinary tract infection
Medication intake—cyclophosphamide and features of adenoviral illness	Hemorrhagic cystitis
A history of pharyngitis or impetigo (2 or 3 weeks earlier)	Poststreptococcal glomerulonephritis (PSGN)
Synpharyngitic hematuria	Immunoglobulin A nephropathy (IgAN)

Red Flag Signs

- Significant proteinuria
- Hypertension with edema
- Persistent gross/glomerular hematuria
- Decreasing glomerular filtration rate (GFR) and rising serum creatinine
- Hematuria in a child with a family history of kidney failure in early adulthood in a first-order relative

Algorithm for Evaluation of Asymptomatic Microscopic Hematuria

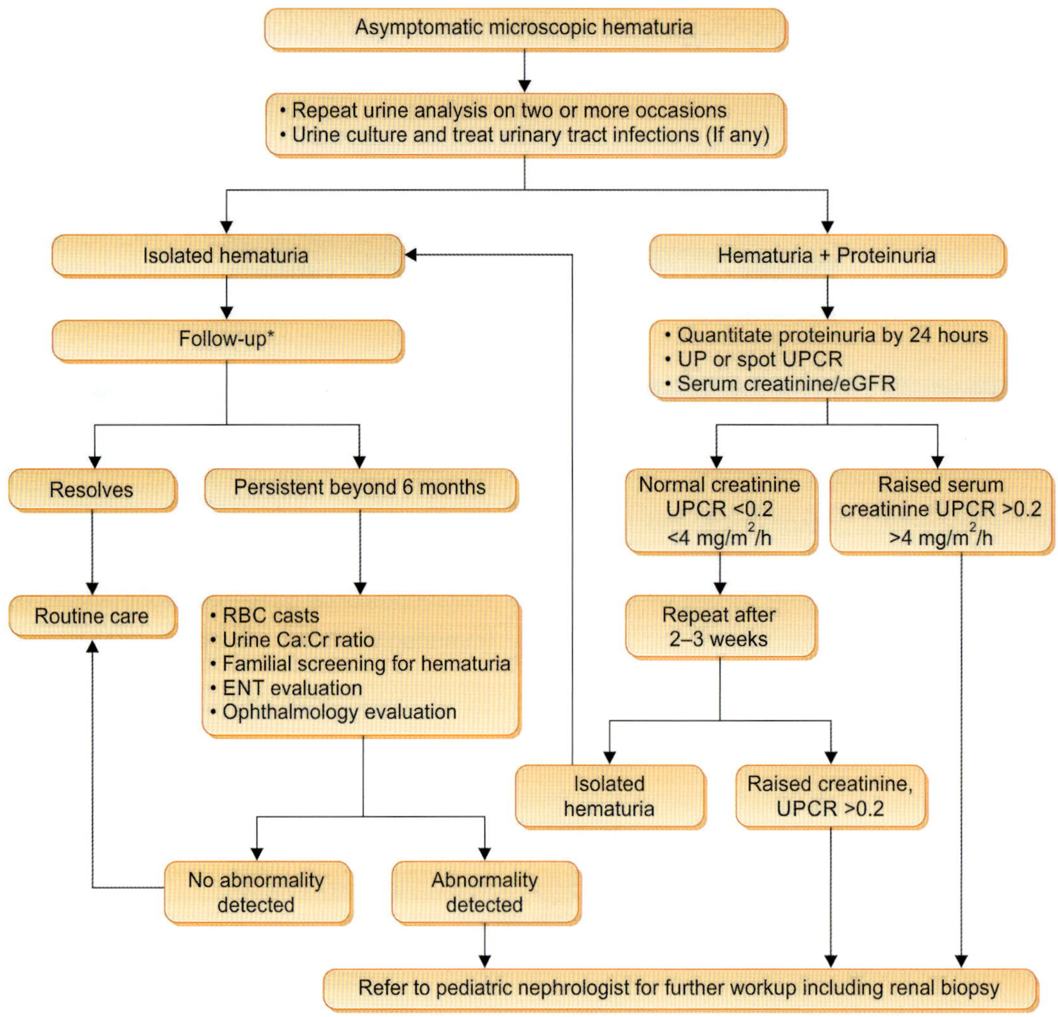

*If anytime during follow-up a patient develops symptoms, work up like symptomatic hematuria

(eGFR: estimated glomerular filtration rate; ENT: ear, nose, and throat; UP: urine protein; UPCR: urine protein to creatinine ratio)

Algorithm for Evaluation of Gross or Symptomatic Microscopic Hematuria

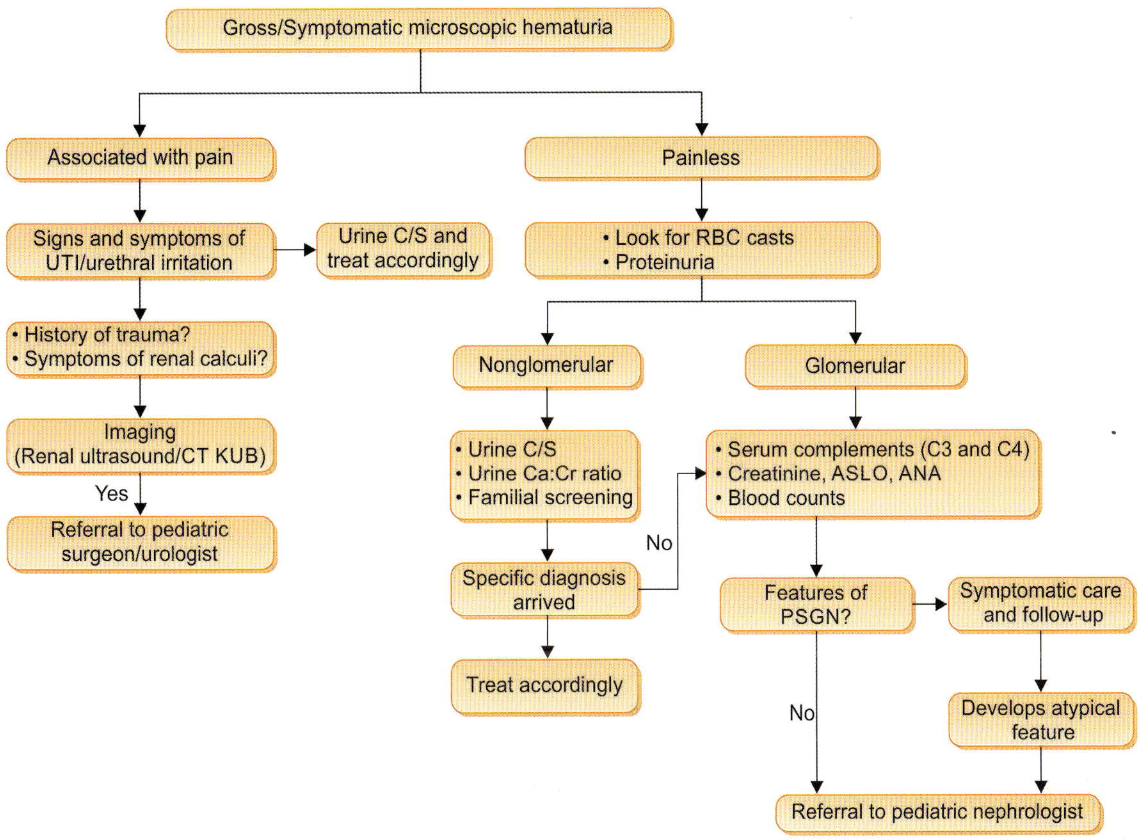

(ANA: antinuclear antibody; ASLO: antistreptolysin O; Ca:Cr: calcium to creatinine ratio; C/S: culture and sensitivity; CT KUB: computed tomography of the kidneys, ureters and bladder; PSGN: poststreptococcal glomerulonephritis; RBC: red blood cells; UTI: urinary tract infection)

Other Investigations

TESTS	DIAGNOSIS
Serum creatinine	To identify renal impairment
Serum complements (C3 and C4)	Low in SLE and PSGN
ANA, ASLO	SLE and PSGN
Familial screening for hematuria	Hereditary nephritis
Kidney biopsy (when indicated)	Helps in diagnosis and prognostication

(ANA: antinuclear antibody; ASLO: antistreptolysin O; PSGN: poststreptococcal glomerulonephritis; SLE: systemic lupus erythematosus)

Cystoscopy

Cystoscopy is rarely indicated in children.

Indications:

- Bladder mass on ultrasound
- Urethral abnormalities due to trauma
- Symptoms suggestive of inflammatory cystitis

Suggested Reading

- Patel HP, Bissler JJ. Hematuria in children. Pediatr Clin North Am. 2001;48:1519-37.
- Phadke KD, Vijayakumar M, Sharma J, Iyengar A; Indian Pediatric Nephrology Group. Consensus statement on evaluation of hematuria. Indian Pediatr. 2006;43:965-73.

Goiter

11

Section Editor: **Kripasindhu Chatterjee**
Section Co-Editors: **Ashim Kumar Ghosh, Atanu Bhadra**
Author: **Vasundhara Chugh**

Introduction

Goiter is a common endocrine disorder characterized by the enlargement of the thyroid gland. Depending on the etiology, children with goiter can be euthyroid, hypothyroid, or hyperthyroid.

Etiology

CONGENITAL	ACQUIRED
• Dyshormonogenesis • Neonatal Graves' disease – Transplacental passage of maternal TSH receptor-stimulating antibodies – Activating mutation of TSH receptor – McCune–Albright syndrome • Thyroglossal duct cysts • Excess iodine exposure to mother or infant • Severe maternal iodine deficiency	• Iodine deficiency • Colloid goiter • Chronic autoimmune (Hashimoto's) thyroiditis • Ingestion of goitrogens • Graves' disease • Thyroid nodules (benign/malignant) • Thyroid infiltrative diseases (cystinosis and histiocytosis) • Subacute granulomatous thyroiditis • Acute suppurative thyroiditis (thyroid gland abscess caused by bacterial infection)

(TSH: thyroid-stimulating hormone)

Red Flag Signs

- *Thyroid nodules on palpation:* Thyroid nodules are less common in children than in adults, but the rate of malignancy is significantly higher in children.
- *Severe thyroid tenderness:* It is seen in acute suppurative thyroiditis and needs urgent treatment.
- *Palpitations and tremors:* These are seen in hyperthyroidism and need treatment with beta-blockers along with antithyroid drugs.
- *Coarse facies, umbilical hernia, macroglossia, prolonged jaundice in neonates:* Signs of congenital hypothyroidism

Investigations

- Thyroid function test
- *Thyroid antibodies*: In children with hypothyroidism or euthyroid status, measurement of anti-thyroid peroxidase and antithyroglobulin antibodies should be done. Children presenting with hyperthyroidism should be checked for thyroid-stimulating hormone (TSH) receptor-stimulating antibodies.
- *Ultrasound*: Performed in cases with thyroid gland asymmetry, thyroid nodules on palpation, and cervical lymphadenopathy
- *Urinary iodine excretion*: Done in selected children to determine iodine deficiency
- *Radionuclide thyroid scan*: Done in children with hyperthyroidism or suspicion of toxic nodules
- *Fine needle aspiration cytology (FNAC)*: Performed if the size of the nodule is >1 cm

Approach

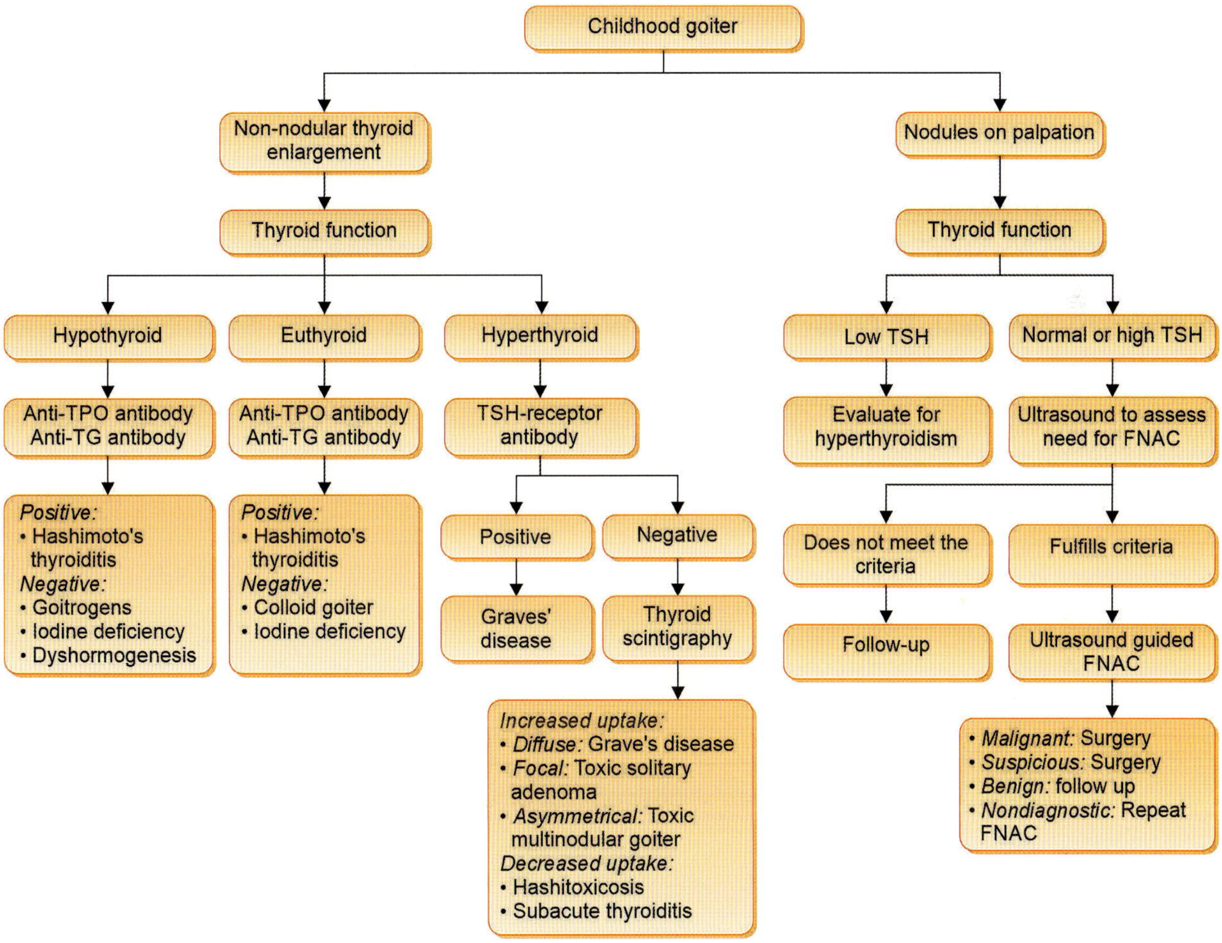

(FNAC: fine-needle aspiration cytology; TG: thyroglobulin; TPO: thyroid peroxidase; TSH: thyroid-stimulating hormone)

Suggested Reading

- Desai MP, Sharma R, Riaz I, Sudhanshu S, Parikh R, Bhatia V. Newborn screening guidelines for congenital hypothyroidism in India: Recommendations of the Indian Society for Pediatric and Adolescent Endocrinology (ISPAE) -Part I: Screening and confirmation of diagnosis. Indian J Pediatr. 2018;85(6):440-53.
- Francis GL, Waguespack SG, Bauer AJ, Angelos P, Benvenga S, Cerutti JM, et al; American Thyroid Association Guidelines Task Force. Management guidelines for children with thyroid nodules and differentiated thyroid cancer. Thyroid. 2015;25(7):716-59.
- Hegedüs L, Bonnema SJ, Bennedbæk FN. Management of simple nodular goiter: current status and future perspectives. Endocr Rev. 2003;24(1):102-32.
- Unnikrishnan AG, Kalra S, Baruah M, Nair G, Nair V, Bantwal G, et al. Endocrine Society of India management guidelines for patients with thyroid nodules: A position statement. Indian J Endocrinol Metab. 2011;15(1):2-8.
- Zimmermann MB, Jooste PL, Pandav CS. Iodine-deficiency disorders. Lancet. 2008;372(9645):1251-62.

Bowlegs

12

Section Editor: **Janani Shankar**
Section Co-Editor: **Arathi Srinivasan**
Author: **Shama Sowdagar**

Introduction

Bowlegs or genu varum is an angular deformity of the knees where the apex of the deformity points away from the midline.

Normal Physiological Development of Lower Extremity

At birth, normal alignment is varus. During infancy, with weight-bearing, the varus increases. After 2 years of age, the alignment progresses to valgus and maximizes by 4 years of age. After 4 years of age, valgus alignment decreases and gradually progresses to slight valgus to neutral by 7 years of age. This is the physiologic adult alignment.

Etiology

Genu varum can be of the following types:

- *Physiological:* The tibiofemoral angle is within 2 standard deviations from mean for any age. A majority of children presenting with bowlegs have physiologic bowing.

  Characteristics include:

  - Age between birth and 2 years
  - Bilateral, symmetric, and painless
  - Normal length/height for age and sex
  - Bowing of both femur and tibia
  - Absence of lateral thrust/protrusion with ambulation during the stance phase
  - Improves with age

- *Pathological*: This type is much less prevalent compared to physiological varus, with a variable frequency.

  Causes include:

  - Blount's disease (tibia vara)—most common
  - Rickets—nutritional/hypophosphatemic/renal disease/celiac sprue and other gastrointestinal disorders
  - Skeletal dysplasias—achondroplasia/pseudoachondroplasia/metaphyseal chondrodysplasia/cartilage hair hypoplasia/multiple epiphyseal dysplasia
  - History of fracture/infection
  - Neoplasia
  - Untreated congenital anomalies and metabolic and rheumatological diseases like juvenile idiopathic arthritis (JIA)

Pointers for Pathological Varus

- Length/height of the child is below the third centile.
- Weight—obesity is a risk factor for adolescent Blount's disease.
- Relevant examination to look for signs suggestive of pathologic varus etiology.
- Gait—look for in-toeing/out-toeing and lateral thrust.
- Symmetrical versus asymmetrical/limb-length shortening
- Site of angulation—femur and tibia (physiologic), knee (ligamentous laxity), and proximal tibia metaphysis (Blount's disease)
- Epiphyseal widening on palpation suggestive of nutritional rickets
- Intercondylar distance between the two medial femoral condyles >6 cm at any age.
- Coxa vara, positive Trendelenburg gait, and limited hip abduction may suggest dysplasias or metabolic disease.

Red Flag Signs

- Severe bowing (defined as >6 cm between the femoral condyles with patella facing forward and medial malleoli together)
- Progressive bowing
- Persistent bowing after 3 years of age
- Asymmetrical or unilateral bowing
- Lateral thrust with ambulation
- Short stature
- History of metabolic disease, lower extremity fracture, infection, or tumor

Investigations

- Radiographs of both legs from hips to ankles with the child standing and patella pointing straight are indicated if pathologic varus is suspected.
- Serum alkaline phosphatase, calcium, phosphorus, 25-hydroxyvitamin D, and 1,25 $(OH)_2$ vitamin D levels should be investigated in appropriate cases.

Approach

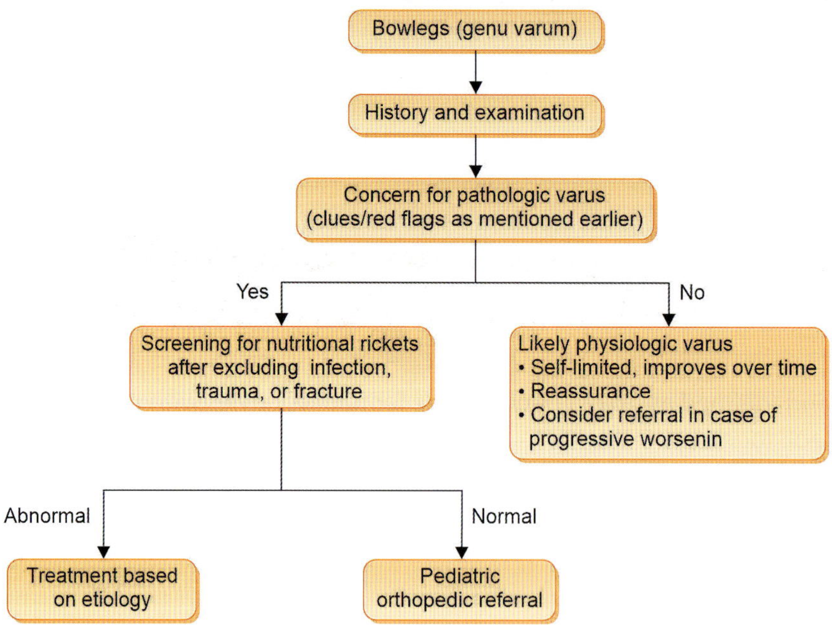

Suggested Reading

- Heath CH, Staheli LT. Normal limits of knee angle in white children—genu varum and genu valgum. J Pediatr Orthop. 1993;13(2):259-62.
- Salenius P, Vankka E. The development of the tibiofemoral angle in children. J Bone Joint Surg Am. 1975;57(2):259-61.
- Sass P, Hassan G. Lower extremity abnormalities in children. Am Fam Physician. 2003;68(3):461-8.
- Schoenecker PL, Rich MM. The lower extremity. In: Morrissy RT, Weinstein SL (Eds). Lovell and Winter's Pediatric Orthopaedics, 6th edition. Philadelphia: Lippincott Williams and Wilkins; 2006. p. 1158.
- Schoenecker PL, Rich MM, Gordon JE. The lower extremity. In: Weinstein SL, Flynn JM (Eds). Lovell and Winter's Pediatric Orthopaedics, 7th edition. Philadelphia: Lippincott Williams and Wilkins; 2014. p. 1261.
- Vogt B, Frommer A, Gosheger G, Toporowski G, Tretow H, Rödl R, et al. Growth modulation through hemiepiphysiodesis: Novel surgical techniques: risks and progress. Orthopade. 2021;50(7):538-47.

Flatfeet

13

Section Editor: **Janani Shankar**
Section Co-Editor: **Arathi Srinivasan**
Author: **Shama Sowdagar**

Introduction

- Flatfoot or pes planus refers to a diminished or absent medial longitudinal arch (MLA). It is relatively common and affects up to 14% of children.
- It may occur in isolation or associated with a hindfoot abnormality called valgus alignment (pes planovalgus).

Normal Physiological Development of Foot

- All infants are born with flatfeet because of physiologic ligamentous laxity and lack of MLA.
- At birth, a fat pad is the dominant visible structure in this region, which slowly decreases as children grow. Normal foot arch develops during the first decade of life, by the age of 5–6 years.

Types

- *Flexible flatfoot:* It is usually physiologic and accounts for 95% of all cases.

  The MLA is present while sitting but disappears with weight-bearing or stance phase of walk. It usually resolves by the age of 10 years but may persist into adolescence and adulthood.
- *Rigid flatfoot:* It is nonphysiologic. There is restriction of subtalar joint motion.

  It is associated with pain and serious underlying pathology.

  Tiptoe walking differentiates rigid from flexible flatfoot by the absence of arch formation, and the heel remains in valgus alignment.

Causes

FLEXIBLE FLATFOOT	RIGID FLATFOOT
Physiological ligamentous and joint laxity	Congenital vertical talus (rocker-bottom foot with equinus heel)
Inherited (positive family history)	Tarsal coalition (peroneal spastic flatfoot syndrome)
Generalized ligamentous laxity (Down syndrome)	Inflammatory arthritis of the subtalar joint [juvenile idiopathic arthritis (JIA), e.g., enthesitis-related arthritis (ERA)]
Familial flatfeet	Accessory navicular bone
Benign hypermobile joint syndrome	Cerebral palsy and other neurodevelopmental disorders

Examination

- Gait assessment with shoes and barefoot including heel and tiptoe walking, and extension of great toe
- Look for hallux valgus, crowding of lesser toes, Achilles valgus, and callosities.
- Signs of inflammation
- Active and passive dorsiflexion of ankle and inversion and eversion of foot
- Look for ligamentous laxity in other joints (Beighton score) and skin laxity.
- Complete neurological examination

Delaying shoe wear until childhood and barefoot walking decrease the propensity for flatfeet.

Red Flag Signs

- Feet, which are painful, stiff, weak, or numb
- Repeated feet or ankle injuries
- Problems with walking or balance
- Late onset of flatfeet
- Unilateral flatfoot
- Persistent flatfeet after 10 years of age

Approach

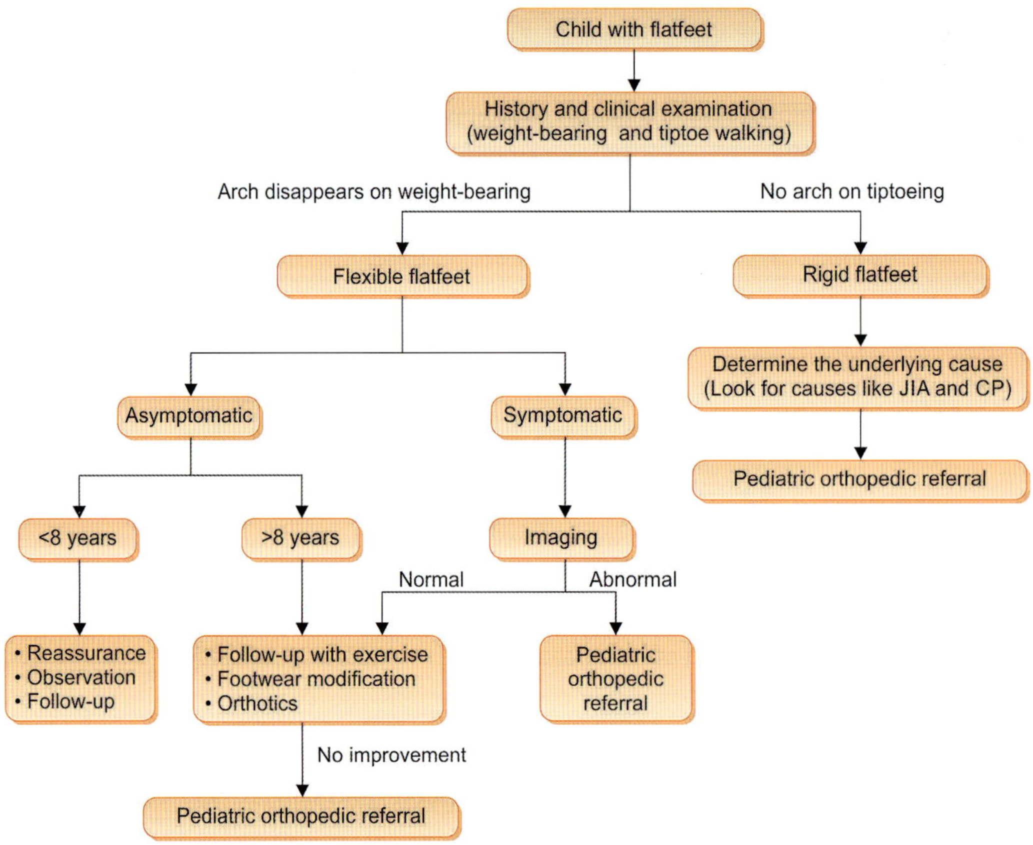

(CP: cerebral palsy; JIA: juvenile idiopathic arthritis)

Suggested Reading

- Carr JB 2nd, Yang S, Lather LA. Pediatric pes planus: A state-of-the-art review. Pediatrics. 2016;137(3):e20151230.
- Dare DM, Dodwell ER. Pediatric flatfoot: Cause, epidemiology, assessment, and treatment. Curr Opin in Pediatr. 2014;26(1):93-100.
- Morley AJM. Knock-knee in children. BMJ. 1957;2(5051):976-9.
- Mortazavi SJ, Espandar R, Baghdadi T. Flatfoot in children: How to approach? Iran J of Pediatr. 2007;17(2).
- Rome K, Ashford RL, Evans A. Non-surgical interventions for paediatric pes planus. Cochrane Database Syst Rev. 2010;(7):CD006311.
- Turner C, Gardiner MD, Midgley A, Stefanis A. A guide to the management of paediatric pes planus. Aust J Gen Pract. 2020;49(5):245-9.
- Vulcano E, Maccario C, Myerson MS. How to approach the pediatric flatfoot. World J Orthop. 2016;7(1):1-7.

Approach to Short Stature

14

Section Editor: **Kripasindhu Chatterjee**
Section Co-Editors: **Ashim Kumar Ghosh, Atanu Bhadra**
Authors: **Hriday De, Debaditya Das**

Definition

- Height 2 standard deviation score (SDS) below the mean for age and sex, height <2 SDS of the target height (TH)
- A significant decrease in height SDS defined as a deflection of at least 0.3 SDS/yr

Etiology

Causes of short stature:

- *Isolated short stature:*
  - Idiopathic short stature (ISS)
  - Familial short stature (FSS)
  - Constitutional delay in growth and puberty (CDGP)
- *Syndromic short stature:*
  - Turner syndrome
  - Noonan syndrome
  - Silver–Russel syndrome
  - Prader–Willi syndrome

- *Disorders of the growth hormone (GH)–insulin-like growth factor (IGF)-I axis:*
  - Growth hormone deficiency (GHD)
  - Growth hormone insensitivity
- *Chronic systemic diseases:*
  - Celiac disease
  - Chronic kidney disease
  - Cardiac conditions
  - Pulmonary diseases
  - Neuromuscular disorders
  - Endocrine conditions
  - Gastrointestinal disorders
  - Protein energy malnutrition
  - Rheumatic disorders
  - Hematological disorders
- *Skeletal dysplasia:*
  - Achondroplasia
  - Hypochondroplasia
- *Small for gestational age babies (SGA)*
- *Psychosocial deprivation*

Red Flag Signs

- Height < –3 SD for age and sex
- Growth velocity <25th percentile
- Abnormal body proportions
- Dysmorphic features
- Abnormal central nervous system (CNS)/eye findings
- Goiter

Clinical Evaluation

Anthropometry

Anthropometry—weight, standing height (stadiometer)/length by infantometer (<2 years), proportion (upper segment: lower segment), head circumference, arm span.

Growth Chart

It is recommended that the measurements should be plotted and evaluated using country specific charts, that is combined World Health Organization/Indian Academy of Pediatrics (WHO/IAP) growth charts.

Growth Velocity

A series of height measurements indicates the growth pace. Poor prognosis for height if below the 25th centile.

T1: Height measured previously. T2: Height measured thereafter

$$\text{Growth velocity (cm/yr)} = \frac{T2 - T1}{\text{Number of months between T2 and T1}} \times 12 \text{ months}$$

Growth Potential

The midparental height (MPH) is used in order to identify FSS. The MPH for boys and girls is determined differently, as follows:

- MPH (Boys) = (Father's height + Mother's height + 13)/2
- MPH (girls) = (Father's height + Mother's height – 13)/2

Midparental height gives us an idea about the growth potential genetically endowed on the child.

Pointers to etiology in clinical evaluation are given in **Table 1.**

TABLE 1: Pointers to etiology in clinical evaluation.

Pointers	*Etiology*
Skull	Large anterior fontanelle—achondroplasia, MPS
Facies	Cherubic facies—GHD, Gargoyle facies—MPS
Eyes	Cataract—intrauterine infections, corneal clouding—MPS
Teeth	Delayed dentition—hypothyroidism, GHD, rickets
Neck, chest	Webbed neck, shield chest—Turner syndrome
Limbs	Deformities in skeletal dysplasia, rickets
Genitalia	Cryptorchidism in hypopituitarism

(GHD: growth hormone deficiency; MPS: mucopolysaccharidoses)

Investigations

FIRST-LINE	SECOND-LINE
CBC, ESR, CRP	Growth hormone stimulation test—at least two growth provocation tests done in suspected isolated GHD (stimulating agent—clonidine/arginine/insulin/glucagon/dopamine/GHRH)
Renal and liver function test	MRI brain
Venous blood gas, electrolytes	Genetic test
Calcium, phosphorus, alkaline phosphatase	
Thyroid function test	
Celiac screen	
• Insulin-like growth factor 1 (IGF1) • IGF-binding protein 3 (IGFBP3) in children <2 years	
Bone age	
Karyotyping in girls with unexplained short stature	

(CBC: complete blood count; CRP: C-reactive protein; ESR: erythrocyte sedimentation rate; GHD: growth hormone deficiency; GHRH: growth hormone-releasing hormone)

Approach to Short Stature

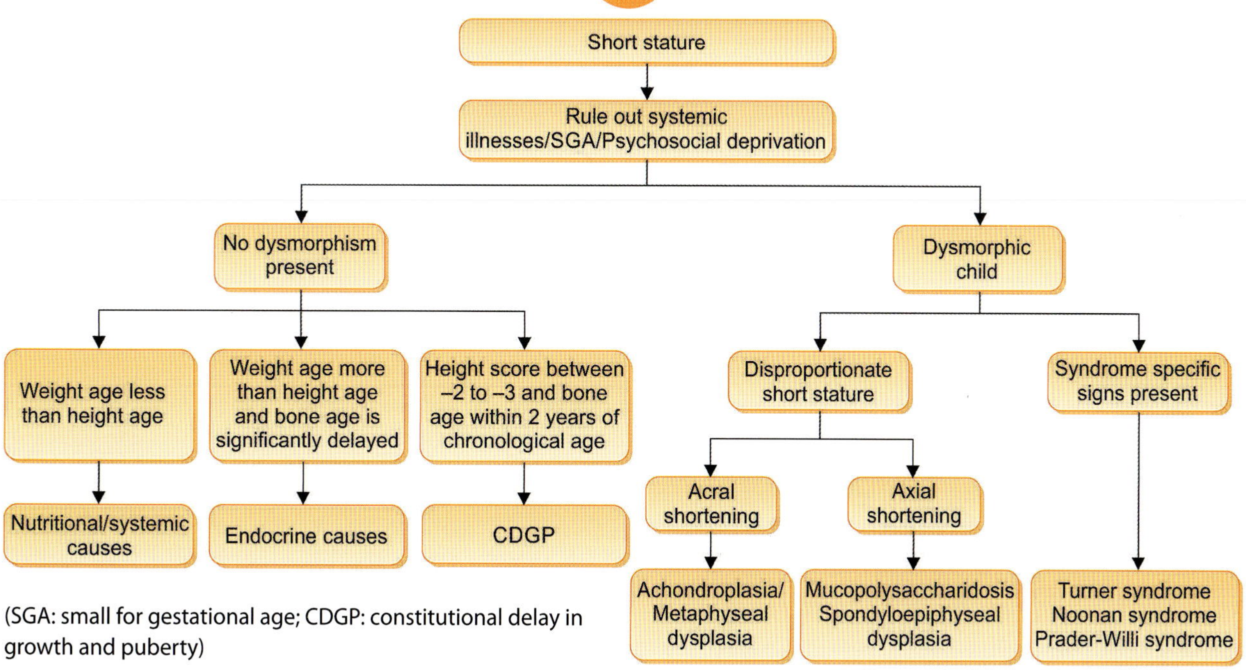

(SGA: small for gestational age; CDGP: constitutional delay in growth and puberty)

Suggested Reading

- Khadilkar V, Bajpai A, Prasad HK. IAP Textbook on Pediatric Endocrinology. New Delhi: Jaypee Brothers Medical Publishers; 2019. pp. 55-65.
- Singh H. Short stature in adolescence. In: Shanthi BL (Ed). IAP Standard Treatment Guidelines 2022. New Delhi: Jaypee Brothers Medical Publishers; 2022. pp. 905-10.
- Sperling M. Sperling Pediatric Endocrinology. Philadelphia, PA: Elsevier; 2021. pp. 314-38.
- Yadav S, Dabas A. Approach to short stature. Indian J Pediatr. 2015;82(5):462-70.

Alopecia and Hair Shaft Disorders

15

Section Editor: **Gnanamurthy Narasimha**
Section Co-Editor: **Nagalatha Chidananda**
Authors: **Sahana M Srinivas, Hania Qamar Khan**

Introduction

- There are three distinct hair types—lanugo (present in utero), vellus, and terminal hair. Each hair has a cycle of growth and shedding. Hair root grows from hair follicle composed of actively dividing cells and progresses to form the hair shaft. Hair stem cells are responsible for continuous regrowth of hair after shedding.
- *Hair loss or alopecia* can be due to insult to any part of hair.
- Alopecia can be broadly classified as scarring or nonscarring, if stem cells are destroyed or preserved respectively.
- Hair shaft disorders can be further classified into disorders with increased hair fragility and without increased hair fragility.

WITH INCREASED HAIR FRAGILITY	WITHOUT INCREASED HAIR FRAGILITY
Congenital trichorrhexis nodosa	Trichonodosis
Monilethrix	Woolly hair
Trichothiodystrophy	Uncombable hair syndrome (Pili trianguli et canaliculi)
Trichorrhexis invaginata (Netherton syndrome)	Trichoptilosis
Menke's kinky hair disease	Pili annulati
Pili torti	Pili bifurcati
Trichorrhexis nodosa	Pili multigemini

Further Examination

- Trichoscopy—using dermatoscope—can magnify 10–200 times. It shows characteristic features of patchy alopecia such as tinea capitis, alopecia areata, and other scarring alopecia
- *Hair pull test:* Pull about 40–50 hairs between the thumb and index finger from different regions of scalp. It is significant if over 10% of hairs are pulled out.
- *Tug test:* Grasp hair between the thumb and index finger near its root and tug with the other hand on the same strand distally. Positive if the hair fractures, indicating fragility.
- *Microscopy:* Examine hair bulb to identify the type of hair lost. Polarized light can identify trichothiodystrophy (alternate light and dark bands).
- Scalp biopsy

Common Causes

HAIR LOSS DISORDERS	CLINICAL FEATURES
Tinea capitis	May be nonscarring or scarring
	Present as black dots, gray patch, or boggy swelling
Alopecia areata (AA)	Smooth patch of hair loss
AA totalis	Diffuse scalp hair loss
AA universalis	Whole body hair loss
Trichotillomania	Focal patches with irregular borders
	Usually over nondominant side of scalp
	Friar tuck—tonsural alopecia
Tractional alopecia	Hair loss at scalp margins due to repeated pulling

Congenital Alopecia

HAIR DISORDERS WITH CONGENITAL ALOPECIA	ALOPECIA	OTHER FEATURES
Transient neonatal hair loss	Occipital	
Congenital triangular alopecia	Frontotemporal patch	—
Atrichia with papules	Absent hair since birth	Diffuse papules
Vitamin D-dependent rickets type II	Diffuse alopecia	Rickets in late childhood
Hair shaft disorders		
Trichorrhexis invaginata	• Alopecia • Erythroderma • Ichthyosis linearis circumflexa	• Atopy • Raised IgE levels
Trichorrhexis nodosa	Trichothiodystrophy	• Photosensitivity • Ichthyosis • Short stature • Neurological impairment
	Argininosuccinic aciduria	Mental retardation
	Citrullinemia	Mental retardation
Pili Torti-180° twist on microscopy	Twisted hair	• Menke's kinky hair disease • Biotin deficiency
Monilethrix	Alternating thickening and thinning of hair strand	Autosomal dominant
Pili annulati—alternate light and dark bands on light microscopy	Microscopy changes	Immunoglobulin A deficiency
Pili multigemini—multiple hair from single follicle	Short irregular hair	Cleidocranial dysostosis
Woolly hair	Tightly curled short and kinked hair	*Naxos syndrome:* • Diffuse palmoplantar keratoderma (PPK) • Right ventricular hypertrophy *Carvajal syndrome:* Striate PPK with left ventricular hypertrophy
Ectodermal dysplasia	Teeth, hair, and nail anomalies	• Hypodontia • Conical teeth • Dry skin • Nail dystrophy • Absent nails • Sparse brittle hair

Red Flag Signs

- Occipital alopecia
- Refractory alopecia areata/alopecia totalis or universalis
- Brittle hair
- Alopecia with erythroderma
- Woolly hair
- *Silvery gray hair:* Could indicate Griscelli syndrome and Chediak–Higashi syndrome

Approach

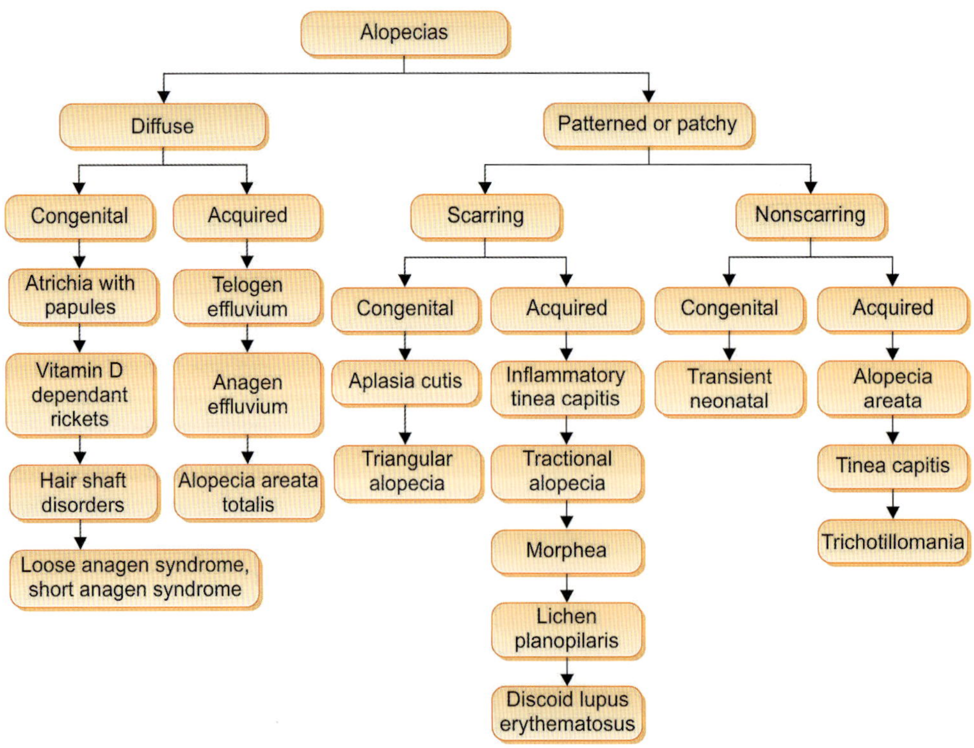

Suggested Reading

- Bhat YJ, Trumboo T, Krishan K. Hair Shaft Disorders in Children - An Update. Indian Dermatol Online J. 2023;14(2): 163-71.
- Srinivas SM. Genotrichoses including hair shaft disorders. In: Chandrashekar BS (Ed). IADVL Textbook of Trichology, 1st edition. New Delhi: Jaypee Brothers Medical Publishers; 2018. p. 231.
- Xu L, Liu KX, Senna MM. A practical approach to the diagnosis and management of hair loss in children and adolescents. Front Med (Lausanne). 2017;4:112.

Self-Stimulatory Behavior in Children

16

Section Editor: **Sumitha Nayak**
Section Co-Editor: **Priya Shivalli**
Author: **Ravishankara Marpalli**

Introduction

Self-stimulatory behavior is repetitive, stereotyped, functionally autonomous behavior seen in normal and developmentally disabled populations. Almost everyone engages in some form of self-stimulating behavior at different times. Some examples include nail biting, and twirling hair around fingers when bored, nervous, or stressed. Self-stimulation, also known as stimming, can become habitual and be done as an unconscious act. Stimming is a coping mechanism that can serve a variety of purposes. Most often, it is a harmless behavior. However, when done at inappropriate times and places, it should be recognized and aborted.

Common stimming behaviors include:

- Nail biting
- Twirling hair around the fingers
- Cracking of knuckles/other joints
- Drumming of fingers
- Tapping of pencil
- Jiggling with foot

In an autistic person, stimming might involve:

- Swaying back and forth (rocking)
- Flapping with the hands/flicking/snapping fingers
- Pacing/walking on tiptoes
- Pulling of the hair
- Repeating words or phrases
- Rubbing the skin/scratching
- Repetitive blinking with the eyes

Red Flag Signs

- Banging head against hard surfaces
- Punching or biting
- Excessive rubbing or scratching on skin
- Scratching over scabs or sores
- Tendency to swallow dangerous items

Benefits

In autistic children, the need for stimming arises to:

- Stimulate the senses/decrease sensory overload
- Adjust to an unfamiliar environment
- Reduce the anxiety and for self-calming
- Express frustration, especially with communication problems
- Avoidance

Approach

- Stimming does not necessarily need to be controlled unless it is causing a problem.
- Do a physical examination and evaluate for existing injuries.
- It is more appropriate to manage stimming rather than attempt to completely control it.
- Encourage the child to self-control themselves.
- Understanding the cause of stimming is useful to control the behavior.

Recommendations to Manage the Behavior **(Flowchart 1)**

- Learn when to intervene and when not to respond to any unsafe behaviors. Advise the family members to learn how they can help.
- Reinforce positive and acceptable behavior
- Provide a safe environment to develop acceptable behavior
- Teach any alternate activities that provide the desired effect to be thought of.
- Teach self-management tools
- Take a multispecialty approach with occupational therapists, educators, and pediatricians.
- Avoid triggers. Try to eliminate/reduce the trigger, lower the stress, and provide a calming environment.
- Try to stick to a routine for daily tasks.
- Encourage acceptable behaviors and self-control.
- Avoid punishments. If we stop one stimming behavior without addressing the reasons behind it, it is likely to be replaced with another, which could be worse.
- Teach an alternate behavior that helps to meet the same needs. For example, hand-flapping can be replaced with squeezing a stress ball or other fine motor activity.

FLOWCHART 1: Algorithm showing the approach to manage self-stimulation behavior (SSB).

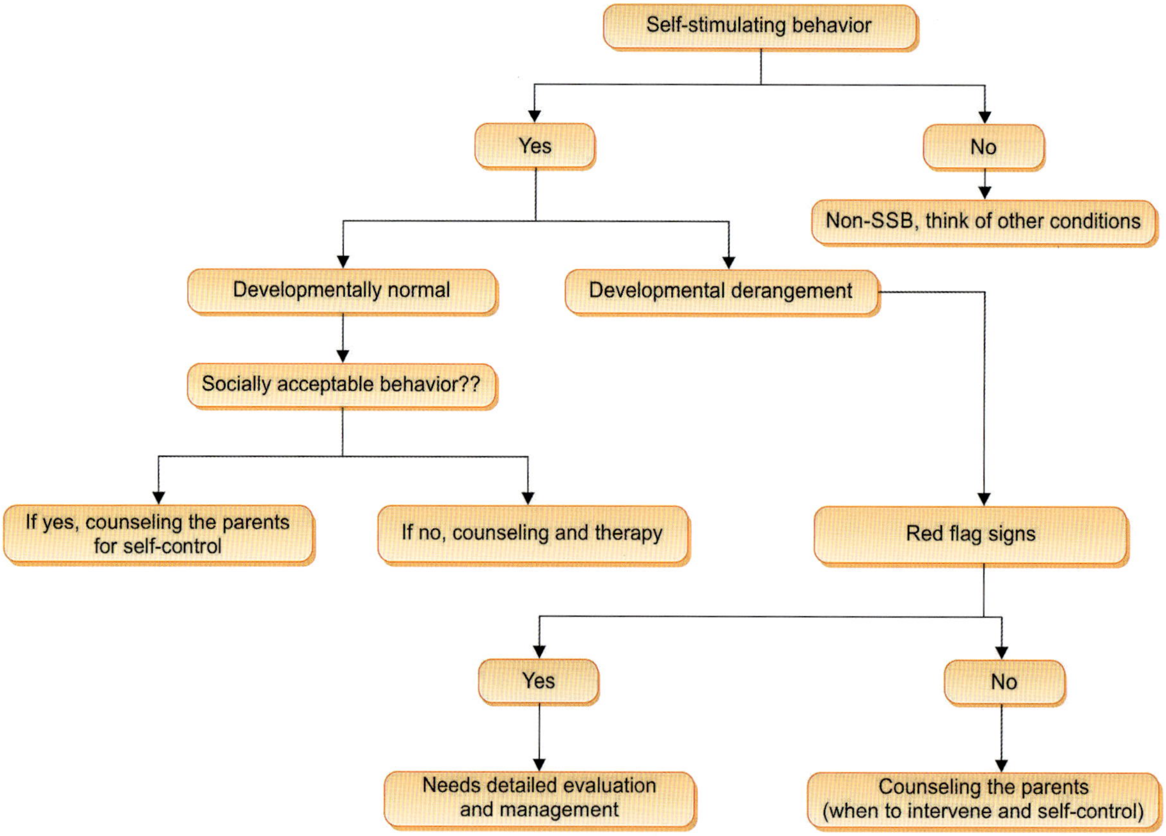

Suggested Reading

- Child Neurology Division, AIIMS, New Delhi (2023). Autism Spectrum Disorder. [online] Available from https://pedneuroaiims.org/autism-spectrum-disorder-diagnosis.html [Last accessed January, 2024].
- Children's Hospital of Philadelphia Research Institute (2020). Stimming: What is it and does it matter? [online] Available from https://www.research.chop.edu/car-autism-roadmap/stimming-what-is-it-and-does-it-matter [ast accessed January, 2024].
- Gutierrez DS, Carugno P. Thumb Sucking. In: StatPearls [Internet]. Treasure Island (FL): StatPearls Publishing; 2023. [online] Available from https://www.ncbi.nlm.nih.gov/books/NBK556112/[Last accessed January, 2024].
- Lovaas I, Newson C, Hickman C. Self-stimulatory behaviour and perceptual reinforcement. J App Behav Anal. 1987;20(1):45-68.

The "ABCs" of Cyanosis

17

Section Editor: **Nehal Patel**
Section Co-Editor: **Jay T Dhirwani**
Authors: **H Ravi Ramamurthy, HS Arora**

Introduction

Cyanosis is the bluish discoloration of the skin, nail beds, and/or mucous membranes.

Types

Cyanosis is of the following types:

- *Peripheral cyanosis (acrocyanosis):* It is limited to extremities. It is relatively common in young infants, and is commonly physiologic.
- *Central cyanosis:* It is present all over the body and noted in mucous membranes and tongue. It indicates a potentially serious and life-threatening disease requiring urgent evaluation.

Note: Cyanosis is visualized depending upon the absolute concentration of reduced hemoglobin, rather than on the partial pressure of arterial oxygen (PaO_2). The ratio of reduced hemoglobin to oxyhemoglobin decides cyanosis. Therefore, patients with anemia will manifest cyanosis at much lower level of PaO_2 when compared to patients with polycythemia.

Etiology, Approach, and Specific Workup of a Neonate with Central Cyanosis

Table 1 displays etiology, approach, and specific workup of neonate with central cyanosis.

TABLE 1: ABC's of cyanosis in neonates.

Location of lesion	*Lesion*	*Associated with respiratory distress*	*Specific differentiating clinical feature*	*Investigation to confirm*
		A. Airway		
Upper airway	Choanal atresia	Yes	Cyanosis reduces on crying and aggravates on rest	CT scan
	Micrognathia, retrognathia, or the Pierre Robin sequence	Yes	Abnormal facies	ENT consultation
	Congenital anomalies of larynx: • Laryngomalacia • Subglottic stenosis • Vocal cord paralysis	Yes	Stridor	ENT consultation
Lower airway	*Tracheal compression:* • Tracheal stenosis • Vascular ring	Yes	Stridor	ENT consultation CT scan and CT angiography
		B. Breathing		
Hypoventilation	*Metabolic:* Hypoglycemia	Hypoventilation	Depressed neurological state	Tandem mass spectroscopy
	Neurological: • Central hypoventilation • Seizures	Hypoventilation	• Altered sensorium • Seizure activity	• EEG • MRI scan brain
	Phrenic nerve palsy	Hypoventilation	Paradoxical breathing	• USG diaphragm • Fluoroscopy
Lung disease	Respiratory distress syndrome	Yes	• Prematurity • Maternal diabetes	Chest radiography
	Pneumonia	Yes	• Premature rupture of membranes • Maternal fever	• Chest radiography • CRP • Blood culture
	Congenital anomalies: • Congenital pulmonary airway malformation (CPAM) • Congenital diaphragmatic hernia (CDH) • Congenital lobar emphysema (CLE)	Yes	History of antenatal diagnosis by fetal scan	• Chest radiography • CT scan chest

Contd...

Contd...

Location of lesion	*Lesion*	*Associated with respiratory distress*	*Specific differentiating clinical feature*	*Investigation to confirm*
		C. Circulation		
Cardiac diseases	*Congenital heart disease:* Cyanotic	No	• Abnormal S2 (single/wide split) • Cardiac murmur	• Chest radiography • Electrocardiogram • Echocardiography • CT angiography
	Persistent fetal circulation (PPHN)	Yes	Sick infant with labile SpO_2	• Chest radiography • Echocardiography
Circulatory/ blood diseases	Methemoglobinemia	No	Cyanosis with normal PaO_2	Hb electrophoresis
	Polycythemia	No	Underlying disease causing hypoxia	• Hemogram • Investigate for secondary causes

(CRP: C-reactive protein; CT: computed tomography; EEG: electroencephalography; ENT: ear, nose, and throat; Hb: hemoglobin; MRI: magnetic resonance imaging; PaO_2: partial pressure of arterial oxygen; SpO_2: peripheral capillary oxygen saturation; USG: ultrasonography)

Flowchart 1 illustrates approach to central cyanosis in neonates.

FLOWCHART 1: Approach to central cyanosis in neonates.

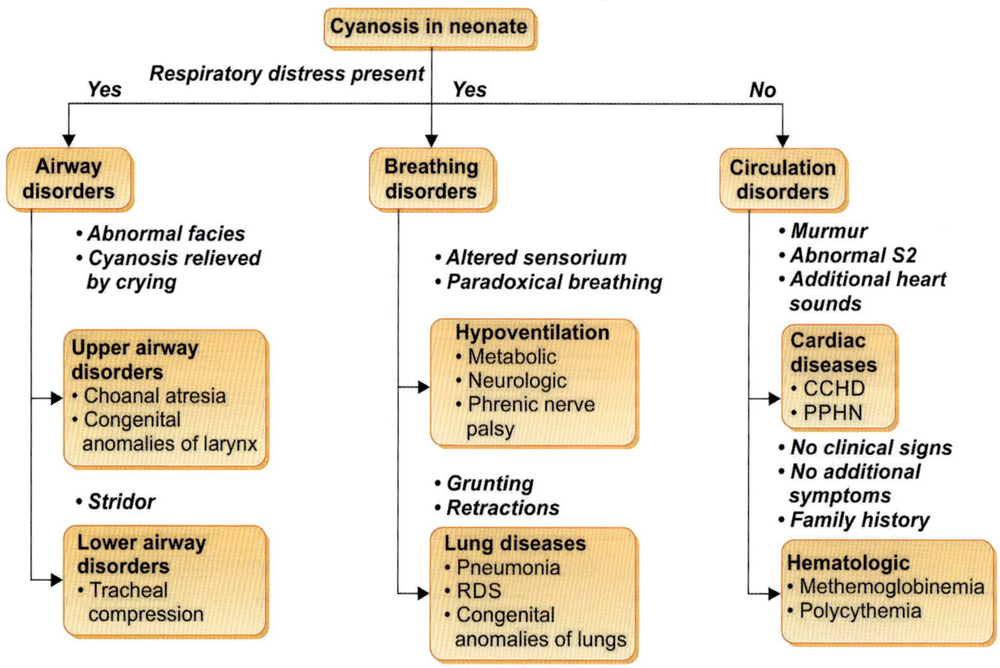

(CCHD: cyanotic congenital heart disease; PPHN: persistent fetal circulation; RDS: respiratory distress syndrome)

Etiology, Stepwise Approach, and Specific Workup of an Older Child with Central Cyanosis

Table 2 shows etiology, approach, and specific workup of older children with central cyanosis.

TABLE 2: ABC's of cyanosis in older children.

Location of lesion	*Lesion*	*Associated with respiratory distress*	*Specific differentiating feature*	*Investigation to confirm*
		A. Airway		
Upper airway	Foreign body	Yes	History of foreign body inhalation	ENT consultation
	Croup	Yes	Stridor	Emergency management
Lower airway	Bacterial tracheitis /Laryngotracheo-bronchitis	Yes	Stridor	Emergency management
		B. Breathing		
Hypoventilation	Accidental drug ingestion (benzodiazepines, opioids, etc.)	Hypoventilation	Depressed neurological state	Toxicological analysis
	Head injuries	Hypoventilation	Altered sensorium Trauma	CT scan/MRI scan brain
	Breath-holding spell	Hypoventilation	Classical history	No investigations required
Thoracic cavity problems	Tension pneumothorax	Yes	Physical findings of pneumothorax	Chest radiography
	Hemothorax	Yes	Trauma	Chest radiography
Lung parenchymal disease	Acute respiratory distress syndrome	Yes	Predisposing event: infection	• Chest radiography • CT scan chest
	Bronchiolitis	Yes	Bilateral lung involvement	Chest radiography
	Pneumonia	Yes	Fever	• Chest radiography • CRP • Blood culture
	Acute severe asthma	Yes	• Expiratory wheezing • "Silent chest" • History of recurrent wheezing	• Chest radiography • Pulmonary function test

Contd...

Contd...

Location of lesion	*Lesion*	*Associated with respiratory distress*	*Specific differentiating feature*	*Investigation to confirm*
		C. Circulation		
Cardiac diseases	Congenital heart disease	No	• Abnormal S2 (single/wide split) • Cardiac murmur • Dysmorphic facies	• Chest radiography • Electrocardiogram • Echocardiography • CT angiography
	Pulmonary hypertension	No	Cyanosis out of proportion to respiratory distress	• Chest radiography • Echocardiography • CT angiography
	Pulmonary thromboembolism	Variable	• Chest pain • Rusty sputum	• Chest radiography • Echocardiography • CT angiography
Circulatory/ blood diseases	Methemoglobinemia	No	Cyanosis with normal PaO_2	Hb electrophoresis
Pulmonary vasculature	Pulmonary arteriovenous malformations	No	Cyanosis without any other clinical findings	• Contrast echocardiography (with agitated saline) to be done by an experienced pediatric cardiologist along with all resuscitative precautions • CT angiography is diagnostic • Cardiac catheterization (diagnostic and therapeutic)

(CRP: C-reactive protein; CT: computed tomography; ENT: ear, nose, and throat; Hb: hemoglobin MRI: magnetic resonance imaging; PaO_2: partial pressure of oxygen)

Flowchart 2 illustrates approach to central cyanosis in older children.

FLOWCHART 2: Approach to central cyanosis in older children.

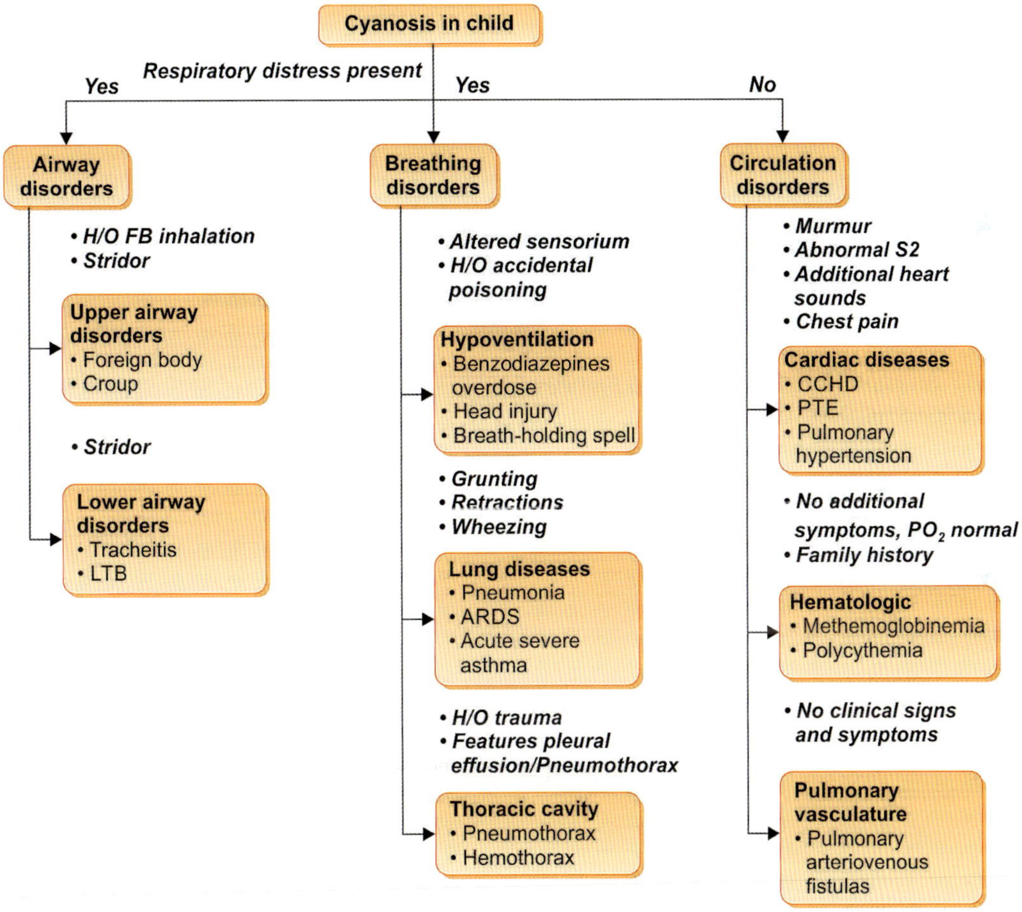

(ARDS: acute respiratory distress syndrome; CCHD: cyanotic congenital heart disease; FB: foreign body; H/O: history of; LTB: laryngotracheobronchitis; PTE: pulmonary thromboembolism)

Red Flags

- Central cyanosis in neonates
- Associated altered sensorium
- Inability to speak in sentences
- Hypercyanotic spell in a known case of cyanotic congenital heart disease

Suggested Reading

- Sasidharan P. An approach to diagnosis and management of cyanosis and tachypnea in term infants. Pediatr Clin North Am. 2004;51(4):999-1021.
- Steinhorn RH. Evaluation and management of the cyanotic neonate. Clin Pediatr Emerg Med. 2008:9(3):169-75.

Hearing Loss

18

Section Editor: **Rupesh Masand**
Section Co-Editor: **Hema Gupta Mittal**
Author: **Prem Kumar P**

Introduction

Hearing loss, or hearing impairment, is a partial or total inability to hear. It is the most common sensory deficit in humans today.

Types

Disabling hearing loss is a hearing loss >30 dB in the better hearing ear in children. Around 360 million people in the world have disabling hearing loss (5.3% of population). Of these, 32 million (9%) are children.

Permanent childhood hearing impairment (PCHI) is a confirmed permanent bilateral hearing impairment of >40 dB hearing level (HL)—averaged over the frequencies of 0.5, 1, 2, and 4 kHz in the better hearing ear, with an incidence of 4/1,000 children.

Classification and Features

Criteria	*Classification*	*Comment*
Causality	Genetic Environmental Multifactorial	Hereditary Nonhereditary
Time of onset	Congenital Acquired	At birth Develops any time after birth
Age of onset	Prelingual Postlingual	Before speech development After speech development
Clinical presentation	Nonsyndromic Syndromic	Hearing loss is the only symptom Hearing loss and other symptoms
Anatomic defect	Conductive Sensorineural Mixed	Dysfunction of outer or middle ear Dysfunction of inner ear or auditory nerve Both conductive and sensorineural components
Severity	Mild Moderate Moderately severe Severe Profound	20–40 dB 41–55 dB 56–70 dB 71–90 dB >90 dB
Frequency loss	Low frequency Mid frequency High frequency	<500 Hz 501–2,000 Hz >2,000 Hz
Ears affected	Unilateral Bilateral Symmetric Asymmetric	One ear affected Both ears affected Both ears affected equally Both ears are not affected equally
Prognosis	Stable Progressive	Severity remains unchanged Severity increases over time

Red Flags

Symptoms	*Signs*
Not responding when called	Malformations of external ear
Watching TV with loud volume	Glue ear
Lack of awareness to usual sounds	Ear discharge
Talking loudly	Tympanic membrane perforations

Causes of Hearing Loss in Children

Conductive hearing loss

- Otitis media with effusion (Glue ear)
- Acute otitis media
- Foreign body
- Wax
- Tympanic membrane perforation
- Ossicular fixation
- Ossicular discontinuity secondary to trauma

Sensorineural hearing loss

- Syndromic disease
- Nonsyndromic genetic hearing loss
- Bacterial meningitis
- Perinatal hypoxic ischemic encephalopathy
- Ototoxic drugs
- Congenital infections-TORCH
- Trauma

Hearing Assessment in Children

Hearing assessment in children is age and ability dependent and can be addressed as follows:

Neonates	• Otoacoustic emissions (OAE) • Automated auditory brainstem response (AABR)
6–8 months	Distraction techniques
9–36 months	Visual reinforcement audiometry (VRA)
24–60 months	Conditioned play audiometry
>60 months	Pure tone audiometry

Newborn Hearing Screening

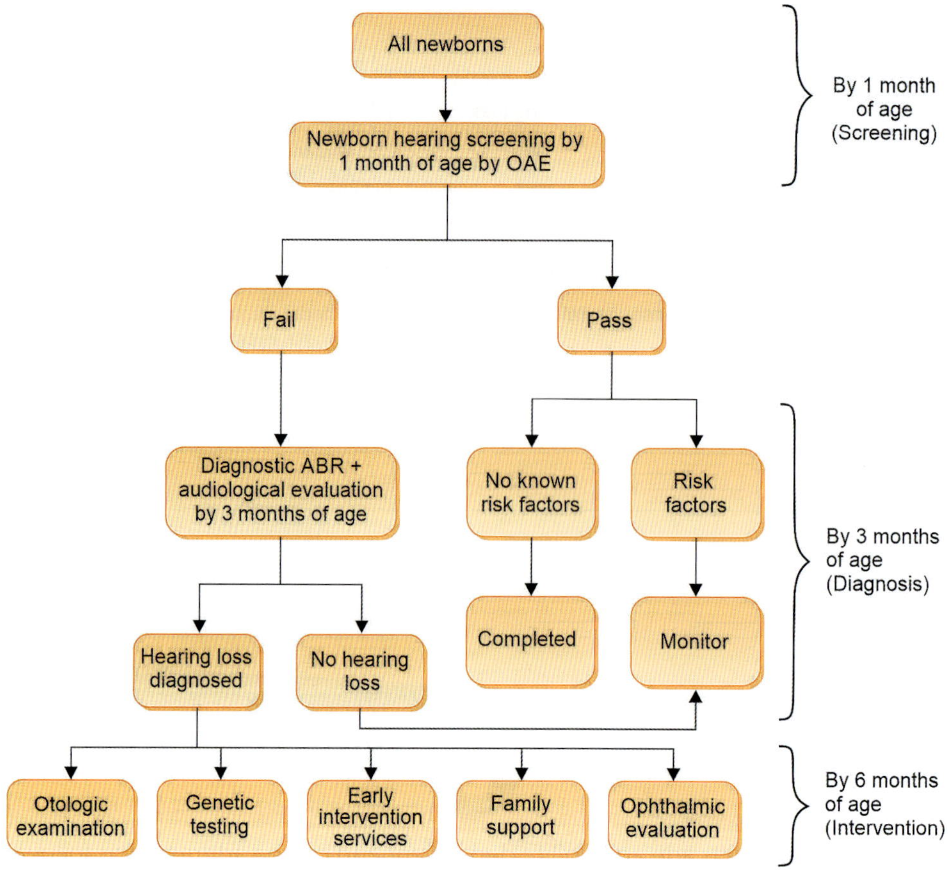

(ABR: auditory brainstem response; OAE: otoacoustic emissions)

If the 1-3-6 rule (screening by 1 month, diagnosis by 3 months and intervention by 6 months) is met, then the 1-2-3 timeline should be aimed.

Approach to a Child with Hearing Loss

Multidisciplinary Approach

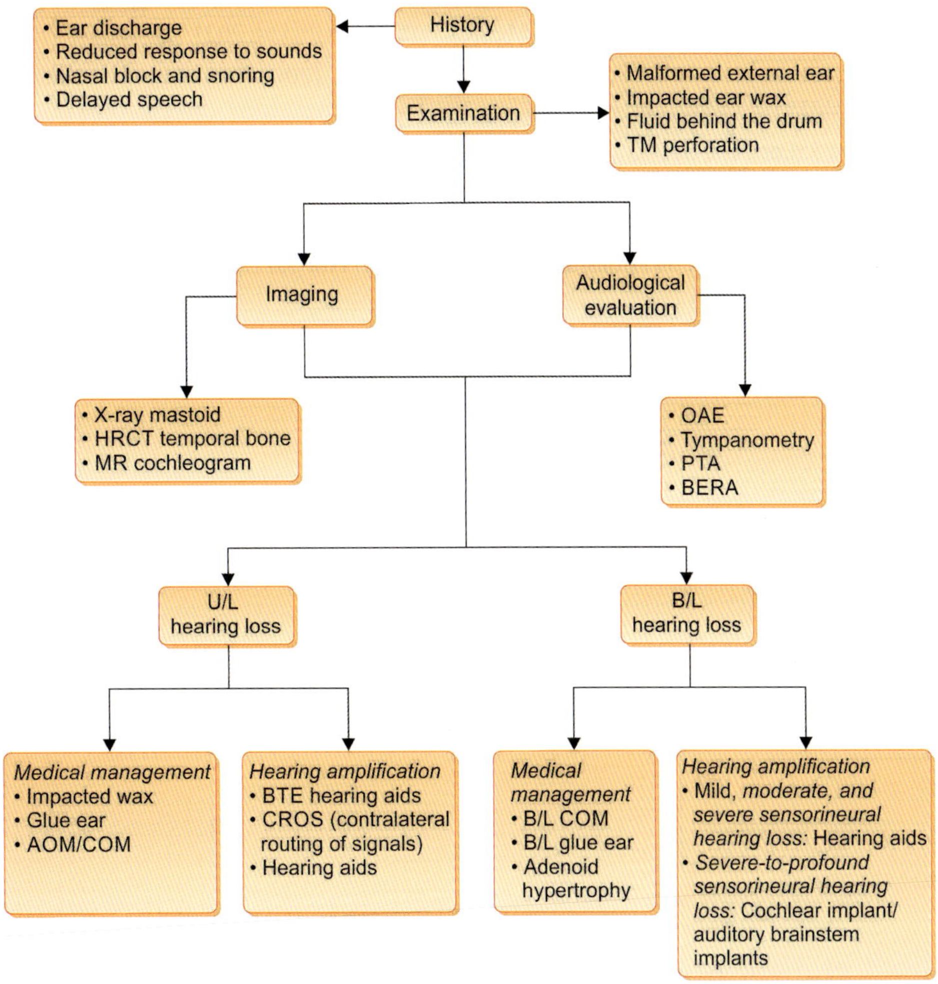

(AOM: acute otitis media; BERA: brainstem auditory evoked response; B/L: bilateral; BTE: behind-the-ear hearing aid; COM: chronic otitis media; HRCT: high-resolution computed tomography; MR: magnetic resonance; OAE: otoacoustic emissions; PTA: pure tone audiometry; U/L: unilateral; TM: tympanic membrane)

Suggested Reading

- Anand V. ENT Head and Neck Diseases Made Easy, 1st edition. New Delhi. Jaypee Brothers Medical Publishers (P) Ltd; 2011.
- Bansal M. Hearing impairments in infants and young children. Diseases of Ear, Nose and Throat, Head and Neck Surgery, 3rd edition. New Delhi: Jaypee Brothers Medical Publishers (P) Ltd; 2021. pp. 166-71.
- Bhargava KB, Bhargava SK, Shah TM. A Short Book of ENT Diseases, 12th edition. Mumbai: National Book Depot; 2022.
- Dhingra PL, Dhingra S (Eds). The deaf child. In: Diseases of Ear, Nose and Throat and Head and Neck Surgery, 8th edition. New Delhi: Elsevier; 2021. pp. 135-40.
- Hazarika P, Nayak DR, Balakrishnan R. Textbook of Ear, Nose and Throat and Head-Neck Surgery, Clinical and Practical, 5th edition. New Delhi: CBS Publishers & Distributors (P) Ltd; 2022.

Anemia in Children

19

Section Editor: **Janani Shankar**
Section Co-Editor: **Arathi Srinivasan**
Author: **Meena Sivasankaran**

Definition

Anemia is a condition where the number of erythrocytes and carriers of oxygen is insufficient to meet metabolic demands. It is defined by hemoglobin (Hb)/hematocrit/red blood cell counts lower than the normal age- and sex-adjusted ranges.

World Health Organization's Classification of Anemia According to the Age and Severity

Table 1 shows classification of anemia according to age and severity as per World Health Organization.

TABLE 1: World Health Organization's classification of anemia according to age and severity.

POPULATION	NONANEMIA*	MILD ANEMIA*	MODERATE ANEMIA*	SEVERE ANEMIA*
6–59 months of age	≥11	10–10.9	7–9.9	<7
5–11 years of age	≥11.5	11–11.4	8–10.9	<8
12–14 years of age	≥12	11–11.9	8–10.9	<8
Nonpregnant women ≥15 years of age	≥12	11–11.9	8–10.9	<8
Pregnant women	≥11	10–10.9	7–9.9	<7
Men ≥15 years of age	≥13	11–12.9	8–10.9	<8

*g/dL.

Diagnostic Guidance Based on History and Physical Examination

Diagnostic guidance based on history and physical examination is given in **Table 2**.

TABLE 2: Diagnostic guidance based on history and physical examination.

HISTORY	
Common causes of anemia based on the age	• *Neonates:* Immune hemolysis and hereditary disorders • *3–6 months:* Hemoglobinopathies • *6 months to 6 years:* Nutritional anemias
Sex	*Glucose-6-phosphate dehydrogenase (G6PD) deficiency:* X linked
Symptoms	• *Fatigue, exercise intolerance:* Suggests anemia • *Changes in urine color, jaundice:* Hemolytic disorder • *Bloody stools, hematemesis, severe epistaxis, and severe menstrual bleeding:* Anemia from blood loss/iron deficiency • *Renal disease, malignancy, or inflammatory disorder:* Anemia of chronic disease
Family history	*Jaundice, gallstone, splenomegaly:* Hereditary hemolytic anemia
Diet history	• *Excess cow's milk intake/Pica/diet with low iron content:* Iron-deficiency anemia • *Vegetarian diet:* Vitamin B_{12} deficiency
Developmental history	*Developmental delay:* Megaloblastic anemia
PHYSICAL EXAMINATION	
Severity of anemia	*Tachypnea, tachycardia, pallor, poor perfusion, systolic ejection heart murmur, distended neck veins, wheezing, and hepatomegaly:* Severe anemia presents with signs of congestive cardiac failure
Growth	*Short stature:* • Fanconi anemia • Chronic hemolytic anemias
Skin	• *Hyperpigmentation:* Fanconi anemia and vitamin B_{12} deficiency • *Petechiae:* Evans syndrome, marrow failure, and leukemia • *Jaundice:* Hemolytic anemia
Face	*Malar and maxillary prominence:* Thalassemia
Eyes	• *Microcornea:* Fanconi anemia • *Tortuous conjunctival and retinal vessel:* Sickle cell disease • *Cataract:* G6PD deficiency
Mouth	*Glossitis:* Vitamin B_{12} deficiency
Hand	• *Triphalangeal thumb:* Pure red cell aplasia • *Hypoplastic thenar eminence:* Fanconi anemia • *Nail abnormality:* Iron deficiency
Spleen	*Splenomegaly:* Hemolytic anemia

Diagnostic Approach to a Child with Anemia and Other Cell Line Abnormalities

Algorithm 1

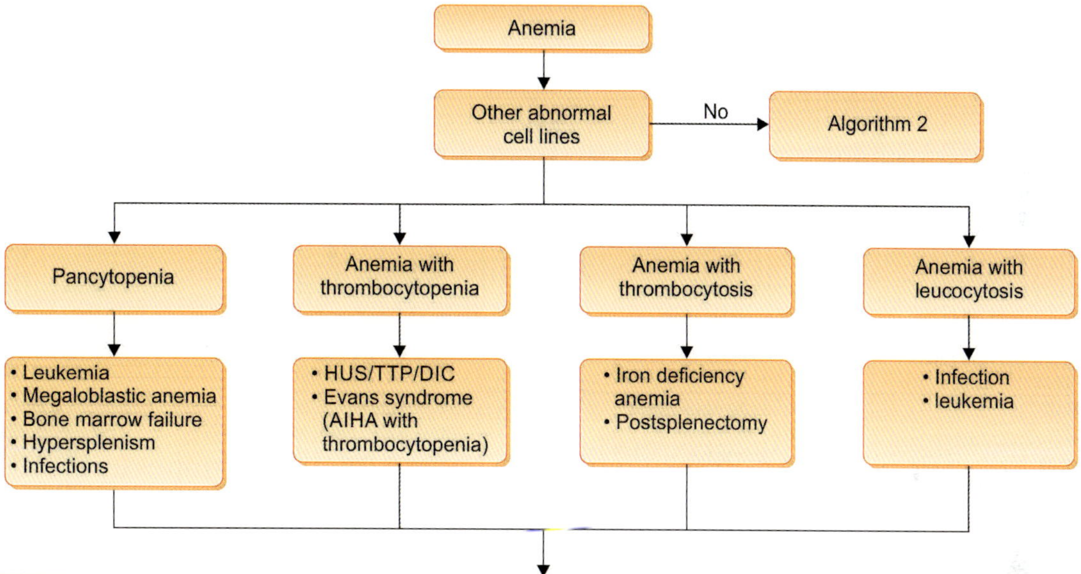

Further investigations based on peripheral smear findings and reticulocyte count	
Blast in the smear: Leukemia	Bone marrow aspiration
Macro-ovalocytes and hypersegmented neutrophils: Megaloblastic anemia	Vitamin B_{12}/folate levels
Pancytopenia with low reticulocyte count: Bone marrow failure	Bone marrow aspiration and biopsy
Evidence of hemolysis and thrombocytopenia: Evans syndrome	LDH, bilirubin, and DCT
Fragmented RBCs and thrombocytopenia	Workup for HUS/TTP/DIC
Microcytic RBCs and thrombocytosis: Iron deficiency	Iron studies (ferritin, serum iron, and total iron binding capacity)

(AIHA: autoimmune hemolytic anemia; DCT: direct Coombs test; DIC: disseminated intravascular coagulation; HUS: hemolytic uremic syndrome; LDH: lactate dehydrogenase; RBC: red blood cells; TTP: thrombotic thrombocytopenic purpura)

Diagnostic Approach to Anemia Based on Mean Corpuscular Volume

Algorithm 2

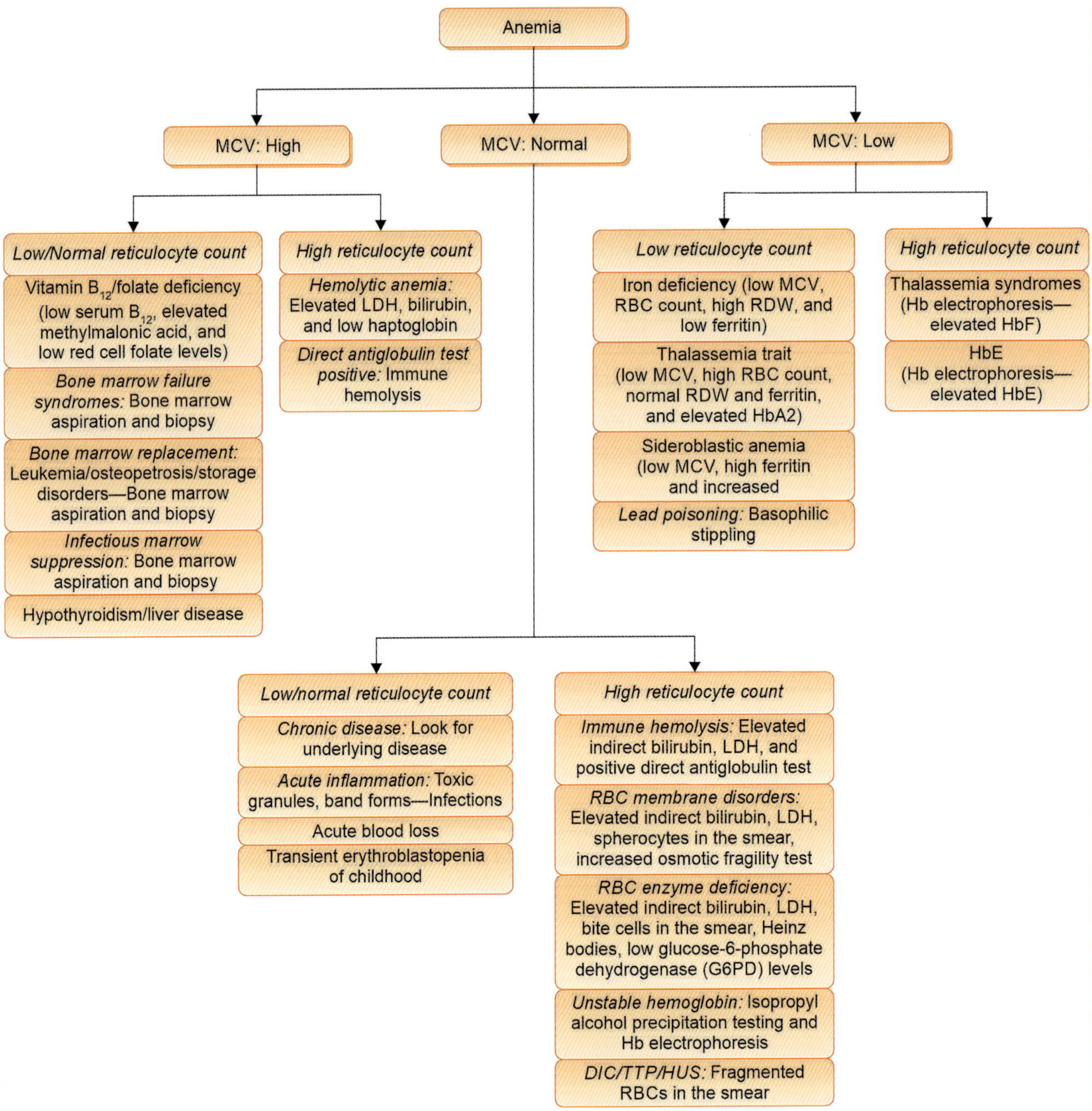

(DIC: disseminated intravascular coagulation; Hb: hemoglobin; HUS: hemolytic uremic syndrome; LDH: lactose dehydrase; MCV: mean corpuscular volume; RBC: red blood cell; RDW: RBC distribution width; TTP: thrombotic thrombocytopenic purpura)

Suggested Reading

- Gallagher PG. Anemia in the pediatric patient. Blood. 2022;140(6):571-93.
- Niss O, Quinn CT. Classification and diagnosis of anemia in children and neonates. Lanzkowsky's Manual of Pediatric Hematology and Oncology, 7th edition. Amsterdam: Elsevier; 2022. pp. 37-59.

Neonatal Seizures

20

***Section Editor:* Nehal Patel**
***Section Co-Editor:* Jay T Dhirwani**
***Authors:* Naveen Parkash Gupta, Sayoni Roy Chowdhury**

Introduction

Neonatal seizures represent a common neurological emergency. The incidence is around 1–5 per 1,000 live births. Majority are acute provoked seizures/acute symptomatic seizures, possibly from systemic illness/central nervous system insult.

Etiology

Etiology of neonatal seizures is given in **Box 1**.

BOX 1: Etiology of neonatal seizures.

Acute provoked (symptomatic) seizures (*most frequent*):
- Hypoxic ischemic encephalopathy (HIE) (*most common cause*)
- *Vascular:* Perinatal arterial ischemic stroke, intracranial/intraventricular hemorrhage, venous thrombosis, etc.
- *Central nervous system infections:* Meningitis, encephalitis [herpes simplex virus (HSV), parechovirus, and rotavirus], intrauterine infections, etc.
- *Metabolic disturbances:* Hypoglycemia, hypocalcemia, hypomagnesemia, etc.
- *Others:* Inborn errors of metabolism, neonatal drug withdrawal, and birth-related head trauma

Unprovoked seizures:
- *Structural:* Lissencephaly, cortical dysplasia, polymicrogyria, etc.
- *Genetic:* Self-limited epilepsies (*KCNQ2/3* and *SCN2A*), developmental and epileptic encephalopathies (*STXBP1*, *BRAT1*, *CDKL5*, and *KCNT1*)
- *Metabolic:* Pyridoxine dependent, pyridoxal 5-phosphate dependent epilepsies, glucose transporter 1 deficiency syndrome, etc.
- Unknown

Hypoxic ischemic encephalopathy, stroke, and hemorrhage account for almost 75% of all neonatal seizures. Neonatal seizures may also directly progress to neonatal epilepsy (severe insult) or evolve into postneonatal epilepsy after a latent period.

Types

Neonatal seizures have been classified by the International League Against Epilepsy (ILAE) task force. The emphasis is on electroencephalography (EEG) to diagnose these seizures.

- *Electroclinical seizure:* When the clinical event is time locked with an EEG-confirmed seizure
- *Electrographic-only seizure:* EEG-confirmed seizure without associated clinical signs
- *Clinical events that have no EEG correlate are not seizures.*

Diagnosis

Video EEG with polygraphic channel recording (cEEG) is the gold standard in neonates. Alternatively, a routine 60-minute EEG can be used.

Amplitude-integrated EEG (aEEG), a simplified setup with two channels of EEG in a filtered and compressed manner, is a useful adjuvant tool when cEEG is not available. The sensitivity and specificity ranges between 25% and 80% with good prognostic value.

Red Flags

- Regular repetitive rhythmic jerking movements of limbs, trunk, and face
- Tonic stiffening of limbs and trunk, sustained eye/head deviation to one side
- A sudden, brief jerk involving one or more limbs or whole body
- Ocular movements (eyelid fluttering, roving eye movements, and eyes rolling up), oral–buccal–lingual movements (smacking, sucking, chewing, and tongue protrusions), and progression movements of limbs (pedaling, roving, and swimming)
- Fluctuations in respiratory rate, heart rate, and blood pressure; vasomotor changes; salivation; and apnea
- Unexplained encephalopathy

Approach

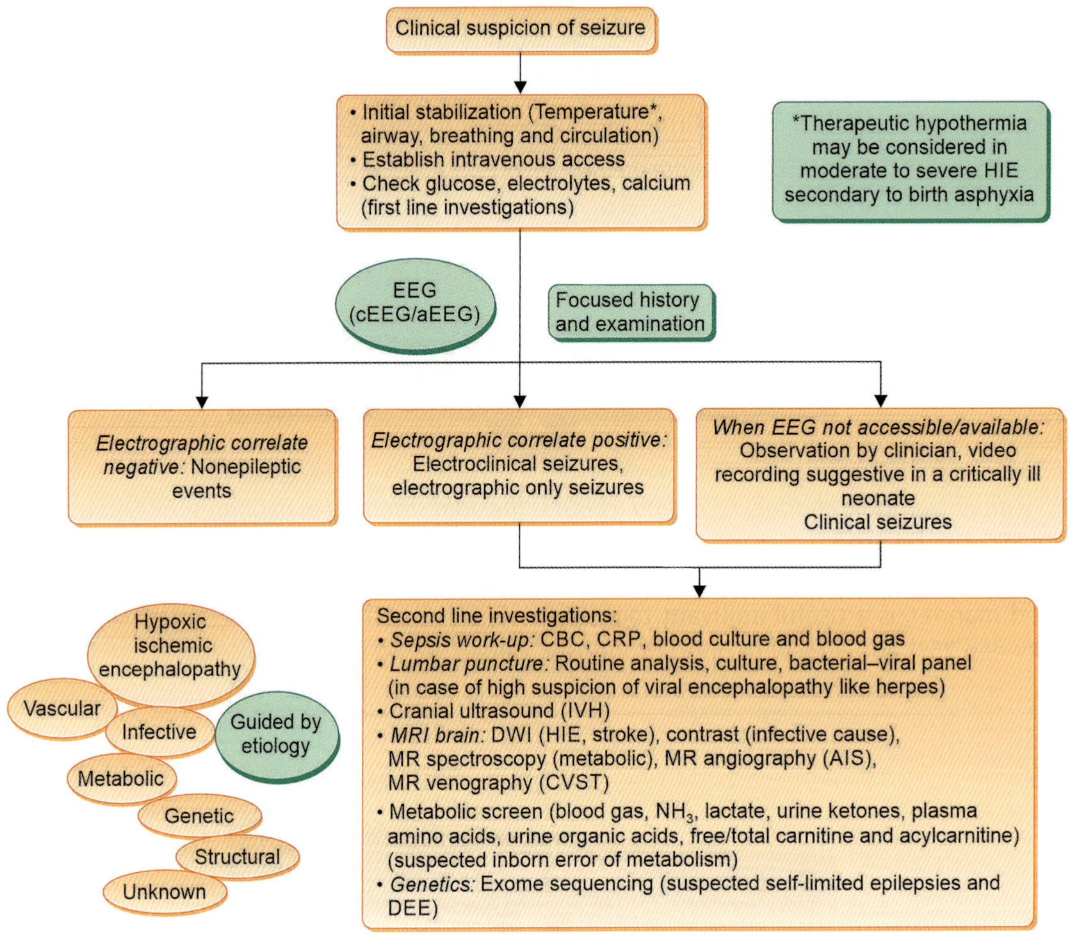

(aEEG: amplitude integrated EEG; AIS: arterial ischemic stroke; CBC: complete blood count; cEEG: conventional EEG; CRP: C-reactive protein; CVST: cerebral venous sinus thrombosis; DEE: developmental and epileptic; DWI: diffusion-weighted imaging; EEG: electroencephalogram; HIE: hypoxic–ischemic encephalopathy; IVH: intraventricular hemorrhage; MR: magnetic resonance; MRI: magnetic resonance imaging)

Suggested Reading

- Kim EH, Shin J, Lee BK. Neonatal seizures: Diagnostic updates based on new definition and classification. Clin Exp Pediatr. 2022;65(8):387-97.
- Panayiotopoulos CP. Neonatal seizures and neonatal syndromes. The Epilepsies: Seizures, Syndromes and Management. Oxfordshire (UK): Bladon Medical Publishing; 2005.
- Pisani F, Spagnoli C, Falsaperla R, Nagarajan L, Ramantani G. Seizures in the neonate: A review of etiologies and outcomes. Seizure. 2021;85:48-56.
- Pressler RM, Cilio MR, Mizrahi EM, Moshé SL, Nunes ML, Plouin P, et al. The ILAE classification of seizures and the epilepsies: Modification for seizures in the neonate. Position paper by the ILAE Task Force on Neonatal Seizures. Epilepsia. 2021;62(3):615-28.
- Volpe JJ, Inder T, Darras B, de Vries L, du Plessis A, Neil J, et al. Neonatal seizure. In: Volpe JJ (Ed). Volpe's Neurology of the Newborn, 6th edition. Amsterdam: Elsevier; 2017. pp. 275-321.e14.
- Zuberi SM, Wirrell E, Yozawitz E, Wilmshurst JM, Specchio N, Riney K, et al. ILAE classification and definition of epilepsy syndromes with onset in neonates and infants: Position statement by the ILAE Task Force on Nosology and Definitions. Epilepsia. 2022;63(6):1349-97.

Vertigo

21

Section Editor: **Rupesh Masand**
Section Co-Editor: **Hema Gupta Mittal**
Authors: **Deepak V Haldipur, Akshay BK**

Introduction

- *Vertigo* is a condition in which a person has the sensation of movement or of surrounding objects moving when they are not. It may be associated with nausea, vomiting, sweating, or difficulty in walking.
- *Disequilibrium* represents a disturbance in balance or coordination such that confident ambulation is impaired.
- *Presyncope* means that the patient senses *impending* loss of consciousness.
- *Light-headedness* refers to a sensation "in the head" that is clearly not vertiginous or presyncopal and that is *not* invariably related to ambulation.
- Prevalence of vertigo in the pediatric age group ranges from 8% to 15%. In otolaryngology clinics, the prevalence of the pediatric vertigo patients constitutes around 0.7%.

Etiology

- Vestibular migraine (VM)
- Benign paroxysmal vertigo of children (BPVC)
- Vestibular neuritis
- Post-traumatic/head trauma
- Otitis media
- Ménière's disease
- Psychogenic vertigo
- Epileptic vertigo
- Unclassified

The most frequent diagnoses are VM, BPVC, and other migraine variants, followed by audiovestibular disorders, psychogenic vertigo, neurological diseases, and post-traumatic vertigo. Less frequent diagnoses (<5%) include motion sickness, cardiovascular diseases, and ophthalmic disorders.

Red Flags

These symptoms should alert to a nonvestibular cause:

- Persistent worsening vertigo or disequilibrium
- Atypical "nonperipheral" vertigo showing vertical nystagmus
- Severe headache, especially early in the morning
- Diplopia
- Cranial nerve palsies
- Dysarthria
- Ataxia, or other cerebellar signs
- Papilledema
- Signs of psychiatric illness

Evaluation

Signs and symptoms to be looked at presentation are given in **Box 1**.

BOX 1: Signs and symptoms to be looked at presentation.

- *Symptoms to be looked at presentation*
  - Headache
  - Vomiting
  - Nausea
  - Hearing loss
  - Tinnitus
- *Signs to be looked at presentation*
  - Spontaneous nystagmus
  - Positive post-head-shaking nystagmus
  - Positional nystagmus
  - Positive head impulse test

Diagnostic Modalities

- Complete otolaryngological and otoneurological physical examination
- *Audiological evaluation:* Pure tone, speech, and impedance audiometry
- Electronystagmography (ENG)

In selective cases:

- Auditory brainstem response (ABR)
- Computerized tomography (CT)
- Magnetic resonance imaging (MRI) is needed in selective cases

Diagnostic Algorithm

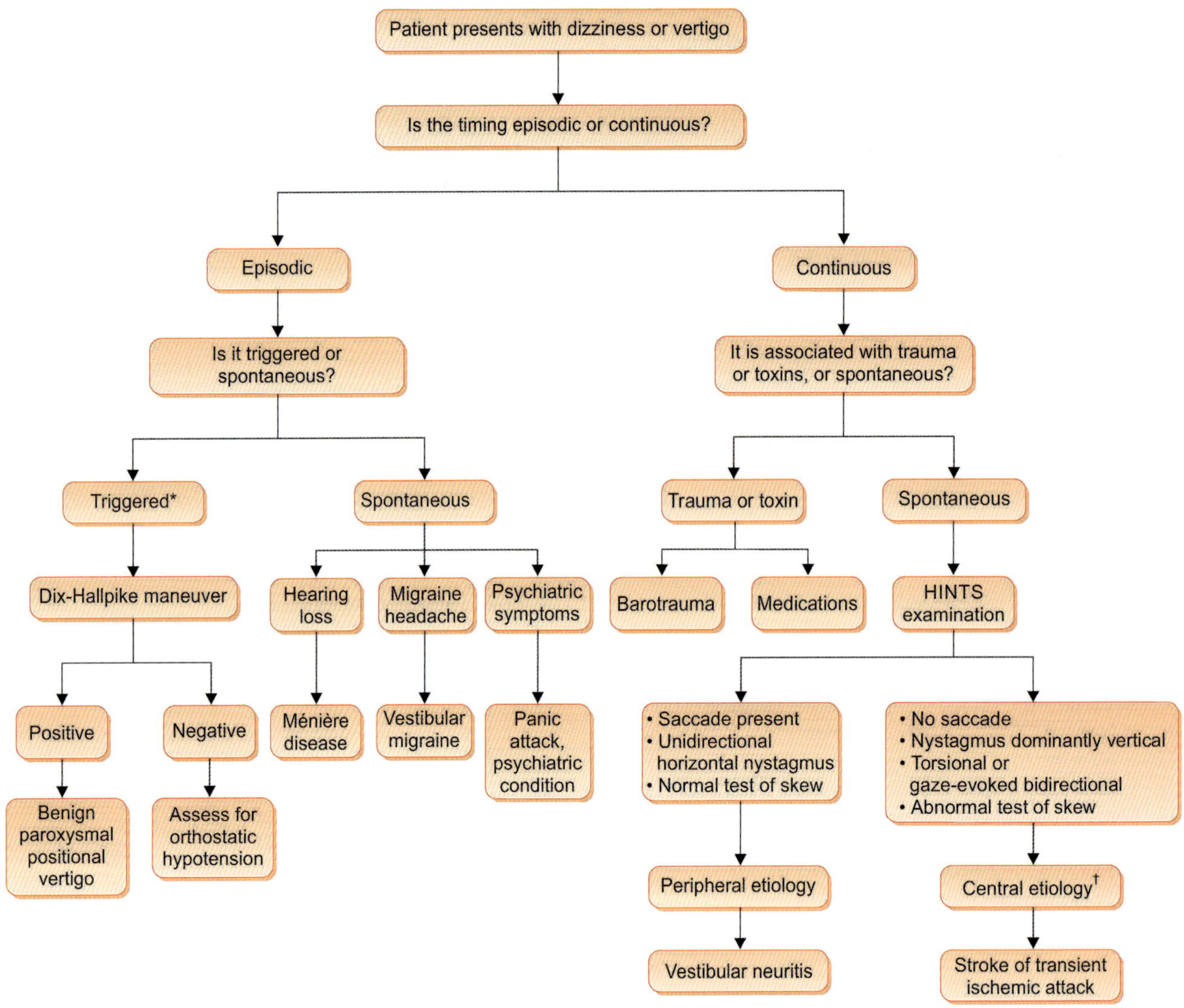

*Exacerbation of symptoms with movement does not aid in determining whether the etiology is peripheral versus central.

†Central causes can also occur with patterns triggered by movement.

(HINTS: head impulse, nystagmus, test for skew)

Suggested Reading

- Gruber M, Cohen-Kerem R, Kaminer M, Shupak A. Vertigo in Children and Adolescents: Characteristics and Outcome. Scientific World J. 2012;2012:1-6.
- Niemensivu R, Pyykkö I, Wiener-Vacher SR, Kentala E. Vertigo and balance problems in the children–an epidemiologic study in Finland. Int J Pediatr Otorhinolaryngol. 2006;70(2):259-65.
- Riina N, Ilmari P, Kentala E. Vertigo and imbalance in children: A retrospective study in a Helsinki University Otorhinolaryngology Clinic. Arch Otolaryngol Head Neck Surg. 2005;131(11):996-1000.
- Swain S, Behera IC, Rajvanshi P. Vertigo in children-A review. Indian J Child Health. 2022;9(5):68-73.
- Swain SK, Achary S, Das SR. Vertigo in pediatric age: Often challenge to clinicians. Int J Cur Res Rev. 2020;12(18): 136-41.
- Weiner-Vacher SR. Vestibular disorders in children. Int J Audiol. 2008;47:578-83.

Undescended Testis or Cryptorchidism

22

***Section Editor:* Gnanamurthy Narasimha**
***Section Co-Editor:* Nagalatha Chidananda**
***Authors:* MM Zameer, Pavithra Nagaraj**

Introduction

- Failure of one or both testes to descend normally into the scrotum is referred to as cryptorchidism.
- The major function of the testis is to produce a sufficient amount of testosterone and sperm to support the development and maintenance of male sexual function, body function, and fertility.
- The incidence is more common in the preterm babies (25–30%).
- Usually unilateral, it can be bilateral in 10–20% cases.

Descent of Testis

Normal testicular descent occurs in two phases:

- *Transabdominal phase (hormonal influence):* 10–23 weeks

  This involves descent from abdomen to the inguinal region. Testosterone induced regression of cranio suspensory ligament and thickening of gubernaculum influenced by insulin like factor 3.
- *Inguinal phase (mechanical/gubernacular influence):* 26–28 weeks

  This phase involves descent into the scrotum influenced by genitofemoral nerve and is calcitonin gene-related peptide (CGRP) induced.

Definitions

- *True undescended testes (UDT):* Testis is on its normal path of descent but is halted on its way to the scrotum.
- *Ectopic testes:* Position of the testis is outside its normal path of descent and outside the scrotum. The most common aberrant position is the superficial inguinal pouch. Others are medial thigh, perineum, and contralateral hemiscrotum.
- *Retractile testes:* Pseudocryptorchidism
  - Testes are normally descended in scrotum in suprascrotal position due to an overactive cremasteric reflex.
  - Testes can be manipulated into the scrotum and remain there at least temporarily.
- *Ascending testis:* Acquired UDT can be because of entrapment after inguinal hernia surgery or spontaneously.

Etiology

A combination of genetics, maternal health, and other environmental factors might disrupt the hormones, physical changes, and nerve activity that influence the development of the testicles.

SRY gene on Y chromosome along with neurohormonal pathways is responsible for normal testicular descent.

Bilateral Cryptorchidism

- Klinefelter syndrome
- Noonan syndrome
- Idiopathic hypogonadotropic hypogonadism (IHH)
- Kallmann syndrome
- *Genetic disorders:* Prader–Labhart Willi syndrome and Laurence–Moon–Biedl syndrome
- *Androgen resistance syndrome:* Reifenstein syndrome
- Mutations in Leydig cell and INSL3/relaxin family peptide receptor 3(RXFP3)

Presentation

- History of *empty scrotum*
- Inguinal hernia due to patent processus vaginalis
- Atypical genitalia

Examination

Examination is done in either standing, squatting, or supine position with legs abducted.

- *Location of the testis:* Retractile/unpalpable

  For retractile testis, pressure to the lower abdomen or by Valsalva maneuver is applied, pushing the testis with one hand on the lower abdomen, with firm strokes from anterior superior iliac spine through the groin to the pubis into the scrotum.
- Associated with inguinal hernia/hydrocele
- Penile size
- Hypospadias (urethra meatus opening)

Investigations

- UDT is a *clinical diagnosis*.
- Ultrasonography (USG) may be beneficial, if suspecting an inguinal testis.
- Magnetic resonance imaging (MRI) value is limited. In case of suspected disorder of sexual development, pelvic MRI can help confirm the presence or absence of Müllerian structures.
- *Diagnostic laparoscopy remains the gold standard in exclusion of intra-abdominal testis.*
- *Karyotype:* Atypical genitalia
- *In older children:* Luteinizing hormone (LH), follicle-stimulating hormone (FSH), human chorionic gonadotropin (hCG) stimulation test in case of bilateral UDT to rule out agonadism.

Complications

Complications are associated with an increased risk of:

- Testicular carcinoma (seminoma)
- Fertility problems
- Impaired sperm production
- *Testicular torsion:* It occurs 10 times more often in UDT than in normal testis.
- *Trauma:* Injured from pressure against the pubic bone
- Psychological stress

Red Flags

- Bilateral UDT
- Associated with hypospadias
- Hard solid mass palpable in the testis points toward testicular malignancy, especially seminoma.
- Associated inguinal hernia

Approach

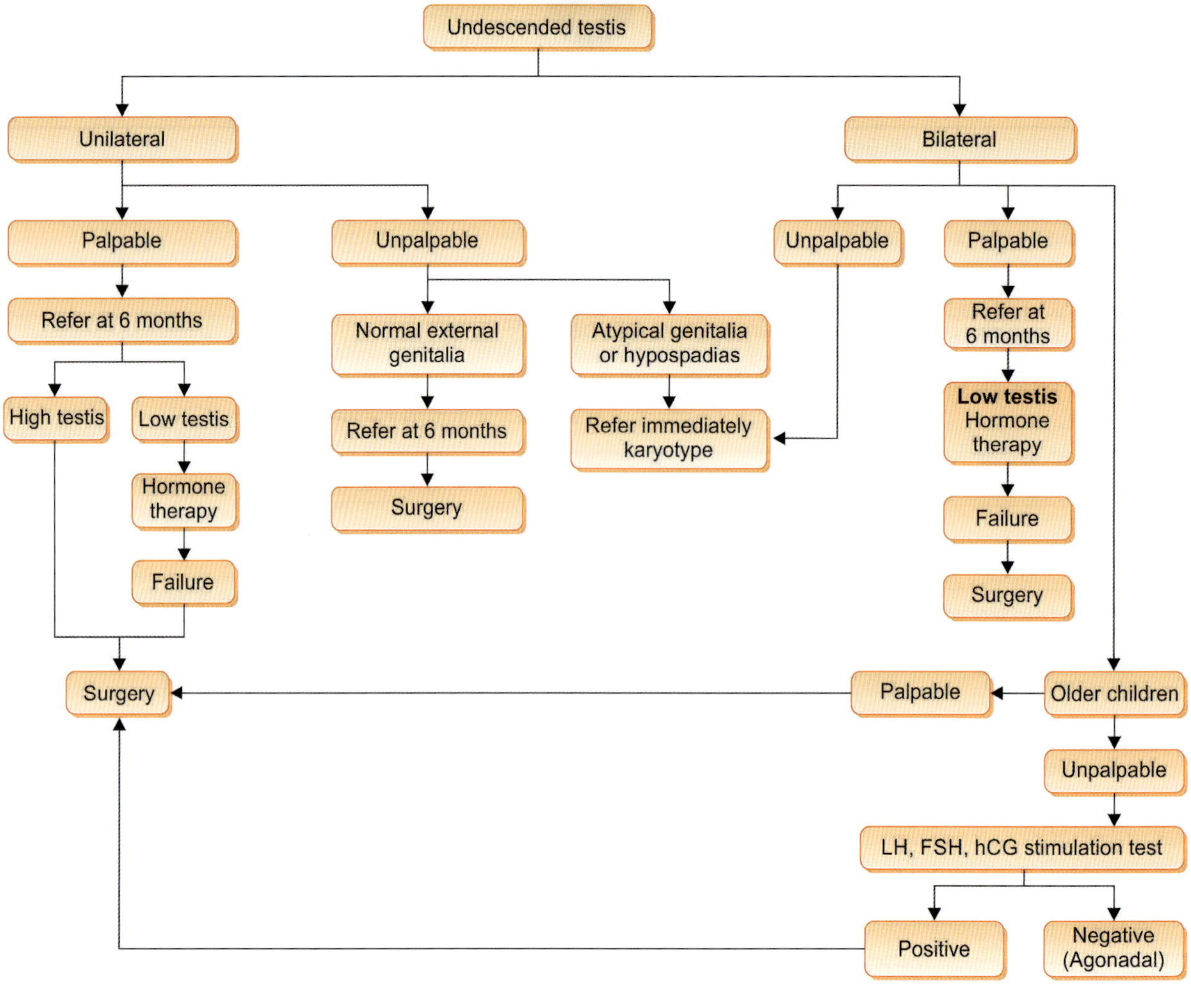

(LH: luteinizing hormone, FSH: follicle-stimulating hormone, hCG: human chorionic gonadotropin)

Suggested Reading

- Cortes D, Holt R, de Knegt VE. Hormonal aspects of the pathogenesis and treatment of cryptorchidism. Eur J Pediatr Surg. 2016;26(5):409-17.
- Lee PA, Coughlin MT. Leydig cell function after cryptorchidism: Evidence of the beneficial result of early surgery. J Urol. 2002;167(4):1824-7.
- Melmed S, Koenig R, Rosen CJ, Auchus RJ, Goldfine AB. Williams Textbook of Endocrinology, 14th edition. Amsterdam, Netherlands: Elsevier; 2020. pp. 678-80.

Tinnitus

23

***Section Editor:* Rupesh Masand**
***Section Co-Editor:* Hema Gupta Mittal**
***Authors:* Deepak V Haldipur, Akshay BK**

Introduction

- Tinnitus is defined as the perception of sounds like buzzing, ringing, roaring, clicking, pulsations, and other noises in the ear/ears/head occurring without an outside acoustic stimulus.
- Tinnitus is a symptom, not a disease, and can arise due to inappropriate activity at any point in the auditory pathway.

Classification

Tinnitus can be classified as being objective or subjective:

- *Objective tinnitus:* It is a sound that the examiner can also hear during testing.
- *Subjective tinnitus:* It is the perception of a sound experienced by the patient for which no source can be found.

The prevalence of tinnitus in children has been studied in several articles with reports ranging from 7.5% to 60%. Tinnitus is more common among children with hearing impairment compared to those with normal hearing.

Etiology

Subjective Tinnitus

- *Otologic:* Hearing loss, Ménière's disease, acoustic neuroma, and ototoxic medications or substances
- *Neurologic:* Multiple sclerosis and head injury
- *Metabolic:* Thyroid disorder, hyperlipidemia, and vitamin B_{12} deficiency
- *Psychogenic:* Depression, anxiety, and fibromyalgia

Objective Tinnitus

- *Vascular:* Arterial bruit, venous hum, arteriovenous malformation, and vascular tumors
- *Neurologic:* Palatal myoclonus, idiopathic stapedial muscle spasm, and patulous Eustachian tube.

Red Flag Signs

- Tinnitus with suicidal ideation
- Sudden onset of focal neurological symptoms
- Acute uncontrolled vestibular symptoms (acute severe vertigo)
- Suspected stroke
- Following a head injury
- Sudden-onset hearing loss (defined as onset over a 72-hour period within the last 30 days)
- Tinnitus causing significant impact upon mental health despite support

Investigations

- Pure tone audiometry
- Speech discrimination scoring
- Tympanometry
- Tinnitus pitch masking (matching the frequency of the tinnitus with a variety of stimuli)
- Tinnitus loudness matching (estimating the loudness of tinnitus with a pure tone or noise)

- Tinnitus minimum masking level (a test in which the amount of sound required to cover the tinnitus is recorded)
- Tinnitus residual inhibition (achieving decreased or absent tinnitus after exposure to a masking tone at the pitch and intensity of the tinnitus)
- *Blood tests:* Thyroid profile, complete hemogram, and lipid profile
- *Pulsatile tinnitus:* Contrast-enhanced computed tomography (CT) or magnetic resonance imaging (MRI) of the brain
- *Nonpulsatile (continuous) tinnitus:* Gadolinium-enhanced MRI

Diagnostic Algorithm

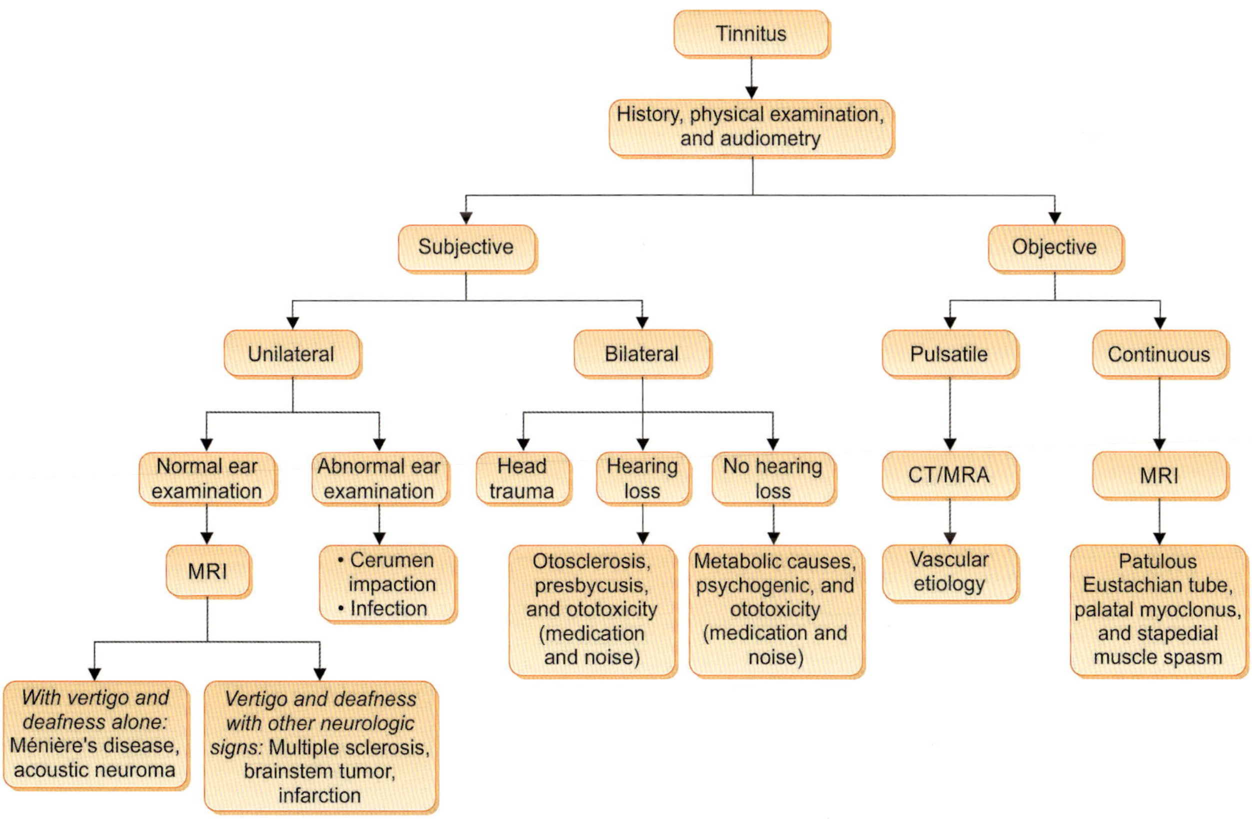

(CT: computed tomography; MRI: magnetic resonance imaging)

Suggested Reading

- Collins RD. Algorithmic Diagnosis of Symptoms and Signs: A Cost-Effective Approach, 3rd edition. Philadelphia (PA): Lippincott Williams & Wilkins; 2013.
- Crummer RW, Hassan GA. Diagnostic approach to tinnitus. Am Fam Physician. 2004;69(1):120-6.
- Dullaart MJ, Kip M, Smit AL, Stegeman I. Treatment of tinnitus in children—A systematic review. Front Neurol. 2021;12:726803.
- Ellis S, Wilson R, Dolan S. Tinnitus: Systematic approach to primary care assessment and management. Br J Gen Pract. 2022;72(717):190-2.
- Raj-Koziak D, Gos E, Swierniak W, Skarzynski H, Skarzynski PH. Prevalence of tinnitus in a sample of 43,064 children in Warsaw, Poland. Int J Audiol. 2021;60(8):614-20.

Fever without Focus

24

Section Editor: B Rajsekhar
Section Co-Editor: Suchitra Pusapati
Authors: AS Kireeti, V Spandana

Definition

When a complete history and physical examination cannot identify a specific source of fever ≥39°C (102.2°F) in a previously healthy, otherwise well-appearing child between 3 months and 3 years of age, the illness is called fever without focus.

Etiology

- It varies with age, and the risk of invasive bacterial infection is more common in young infants. About 1–30% of them may have some form of serious bacterial infection (SBI).
- A majority have a self-limiting viral etiology.
- *Postvaccination fever:* It may last for 2–3 days from the day of vaccination.
- *Other common causes:* Clinically occult pneumonia, urinary tract infection (UTI—most common), and bacteremia.
- Occult bacteremia refers to the isolation of a bacterial pathogen in a blood culture done in an otherwise well-appearing febrile child.
- *Rarely:* Osteomyelitis and septic arthritis

Red Flags

- Tachypnea, respiratory distress, and other signs of pneumonia
- Bony tenderness/painful joint movements
- Tenderness in costovertebral angle or suprapubic region for UTI
- *Skin manifestations:* Viral exanthem, petechiae, cellulitis, etc.

Approach

Approach to fever without focus in children aged 3–36 months is illustrated in **Flowchart 1**.

FLOWCHART 1: Approach to fever without focus in either unimmunized or incompletely immunized children aged 3–36 months.

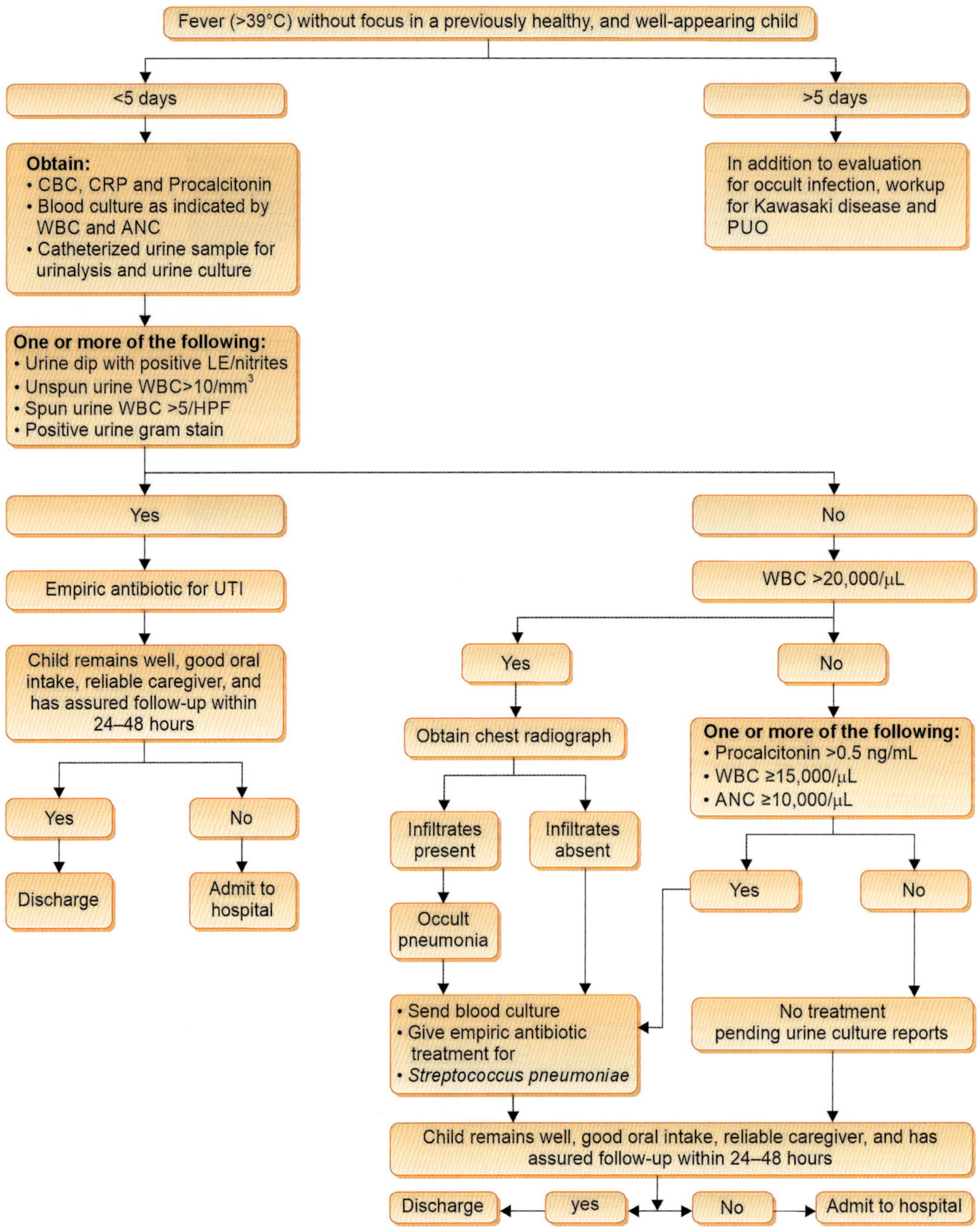

(ANC: absolute neutrophil count; CBC: complete blood count, CRP: C-reactive protein; HPF: high power field; LE: leukocyte esterase; PUO: pyrexia of unknown origin; UTI: urinary tract infection; WBC: white blood cell count)

Flowchart 2 illustrates approach to fever in a fully immunized child aged 6–36 months.

FLOWCHART 2: Approach to fever without focus in a fully immunized child of age 6–36 months.

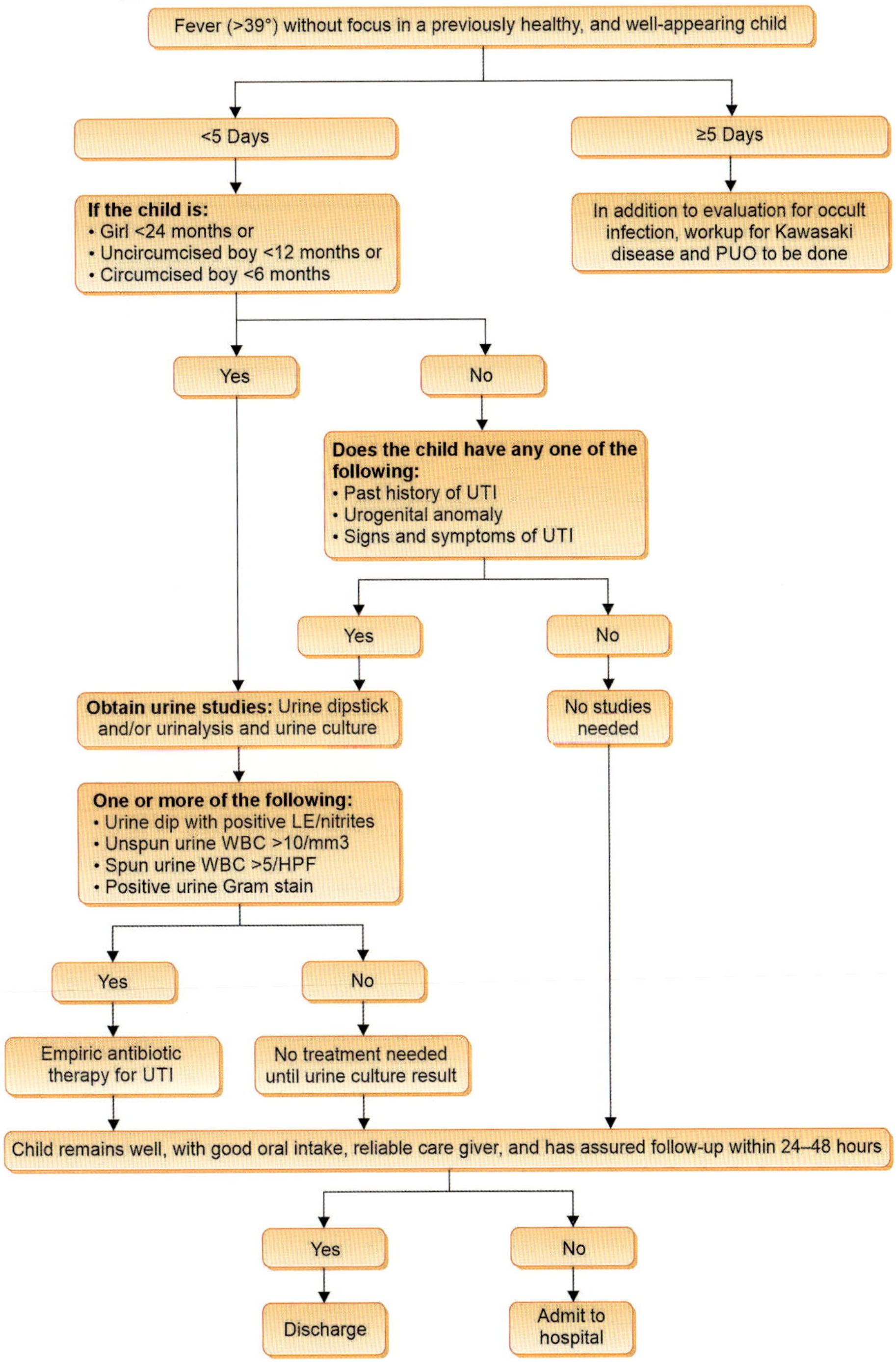

(HPF: high power field; LE: leukocyte esterase; PUO: pyrexia of unknown origin; UTI: urinary tract infection; WBC: white blood cell count)

Flowchart 3 displays blood culture follow-up in children aged 3–36 months.

FLOWCHART 3: Blood culture follow-up in children 3–36 months of age.

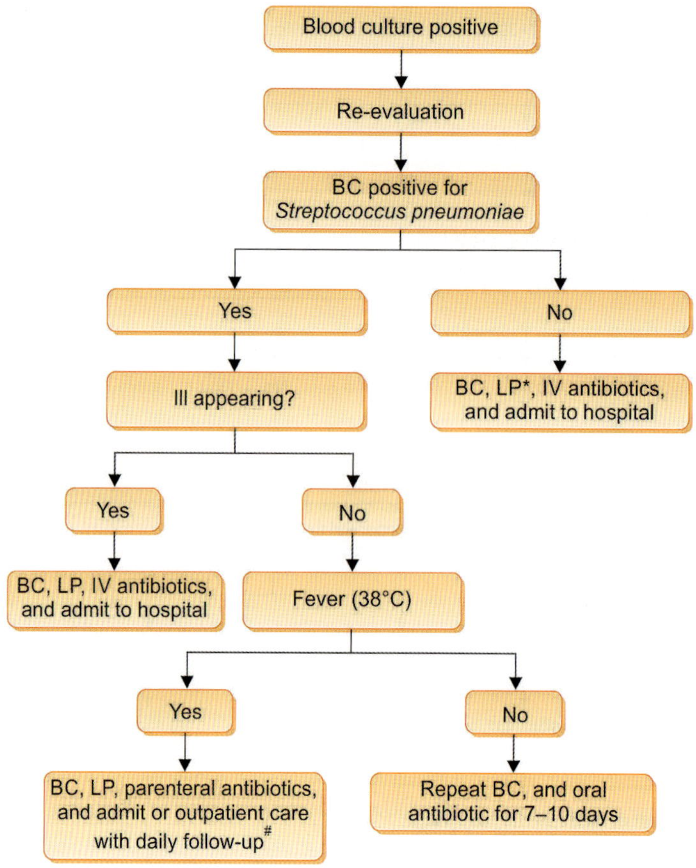

(BC: blood culture; IV: intravenous; LP: lumbar puncture)

*Well children with blood culture positive for *Escherichia coli* or *Staphylococcus aureus* do not need a lumbar puncture; for other pathogens, which are encountered rarely, the decision should be individualized.

#Outpatient care is only appropriate in children without evidence of meningitis on cerebrospinal fluid (CSF) analysis.

Suggested Reading

- Baraf LJ. Management of fever without source in infants and children. Ann Emerg Med. 2000;36(6):602-14.
- DePorre AG, Aronson PL, McCulloh RJ. Facing the ongoing challenge of the febrile young infant. Crit Care. 2017; 21(1):68.
- Greenhow TL, Hung YY, Herz A. Bacteremia in children 3 to 36 months old after introduction of conjugated pneumococcal vaccines. Pediatrics. 2017;139(4):e20162098.
- National Institute for Health and Care Excellence. (2021). Fever in under 5s: Assessment and initial management NICE guideline [NG143]. [online] Available from https://www.nice.org.uk/guidance/ng143 [Last accessed February, 2024].
- Shaw KN, Gorelick M, McGowan KL, Yakscoe NM, Schwartz JS. Prevalence of urinary tract infection in febrile young children in the emergency department. Pediatrics. 1998;102(2):e16.

Tics

25

***Section Editor:* Sumitha Nayak**
***Section Co-Editor:* Priya Shivalli**
***Author:* Mrutunjay Dash**

Definition

- Tics are brief and sudden movements or sounds that may be indistinguishable from physiological actions but appear repetitive, often disruptive, and are not embedded in a certain context but can be inhibited on demand.
- Tics are classified as a hyperkinetic movement disorder; however, different from other hyperkinesias, they are typically preceded by a premonitory sensation known as the "premonitory urge".

Classification

Classification of tics disease is illustrated in **Table 1**

TABLE 1: Classification of tics in children.

	MOTOR TICS	VOCAL TICS
Simple	• Eye blinking • Eye rolling • Grimacing (pulling faces) • Shoulder shrugging • Limb and head jerking/head nodding • Abdominal tensing	• Whistling • Throat clearing • Sniffing • Coughing • Tongue clicking • Grunting • Animal sounds
Complex	• Jumping • Twirling • Touching objects and other people • Obscene movements or gestures (copropraxia) • Repeating other people's gestures (echopraxia)	• Nonobscene socially inappropriate (NOSI) behavior (e.g., remarking about a person's weight or inappropriately touching someone) • Involuntary swearing (coprolalia) • Repeating a sound, word, or phrase (echolalia)

Red Flags

- Severe tics during early childhood
- *Point to:* Presence of common neuropsychiatric comorbidities, attention-deficit hyperactivity disorder (ADHD) (50–80%), obsessive-compulsive disorder (OCD) (22–44%), learning difficulties (20–30%), anxiety (20%), and sleep problems (64%).
- ADHD precedes the tic disorders and OCD usually follows tics.

Approach

- Detailed history, including age of onset, duration of tics, pattern, rhythm, family history, premonitory urge, associated comorbid conditions, absence of any significant cause, absence of movement disorders (athetosis, chorea, ballismus, myoclonus, etc.)
- Postviral encephalitis
- History of ingestion of any stimulant medications, Presence of pathological Huntington's chorea to be ruled out

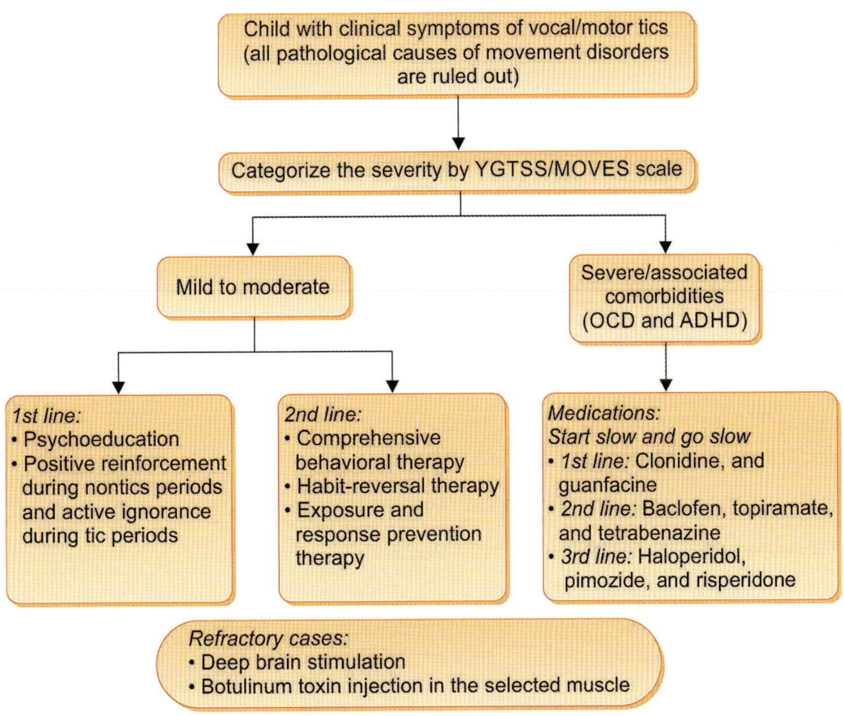

(ADHD: attention-deficit/hyperactivity disorder; MOVES: motor tic, obsessions, and compulsions, vocal tic evaluation survey; OCD: obsessive-compulsive disorder; YGTSS: Yale Global Tic Severity Scale)

Scales to Grade

Yale Global Tic Severity Scale (YGTSS) **(Table 2)**

TABLE 2: Yale Global Tick Severity Scale.

	NUMBER 0–5	FREQUENCY 0–5	INTENSITY 0–5	COMPLEXITY 0–5	INTERFERENCE 0–5	TOTAL
Motor tics						
Vocal tics						

Note: Scoring:

1 = None, 10 = minimal, 20 = mild, 30 = moderate, 40 = marked, 50 = severe

Another scoring used is:

Motor tic, obsessions and compulsions, vocal tic evaluation survey (MOVES): This is a self-report scale for the symptoms in five subscales: Motor tics, vocal tics, obsessions, compulsions, and associated symptoms (echolalia, echopraxia, coprolalia, and copropraxia).

Management

- No specific laboratory tests
- If risk factors like dysmorphic facies, febrile seizure, unusual deterioration, and suspected chromosomal anomalies occur, do neuroimaging, electroencephalogram (EEG), and exome sequencing.
- Group A streptococcal infection to be ruled out if suspected pediatric autoimmune neuropsychiatric disorders associated with Streptococcus (PANDAS)
- Medication is the cornerstone along with behavioral therapy for severe tics.
- Motor tics respond better to medication than vocal tics.

Suggested Reading

- Ganos C, Martino D, Pringsheim T. Tics in the pediatric population: Pragmatic management. Mov Disord Clin Pract. 2017:4(2):160-72.
- Jain R, Pandey S, Raghav S. Movement disorders in children. Indian Pediatr. 2021;58(9):861-70.
- Rossi PJ, Opri E, Shute JB, Molina R, Bowers D, Ward H, et al. Scheduled, intermittent stimulation of the thalamus reduces tics in Tourette syndrome. Parkinsonism Relat Disord. 2016:29:35-41.
- Ueda K, Black KJ. A comprehensive review of tic disorders in children. J Clin Med. 2021;10(11):2479.
- Weisman H, Qureshi IA, Leckman JF, Scahill L, Bloch MH. Systematic review: Pharmacological treatment of tic disorders: efficacy of antipsychotic and alpha-2 adrenergic agonist agents. Neurosci Biobehav Rev. 2013:37(6):1162-71.
- Yadegar M, Guo S, Ricketts EJ, Zinner SH. Assessment and management of tic disorders in pediatric primary care settings. Curr Dev Disord Rep. 2019;6(3):159-72.

Abnormal Gait

26

Section Editor: **Janani Shankar**
Section Co-Editor: **Arathi Srinivasan**
Authors: **Sandeep PS, R Venkateswari**

Introduction

- Abnormal gait refers to an unusual walking pattern.
- It is a common complaint in children.
- Limping is a common cause of abnormal gait. It can range from simple benign reasons, such as ill-fitting shoes, and sprain to devastating ominous causes like malignancy or septic arthritis.
- Normal variants of gait are given in **Box 1**.

BOX 1: Normal variants of gait.

- Toe walking is common till 3 years of age. Mature adult gait develops between 3 and 4 years of age.
- Bowing of legs is common during the early toddler age group and is normal up to 2 years of age.
- Knock-knees are common, associated with intoeing, and can be seen till 7 years of age.

- Types of abnormal gait:
  - Antalgic gait
  - Nonantalgic gait

Causes by Anatomical Origin

More and less common causes by anatomical origin are given in **Table 1**.

TABLE 1: Causes by anatomical origin.

	ANATOMICAL ORIGIN	MORE COMMON	LESS COMMON
	Muscles and ligaments	• Sprain/strain • Sports injury • Viral myositis	Juvenile dermatomyositis
	Bones	• Trauma/fractures • Toddler abuse • Growing pain • Vitamin D3 deficiency • Osteomyelitis • Leukemia • Limb length discrepancy	• Caffey's disease • Osteosarcoma • Ewing sarcoma
	Neurological	• Cerebral palsy • Guillain–Barré syndrome	• Polio • Spinal cord discitis
4	Vaso-occlusive	• Henoch–Schönlein purpura	Deep vein thrombosis
	Hematological	• Sickle cell arthropathy • Hemarthrosis due to hemophilia	
	Single joint	• *Hip:* Transient synovitis and SCFE • *Knee:* Reactive arthritis, septic arthritis, and tuberculosis	Tumor Oligoarticular JIA
	Multiple joints	• Acute • Rheumatic fever • Polyarticular/oligoarticular JIA	SLE

(JIA: juvenile idiopathic arthritis; SCFE: slipped capital femoral epiphysis; SLE: systemic lupus erythematosus)

Age calendar can guide to common problems:

- *At birth:* Developmental dysplasia of the hip
- *0–5 years:* Infection
- *5–10 years:* Perthes disease
- *10–20 years:* Slipped capital femoral epiphysis

Red Flags

- Duration of symptoms >7 days
- Acute-onset severe localized joint pain
- Complete inability to weight bear/walk
- Nocturnal bone pain
- *Systemic signs:* Fever, chills, weight loss, organomegaly, and enlarged nodes
- Petechiae or purpura in the back or lower limbs

Clinical Pointers

- *Associated abdominal pain:* Acute abdomen, Henoch–Schönlein purpura, and psoas abscess
- *Fever, anorexia, weight loss, and night sweats:* Infection and malignancy
- *Pain that worsens at night:* Malignancy
- *Pain that improves with activity:* Rheumatological cause
- *History of bleeding disorder:* Hemarthrosis in hemophilia
- *History of preceding pharyngitis with polyarthralgia:* Rheumatic fever
- *Burning or radiating pain:* Neuropathic pain

Types of nonantalgic gait are given in **Flowchart 1**.

FLOWCHART 1: Nonantalgic gait.

- Nonantalgic gait
  - *Steppage gait:* Hip and knee joints flex excessively in the stance phase
    Example: Foot drop in peripheral nerve pathology
  - *Trendelenburg gait:* Hip tilted downward in the unaffected side during the stance phase
    Example: DDH and hip pathologies
  - *Circumduction gait:* Hyperextension of knee followed by circumduction or abduction of the unaffected leg to clear the ground
    Example: Hemiplegia and limb length discrepancy
  - *Equinus gait:* Inability to dorsiflex the foot with spasticity of the tendon Achilles
    Example: Cerebral palsy and CTEV

(CTEV: congenital talipes equinovarus; DDH: developmental dysplasia of the hip)

The approach to antalgic gait is shown in **Flowchart 2**.

FLOWCHART 2: Approach to the management of antalgic gait.

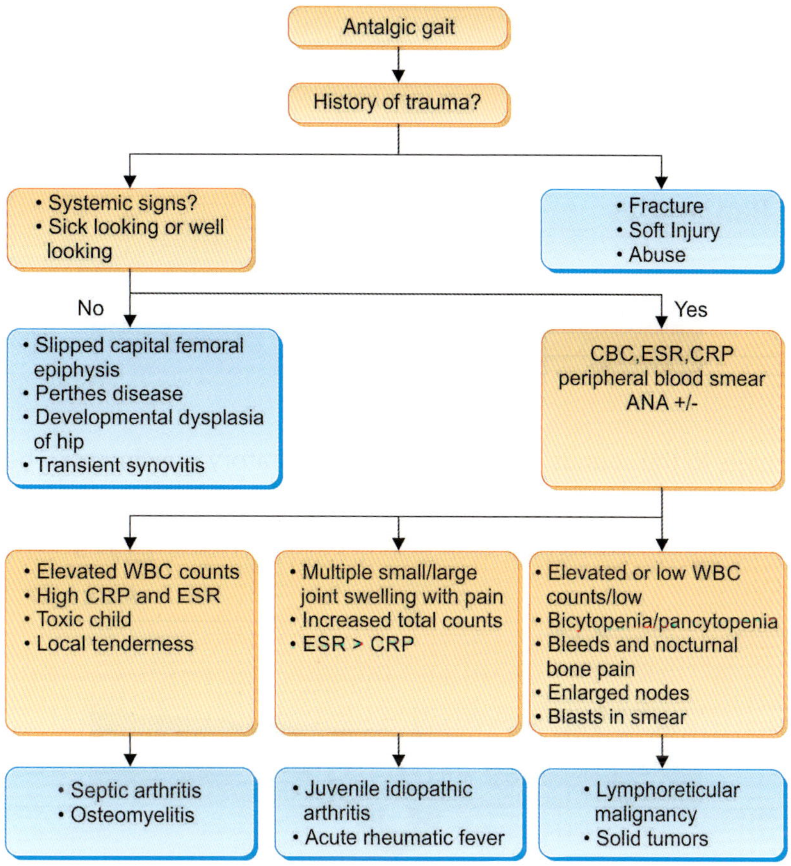

(ANA: antinuclear antibody; CBC: complete blood count; CRP: C-reactive protein; ESR: erythrocyte sedimentation rate; WBC: white blood cells)

Suggested Reading

- Morancie NA, Helton MR. Evaluating the Child with a Limp. Am Fam Physician. 2023;107(5):474-85.
- Sawhney S, Aggarwal A (Eds). Pediatric Rheumatology: A Clinical Viewpoint. Singapore: Springer Verlag; 2017.

Noisy Breathing

27

***Section Editor:* Rupesh Masand**
***Section Co-Editor:* Hema Gupta Mittal**
***Author:* Rashmi Ranjan Das**

Introduction

- Noisy breathing refers to the sounds produced during respiratory movements. These are secondary to partial blockage/narrowing at some point in the respiratory tract.
- Noisy breathing is a common problem in children, especially in younger age groups, and may be due to various reasons.

Etiology

Etiology depends on the type of sounds produced:

- *Snuffle from anterior part of nose:* Nasal block
- *Snoring from posterior part of nose or nasopharynx:* Adenoid hypertrophy
- *Stridor from large/central airways like larynx and trachea*: Infection (croup), airway malacia (laryngomalacia and tracheobronchomalacia), subglottic pathology (stenosis and hemangioma), and tracheal compression (externally by a vascular ring or sling or lymph node and internally by any foreign body or mass)
- *Wheeze from large and medium-sized airways like bronchi:* Bronchiolitis, asthma, foreign body, or any compression (internally or externally)
- *Rattle from small airways like terminal bronchioles:* Secondary to fluid or secretions (e.g., bronchiolitis)
- *Grunting from small airways like respiratory bronchioles and alveoli:* Secondary to fluid or secretions (e.g., pneumonia and pulmonary edema)

Red Flags

SYMPTOMS	SIGNS
• Choking during feeding • Difficulty in sleeping at night • Apnea or cyanosis • Poor weight gain • Rapid worsening of symptoms • Exercise intolerance	• Severe respiratory distress/apneic episodes • Pallor, cyanosis • Sick looking and lethargic • Failure to thrive • Hypoxia or hypercarbia with CO_2 narcosis • Syndromic child • Acute onset and rapid progression • Markedly decrease air entry or silent chest

Approach (Flowchart 1)

Noisy Breathing

Enquire: Age of onset, phase (inspiratory or expiratory or biphasic), acute or persistent, continuous or intermittent, heard during sleep or awake state, mouth breathing during sleep, aggravating and relieving factors, voice involvement or abnormal cry, feeding difficulties, sleeping difficulties, and poor weight gain.

Examination of a child with noisy breathing is given in **Box 1**

BOX 1: Examination of a child with noisy breathing.

PHYSICAL EXAMINATION FINDINGS	RESPIRATORY SYSTEM EXAMINATION FINDINGS	SYSTEMIC EXAMINATION (EXCEPT RESPIRATORY)
General look (sick or well looking), vital parameters, anthropometry, craniofacial anomalies, neuromuscular weakness, skin hemangioma, and allergic markers	• Observe the child and listen to the sound • *Inspection:* Nasal and oral cavity, tracheal position, and chest deformity • *Auscultation:* Air entry, classify the sounds on auscultation (character and phase of respiration during which it is heard and any combinations of sound present)	Neuromuscular weakness, murmurs

FLOWCHART 1: Approach to noisy breathing.

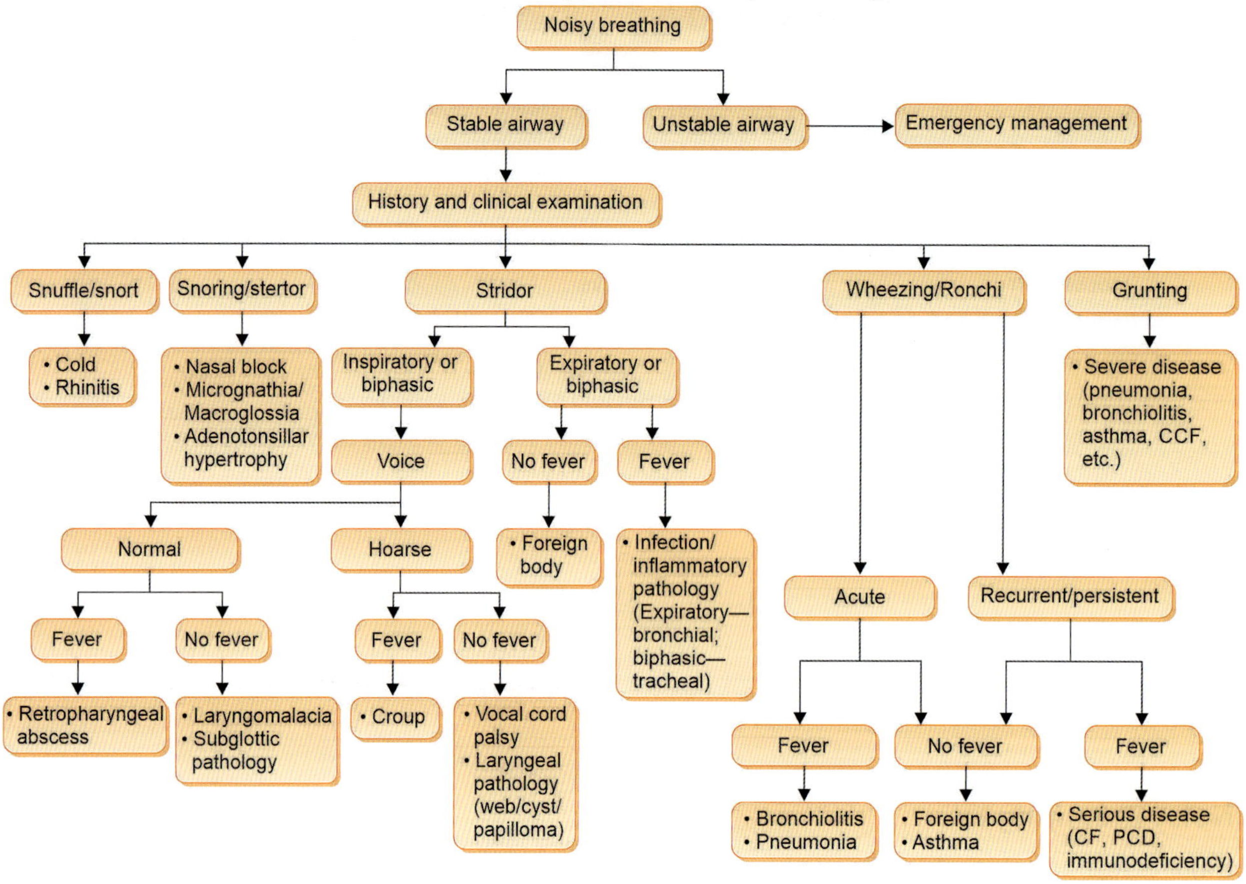

(CF: cystic fibrosis; CCF: congestive cardiac failure; PCD: primary ciliary dyskinesia)

Relevant Investigations

Relevant investigations are given in **Box 2.**

BOX 2: Investigations.

Depending on the type of noisy breathing, the following examinations are done:

- Nasal speculum examination
- Chest X-ray (parenchymal or mediastinal pathology or foreign body)
- Oral cavity examination with a spatula
- X-ray neck lateral view (adenoid hypertrophy and foreign body)
- Fiberoptic laryngoscopy (from ENT) to confirm laryngomalacia or cause of voice change or abnormal cry (if present)
- *CT chest*: Ideally, contrast CT should be done (HRCT not helpful).
- Bronchoscopy (visualize the airway pathology and remove foreign body)—can refer the patient to a higher center

(ENT: ear, nose and throat; CT: computed tomography; HRCT: high-resolution computed tomography)

Diagnostic Pointers

- *Stridor:*
  - *Well-looking infant, onset at around 4–8 weeks, relieved during prone position/sound getting aggravated during crying or periods of upper respiratory infections:* Laryngomalacia
  - *Acute with barking cough:* Croup
  - *Skin hemangioma:* Subglottic hemangioma
  - *History of multiple intubations:* Subglottic stenosis
  - *Biphasic stridor:* Vascular ring or sling or lymph node or mass
  - *Acute onset with or without choking episodes:* Foreign body
- *Wheeze:*
  - *Acute onset (monophonic) with/without choking episodes:* Foreign body
  - *Skin hemangioma:* Subglottic hemangioma
  - *Allergy history or allergic markers or response to bronchodilators:* Allergic wheeze (under 5 years) or asthma (older kids)
  - *With crackles:* Acute presentation (bronchiolitis and pneumonia), and recurrent or chronic presentations (immunodeficiency and ciliary disorders like cystic fibrosis)
  - *Red flag signs present:* Atypical wheezers (not due to asthma)
- *Snoring:*
  - *Well-looking child, obese/overweight, allergic rhinitis, and mouth breathing during sleep:* Adenoid hypertrophy
  - *Syndromic/dysmorphic child:* Musculoskeletal problem (e.g., Down syndrome)
- *Grunting:* Indicates respiratory failure and usually sick child (e.g., severe bronchiolitis or pneumonia, and acute pulmonary edema)

Suggested Reading

- Chang AB (Ed). Common Respiratory Symptoms and Illnesses: A Graded Evidence-Based Approach, An Issue of Pediatric Clinics, 1st edition. Amsterdam: Elsevier Publishing; 2009.
- Hirschberg J, Szende T, Koltai PJ, Illényi A (Eds). Pediatric Airway: Cry, Stridor and Cough. San Diego: Plural Publishing; 2009.

Grunting

28

Section Editor: **Nehal Patel**
Section Co-Editor: **Jay T Dhirwani**
Authors: **Ashish Mehta, Vishal Gohil**

Introduction

Grunting is a very common sign noted after newborn delivery. It occurs when the newborn exhales against a partially closed glottis. It produces a mean increase in PaO_2 and a mean decrease in $PaCO_2$ and improves with oxygenation and ventilation.

These effects are less pronounced when there are parenchymal lung diseases like hyaline membrane disease (HMD) and respiratory distress syndrome (RDS).

It is a compensatory mechanism to achieve respiratory adaptation in the face of an overdistended circulatory system.

Grunting is a protective form of breathing resulting in improved alveolar ventilation.

Grunting is part of respiratory distress assessment in term **(Table 1)** and in preterms **(Table 2)**.

In the scoring system, 0 indicates no grunt, 1 = expiratory grunt heard with a stethoscope only, and 2 = expiratory grunt heard with the naked ear. Grunting should not be ignored in neonates.

TABLE 1: Downes' score.

SCORE	RESPIRATORY RATE	CYANOSIS	AIR ENTRY	GRUNT	RETRACTION
0	<60/min	Nil	Normal	None	Nil
1	60–80/min	In-room air	Mild?	Auscultation with stethoscope	Mild
2	>80/min	In >40%	Marked?	Audible with naked ear	Moderate

TABLE 2: Silverman–Anderson retraction score.

SCORE	UPPER-CHEST RETRACTION	LOWER-CHEST RETRACTION	XIPHOID RETRACTION	NASAL DILATATION	GRUNT
0	Synchronized	None	None	None	None
1	Lag on inspiration	Just visible	Just visible	Minimal	Stethoscope only
2	Seesaw	Marked	Marked	Marked	Naked ear

Etiology

- *Parenchymal involvement:*
  - HMD
  - Meconium aspiration syndrome (MAS)
  - Transient tachypnea of the newborn (TTNB)
  - Congenital or acquired pneumonia
  - Air leak
- *Parenchymal + cardiovascular involvement:* Persistence pulmonary hypertension of the newborn (PPHN)
- *Congenital anomalies:*
  - *Upper airway:* Choanal atresia
  - *Gut:* Congenital diaphragmatic hernia (CDH), tracheoesophageal fistula (TEF)
  - *Lung:* Lobar emphysema, congenital cystic adenomatoid malformation, and cysts
  - Congenital heart disease
- *Nonparenchymal causes:*
  - *Hematological causes:* Severe anemia and polycythemia
  - Neurological cause [intracerebral hemorrhage (ICH), intraventricular hemorrhage (IVH), and stroke]
  - *Metabolic cause:* Inborn errors of metabolism (IEM)

FLOWCHART 1: Etiology of respiratory distress according to age.

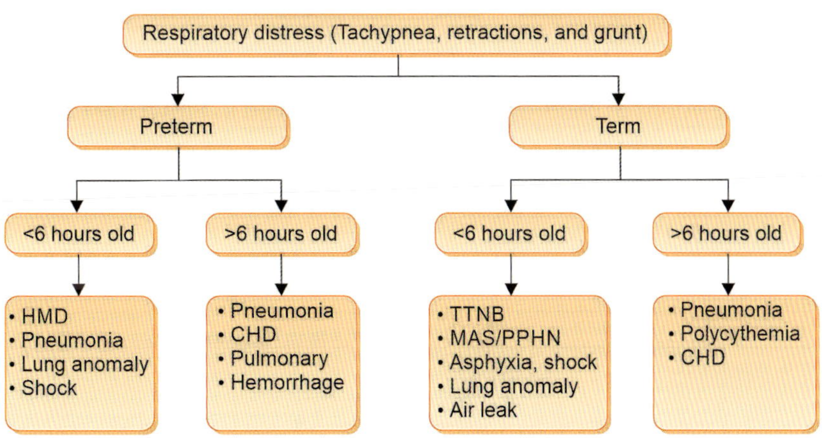

(CHD: congenital heart defects; HMD: hyaline membrane disease; MAS: meconium aspiration syndrome; TTNB: transient tachypnea of the newborn; PPHN: persistence pulmonary hypertension of the newborn)

Red Flags

Using Silverman–Anderson score for:

- Preterm infants
- <6 hours of life
- >6 hours of life
- >3 score

Use Downes' score for:

- Term infants,
- In term infants, score >5 irrespective of age

Investigation

- Chest X-ray
- Lung ultrasound
- Arterial blood gas (ABG)
- Blood investigation
- TABC assessment including saturation (SpO_2)

Approach

An approach to the management of children with grunting is given in **Flowchart 2**.

FLOWCHART 2: Algorithm for approach to grunting in children.

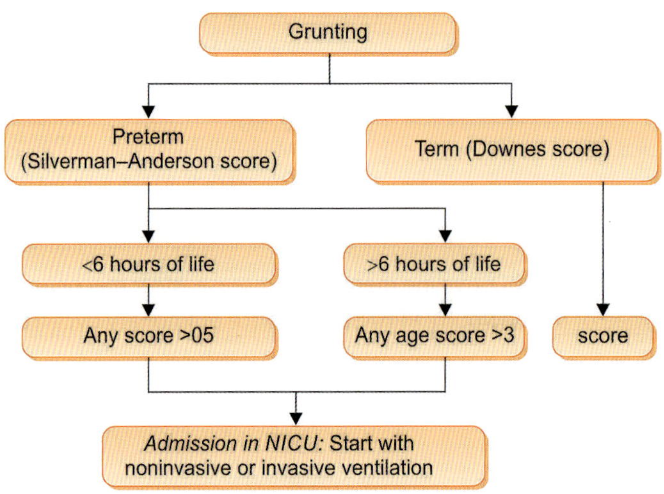

(NICU: neonatal intensive care unit)

Conclusion

A number of studies support an association of grunting with serious illness in older infants but this may not be applicable to all newborns. As per the scoring system, any preterm with score > 0 after birth must be admitted to a neonatal intensive care unit (NICU) to escalate treatment. But for term neonates, it is difficult to answer "How long should a general pediatrician in a well-baby nursery observe a newborn, term or near-term infant with grunting with or without distress before intervening?". Based on all the literature, if only grunting without distress is present, the term neonate must be observed until it disappears. If there is grunting with distress and score >5, a term neonate must be admitted to the NICU to escalate treatment. If any grunting lasts >6 hours irrespective of term or preterm, the neonate must be admitted to the NICU for further management.

Suggested Reading

- DK Guha (Ed). NNF Recommended Basic Perinatal-Neonatal Nomenclature. Guha's Neonatology: Principles and Practice, 1st edition. New Delhi: Jaypee Brothers Medical Publishers (P) Ltd; 1998. pp. 131-2.
- Mathai SS, Raju C, Kanitkar C. Management of respiratory distress in the Newborn. Med J Armed Forces India. 2007;63(3):269-72.
- Silverman WA, Anderson DH. A controlled clinical trial on effects of water mist on obstructive respiratory signs, death rate and necropsy findings among premature infants. Pediatrics. 1956;17(1):1-10.
- Wood DW, Downes JJ, Lecks HI. A clinical scoring for the diagnosis of respiratory failure. Preliminary report on childhood status asthmaticus. Am J Dis Child. 1972;123(3):227-8.
- Yost GC, Young PC, Buchi KF. Significance of Grunting Respirations in Infants Admitted to well-baby Nursery. Arch Pediatr Adolesc Med. 2001;155(3):372-5.

Hemoptysis

29

Section Editor: **Rupesh Masand**
Section Co-Editor: **Hema Gupta Mittal**
Authors: **Jagdish Prasad Goyal, Sathya Srivatsav**

Introduction

- Hemoptysis is the expectoration of blood or the presence of blood in the sputum.
- Sputum expectoration is uncommon in young children; the blood is usually swallowed before being coughed.
- It is important to identify true hemoptysis from hematemesis or upper airway bleeding **(Table 1)**.
- Frank hemoptysis is rare, usually self-limiting, and can be potentially life-threatening.

TABLE 1: Difference between hemoptysis versus hematemesis.

PARAMETER	HEMOPTYSIS	HEMATEMESIS
Major symptom	Cough	Vomiting
Past history	Lung disease	Hepatic/GI pathology
Appearance	Frothy, pink, or red	Dark red/brown, mixed with food particles
pH	Alkaline	Acidic

(GI: gastrointestinal)

Etiology

The etiology of hemoptysis is given in **Box 1**.

BOX 1: Etiology of hemoptysis.

• *Infections* Pneumonia, lung abscess, and tracheobronchitis
• *Diffuse alveolar hemorrhage:* Idiopathic pulmonary hemosiderosis, vasculitis, coagulopathy, and celiac disease
• *Bronchiectasis:* Postinfectious—tuberculosis, aspergillosis, and cystic fibrosis • Non-cystic fibrosis bronchiectasis—primary ciliary dyskinesia, ABPA, aspiration syndromes, and immunodeficiencies
• *Tumors:* Bronchial adenoma and carcinoid
• *Trauma* Foreign body aspiration, contusion, and iatrogenic
• *Cardiac:* Pulmonary venous obstructive disease, pulmonary hypertension, and mitral stenosis
Vascular: Pulmonary thromboembolism and pulmonary AVM

(ABPA: allergic bronchopulmonary aspergillosis; AVM: arteriovenous malformations)

Red Flags

Symptoms

- Sudden onset cough
- Massive hemoptysis (>200 mL)
- Frothy sputum
- Stridor
- Fast breathing
- Chest pain

Signs

- Worsening pallor
- Cyanosis
- Altered sensorium
- Elevated jugular venous pressure (JVP), hepatomegaly, and pedal edema
- *Unilateral findings:* Reduced air entry and monophonic wheeze
- Bruises in chest/neck

Approach (Flowchart 1)

- *History:* Timing and quantity of blood, trauma, previous bleeding, other site bleeding, associated symptoms like fever, fatigue, sore throat, cough, recent choking episode, loss of weight and appetite, shortness of breath, and chest pain (localized or generalized)
- *Physical examination:*
  - *Bruises around neck or chest and crepitus*: Trauma/airway disruption/lung contusion
  - *Skin hemangiomas/telangiectasias:* Arteriovenous malformations (AVM)
  - *Oral cavity:* Bleeding and missing tooth
  - *Clubbing:* Chronic suppurative lung disease, AVM, and heart disease
  - *Abnormal focal breath sounds:* Infection, foreign body, and localized airway/parenchymal bleeding

FLOWCHART 1: Suggested algorithm for evaluation of hemoptysis in children.

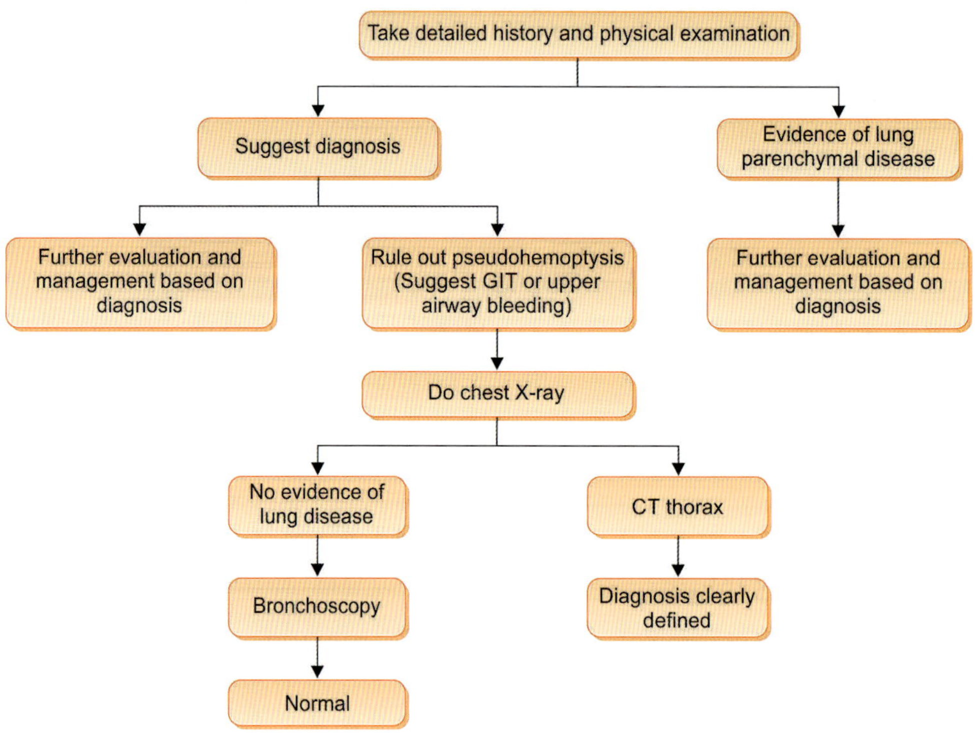

Severity of Hemoptysis

- *Scant:* <5 mL (streaks of blood)
- *Mild to moderate:* >5–200 mL within 24 hours (no hemodynamic instability)
- *Life-threatening or massive:* >200 mL or 8 mL/kg of blood over 24 hours with hemodynamic instability.

Investigations

- *Infective workup:* Complete blood count (CBC), erythrocyte sedimentation rate (ESR), C-reactive protein (CRP), sputum culture, acid-fast bacteria (AFB) staining, and cartridge-based nucleic acid amplification test (CBNAAT)
- *Coagulation studies:* Prothrombin time (PT)/international normalized ratio (INR), activated partial thromboplastin time (APTT), and D-dimer
- *Urinalysis:* Microscopy
- *Imaging:* To identify the immediate source of the bleeding, aid in diagnosis, and roadmap before intervention
  - *Chest X-ray (CXR):* 50% can have normal X-ray; helpful in screening for infection, foreign body, bronchiectasis, and cavity
  - *Computed tomography (CT):* Depiction of underlying disease and visualization of thoracic vasculature (AVM, aneurysms, and infarcts)
- *Bronchoscopy:*
  - Flexible, preferred for diagnostic bronchoscopy once bleeding is controlled; direct inspection of airways for the presence of blood
  - *BAL:* Hemosiderin-laden macrophages—subacute/chronic bleed, infective workup
  - Rigid bronchoscopy for profuse bleeding, interventions
- *Lung biopsy:* Helpful in autoimmune systemic disorders/persistent, unexplained hemoptysis

FLOWCHART 2: Algorithm to differentiate hemoptysis of lower respiratory causes from other causes.

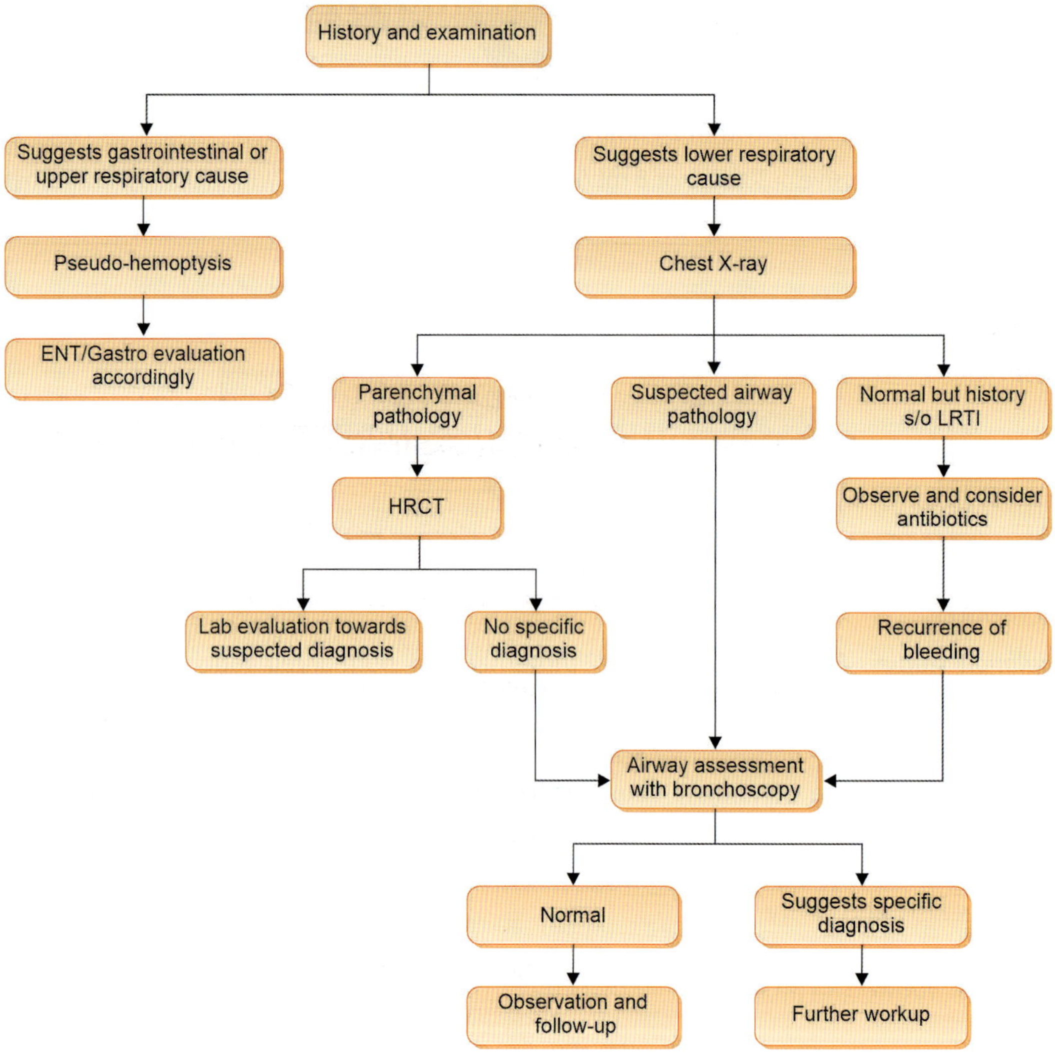

Suggested Reading

- De Silva C, Mukherjee A, Jat KR, Lodha R, Kabra SK. Pulmonary hemorrhage in children: etiology, clinical profile and outcome. Indian J Pediatr. 2019;86(1):7-11.
- Gaude GS. Hemoptysis in children. Indian Pediatr. 2010;47(3):245-54.
- Godfrey S. Pulmonary hemorrhage/hemoptysis in children. Pediatr Pulmonol. 2004;37(6):476-84.
- Lodha R, Kabra SK (Eds). Pulmonary hemorrhage. Essential Paediatric Pulmonology, 4th edition. New Delhi: Jaypee Brothers Medical Publishers (P) Ltd; 2023. pp. 263-8.
- Vijayasekaran D, Gowrishankar NC, Balaji BS, Kalpana S, Nedunchelian K. Etiology of hemoptysis in children and adolescents-multicentric retrospective data (2012-2021) from Chennai. Indian Pediatr. 2023;60(4):290-3.

Inborn Errors of Immunity

30

***Section Editor:* B Rajsekhar**
***Section Co-Editor:* Suchitra Pusapati**
***Author:* Veeraraja Basavanthappa Sathenahalli**

Introduction

- Inborn errors of immunity (IEIs), known as primary immunodeficiency disorders (PIDs), are inherited disorders caused by germline mutation in single genes. They cause increased susceptibility to infections, allergies, autoimmune, autoinflammatory, nonmalignant lymphoproliferative and malignant manifestations.
- The estimated prevalence is 4–10/100,000 live births/yr.
- They require early identification for life-changing and/or lifesaving intervention.

Etiology

Monogenic germline mutations causing impairment of innate and acquired immunity predispose to recurrent infections and other noninfectious manifestations. The detected number of IEIs have reached 490 from 190 due to accessibility and affordability of next-generation sequencing.

The International Union of Immunological Societies (IUIS) Inborn Errors of Immunity Committee (IEIC) has classified IEIs as given in **Table 1**.

TABLE 1: Classification.

	DISEASE
1.	Combined immunodeficiencies
2.	Combined immunodeficiencies with syndromic features
3.	Predominantly antibody deficiencies
4.	Diseases of immune dysregulation
5.	Congenital defects of phagocytes
6.	Defects in intrinsic and innate immunity
7.	Autoinflammatory diseases
8.	Complement deficiencies
9.	Bone marrow failure
10.	Phenocopies of inborn errors of immunity

Warning Signs

The Jeffrey Modell Foundation (JMF) together with immunologists has compiled a list of 10 warning signs of IEI. Four additional signs are also proposed to include noninfectious signs of IEI **(Box 1)**.

BOX 1: Warning signs.

- Four/more new ear infections within 1 year
- Two/more serious sinus infections within 1 year
- Two/more months on antibiotics with little effect
- Two/more episodes of pneumonia within 1 year
- Failure to thrive
- Recurrent abscesses of deep skin/internal organs
- Persistent oral candidiasis/fungal skin infections
- Intravenous antibiotics to clear infections
- Two/more deep-seated infections, including septicemia
- A family history of IEI

Additional warning signs:

- Severe eczema
- Allergies
- Hematologic and oncologic disorders
- Autoimmunity

Types and Manifestations of Inborn Errors of Immunity

Types of IEI, their manifestations, and tests are given in **Table 2**.

TABLE 2: Types and manifestations of IEI.

CLINICAL MANIFESTATIONS	SUSPECTED IEI	TESTS
• Early onset of severe, disseminated infections • Absent thymus • Dysmorphic features • Failure to thrive • Reaction to BCG vaccine	• Combined T- and B-cell immunodeficiencies • SCID • Syndromic combined immunodeficiencies	CBC, lymphocyte count—TBNK profile (CD3, CD4, CD8, CD19, CD20, CD16, and CD56) Immunoglobulin levels
• Onset >6 months • Absence of tonsils/adenoids • Lymphoproliferation • Severe and/or recurrent bacterial infections, particularly encapsulated respiratory microorganisms	Predominantly antibody defects	CBC, Immunoglobulin measurements including subtypes, B-lymphocyte count (CD19 and CD20),

Contd...

Contd...

CLINICAL MANIFESTATIONS	SUSPECTED IEI	TESTS
• Early onset granulomas • Recurrent skin infections (staphylococcal/fungal) • Deep abscesses • Delayed umbilical cord fall	Numeric/functional phagocyte diseases	• CBC with WBC morphology • Neutrophil oxidative burst assay (DHR) • Adhesion molecule assays (CD11b/CD18)
• Bacterial, encapsulated microorganisms of the respiratory tract, articular, meninges, and sepsis • Manifestations of autoimmunity, lupus-like glomerulopathy	Complement defects	• CH50 activity • AH50 activity • C3 and C4 assay
• Nonsignificant, nonsevere, and nonrecurring • Cutaneous/invasive fungal infections, mainly *Candida* species, with/without cutaneous staphylococcus infections with autoimmune endocrinopathies	Autoinflammatory diseases	Inflammatory activity test Autoantibodies

(BCG: Bacillus Calmette–Guérin; CD: cluster of differentiation; CBC: complete blood count; IEI: inborn errors of immunity; SCID: severe combined immunodeficiency; WBC: white blood cells)

Approach to Genetic Evaluation of Inborn Errors of Immunity

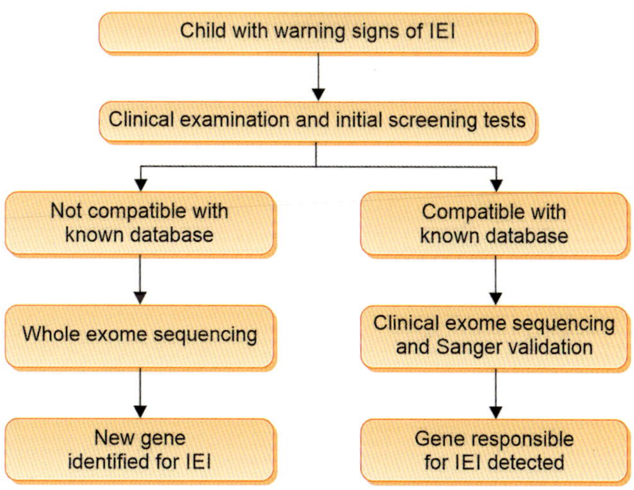

(IEI: inborn errors of immunity)

Suggested Reading

- Notarangelo LD, Bacchetta R, Casanova JL, Su HC. Human inborn errors of immunity: An expanding universe. Sci Immunol. 2020;5(49):eabb1662.
- Reilly L, Emonts M. Recurrent or unusual infections in children–when to worry about inborn errors of immunity. Ther Adv Infect Dis. 2023;10:20499361231162978.
- Tangye SG, Al-Herz W, Bousfiha A, Cunningham-Rundles C, Franco JL, Holland SM, et al, The Ever-Increasing Array of Novel Inborn Errors of Immunity: An Interim Update by the IUIS Committee. J Clin Immunol. 2021;41(3):666-79.
- Tangye SG, Al-Herz W, Bousfiha A, Cunningham-Rundles C, Franco JL, Holland SM, et al, Human inborn errors of immunity: 2022 update on the Classification from the International Union of Immunological Societies Expert Committee. J Clin Immunol. 2022;42(7):1473-507.

Back Pain

31

Section Editor: **Janani Shankar**
Section Co-Editor: **Arathi Srinivasan**
Author: **Palash Das**

Introduction

- Mechanical lower back pain is the most common cause of pain in the back, especially in adolescents.
- Watching television for long hours, heavy backpacks, uncomfortable school desks, and musculoskeletal trauma are the most common causes of back pain.

History

- *Pain:* Severity, site, radiation, nighttime worsening of pain, and relieving factors
- Worsened by coughing or straining
- Worsen on rest or exercise
- *Onset:* Acute or insidious and slowly progressive
- *History:* Trauma, lifting weights, exercise, and sports
- *Systemic signs:* Fever, weight loss, and uveitis
- *Associated features:* Psoriasis and inflammatory bowel disease
- *Neurological symptoms:* Bladder bowel involvement, gait instability, tingling sensation, numbness over limbs, etc.

Examination

- *Inspection:* The spine for redness, deformity, swelling, and sacral tuft hair or dimples
- Kyphosis or scoliosis
- *Palpation:* Tenderness, gibbus, pain in sacroiliac joints, etc., and pain at iliac crest
- *Neurological examination:* Reflexes, dermatomal sensory loss, anal reflex, spasticity, ataxia, etc.
- *Specific tests:*
  - Range of motion of the spine
  - *FABER:* Flexion ABduction and External Rotation of ipsilateral leg. Press on the ipsilateral knee to elicit tendernees of sacro-iliac joint of same side – suggests sacroiliitis.
  - *Straight leg raising test:* Sciatica
  - *Thomas test:* Keeping the patient in the supine position, the examiner uses both hands to bring one knee to the chest. The test is positive if the contralateral leg lifts off the table, suggestive of tightness of hip flexors in cases of lumbar disc prolapse.
  - *Stork test*: The patient stands on one leg and hyperextends the lumbar spine; ipsilateral pain suggests spondylolysis.
  - *Valsalva maneuver*: Increase in pain suggests intradural tumors or spinal stenosis.

Etiology

Etiology of back pain in children is given in **Box 1.**

BOX 1: Acute back pain and chronic back pain in children.

Acute back pain:
- Herniated disc
- *Tumor:* Ewing sarcoma, metastatic leukemia, osteosarcoma, osteoma, Langerhans cell histiocytosis, etc.
- *Trauma:* Vertebral fracture
- *Infection:* Spinal abscess, extraspinal like pyelonephritis, and paraspinal abscess
- Muscle strain

Chronic back pain:
- Vertebral osteomyelitis/tubercular osteomyelitis
- Epidural abscess
- Septic sacroiliitis
- Neoplasm
- Syringomyelia
- Tethered cord
- Transverse myelitis

Red Flag Signs

- Nighttime pains
- Awakening from sleep due to pain
- Persistent pain >4 weeks
- Neurological deficits
  - Calf hypertrophy, spasticity, and extensor plantar
  - *Bowel/bladder involvement:* Incontinence/retention, absent anal reflex
- *Gibbus/spine tenderness:* Malignancy, osteomyelitis, and fracture
- *Worsening on straining or Valsalva:* Syringomyelia, and intraspinal tumor
- History of major trauma
- History of malignancy
- *Pain worsened after rest:* Inflammatory pathology

Relevant Investigations

- Magnetic resonance imaging (MRI) spine
- *If spondylosis:* X-ray anteroposterior (AP) and lateral
- *CT scan:* Bone architecture
- *Laboratory tests:* Complete blood count (CBC), erythrocyte sedimentation rate (ESR), and C-reactive protein (CRP), to rule out osteomyelitis and inflammatory pathology
- Human leukocyte antigen B27 (HLA-B27), rheumatoid arthritis (RA) factor, antinuclear antibody (ANA), if history warrants

Approach

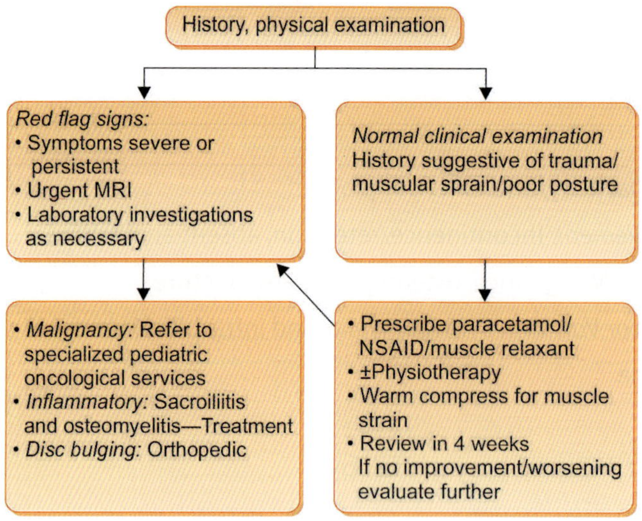

(MRI: magnetic resonance imaging; NSAID: nonsteroidal anti-inflammatory drug)

Suggested Reading

- Achar S, Yamanaka J. Back pain in children and adolescents. Am Fam Physician. 2020;102(1):19-28.
- Kandwal P, Vijayaraghavan G, Goswami A, Jayaswal A. Back pain in children-How sinister? Indian J Pediatr. 2016;83(8):834-43.
- Lamb M, Brenner JS. Back pain in children and adolescents. Pediatr Rev. 2020;41(11):557-69.

Proteinuria

32

Section Editor: **Gnanamurthy Narasimha**
Section Co-Editor: **Nagalatha Chidananda**
Authors: **Hamsa V, Nivedita Kamath**

Definition

- Proteinuria is urine protein excretion higher than normal values.
- Normal values for urinary total protein excretion are <240 mg/m^2/day in children <6 months of age and <150 mg/m^2/day in older children.
- Approximately half of normal urine protein is Tamm-Horsfall protein/uromodulin.
- The rest is albumin and low-molecular-weight plasma proteins.
- Routine urine testing in school-going children may reveal proteinuria in up to 10% and decreases to 0.1% with repeated testing.

Measurement of Proteinuria

- *Urine dipstick method for estimation:* This test semiquantitatively estimates the albumin concentration using chemically impregnated strips containing a pH-sensitive colorimetric indicator. It is reported as negative, trace (10–29 mg/dL), 1+ (30–100 mg/dL), 2+ (100–300 mg/dL), 3+ (300–1,000 g/dL), and 4+ (>1,000 mg/dL).
- *Urine protein to creatinine ratio:* It is a simple measure to quantify proteinuria in a spot sample.
- *24-hour urine protein estimation:* It is the gold standard for the estimation but is cumbersome and time-consuming and may be used only in select situations.

Interpretation of Proteinuria (Table 1)

Interpretation of proteinuria is given in **Table 1**.

TABLE 1: Interpretation of proteinuria.

PROTEINURIA	URINE PROTEIN CREATININE RATIO (PCR) (mg/mg)	24-HOUR URINE ESTIMATION
Normal	• <0.5 for <2 years of age • <0.2 for >2 years of age	≤4 mg/m^2/h
Subnephrotic	0.2–2	4–40 mg/m^2/h
Nephrotic	>2	>40 mg/m^2/h

Etiology

- *Transient proteinuria:* Febrile illness, seizures, dehydration, stress, and strenuous exercise
- *Orthostatic/postural proteinuria:* Benign condition diagnosed by normal protein excretion in a spot, first-morning urine sample; increased protein excretion at least 4–6 hours after the patient has been upright
- *Persistent proteinuria:* Secondary to glomerular or tubular cause

  Glomerular proteinuria associated with glomerular disease, majorly albumin, is the most common cause in children.
- *Tubular proteinuria:* Reduced reabsorption of freely filtered low molecular weight proteins; seen in a variety of tubulointerstitial diseases and proximal tubular dysfunction

Causes of Persistent Proteinuria

Causes of persistent proteinuria are given in **Box 1.**

BOX 1: Various causes of proteinuria.

GLOMERULAR PROTEINURIA	TUBULAR PROTEINURIA
Primary glomerular diseases: • Minimal change disease • Focal segmental glomerulosclerosis • IgA nephropathy • Membranoproliferative glomerulonephritis • Membranous nephropathy *Secondary glomerular diseases:* • Infections (hepatitis B and C, HIV, malaria, CMV, and poststreptococcal) • IgA vasculitis and systemic lupus erythematosus • ANCA vasculitis • Alport syndrome • Diabetes • Hypertension • Reflux nephropathy • *Malignancies:* Lymphoma	*Inherited:* • Lowe syndrome • Dent's disease • Galactosemia • Glycogen storage diseases • Tyrosinemia • Hereditary fructose intolerance • Wilson's disease *Acquired:* • Acute tubular necrosis • Acute interstitial nephritis • Toxins • Drugs • Pyelonephritis

(ANCA: antineutrophil cytoplasmic antibody; CMV: cytomegalovirus; HIV: human immunodeficiency virus; IgA: immunoglobulin A)

Evaluation

- *History:* Oliguria, hypertension, skin lesions, joint symptoms, recent infections, and drug intake. Blood pressure to be measured.
- *Examination*: Signs of edema, flank pain, fluid overload, organomegaly, rashes, anemia, joint swelling, and symptoms of rickets

Investigation

Urinalysis also provides information about hematuria, pyuria, and casts.

- *Laboratory tests:* Renal function tests, complete blood count, serum albumin, serum cholesterol, and complement 3 and 4 levels.
- *Further tests:* Anti-streptolysin O titers, hepatitis B and C tests, and more specific laboratory studies guided by history and physical examination
- *In secondary causes:* Investigations to rule out underlying causes

Red Flag Signs

These could indicate the need for renal biopsy:

- Elevated serum creatinine concentration
- Persistent macroscopic/microscopic hematuria
- Associated hypertension
- Persistent hypocomplementemia
- Steroid-resistant nephrotic syndrome
- Family history of chronic renal disease or end-stage renal disease
- Persistent hypocomplementemia beyond 6 weeks

Approach

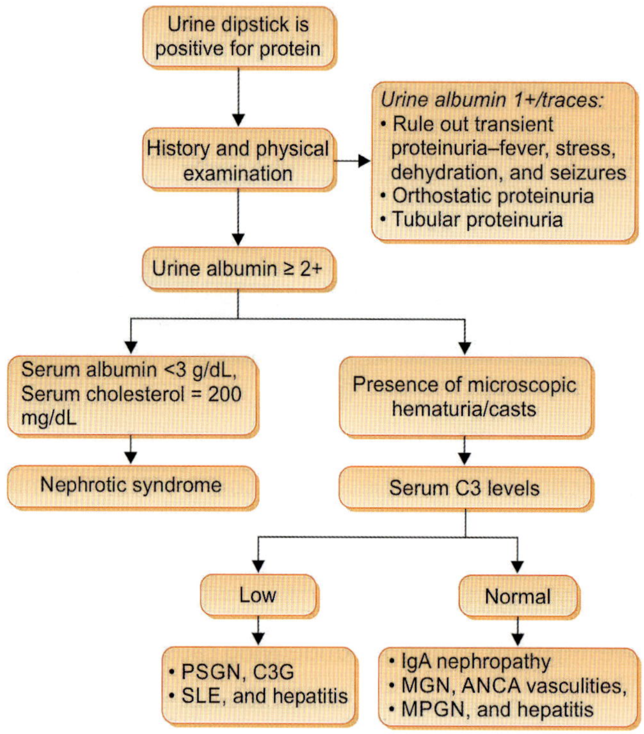

(ANCA: antineutrophil cytoplasmic antibody; C3G: C3 glomerulopathy; IgA: immunoglobulin A; MGN: membranous nephropathy; MPGN: membranoproliferative glomerulonephritis; PSGN: poststreptococcal glomerulonephritis; SLE: systemic lupus erythematosus)

Suggested Reading

- Jang KM, Cho MH. Clinical approach to children with proteinuria. Child Kidney Dis. 2017;21:53-60.
- Leung AK, Wong AH, Barg SS. Proteinuria in children: Evaluation and differential diagnosis. Am Fam Physician. 2017;95(4):248-54.
- Ranch D. Proteinuria in children. Pediatr Ann. 2020;49(6):e268-72.
- Viteri B, Reid-Adam J. Hematuria and proteinuria in children. Pediatr Rev. 2018;39(12):573-85.

Neonatal Jaundice

33

Section Editor: **Nehal Patel**
Section Co-Editor: **Jay T Dhirwani**
Authors: **Kunal P Ahya, Prathik Bandiya**

Introduction

- Neonatal jaundice is defined as yellowish discoloration of skin.
- It is physiological in a majority of the neonates. Over 80% have some degree of jaundice during their neonatal period.
- Physiological jaundice is characterized by onset after 24–72 hours of life, maximum between 4th and 5th day in term babies and on the 7th day in preterm babies. Levels will not exceed 15 mg/dL and is undetectable after 2 weeks.

Red Flag Signs

- Jaundice in the first 24 hours of life
- Staining on the palms and soles [total serum bilirubin (TSB) > 15 mg/dL]
- TSB increasing by >5 mg/dL/day or 0.5 mg/dL/h
- Jaundice persisting >2 weeks in term and >3 weeks in preterm babies
- Acute bilirubin encephalopathy

Etiology

The etiology of unconjugated hyperbilirubinemia is given in **Table 1**.

TABLE 1: Etiology of unconjugated hyperbilirubinemia.

DEFECTS	CAUSE
Isoimmunization	• Rh incompatibility • ABO incompatibility • Other blood group incompatibility
Enzyme and biochemical defects	• Glucose-6-phosphate dehydrogenase deficiency • Pyruvate kinase deficiency • Hexokinase deficiency • Congenital erythropoietic porphyria • Rare biochemical defects
Membrane defects and structural abnormalities of erythrocytes	• Hereditary spherocytosis • Hereditary elliptocytosis • Infantile pyknocytosis
Sepsis	• Bacterial and viral
Sequestered blood	• Large ecchymoses, subdural hematoma and cephalohematoma, and hemangioma
Defects in conjugation	• Crigler–Najjar syndrome, Gilbert syndrome, etc.
Others	• Polycythemia, hypothyroidism, breastfeeding jaundice, and breast milk jaundice

Clinical Assessment

- Neonatal jaundice progresses in cephalocaudal direction. The visual estimation approximately guides the bilirubin level **(Fig. 1)**. Every neonate should be assessed clinically for jaundice once every 12 hours till discharge. If jaundice appears in the first 24 hours, serum bilirubin should be estimated.
- In units where facility of transcutaneous bilirubin (TcB) estimation is available, TcB estimation is used for monitoring and TSB should be done if TcB is within 3 mg/dL of phototherapy treatment threshold/if TcB is ≥15 mg/dL.

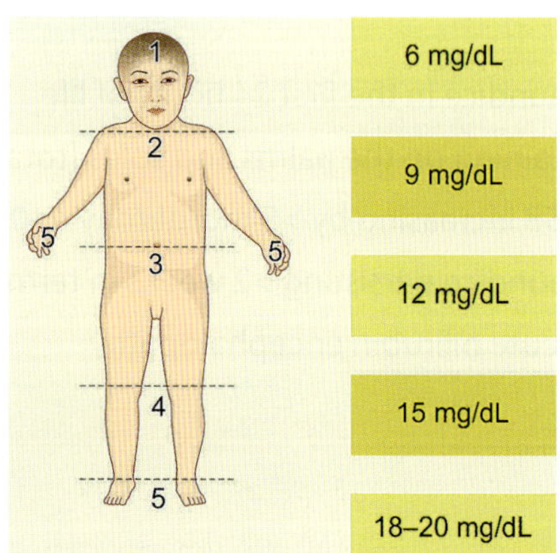

FIG. 1: Visual estimation of jaundice (Kramer, 1969).

Prolonged Jaundice

Persistence of significant jaundice for >2 weeks in term neonates and >3 weeks in preterm neonates is called prolonged jaundice.

Conjugated Hyperbilirubinemia

- Conjugated hyperbilirubinemia refers to direct bilirubin >1 mg/dL (if total bilirubin is <5 mg/dL) or >20% of the total (if total bilirubin is >5mg/dL).
- It needs to be further investigated, as urgent diagnosis and treatment improve the outcome, especially in biliary atresia.

Evaluation

Evaluation is to be done based on the factors given in **Box 1**

BOX 1: Factors to be considered for evaluation.

- Gestational age
- Mother's blood group
- Postnatal age
- Birth weight and current weight
- Hypothyroidism
- Presence of neurotoxicity risk factors
- Signs of bilirubin encephalopathy

Once values are available, plot the values in the American Academy of Pediatrics (AAP) chart for phototherapy, exchange transfusion, and decide about the management accordingly. Various mobile apps like BiliApp, BiliMate, NeonatAI, etc. are available, which help in deciding about the treatment.

Workup for Causes

- Hemoglobin, reticulocyte count, peripheral smear—evidence of hemolysis
- Blood group—Mother and baby
- Glucose-6-phosphate dehydrogenase (G6PD)
- Direct Coombs test (DCT)
- Thyroid-stimulating hormone (TSH)

Approach

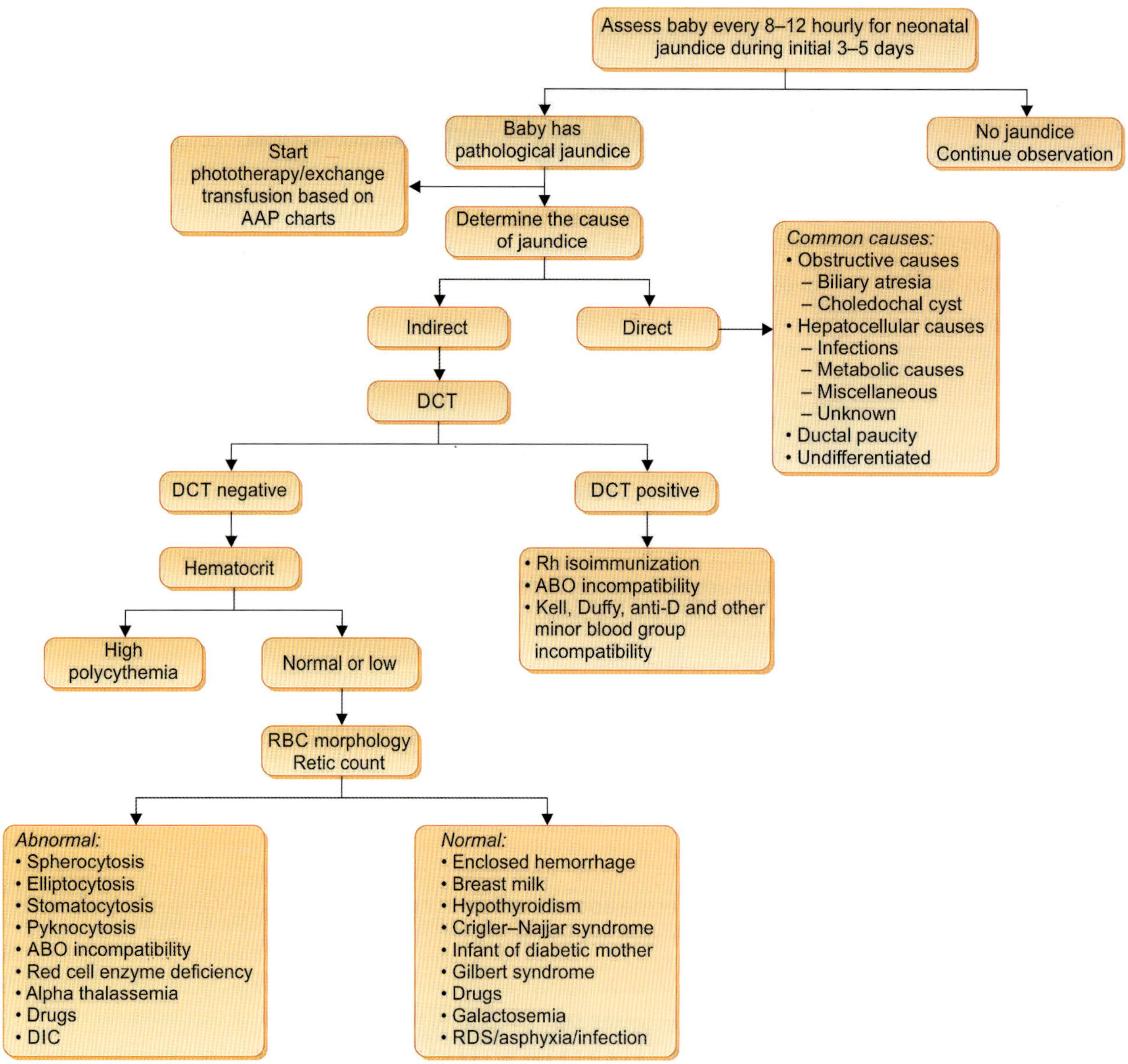

(AAP: American Academy of Pediatrics; DCT: direct Coombs test; DIC: disseminated intravascular coagulation; RBC: red blood cells; RDS: respiratory distress syndrome)

Suggested Reading

- Bansal A. Management of Hyperbilirubinemia. In: Sachan R, Kumar A (Eds). Handbook of Neonatal Clinical Practice, 1st edition. New Delhi: Jaypee Brothers Medical Publishers (P) Ltd; 2023. pp. 129-35.
- Kemper AR, Newman TB, Slaughter JL, Maisels MJ, Watchko JF, Downs SM, et al. Clinical practice guideline revision: Management of hyperbilirubinemia in the newborn infant 35 or more weeks of gestation. Pediatrics. 2022;150(3):e2022058859.
- Neonatal Jaundice. In: Agarwal R, Deorari A, Paul V, Sankar MJ, Sachdeva A (Eds). AIIMS Protocols in Neonatology, 2nd edition. Delhi: Noble Vision; 2019. pp. 217-33.
- Watchko JF. Neonatal indirect hyperbilirubinemia and kernicterus. In: Gleason CA, Devaskar SU (Eds). Avery's Diseases of the Newborn, 9th edition. Philadelphia, USA: Elsevier Saunders; 2012. pp. 1123-42.

Vaginal Bleeding in Neonates

34

Section Editor: **Nehal Patel**
Section Co-Editor: **Jay T Dhirwani**
Authors: **Biraj Thakker, Nihaz Naha**

Introduction

Neonatal vaginal bleeding is often a benign condition, typically in female newborns. This bleeding is often mild and resolves without intervention.

Etiology

- *Physiological hormonal withdrawal:* Maternal estrogen stimulates the growth of the female fetus's endometrial lining during intrauterine life. During the first week of life, as this hormonal support wanes, some neonates produce endometrial slough resulting in a few days of bloody mucoid discharge/light vaginal bleeding. This is self-limited, requiring no treatment.
- *Infections:*
  - Bacterial vaginosis
  - Group B streptococcus
  - Herpes simplex virus
  - Candidiasis and other fungal infections
- *Trauma:*
  - Birth trauma
  - Rough handling/aggressive cleaning of the genital area causing irritation
- *Structural anomalies:* Vaginal septum and various congenital structural anomalies
- *Hematological disorders:*
  - Vitamin K deficiency, hemophilia, Von Willebrand disease, and other abnormalities of the clotting cascade.
  - Thrombocytopenia and platelet function disorders.
- *Congenital adrenal hyperplasia (CAH):* The salt-wasting form of CAH causes excessive androgen production, virilization, and abnormal bleeding.
- *Tumors:* Sarcoma botryoides and cervical adenocarcinoma secondary to diethylstilbestrol (DES) exposure.
- Sexual abuse
- Vaginal foreign bodies

Red Flag Signs

- Continuous/heavy bleeding
- Abnormal discharge/odor
- Signs of distress
- Pale appearance
- Abdominal distension
- Breast development

Approach

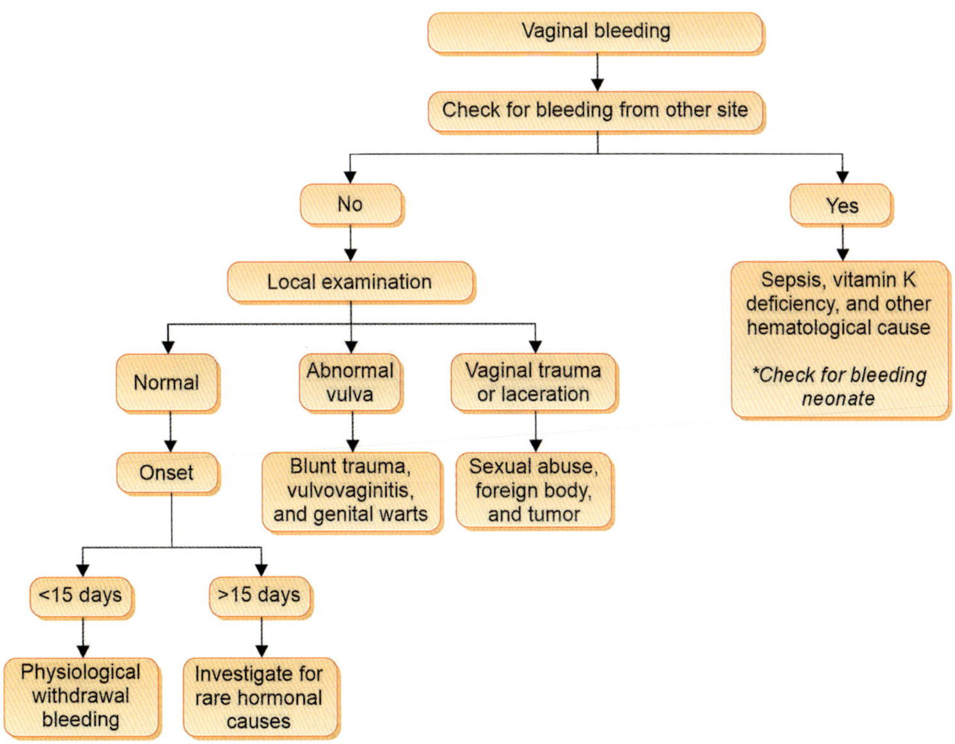

*Investigate further for bleeding disorders.

Detailed Evaluation

- *Assessment and history:*
  - General condition and stability
  - Detailed maternal history, including prenatal care, medications, labor, and delivery details
- *Physical examination:*
  - General examination focusing on the genital area
  - Assess for signs of trauma, abnormal anatomy, and lesions
- *Laboratory investigations:*
  - Routine blood tests, including complete blood count (CBC)
  - Coagulation studies [prothrombin time (PT), partial thromboplastin time (aPTT)] to evaluate clotting factors
  - Hormonal assessments as appropriate
- *Imaging studies:* Ultrasound to visualize the pelvic area and identify structural abnormalities and masses
- *Cultures:* Cultures/swabs to identify potential pathogens, if evidence of infection
- Consultation and further evaluation
- *Treatment and follow-up:*
  - Treatment based on the diagnosis
  - Follow-up visits to monitor progress and ensure resolution

Suggested Reading

- Brosens I, Benagiano G. Clinical significance of neonatal menstruation. Eur J Obstet Gynecol Reprod Biol. 2016; 196:57-9.
- Habiba M, Heyn R, Bianchi P, Brosens I, Benagiano G. The development of the human uterus: Morphogenesis to menarche. Hum Reprod Update. 2021;27(1):1-26.
- Hill NC, Oppenheimer LW, Morton KE. The aetiology of vaginal bleeding in children. A 20-year review. Br J Obstet Gynaecol. 1989;96(4):467-70.
- Shaw KN, Bachur RG, Chamberlain J, Lavelle J, Nagler J, Shook J (Eds). Vaginal bleeding. Fleisher and Ludwig's Textbook of Pediatric Emergency Medicine, 8th edition. Philadelphia: Wolters Kluwer; 2021. pp. 533-42.
- Vogiatzi MG, Pitt M, Oberfield S, Alter CA. Menstrual bleeding as a manifestation of mini-puberty of infancy in severe prematurity. J Pediatr. 2016;178:292-95.

Dysuria

35

Section Editor: **Gnanamurthy Narasimha**
Section Co-Editor: **Nagalatha Chidananda**
Authors: **Shalini Sharma, Keyur Mahajan**

Introduction

- Dysuria is defined as pain and/or burning associated with micturition.
- It is a common symptom reported by most children at least once during childhood.
- Common manifestations, which should lead us to suspect dysuria age wise, include:
  - *Infants and toddlers:* Crying during micturition or during diaper changes, excessive fussiness or irritability, and poor feeding
  - *School-aged children:* Complaints of pain or burning during micturition, increased frequency of urination, rubbing or tugging at the genitals, or regression in toilet training including bedwetting
  - *Adolescents:* Painful and/or frequent urination, changes in toilet habits, mood swings or change in behavior
- Dysuria is a symptom rather than a diagnosis and can be caused by various infectious and noninfectious causes.

Causes

Causes of dysuria may be classified as infectious and noninfectious **(Table 1)**.

TABLE 1: Causes of dysuria.

	INFECTIOUS CAUSES	NONINFECTIOUS CAUSES
Infants and toddlers	• *Cystitis and lower urinary tract infection (UTI):* – Most common cause – May have associated fever and lower abdominal and suprapubic pain/tenderness – Occurs during early childhood and children of both sexes are equally prone to UTIs	• *Structural abnormalities:* Congenital abnormalities of the urinary tract, for example, urethral strictures, vesicoureteral reflux, or labial adhesions

Contd...

Contd...

	INFECTIOUS CAUSES	NONINFECTIOUS CAUSES
	• *Pyelonephritis:* Infection of the upper genitourinary tract, presents as high-grade fever, and flank pain/tenderness • *Investigations*: Urine routine examination, urine culture examination and ultrasound of kidney, ureter, and bladder (KUB) • *Diaper dermatitis*: Bacterial or fungal skin infections of the perineal region causing discomfort during micturition	• *Investigations*: Ultrasound KUB, uroflow, retrograde urethrogram for urethral strictures, and micturating cystourethrogram (MCU) for vesicoureteral reflux
	• *Balanitis and balanoposthitis:* Bacterial infection of the distal penis and preputial skin • *Vulvovaginitis and cervicitis:* Can rarely occur in prepubertal girls	• Lichen sclerosus • *Psychogenic:* Children may complain of dysuria as a psychosomatic response to anxiety
Adolescents	• *Urethritis secondary to sexually transmitted infections (STI) and pelvic inflammatory disease (PID):* Dysuria, local inflammation, discharge • *Neisseria gonorrhoeae and Chlamydia trachomatis* are common pathogens • *Investigations:* Urine routine and culture examination	• *Chemical urethritis:* Local irritants like detergents and other topical products can cause allergies or irritation of the skin/mucosa, characterized by local erythema without discharge • Nephrolithiasis
	• *Vulvovaginitis and cervicitis*: Common in adolescents, may be associated with vaginal discharge that may be scanty, thick, and green in gonorrhea or cheesy white in *Candida* • Group A *Streptococcus* and *Shigella* species are uncommon nonsexual causes.	• *Behcet's syndrome:* Autoimmune systemic vasculitis, recurrent oral and genital ulcerations and chronic relapsing uveitis • *Classic triad of reactive arthritis*: Conjunctivitis, arthritis, and urethritis
	Herpes simplex infection causes ulcers/sores	

Red Flag Signs

- High-grade fever/toxic appearance
- Signs of sepsis and hemodynamic instability
- Severe low back pain
- Suspicion of multisystem involvement
- Suspicion of child abuse and sexually transmitted infections (STI) in prepubertal children

Approach to Child with Dysuria

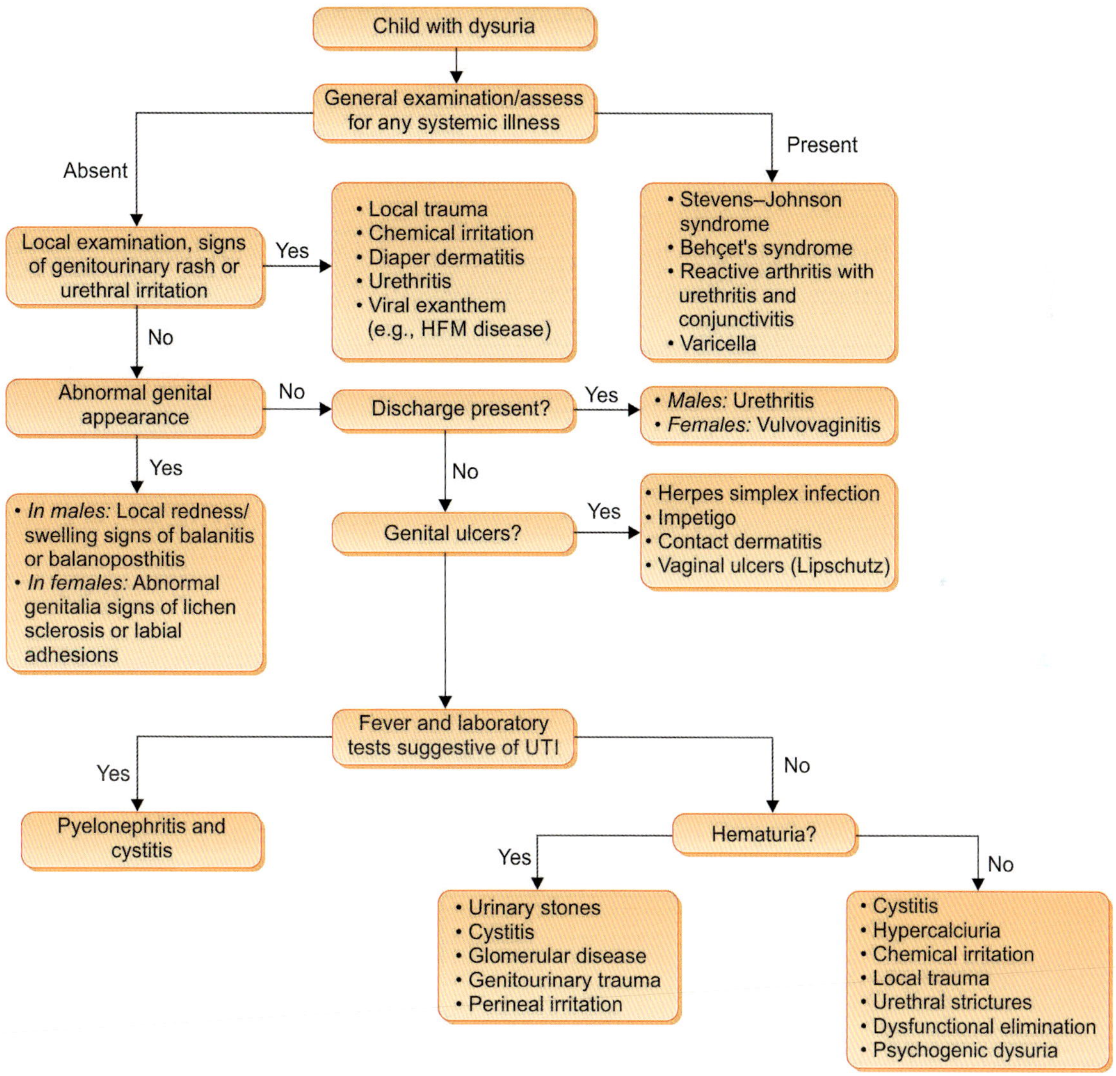

(HFM: hand-foot-and-mouth; UTI: urinary tract infection)

Suggested Reading

- Feemster K. Dysuria. In: Shah SS (Ed). Pediatric Practice: Infectious Disease. New York, US: McGraw Hill; 2009.
- Kliegman RM, Toth H, Bordini BJ, Basel D. Nelson Pediatric Symptom-Based Diagnosis: Common Diseases and their Mimics. Amsterdam, Netherlands: Elsevier; 2022.
- Mehta A, Williams V, Parajuli B. Child with Dysuria and/or Hematuria. Indian J Pediatr. 2017;84(10):792-8.
- Michels TC, Sands JE. Dysuria: Evaluation and differential diagnosis in adults. Am Fam Physician. 2015;92(9):778-86.
- Najar MS, Saldanha CL, Banday K. Approach to urinary tract infections. Indian J Nephrol. 2009;19(4):129-39.
- Robson AM, Pediatric Perspectives. Am J Kidney Dis. 1983;3(3):235-8.

Thumb Sucking

36

***Section Editor:* Sumitha Nayak**
***Section Co-Editor:* Priya Shivalli**
***Author:* Sumitha Nayak**

Introduction

- Thumb sucking is a behavioral disorder that serves as an adaptive function by providing stimulation or self-soothing. Besides the thumb, other fingers of the hands and toes, blankets, pacifiers, etc. are also used for providing comfort and are considered as non-nutritive sucking.
- This habit is common in infancy and usually stops spontaneously by 2–4 years.

Etiology

There is no definite etiology for this behavioral disorder. However, some possible reasons include:

- Habitual causes
- Psychological, especially a lack of self-confidence
- Loneliness
- Emotional insecurity
- Sense of neglect
- Oppressive or over-controlling parents
- Attention-seeking strategy
- Family discord
- Associated with other disabilities, for example, autism spectrum disease, attention-deficit/hyperactivity disorder (ADHD), anxiety neurosis, etc.

This disorder is closely related to the psychoemotional maturity of the child.

Some studies show that thumb sucking stimulates the nasopalatal receptors that ease the psychological and physical tension in the child.

Red Flag Signs

Persistence of the habit beyond 4 years alert to the possibility of several conditions:

- Dental problems
  - Asymmetrical anterior open bite
  - Proclination of mandibular incisors
  - Decreased overbite
  - Posterior crossbite
- Permanent damage to digits/finger
- Speech delay
- Other speech disorders

Approach

- A thorough history including the frequency, duration, and intensity of thumb sucking
- Physical examination to look for blisters on the affected thumb
- Sucking pads or callus formation on the involved thumb/finger due to hyperkeratosis
- Delayed eruption of upper and lower incisors resulting in open bite/increased overbite
- Examination of the oral cavity around 12 months of age
- Look for the oral soft tissues, palate, alveolar ridges, and any erupted/erupting teeth
- Counseling the child and the parents for change in behavior
- Application of nasty-tasting substances on the finger may be useful to break the habit
- Referral to orthodontist and use of orthodontic appliances
- Occasionally, there may be a need for orthographic surgery.
- Orofacial myofunctional therapy to re-educate muscles involved in swallowing, speech, and resting posture
- Newer techniques include the use of alarms that ring when the child places the thumb/finger in the mouth.

The approach to the management of a child with thumb sucking is illustrated in **Flowchart 1.**

FLOWCHART 1: Approach to manage a child with thumb sucking.

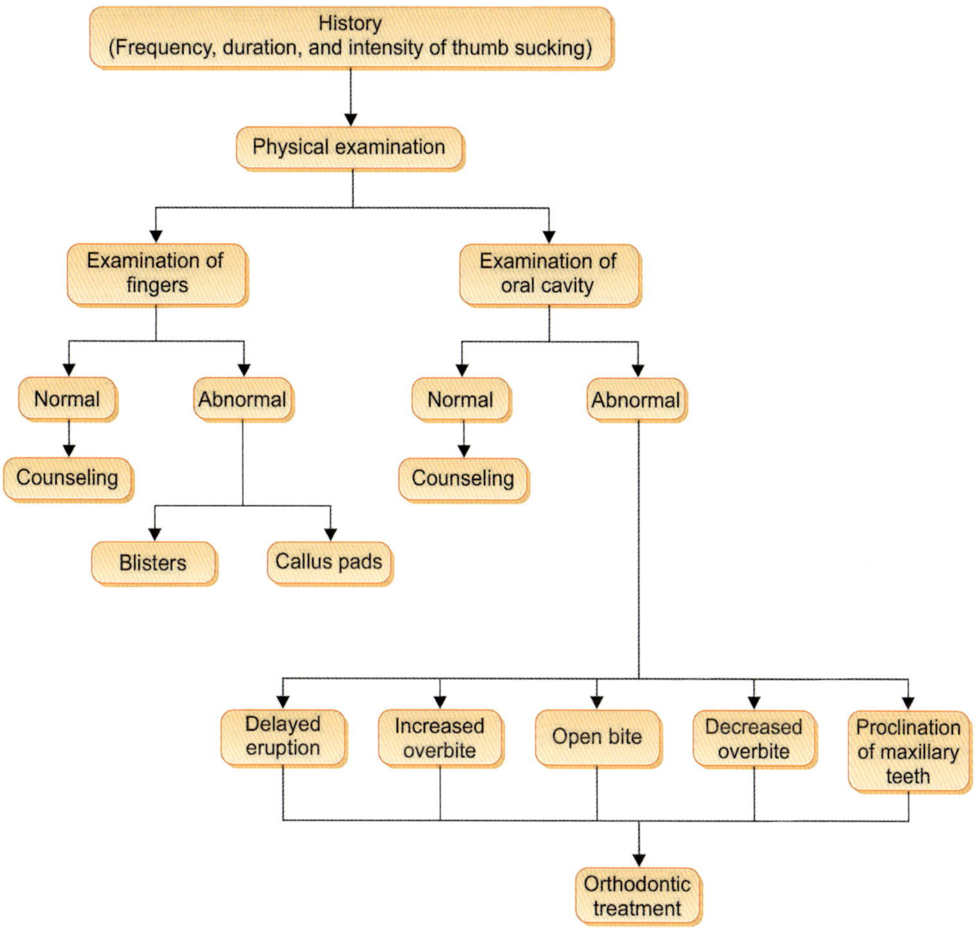

Suggested Reading

- Indian Academy of Pediatrics. (2022). Guidelines for parents. Thumb sucking, temper tanrums and PICA. [online] Available from https://iapindia.org/pdf/IAP-Parental-Guideline-Thumb-sucking-Temper-Tantrums-and-PICA.pdf [Last accessed March 2024].
- Guiterrez DS, Carugno P. Thumb sucking. In: StatPearls [Internet]. Treasure Island (FL): StatPearls Publishing; 2024. [online] Available from https://www.ncbi.nlm.nih.gov/books/NBK556112/ [Last accessed on March, 2023].
- Shetty RM, Shetty M, Shetty NS, Deoghare A. Three-alarm system: Revisited to treat thumb sucking habit. Int J Clin Pediatr Dent. 2015;8(1):82-6.

Hepatomegaly

37

Section Editor: **B Rajsekhar**
Section Co-Editor: **Suchitra Pusapati**
Author: **Kalpana Panda**

Introduction

- Hepatomegaly is an increase in liver size beyond age and gender-appropriate norms.
- It maybe due to intrinsic liver disease or as a hepatic manifestation of systemic illness.
- Palpable liver 1–2 cm liver below the right costal margin is usually appreciable in children. Thoracic/pulmonary pathology might push a normal-sized liver downward. A palpable liver >3.5 cm in newborns and >2 cm in children, below the right costal margin indicates enlargement. It is imperative to measure the liver span. Average liver span is 5–6.5 cm (infants), 6–7 cm (1–5 years of age), 7–9 cm (5–10 years of age), and 8–10 cm (10–15 years of age).

Etiology

- *Inflammation:*
  - Infections
  - Autoimmune
  - Drug
- *Storage:*
  - Glycogen storage diseases
  - Lipid storage (Gaucher/Niemann–Pick/Wolman disease)
  - Iron—Hemochromatosis and copper—Wilson disease

- *Infiltration:*
  - Hepatic tumors
  - Metastasis
  - Cysts
- *Congestive:*
  - Congestive heart failure
  - Constrictive pericarditis
  - Budd–Chiari syndrome
  - Veno-occlusive disease
- *Biliary tract obstruction:*
  - Biliary atresia
  - Choledochal cyst
  - Stricture/stone in the common bile duct

Red Flag Signs

- *History/Symptoms:*
  - Consanguinity/spontaneous abortions/sudden infant deaths
  - Recurrent vomiting, diarrhea, failure to thrive, and recurrence in catabolic stress
  - Developmental delay, seizures, and hypoglycemia
  - Excessive irritability/refusal to feed/gross abdominal distension/bleeding
  - Waxing/waning pattern jaundice
  - Excessive pruritus
  - Obesity
- *Signs:*
  - Short stature, dysmorphism, cataract, rachitic features, hypotonia, and pedal edema
  - Clubbing, spider naevi, facial telangiectasia, and gynecomastia
  - Firm-to-hard, nodular liver; sharp/irregular margin; left lobe > right lobe
  - Presence of ascites/hepatic encephalopathy/dilated tortuous abdominal veins
  - Kayser-Fleischer (KF) ring
  - Xanthomas and scratch marks
  - Acanthosis, central adiposity, and hypertension

Approach

The approach to the management of neonates/infants is illustrated in **Flowchart 1**.

FLOWCHART 1: Approach for management of neonates/infants.

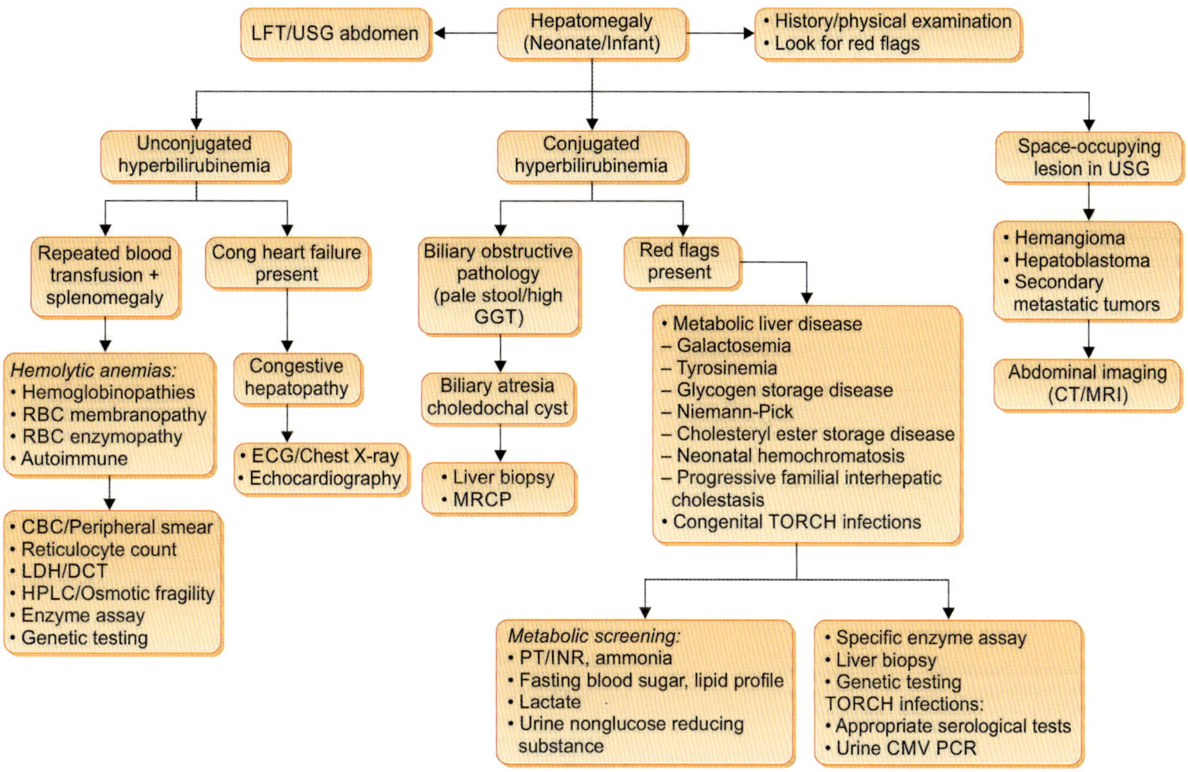

[CBC: complete blood count; CMV: cytomegalovirus; CT: computed tomography; DCT: direct Coombs test; ECG: electrocardiogram; GGT: gamma-glutamyl transferase; HPLC: high-performance liquid chromatography; INR: international normalized ratio; LDH: lactate dehydrogenase; LFT: liver function tests; MRI: magnetic resonance imaging; MRCP: magnetic resonance cholangiopancreatography; PCR: polymerase chain reaction; PT: prothrombin time; RBC: red blood cells; TORCH: toxoplasmosis, others (syphilis, hepatitis B), rubella, cytomegalovirus, herpes simplex; USG: ultrasonography]

The approach to the management of children >1 year of age is illustrated in **Flowchart 2**.

FLOWCHART 2: Approach to management of children >1 year of age with hepatomegaly.

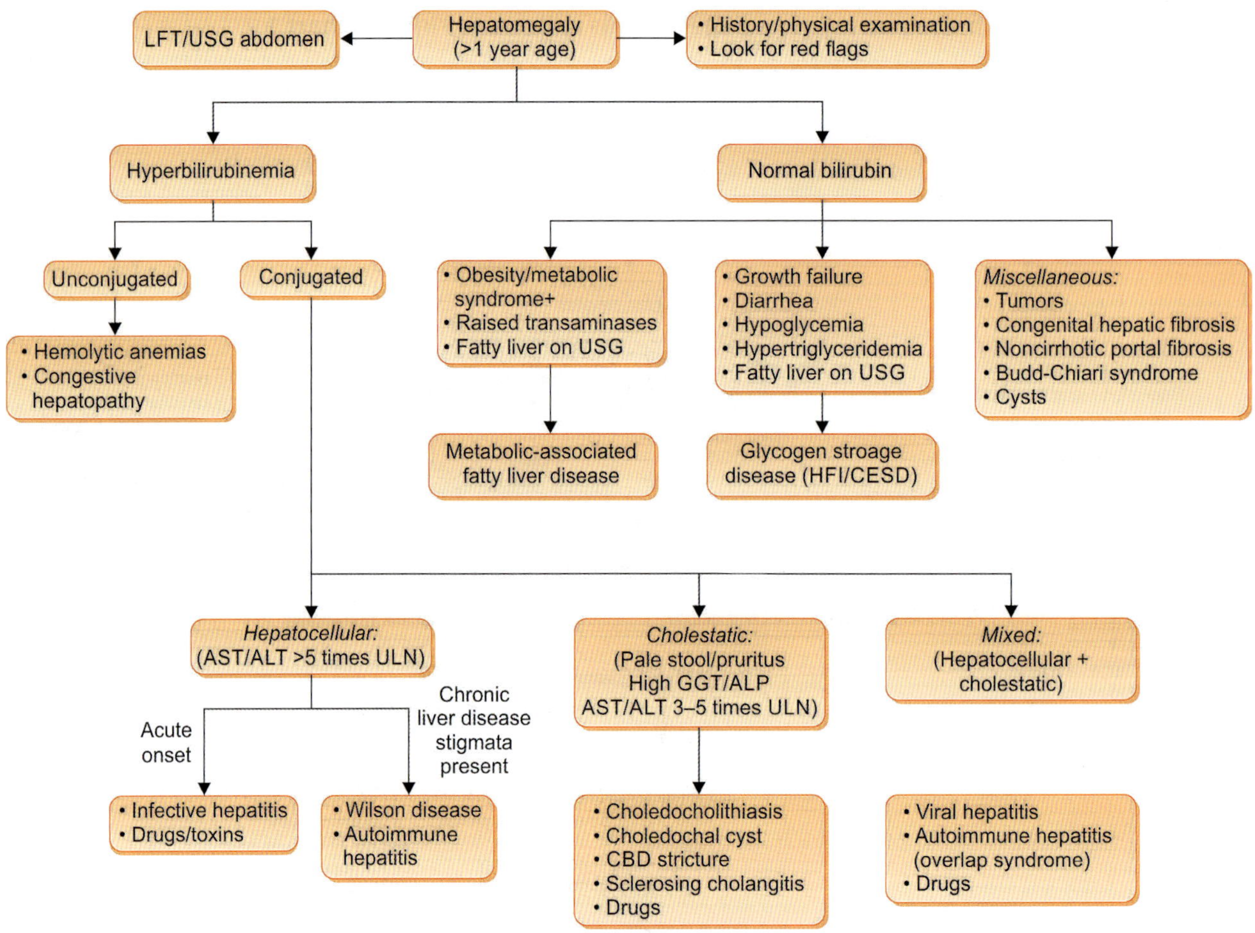

(ALT: alanine aminotransferase; ALP: alkaline phosphatase; AST: aspartate aminotransferase; CBD: common bile duct; CESD: cholesteryl ester storage disease; GGT: gamma-glutamyl transferase; HFI: hereditary fructose intolerance; LFT: liver function test; ULN: upper limit of normal; USG: ultrasonography)

Suggested Reading

- Alam S, Sood V. Metabolic liver disease: When to suspect and how to diagnose? Indian J Pediatr. 2016;83(11):1321-33.
- Gupta P, Menon P, Ramji S, Lodha R. PG Textbook of Pediatrics, 3rd edition. New Delhi: Jaypee Brothers Medical Publishers (P) Ltd; 2022.
- Kliegman RM, St Geme III JW, Blum NJ, Shah SS, Tasker RC, Wilson MK et al. Nelson Textbook of Pediatrics, 21st edition. Philadelphia: Elsevier; 2019.
- Wolf AD, Lavine JE. Hepatomegaly in neonates and children. Pediatr Rev. 2000;21(9):303-10.

Abdominal Pain

38

***Section Editor:* B Rajsekhar**
***Section Co-Editor:* Suchitra Pusapati**
***Author:* Lalit Bharadia**

Introduction

Abdominal pain is one of the most common complaints in childhood. It frequently requires urgent evaluation in the office/emergency department.

Abdominal pain can be classified into the following types:

- *Acute abdominal pain* (**Flowchart 1**)
  - Common complaint in childhood
  - Most Common nonsurgical condition is gastroenteritis, while the most common surgical condition is appendicitis
  - The child's age and the associated symptoms help to reach a diagnosis.
- *Chronic abdominal pain* **(Flowchart 2)**:
  - Intermittent or constant pain for at least 2 months
  - Accounts for almost 50% of visits to a pediatric gastroenterologist
  - It maybe organic in 10–20%, functional in 75–80%, and psychogenic in 5%.
- *Recurrent abdominal pain (RAP):* It is defined as:
  - Three/more episodes
  - Over a period of 3/more months
  - Severe enough to affect day-to-day activities
- *Functional abdominal pain (FAP):* Rome criteria defines FAP as follows:
- Lasting more than 8 weeks
- At least four times/month
- Unexplained by another medical condition on appropriate evaluation

FLOWCHART 1: Acute abdominal pain.

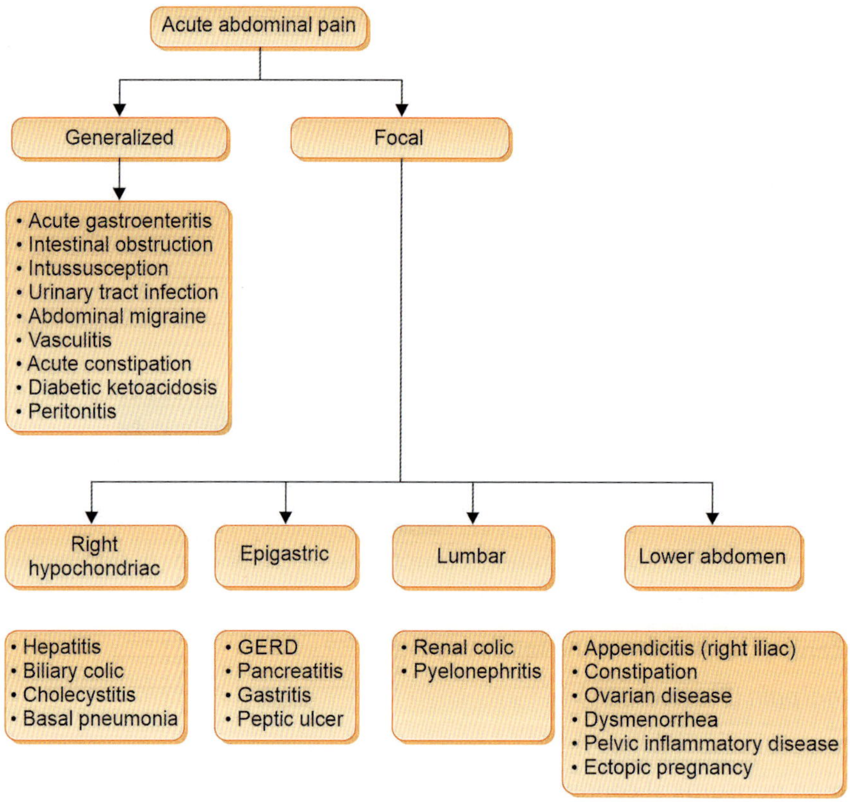

(GERD: gastroesophageal reflux disease)

Etiology of Chronic Abdominal Pain

Etiology of chronic abdominal pain includes:

- *Gastrointestinal:* 70–80%
- *Genitourinary:* 20%
- *Extra abdominal:* 5%

FLOWCHART 2: Chronic abdominal pain.

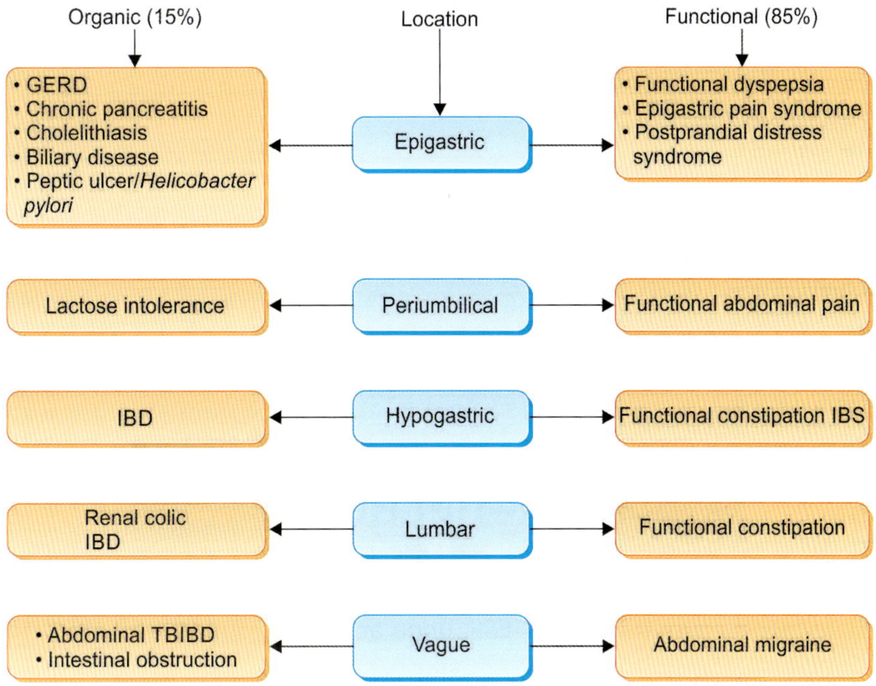

(IBD: inflammatory bowel disease; IBS: irritable bowel syndrome; GERD: gastroesophageal reflux disease syndrome; TB: tuberculosis)

Red Flag Signs in Chronic Abdominal Pain

- *Symptoms:*
  - Onset <5 years of age
  - Weight loss
  - Unexplained fever
  - Nocturnal pain
  - Gastrointestinal (GI) bleeding
  - Joint pain/rash/significant vomiting
  - Pain farther from the umbilicus

- *Signs:*
  - Weight or height <3rd centile
  - Significant pallor
  - Icterus
  - Localized tenderness
  - Perianal disease
  - Raised C-reactive protein (CRP)/Erythrocyte sedimentation rate (ESR)
  - Organomegaly

Investigations

- *Level I:* Complete blood count (CBC), CRP, ESR, urine and stool routine with stool occult blood, and ultrasound abdomen
- *Level II:* In selected cases, fecal calprotectin, endoscopy and biopsies, contrast-enhanced (computed tomography) CT abdomen, and urine for porphobilinogen

Suggested Reading

- Berger MY, Gieteling MJ, Benninga MA. Chronic abdominal pain in children. BMJ. 2007;334(7601):997-1002.
- Ganesh R, Arvind Kumar R, Suresh N, Sathiyasekeran M. Chronic abdominal pain in children. Natl Med J India. 2010;23(2):94-9.
- Hyams JS, Lorenzo CD, Saps M, Shulman RJ, Staiano A, van Tilburg M. Childhood functional gastrointestinal disorders: Child/adolescent. Gastroenterol. 2016;150(6):1456-68.

Splenomegaly

39

Section Editor: **B Rajsekhar**
Section Co-Editor: **Suchitra Pusapati**
Author: **M S Viswanathan**

Introduction

- Significant splenomegaly refers to the spleen palpable at least 1 cm below the costal margin in a child >6 months of age.
- In 30% of newborns, 15% of infants <6 months, palpable spleen is a normal variant. In older children, the palpable spleen is always abnormal.
- The longest craniocaudal diameter should be quantitatively defined by ultrasound. As a rule of thumb, until puberty the formula to assess spleen size is: Spleen length (cm) = 6 cm + 1/3 cm per year of age **(Fig. 1)**.

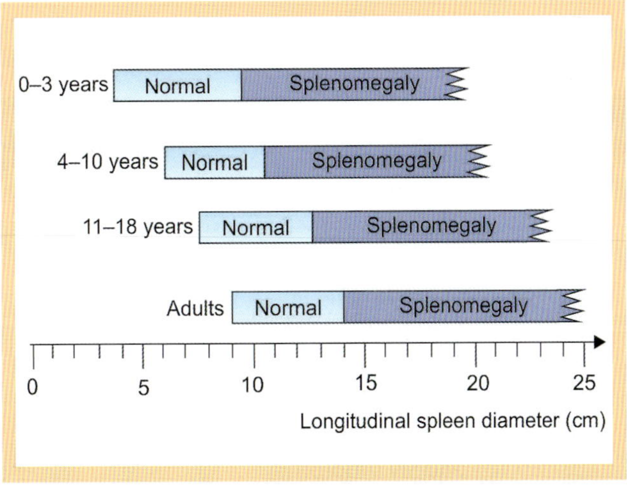

FIG. 1: Longitudinal diameter of spleen size by ultrasound examination and age in Caucasians.

- Types of splenomegaly are given in **Table 1**.

TABLE 1: Types of splenomegaly.

MILD	MODERATE	MASSIVE
Spleen just palpable/enlarged up to 3 cm	Spleen enlarged 4–7 cm (up to umbilicus)	Spleen enlarged >7 cm (beyond umbilicus)
• Acute, subacute, or chronic infections such as malaria, typhoid, septicemia, miliary tuberculosis, leptospirosis, and HIV. • *Viral illness:* EBV, CMV, etc. • Portal hypertension (early stage) • Congestive cardiac failure • Infective endocarditis • Iron deficiency anemia • Acquired hemolytic anemia • Acute leukemia • Hereditary spherocytosis • Idiopathic thrombocytopenic purpura (ITP) • *Immunological mediated diseases:* Juvenile rheumatoid arthritis (JRA), SLE, HLH • Hyperthyroidism	• Viral hepatitis • Malaria, and visceral leishmaniasis • Portal hypertension with congestive splenomegaly • Human immunodeficiency virus (HIV) • Chronic hemolytic anemias such as thalassemia trait • Acute leukemia • Malignant lymphoma • Polycythemia vera • Amyloidosis	• Portal hypertension due to extrahepatic portal venous obstruction (EHPVO) • Cirrhosis • Chronic hemolytic disease or hemolytic anemia, thalassemia major, elliptocytosis, and spherocytosis • Storage disorders such as adult Gaucher's disease and Niemann–Pick disease • *Tropical splenomegaly syndrome*: Chronic malaria • Visceral leishmaniasis • Splenic cyst (hydatid cyst) or tumor • Chronic myeloid leukemia (CML) • Amyloidosis • Idiopathic myelofibrosis and myelosclerosis

(CMV: cytomegalovirus; EBV: Epstein–Barr virus; HLH: hemophagocytic lymphohistiocytosis; SLE: systemic lupus erythematosus)

TABLE 2: Splenomegaly with other organomegaly/system involvement.

HEPATOMEGALY	CENTRAL NERVOUS SYSTEM (CNS) INVOLVEMENT	RENAL INVOLVEMENT
• *Infections:* Intrauterine infections [TORCH (toxoplasmosis, others (syphilis, hepatitis B), rubella, cytomegalovirus, herpes simplex) infections], septicemia, and neonatal hepatitis • *Bacterial:* Disseminated tuberculosis, bacterial endocarditis, and liver abscess • *Viral:* Infective hepatitis (acute and chronic) and infectious mononucleosis • *Fungal:* Histoplasmosis • *Protozoal*: Malaria and kala-azar	• Neonatal hepatitis with intrauterine infection with CNS manifestations • Cerebral malaria • Septicemia with meningitis • Mucopolysaccharidosis • (Hurler syndrome, Hunter's syndrome, Sanfilippo syndrome, and Sly syndrome) • Mucolipidosis • GM1 and GM2 gangliosidosis • Infantile Gaucher's disease • Niemann–Pick disease type A	• Leukemia with renal infiltration • Congenital hepatic fibrosis • Zellweger syndrome • Type I tyrosinemia • Wiedemann–Beckwith syndrome

Contd...

Contd…

HEPATOMEGALY	CENTRAL NERVOUS SYSTEM (CNS) INVOLVEMENT	RENAL INVOLVEMENT
• *Parasitic:* Hydatid cyst (*Echinococcus granulosus*) • Chronic liver disease with portal hypertension • *Congestive causes:* Congestive cardiac failure, hepatic vein thrombosis, Budd–Chiari syndrome, and constrictive pericarditis • *Hematological–hemolytic anemia:* Hemolytic causes usually manifest after 6 months of age • *Metabolic diseases:* Wilson, tyrosinemia, galactosemia, and cystic fibrosis • *Storage/infiltrative disorders:* Gaucher's disease, glycogen storage disease (IV), mucopolysaccharidosis, mucolipidosis, hemochromatosis, and amyloidosis • *Malignancy:* Leukemia and lymphoma	• Wolman disease	

Red Flag Signs

- Faltering growth
- Weight loss
- Feeding difficulties
- Hepatomegaly and abdominal masses
- Abnormal stooling patterns
- Developmental or neurologic abnormalities
- *Musculoskeletal abnormalities:* Pain, limited movements, arthritis, or abnormal bone development
- Pruritus, pallor, icterus, lymphadenopathy, and rash
- Abnormal vital signs
- Ophthalmologic abnormalities (uveitis, iritis, opacification, and vascular occlusion)

Approach

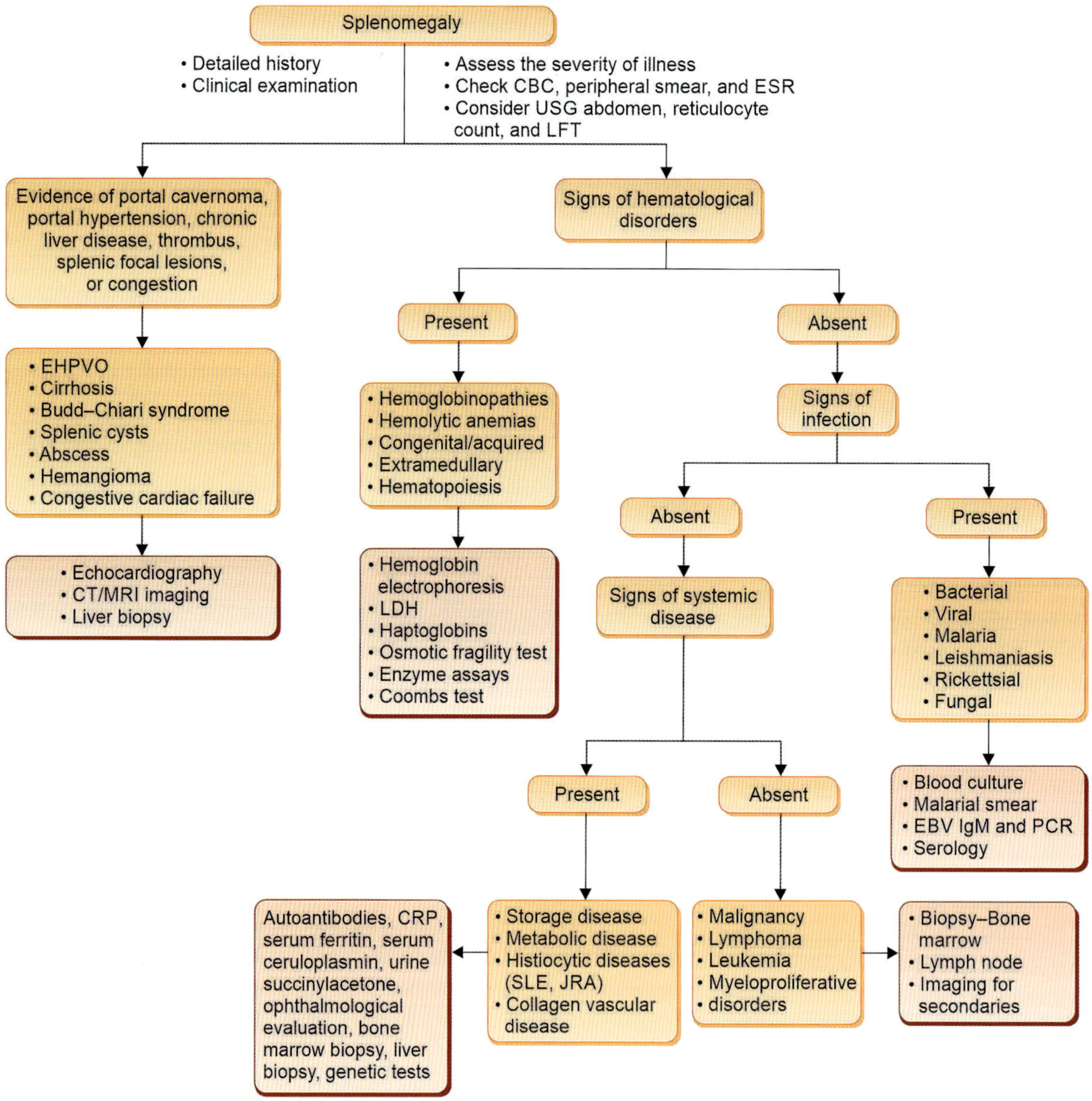

(CBC: complete blood count; CRP: c-reactive protein; CT: computed tomography; EHPVO: extrahepatic portal venous obstruction; ESR: erythrocyte sedimentation rate; EBV: Epstein–Barr virus; IgM: immunoglobulin M; JRA: juvenile rheumatoid arthritis; LDH: lactate dehydrogenase; LFT: liver function tests; MRI: magnetic resonance imaging; PCR: polymerase chain reaction; SLE: systemic lupus erythematosus; USG: ultrasound)

Suggested Reading

- Allan R, Downey P, Kate Paddick K, Cheung G. Normal sonographic measurements and guidelines for EIF, CPC, fetal renal dilatation, markers for chromosomal abnormalities, and fetal abnormalities. Revised Version, November 2014, Page 4 Division of Medical Imaging, Flinders Medical Centre, South Australia http://www.users.on.net/$\sim$cardal/Normal_Sonographic_Measurements and_markers_guidelines_Nov_2014_final.pdf Assessed April 2021.
- Kamble MB, Meena KB, Meena VK. Splenomegaly in children. Int J Contemp Pediatr 2019;6:1552-6.
- Louka, Eleni & Hall, Georgina. (2022). Abnormalities of the spleen: a systematic approach to a child with enlarged spleen and splenic dysfunction. Paediatrics and Child Health. 32. 10.1016/j.- paed.2022.02.006.
- Pelizzo G, Guazzotti M, Klersy C, Nakib G, Costanzo F, Andreatta E, et al. Spleen size evaluation in children: time to define splenomegaly for pediatric surgeons and pediatricians. PLoS ONE. (2018) 13:e0202741.
- Suttorp M, Classen CF. Splenomegaly in Children and Adolescents. Front Pediatr. 2021 Jul 9;9:704635.

Rectal Bleeding

40

Section Editor: **B Rajsekhar**
Section Co-Editor: **Suchitra Pusapati**
Author: **Rakesh Mishra**

Introduction

- Rectal bleeding is less common in children than in adults. Despite being due to benign causes most often, it is a cause of panic and anxiety in parents.
- The bleeding may be bright red called hematochezia or black and tarry called melena. The causes of this may be congenital or acquired and need investigation and appropriate management.
- Bleeding per rectum in children is less common than in adults.
- It can cause a great deal of anxiety amongst parents, and thus requires appropriate assessment, explanation, and reassurance. The vast majority of rectal bleeding in children is benign but it may indicate serious underlying pathology.
- Bleeding per rectum may be in the form of passage of bright red/dark red blood (hematochezia) or black tarry stools (malaena). It may occur due to congenital as well as acquired causes and may require medical or surgical management.

Etiology

The etiology of rectal bleeding in a child is given in **Table 1.**

TABLE 1: Age related causes of bleeding per rectum in children.

Up to 2 years of age	2–5 years of age	6–15 years of age
Anal fissure	Anal fissure	Anal fissure
Necrotizing enterocolitis	Intussusception	Polyps
Milk allergy	Polyps	Infectious enterocolitis
Polyps	Infectious enterocolitis	Inflammatory bowel disease

Contd...

Contd...

Up to 2 years of age	2–5 years of age	6–15 years of age
Intussusception	Meckel diverticulum	Henoch–Schönlein purpura
Hirschsprung disease-related enterocolitis	Bleeding diathesis	Hemolytic uremic syndrome
Meckel diverticulum	Henoch–Schönlein purpura	Bleeding diathesis
Infectious enterocolitis	Hemolytic uremic syndrome	Angiodysplasia
Duplication cyst	Angiodysplasia	Lymphonodular hyperplasia
Bleeding diathesis	Lymphonodular hyperplasia	Extrahepatic portal venous obstruction
	Extrahepatic portal venous obstruction	NSAID use, steroids/aspirin
	NSAID use, steroids/aspirin	

(NSAID: nonsteroidal anti-inflammatory drugs)

Unusual Causes

- Sexual abuse
- Hirschsprung's enterocolitis
- Solitary rectal ulcer syndrome
- Vascular lesions
- Henoch–Schönlein purpura
- Hemolytic uremic syndrome
- Acquired thrombocytopenia

Red Flag Signs

Red flag signs include:

- Any rectal bleeding in infants <2 months of age
- Massive bleeding
- Fever/shock/tachypnea/tachycardia
- Abdominal pain/distension
- Currant jelly stools
- Signs of intestinal obstruction
- Weight loss
- Significant anemia

Approach

History

- Acute/chronic
- Melena/Hematochezia
- Quantity of bleeding
- *Associated Symptoms:* Vomiting, fever, loose stools (infectious cause)/straining, large fecal mass, and painful defecation (constipation—fissure in ano)
- Signs of obstruction, bowel sounds, and distension

Investigations

- Routine complete blood count (CBC), liver function tests (LFT), and prothrombin time (PT)/activated partial thromboplastin time (aPTT)
- Ultrasound abdomen
- Colonoscopy
- Meckel's scan (radionuclide)
- Computed tomography (CT) enteroclysis

The approach to the management of a child with rectal bleeding is given in **Flowchart 1.**

FLOWCHART 1: Approach to management of a child with rectal bleeding.

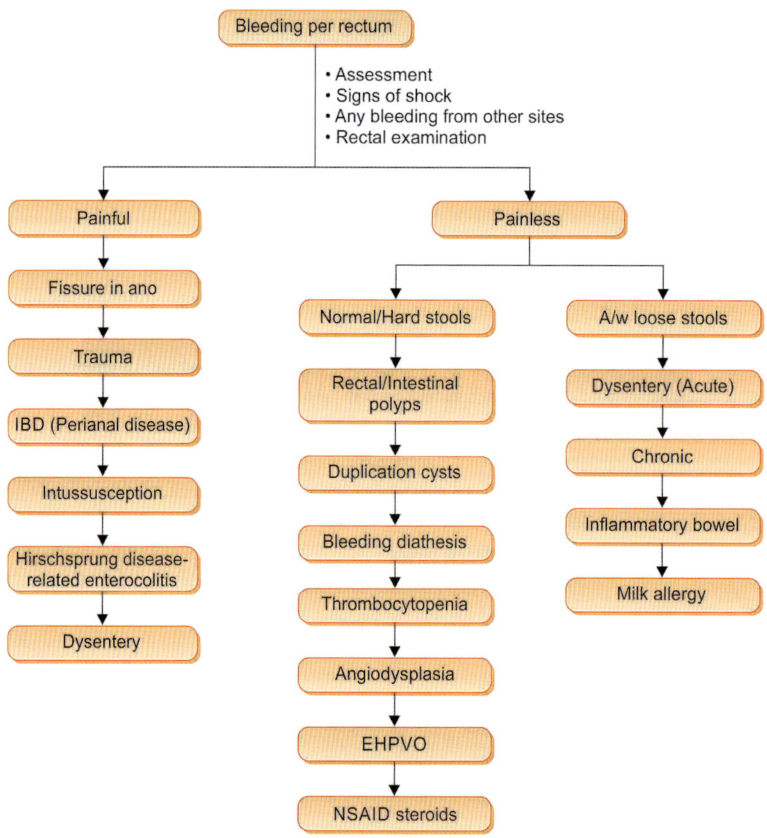

(A/w: associated with; EHPVO: extrahepatic portal vein obstruction; IBD: inflammatory bowel disease; NSAID: nonsteroidal anti-inflammatory drug)

Suggested Reading

- Chandel K, Jain R, Bhatia A, Saxena AK, Sodhi KS. Bleeding per rectum in pediatric population: A pictorial review. World J Clin Pediatr. 2022;11(3):270-88.
- Mushtaq F, Tudor G, El-Hadi S, Rectal bleeding in children: Causes and investigations. Paediatrics and Child Health. 2014;24(11):491-500.
- Wolfram W. Medscape. (2023). Pediatric Gastrointestinal Bleeding. [online] Available from https://emedicine.medscape.com/article/1955984-overview?form=fpf#a5 [Last accessed March, 2023].

Syncope

41

***Section Editor:* Nehal Patel**
***Section Co-Editor:* Jay T Dhirwani**
***Authors:* Neeraj Aggarwal, Shreepal Jain**

Definition

- Syncope is defined as a transient loss of consciousness (TLOC) due to cerebral hypoperfusion, characterized by a rapid onset, short duration, and spontaneous complete recovery.
- Presyncope describes a state that resembles the prodrome of syncope, but is not followed by loss of consciousness.
- The majority of the episodes in pediatric age group are benign in nature but a small percentage of cases can be of cardiac etiology and lethal.

Etiopathogenesis

Reflex (neutrally mediated) syncope (80% cases)	*Cardiac syncope* *Common causes are as follows:*	*Orthostatic hypotension (OH)*
Most common is the neurocardiogenic syncope (vasovagal syncope), it is mostly preceded by a prodrome and followed by quick and complete recovery. Provocative events may include emotional stress such as fear, anxiety, pain (e.g., vaccination), blood phobia (e.g., blood sampling) or sudden change in posture. Precipitating states may include anemia, dehydration, hunger, physical exhaustion, and a crowded or poorly ventilated environment (like rock concerts/church). • Other types include situational syncope (e.g., cough/sneeze, micturition, defecation, laughing, post exercise, etc.) • Carotid sinus syndrome (e.g., shaving with extended neck) • Nonclassical forms are rare (without prodromes and/or without apparent triggers, and/or atypical presentation)	*Outflow obstructions (aortic/ pulmonary stenosis):* • Cardiomyopathy (e.g., hypertrophic obstructive cardiomyopathy) • Pulmonary hypertension or Eisenmenger syndrome • Cardiac masses (atrial myxoma, tumors, etc.), pericardial disease/ tamponade, congenital anomalies of coronary arteries, and prosthetic valve dysfunction • Arrhythmias including bradycardia (sinus node dysfunction/ atrioventricular conduction system disease)/tachycardia (supraventricular or ventricular like Long QT syndrome)	• *Drug-induced OH:* Diuretics, vasodilators, etc. • *Volume depletion-related OH:* Diarrhea, vomiting, and hemorrhage • *Neurogenic OH:* Autonomic failure, diabetes, amyloidosis, etc. *Note:* It may be exacerbated by venous pooling during exercise/after meals (postprandial hypotension) and after prolonged bed rest/deconditioning

Mimics

Conditions that may present like syncope:

- *Generalized seizures:* No prodrome; urinary/fecal incontinence is common and longer postictal phase.
- *Complex partial seizures and absence of epilepsy:* Actively upright child, i.e., sitting or standing (no falls) yet unresponsive and later amnesia
- *Psychogenic pseudosyncope:* Duration of apparent level of consciousness (LOC) lasting many minutes to hours, up to several times a day
- *Transient ischemic attack (TIA)/subclavian steal syndrome:* Focal neurological signs
- *Metabolic disorders/intoxication:* Impaired consciousness

Reflex Syncope

- *Vasovagal syncope:* If precipitated by pain, fear, or standing; is associated with a typical progressive prodrome (pallor, sweating, and/or nausea)
- *Situational reflex:* During or immediately after specific triggers
- *Syncope due to orthostatic hypotension (OH):* Occurs while standing; concomitant significant OH

Cardiac Syncope

- *Arrhythmic syncope:* Electrocardiogram (ECG) abnormality/palpitation preceding syncope
- *Structural cardiopulmonary disorders:* Prolapsing atrial myxoma, left atrial ball thrombus, severe aortic stenosis, pulmonary embolus, and acute aortic dissection
- Unexplained with no history of cardiac disease/family history of sudden death/no supine syncope/syncope during sleep, noise or exercise, no unusual triggers and normal ECG rules out cardiac syncope

Red Flag Signs

- Little or no prodrome
- Prolonged loss of consciousness (longer than 5 minutes)
- Exertion or exercise-induced syncope
- Syncope in a supine position/sleep or with loud noise
- Chest pain or palpitations
- History of cardiac disease/pacemaker implant/cardiac surgery
- Familial history of long QT syndrome, cardiomyopathy, deafness, or sudden cardiac death in early age

Evaluation

- Careful history
- Physical examination [including supine and standing blood pressure (BP)]
- Electrocardiogram

Diagnostic Workup

- *Orthostatic challenge by:*
  - Active standing
  - Head-up tilt test (HUTT)
  - 24-hour ambulatory BP monitoring (ABPM)
- *ECG monitoring:* Holter, smartphone, and invasive loop recorder (ILR)
- Echocardiogram
- Home video recording
- *Active standing*: Intermittent determination of manual BP and heart rate (HR) in supine and active standing for 3 minutes. OH is confirmed when a fall in systolic BP from baseline value ≥20 mm Hg/ diastolic BP ≥10 mm Hg that reproduces symptoms while testing.

- *Head-up tilt test:* To be considered in patients with suspected reflex syncope, OH, postural tachycardia syndrome (PoTS), or psychogenic pseudosyncope. A negative response does not exclude reflex syncope.
- *ABPM:* It is done to detect and monitor the degree of OH and supine hypertension in daily life in suspected autonomic failure.
- *Prolong ECG monitoring (invasive and noninvasive) and echocardiography: These are done* in high-risk cases/atypical syncope/suspected cardiac syncope.
- *Video recording in suspected syncope:* This is done especially for psychogenic pseudosyncope having a high frequency and long duration of attacks.

History

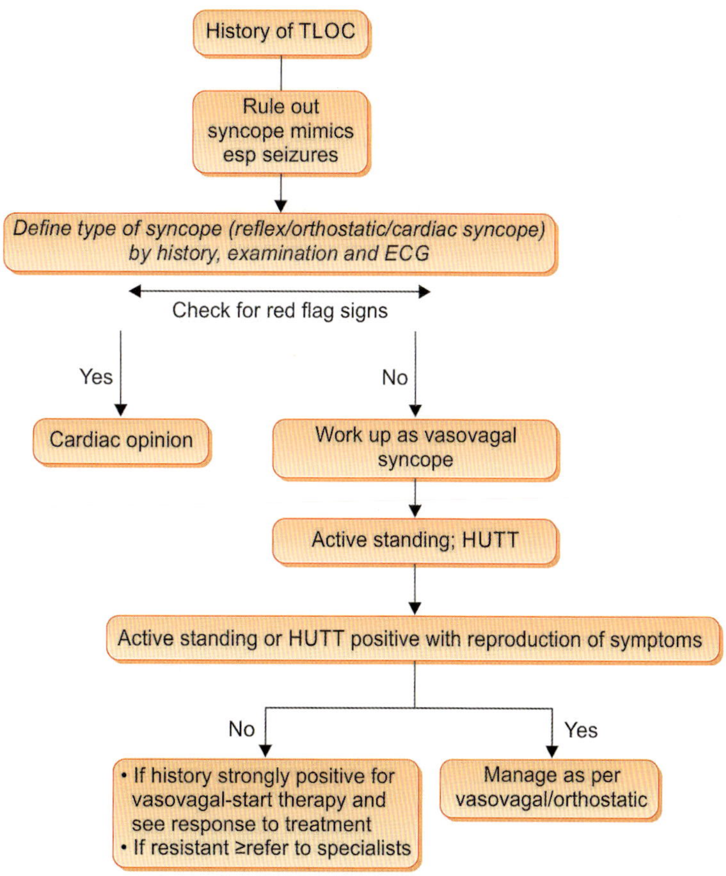

Suggested Reading

- Brignole M, Moya A, de Lange FJ, Deharo JC, Elliott PM, Fanciulli A, et al; ESC Scientific Document Group. 2018 ESC Guidelines for the diagnosis and management of syncope. Eur Heart J. 2018;39(21):1883-1948.
- Goldberger ZD, Petek BJ, Brignole M, Shen WK, Sheldon RS, Solbiati M, et al. ACC/AHA/HRS versus ESC guidelines for the diagnosis and management of syncope: JACC Guideline Comparison. J Am Coll Cardiol. 2019;74(19): 2410-23.
- Schunk PC, Ruttan T. Pediatric Syncope: High-Risk Conditions and Reasonable Approach. Emerg Med Clin North Am. 2018;36(2):305-21.
- Varosy PD, Chen LY, Miller AL, Noseworthy PA, Slotwiner DJ, Thiruganasambandamoorthy V. Pacing as a treatment for reflex-mediated (vasovagal, situational, or carotid sinus hypersensitivity) syncope: A systematic review for the 2017 ACC/AHA/HRS Guideline for the evaluation and management of patients with syncope: A report of the American College of Cardiology/American Heart Association Task Force on Clinical Practice Guidelines and the Heart Rhythm Society. Circulation. 2017;136(5):e123-e135.
- Zavala R, Metais B, Tuckfield L, DelVecchio M, Aronoff S. Pediatric Syncope: A Systematic Review. Pediatr Emerg Care. 2020;36(9):442-5.

Childhood Obesity

42

Section Editor: **Kripasindhu Chatterjee**
Section Co-Editors: **Atanu Bhadra, Ashim Kumar Ghosh**
Author: **Ganesh Jevalikar**

Introduction

- Obesity is an excess accumulation of body fat and can be a presenting complaint/associated with concerns like micropenis, polycystic ovary syndrome (PCOS), respiratory complaints, etc.
- Evaluation is essential to differentiate nutritional from non-nutritional obesity, early diagnosis of comorbid conditions as well as complications of obesity.

Etiology

- Childhood obesity is mostly caused by calorie intake more than expenditure.
- Pathophysiology of "nutritional" obesity is complex and mediated by several genetic, hormonal, metabolic, and neurological factors.
- Non-nutritional causes of obesity are listed in **Table 1**.

TABLE 1: Etiology of non-nutritional obesity.

Etiology	*Examples*
Endocrine conditions	Hypothyroidism, Cushing syndrome, growth hormone deficiency, and pseudohypoparathyroidism
Syndromes with obesity	• Prader–Willi (typical facial features, hypotonia, failure to thrive in infancy, and delayed milestones) • Bardet–Biedl (polydactyly, retinitis pigmentosa, and hypogonadism) • Alström (retinal dystrophy, sensorineural hearing loss, and cardiomyopathy)
Monogenic obesity	Mutations in leptin and leptin receptor, pro-opiomelanocortin (POMC) and melanocortin-4 receptor (MC4R)
Hypothalamic obesity	• Hypothalamic tumors, radiation, infiltrative disorders, and sequelae of infections • ROHHADNET (Rapid onset obesity, hypothalamic dysfunction, hypoventilation, autonomic dysfunction, and neuroendocrine tumor syndrome)
Drugs	Glucocorticoids, atypical antipsychotics, and valproate

Red Flag Signs of Non-nutritional Obesity

- Early onset (<5 years of age)
- Short stature/poor growth velocity
- Dysmorphism/developmental delay
- Rapidly progressive obesity
- Hyperphagia, polyuria, polydipsia, and symptoms of raised intracranial pressure
- Deafness and night blindness
- Intake of medications associated with obesity

Evaluation

History

- Detailed diet and lifestyle (exercise, screen time, and sleep patterns) of the child and family
- Birth weight and milestones
- Family history of obesity and metabolic syndrome
- History of pathological causes of obesity (see under red flag signs)
- *History of complications:* Polyuria, sleep apnea, psychological disorders, gynecomastia, PCOS, bone and joint pains, gastroesophageal reflux, and respiratory problems

Examination

- Height, weight, and body mass index (BMI) plotted on ethnicity-specific growth charts [diagnosis based on World Health Organization (WHO) weight-for-length charts for children <5 years of age and Indian Academy of Pediatrics (IAP) BMI charts for children >5 years of age]
- Waist circumference
- Blood pressure
- Signs of insulin resistance (acanthosis and skin tags)
- Pubertal assessment
- Hirsutism
- *Fundus examination:* Rule out benign intracranial hypertension

Investigations

- *Nutritional obesity:*
  - Blood glucose—fasting and 2 hour post 1.75 gm/kg of anhydrous glucose (maximum 75 gram), glycated hemoglobin (HbA1c), serum glutamic pyruvic transaminase (SGPT), fasting lipids, and other investigations as indicated clinically
  - Ultrasonography (USG) abdomen for fatty liver
  - Sleep studies in suspected sleep apnea
- Non-nutritional obesity

Approach for Evaluation and Management of Obesity in Children

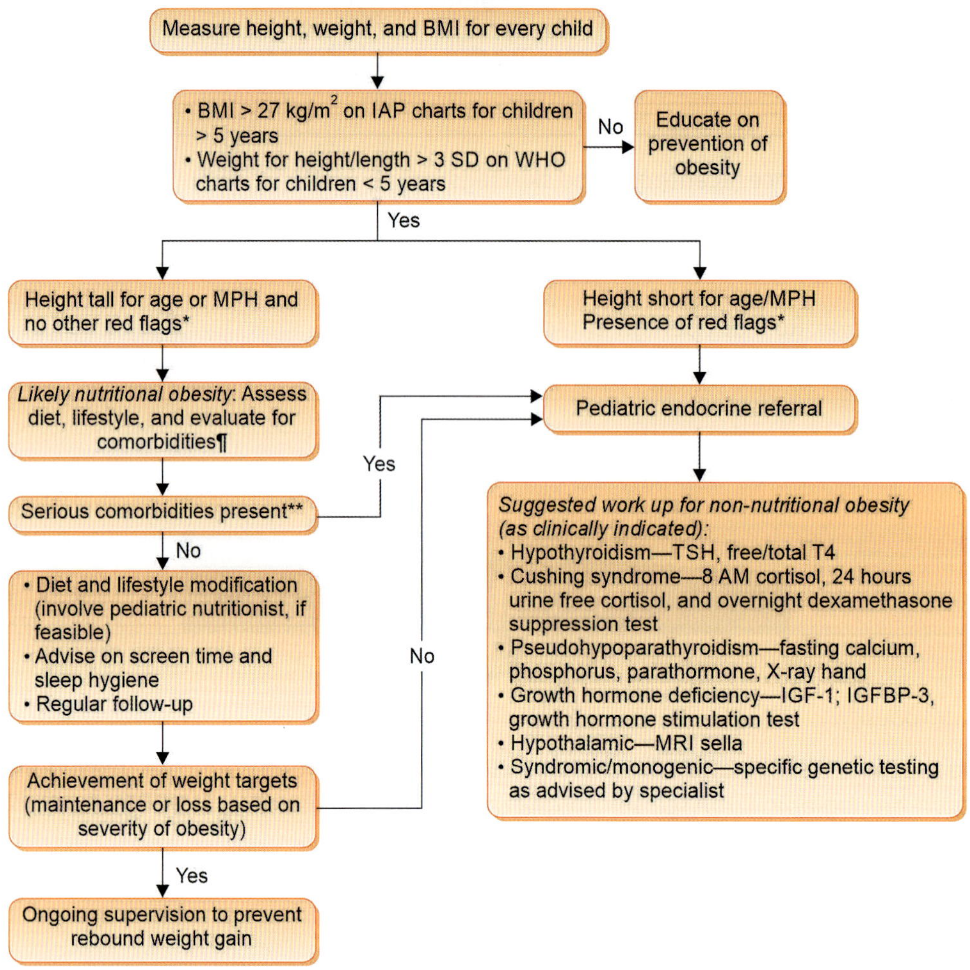

**Red flags for non-nutritional obesity:* Short stature/growth failure, developmental delay, early onset obesity, rapidly progressive weight gain, hyperphagia, hearing/vision abnormalities, and dysmorphism

¶*Evaluation for comorbidities in obesity*: Measure BP, oral glucose tolerance test, HbA1c, ALT, fasting lipid profile, and others as clinically indicated

***Examples of significant comorbidities:* Diabetes, hypertension, fatty liver, polycystic ovary syndrome, psychiatric issues, and bone deformities

(ALT: alanine aminotransferase; BMI: body mass index; BP: blood pressure; HbA1c: glycated hemoglobin; IAP: Indian Academy of Pediatrics; IGF-1: insulin-like growth factor-1; IGFBP-3: insulin-like growth factor binding protein-3; MPH: midparental height; MRI: magnetic resonance imaging; SD: standard deviations TSH: thyroid stimulating hormone; WHO: World Health Organization)

Suggested Reading

- Khadilkar V, Shah N, Harish R, Ayyavoo A, Bang A, Basu S, et al. Indian Academy of Pediatrics Revised Guidelines on Evaluation, Prevention and Management of Childhood Obesity. Indian Pediatr. 2023;60:1013-31.
- Ranjani H, Mehreen TS, Pradeepa R, Anjana RM, Garg R, Anand K, et al. Epidemiology of childhood overweight & obesity in India: A systematic review. Indian J Med Res. 2016;143:160-74.
- Seth A, Dabas A. Obesity and overweight: The Epidemic and Management. In: Desai M, Menon PSN, Bhatia V, Seth A (Eds). Pediatric Endocrine Disorders, 4th edition. Hyderabad, India: Universities Press; 2022. pp. 441-51.
- Styne DM, Arslanian SA, Connor EL, Farooqi IS, Murad MH, Silverstein JH, et al. Pediatric obesity: Assessment, treatment, and prevention: an endocrine society clinical practice guideline. J Clin Endocrinol Metab. 2017;102: 709-57.
- Sudhanshu S, Bhatia V. Obesity and Overweight: Monogenic and Syndromic Disorders. In: Desai M, Menon PSN, Bhatia V, Seth A (Eds). Pediatric Endocrine Disorders, 4th edition. Hyderabad, India: Universities Press;2022. pp. 452-60.

Gonadal Underdevelopment

43

Section Editor: **Kripasindhu Chatterjee**
Section Co-Editors: **Atanu Bhadra, Ashim Kumar Ghosh**
Author: **Chirantap Oza**

Introduction

- Gonadal underdevelopment may present either during infancy or puberty.
- In infancy, this presentation is referred to as "disorders of sex development" (DSD).
- This is defined as "congenital conditions in which development of chromosomal, gonadal, or anatomical sex is atypical".
- It includes conditions like atypical genital appearance; penis with bilateral cryptorchidism; unilateral cryptorchidism with hypospadias; severe hypospadias (penoscrotal, scrotal, or perineal) with or without micropenis; clitoromegaly and/or palpable gonad; and asymmetry in size, pigmentation, and rugosity of labioscrotal folds.

Etiology

- *Sex chromosome DSD:*
  - 47,XXY (Klinefelter syndrome)
  - 45,X (Turner syndrome)
  - 45,X/46,XY [mixed gonadal dysgenesis (MGD)]
  - 46,XX/46,XY (chimerism—ovotesticular DSD)

- *46XY DSD*
  - Disorders of testis development like complete gonadal dysgenesis (CGD)
  - Disorders in androgen synthesis or action like luteinizing hormone (LH) receptor mutations, mutations of genes coding for enzymes in steroidogenesis pathway (StAR protein, CYP11A1, HSD3B2, CYP17, POR, HSD17B3, and SRD5A2)
  - End organ resistance like androgen insensitivity syndrome
- *46XX DSD*
  - Disorders of ovarian development like XX testicular DSD and gonadal dysgenesis
  - Disorders of androgen excess like congenital adrenal hyperplasia due to mutation of HSD3B2, CYP21A2, POR, and CYP11B1
  - Placental aromatase deficiency and maternal virilizing tumors or androgenic drugs.

Red Flag Signs

- *Hyperpigmentation:* It is caused due to congenital adrenal hyperplasia (CAH), leading to severe hypoglycemia, hyponatremia, hyperkalemia, hypovolemia, shock, and death due to adrenal crisis.
- *Asymmetric genitalia:* Suggests ovotesticular DSD or MGD requiring exploratory laparoscopy and biopsy for diagnosis and prognosis
- *Syndromic features:* Skeletal dysplasia, aniridia, mental retardation, growth retardation, etc.
- *Children with Y chromosomal material and intra-abdominal gonads:* High risk for malignancy

Approach

- *History*:
  - History of maternal drug use like androgens/maternal hirsutism/virilization
  - Virilization during the pregnancy (aromatase deficiency)
  - *Family history:* Infertile nonmenstruating maternal female relatives with scant or absent pubic and axillary hair (androgen insensitivity)
  - Consanguinity (5α-reductase deficiency)
  - Prenatal findings
- *Physical Examination:*
  - External genitals symmetric/asymmetric and palpable
  - Score and interpret the external genitalia by external masculinization score **(Table 1)** or Prader staging **(Fig. 1)**.
  - *Associated anomalies:* Dysmorphism, campomelic dysplasia (SOX9), aniridia (WT1), etc.

TABLE 1: External masculinization score.

FEATURE	SCORE FOR YES/NO
• Scrotal fusion	3/0
• Micropenis	0/3
Urethral meatus	
• Normal	3
• Glandular	2
• Penile	1
• Perineal	0
Left and right gonad (score for each)	
• Scrotal	1.5
• Inguinal	1
• Abdominal	0.5
• Absent	0

Note: A score less than 10 out of 12 warrants evaluation.

- *Investigations:*
  - *Imaging:* Ultrasound/magnetic resonance imaging (MRI) pelvis to identify Müllerian structures and localization of gonads
  - Karyotype [fluorescence in situ hybridization (FISH) for sex reversal Y (SRY) gene—faster results]
  - *Biochemistry (after 48 hours of life):* Testosterone, dihydrotestosterone (DHT), LH, follicle-stimulating hormone (FSH), 17-hydroxyprogesterone (17-OHP), androstenedione, 17-hydroxypregnenolone, dehydroepiandrosterone sulfate (DHEAS), renin, and electrolytes

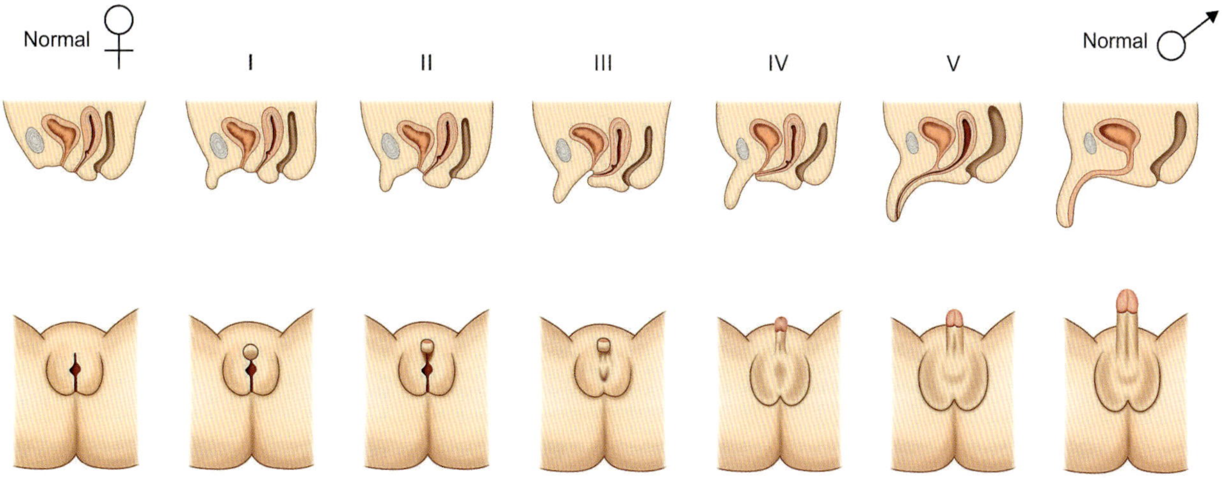

FIG. 1: Differential virilization of the external genitalia using the staging system of Prader.

FLOWCHART 1: Approach to children with gonadal underdevelopment.

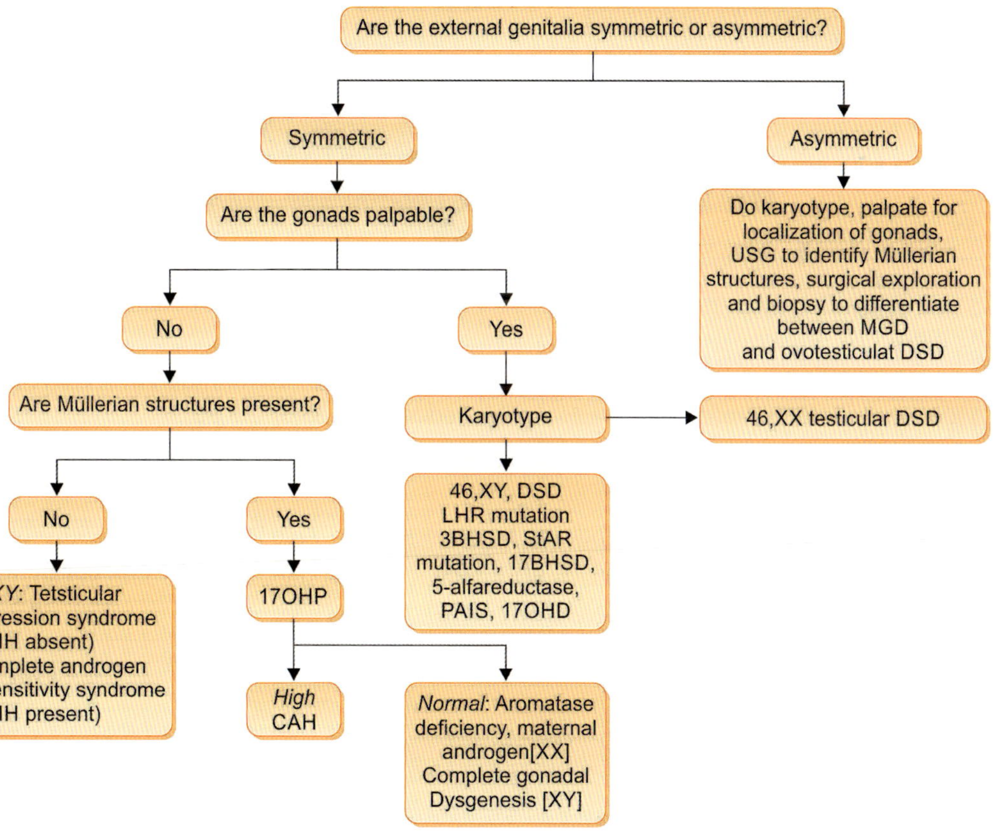

(17OHD: 17-alpha-hydroxylase deficiency; 17OHP: 17-hydroxyprogesterone; AMH: anti-Müllerian hormone; BHSD: beta–hydroxysteroid dehydrogenase; CAH: congenital adrenal hyperplasia; MGD: mixed gonadal dysgenesis; LHR: luteinizing hormone receptor; PAIS: partial androgen insensitivity syndrome; USG: ultrasonography)

The mean and standard deviation (SD) of anthropometric parameters of the external genitalia of

Indian newborns are given in **Table 2**.

TABLE 2: Mean and standard deviation (SD) of anthropometric parameters of the external genitalia of Indian newborns.

PARAMETER	MEAN	SD
Stretched penile length in cm	3.6	0.4
Penile width in cm	1.14	0.007
Clitoris length in mm	3.1	1.54
Anogenital ratio	0.342	0.07

Suggested Reading

- Ahmed SF, Khwaja O, Hughes IA. The role of a clinical score in the assessment of ambiguous genitalia. BJU Int. 2000;85:120-4.
- Lee PA, Nordenström A, Houk CP, Ahmed SF, Auchus R, Baratz A, et al. Global disorders of sex development update since 2006: Perceptions, approach and care. Horm Res Pediatr. 2016;85(3):158-80.
- Mondal R, Chatterjee K, Samanta M, Hazra A, Ray S, Sabui TK, et al. Clitoral length and anogenital ratio in Indian newborn girls. Indian Pediatr. 2016;53:299-303.
- Ogilvy-Stuart AL, Brain CE. Early assessment of ambiguous genitalia. Arch Dis Child. 2004;89(5):401-7.
- Vasudevan G, Manivarmane B, Bhat BV, Bhatia BD, Kumar S. Genital standards for south Indian male newborns. Indian J Pediatr. 1995;62:593-6.

Enuresis

44

Section Editor: **Sumitha Nayak**
Section Co-Editor: **Priya Shivalli**
Author: **Poornima RN**

Introduction

- As per normal development, children learn to be dry by day at around 2 years of age, dry by night at around 3 years of age.
- They are able to independently attend their toilet needs by the age of 4 years.

Classification

Enuresis can be classified into:

- *Primary:* Not been dry for at least 6 months after 5 years of age
- *Secondary:* Onset after a period of nocturnal dryness of at least 6 months
- *Monosymptomatic:* Absence of daytime lower urinary tract symptoms like frequency, urgency, etc.
- *Nonmonosymptomatic:* Presence of daytime lower urinary tract symptoms

Etiology

The etiology of enuresis involves:

- Congenital abnormality of the urinary tract
- Urinary tract infection (UTI)
- Neurological disorders (neurogenic/neuropathic bladder)
- Delayed bladder maturation and decreased bladder capacity
- Detrusor overactivity/areflexia
- Developmental delay/birth asphyxia
- Diabetes mellitus
- Recurrent UTI [vesicoureteral reflux (VUR) and posterior urethral valves (PUV)]
- Poor arousal from sleep
- Decreased vasopressin release

Risk Factors

Risk factors for enuresis include the following:

- Constipation
- Unusual stress/emotional problems [attention-deficit/hyperactivity disorder (ADHD) and learning disabilities]
- Low socioeconomic status
- Sibling birth
- Family history of enuresis
- Parental divorce

Differential Diagnosis with Investigation

CONDITION	SYMPTOMS/SIGNS	INVESTIGATION
Congenital abnormality of the urinary tract	Recurrent UTI, incontinence, and hydronephrosis	USG KUB and VCUG
Constipation	Hard stools, fecal incontinence, and rectal bleeding	Abdominal X-ray and USG
Diabetes mellitus	Polydipsia, polyuria, and weight loss	FBS, urine analysis, and HBA1c
Detrusor overactivity and areflexia	Daytime urinary frequency, urgency, and incontinence	USG KUB and urodynamic studies
Emotional disturbances	Depression and or defiant activity	Clinical diagnosis
Neurological disorder	Sacral deformity, spina bifida, and daytime voiding dysfunction	Xray spine and MRI spine
UTI	Fever, dysuria, and abdominal pain	Urine analysis and urine culture
VUR	Voiding symptoms and abdominal pain	Renal USG
Chronic kidney disease	Edema of face, hands and feet, and polyuria	RFT and Renal USG
Posterior urethral valve	Urethral obstruction and incontinence	Renal USG
Neurogenic bladder	Spontaneous bladder contraction incontinence	Urodynamic study

(FBS: fasting blood sugar; HBA1c: glycated hemoglobin; KUB: Kidney, ureters, and bladder; MRI: magnetic resonance imaging; RFT: renal function tests; USG: ultrasonography; UTI: urinary tract infection; VCUG: voiding cystourethrogram, VUR: vesicoureteral reflux)

Red Flag Signs

- Recurrent UTI
- Genital or rectal pain and discharge
- Daytime incontinence
- Dysuria and hematuria
- Snoring and daytime sleeping
- Fecal soiling
- Neurological abnormalities

Approach

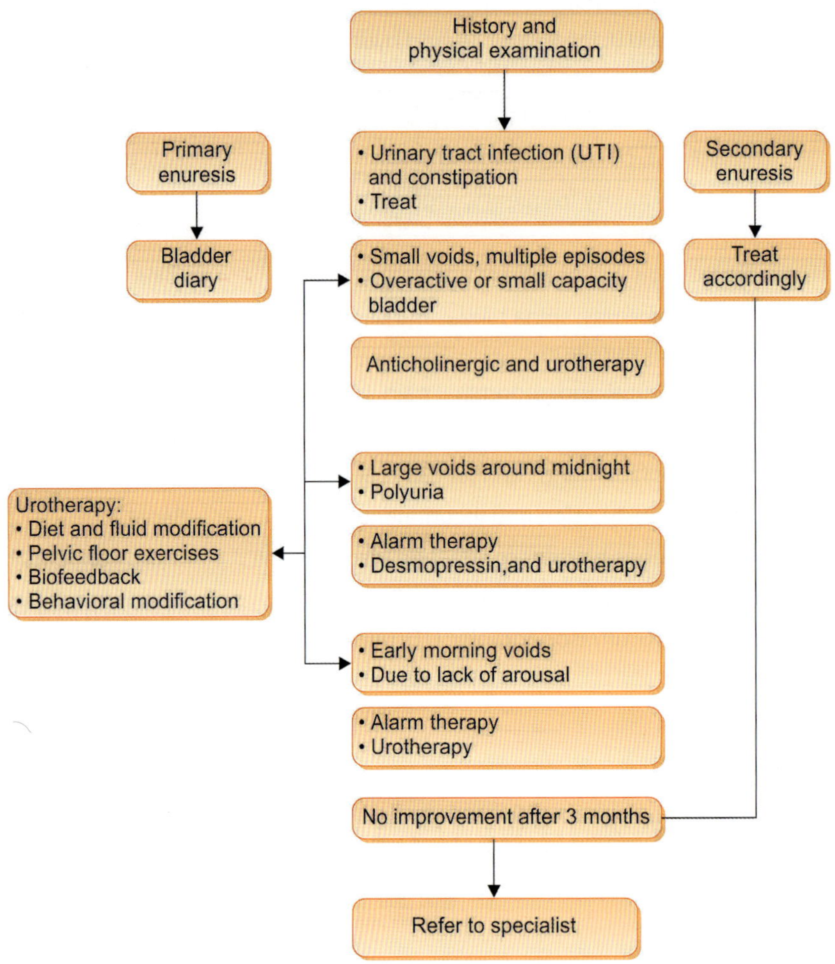
History and physical examination
• Urinary tract infection (UTI) and constipation
• Treat
Primary enuresis
Bladder diary
Secondary enuresis
Treat accordingly
• Small voids, multiple episodes
• Overactive or small capacity bladder
Anticholinergic and urotherapy
• Large voids around midnight
• Polyuria
• Alarm therapy
• Desmopressin,and urotherapy
Urotherapy:
• Diet and fluid modification
• Pelvic floor exercises
• Biofeedback
• Behavioral modification
• Early morning voids
• Due to lack of arousal
• Alarm therapy
• Urotherapy
No improvement after 3 months
Refer to specialist

Suggested Reading

- Gomez Rincon M, Leslie SW, Lotfollahzadeh S. Nocturnal Enuresis. In: StatPearls [Internet]. Treasure Island (FL): StatPearls Publishing; 2024. [online] Available from: https://www.ncbi.nlm.nih.gov/books/NBK545181/[Last accessed April,2014].
- Reddy NM, Malve H, Nerli R, Venkatesh P, Agarwal I, Rege V. Nocturnal enuresis in India: Are we diagnosing and managing correctly? Indian J Nephrol. 2017;27(6):417-26.
- Sarabi M, Nikpasand N, Mahmoudabadi E, Torshizian A, Ghodsi A, Azarfar A. Comprehensive Review of Nocturnal Enuresis in Children. J Pediatr Rev. 2022;10(3):227-38.
- Vande Walle J, Rittig S, Tekgül S, Austin P, Yang SS, Lopez PJ, et al. Enuresis: Practical guidelines for primary care. Br J Gen Pract. 2017;67:328-9.

Acute Red Eye

45

***Section Editor:* Sumitha Nayak**
***Section Co-Editor:* Priya Shivalli**
***Author:* Priya Shivalli**

Introduction

- A red eye in a child can occur suddenly and acutely.
- It is a common ocular presentation in general practice.
- It is a nonspecific ocular sign encountered in emergency and outpatient settings.
- It can arise from a wide spectrum of pathologies and involve various ocular structures.

Etiology

- Conjunctiva
  - *Infectious conjunctivitis:* Neonatal and post neonatal
  - Chemicals and irritants
  - Allergic conjunctivitis
  - Subconjunctival hemorrhage
- *Trauma:* Corneal abrasion, foreign body, hemorrhage, burns, blunt or penetrating injury, contact lens problems, and child abuse
- *Lid disorders:* Hordeolum, blepharitis, and chalazion
- Nasolacrimal duct obstruction, including dacryocystitis
- Preseptal and orbital cellulitis
- *Cornea:* Corneal ulcer/abrasion and keratitis
- Iritis/uveitis
- Allergic reactions
- Angle-closure glaucoma

Red Flag Signs

- Staining of the cornea
- Corneal haze/opacity
- Abnormal red reflex
- Photophobia
- Lid swelling
- Associated new onset squint
- Reduced visual acuity
- Failure to improve by 2 weeks
- Contact lens use
- Abnormal pupillary reaction
- Difficulty in examination
- High-velocity injury

Approach

History

Time course of the redness, eye pain, vision impairment, eye trauma, photophobia, sensation of foreign body, itch, discharge, contact lens wear, fever, systemic features of inflammation [E.g., suggestive of Kawasaki disease and pediatric inflammatory multisystem syndrome-temporally associated with SARS-CoV-2 (PIMS-TS)]

Other factors to consider:

- In a neonate, consider birth history and history of maternal sexually transmitted infections (STI)
- Vomiting/coughing
- Rheumatological/autoimmune conditions or family history
- Anticoagulant/antiplatelet treatment

Examination

Signs and symptoms and diagnoses to consider for acute red eye are given in **Table 1**.

TABLE 1: Examination for acute red eye.

SIGNS AND SYMPTOMS	DIAGNOSIS TO CONSIDER
Pain, photophobia, and watery discharge	• Foreign body • Traumatic corneal ulcer • Herpetic ulcer • Acute angle-closure glaucoma • Corneal abrasion
Purulent discharge	• Bacterial conjunctivitis • Infectious keratitis • Endophthalmitis
Itchiness, eyelid swelling and redness, and watery discharge	• Allergic conjunctivitis • Viral conjunctivitis
Dull, aching eye pain	• Iritis • Scleritis
Subconjunctival hemorrhage	• Trauma • Vigorous coughing/vomiting
Focal conjunctival injection	• Trauma • Episcleritis

An algorithmic approach to the acute red eye is given in **Flowchart 1**.

FLOWCHART 1: Algorithmic approach to the management of acute red eye.

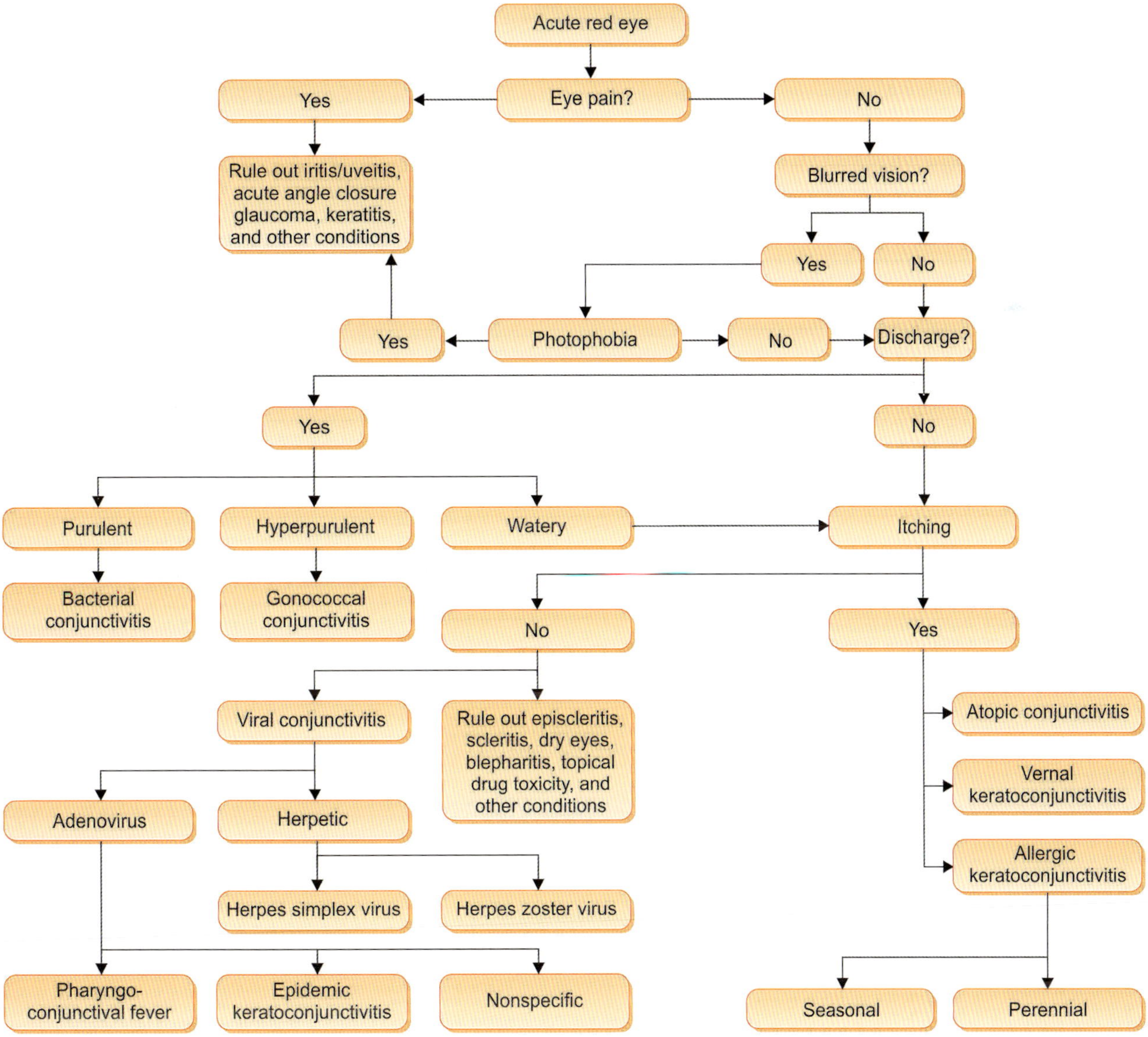

Suggested Reading

- Kliegman RM, St. Geme JW III. Disorders of the Eye. Nelson Textbook of Pediatrics, 21st edition. Amsterdam: Elsevier; 2020.
- Lu SJ, Lee GA, Gole GA. Acute red eye in children: A practical approach. Aust J Gen Pract. 2020;49(12):815-22.
- The Royal Children's Hospital Melbourne. (2022). Clinical Practice Guidelines: Acute red eye. [online] Available from https://www.rch.org.au/clinicalguide/guideline_index/acute_red_eye/[Last accessed April,2024].

Gynecomastia

46

Section Editor: **Kripasindhu Chatterjee**
Section Co-Editors: **Atanu Bhadra, Ashim Kumar Ghosh**
Authors: **Santanu Deb, Hunsi Giri**

Definition

- Gynecomastia is defined as an enlargement of the male breast due to benign proliferation of the glands, ducts, and stromal components including fat.
- It is commonly seen in adolescent males, and clinically detected when the diameter of glandular tissue exceeds 0.5 cm.

Types

- Gynecomastia can be of the following types:
  - Unilateral or bilateral
  - Physiological (>95%) or pathological (<5%)
- Pubertal gynecomastia is almost always physiological.
- Three well-defined periods of occurrence are as follows:
  - Neonates
  - Puberty
  - Older adults

Neonatal Gynecomastia

This may occur in 60–90% of male newborns. The diameter of the breast bud measures 1–2 cm in the first few weeks of life. Occasionally significant enlargement may occur. Postnatally, falling level of maternal estrogen is thought to trigger prolactin secretion in the pituitary of the newborn. Resultant prolactinemia stimulates neonatal breasts and causes milk secretion in 5–20% of newborns.

Pubertal Gynecomastia

- *Etiology:* This occurs due to a relative imbalance between estrogen and testosterone levels during puberty. Onset is between 10–12 years of age and peaking between 13–14 years of age due to fall in adult.
- After about 18 months, involution begins and is completed by 16–17 years of age due to achievement of adult androgen–estrogen ratios.

Pathological Gynecomastia

- When gynecomastia is unilateral and eccentric in position (not concentric below areola)—Differentiate from neurofibroma, lipoma and lymphangioma.
- Breast cancer is usually not a differential in this age group.
- *Bilateral:*
  - Chronic liver disease
  - Refeeding syndrome following severe acute malnutrition
  - Klinefelter's syndrome
  - *Gonadal dysfunction:* Primary or secondary
  - Hyperthyroidism
  - *Neoplasms:* Testicular tumors or adrenal tumors
  - *Drugs:*
    - *Hormones:* Androgens, anabolic steroids, estrogen agonists, and antiandrogens
    - Isoniazid, ketoconazole, metronidazole
    - Cimetidine
    - *Cancer chemotherapeutics:* Alkylating agents
    - Captopril and digoxin
    - Diazepam and tricyclic antidepressants
    - Alcohol and Marijuana
    - Penicillamine

Pseudogynecomastia

This is caused by breast enlargement due to the deposition of fat and not breast gland tissue in obesity.

Red Flag Signs

- Prepubertal
- Worsening/deviation during the observation period—pathological gynecomastia
- Syndromic
- Painful
- Discharge

Approach

History

- Pubertal history
- Family history of male relatives with gynecomastia
- Family history of infertility
- Chromosomal disorders
- History of liver or renal disease
- Drug/substance abuse history
- Exposure to herbal and cosmetic products that may contain phytoestrogens
- Past history of mumps

Examination

- Confirm gynecomastia by palpation of glandular tissue >0.5 cm. Look for overlying skin conditions and discharge.
- Gynecomastia with galactorrhea—hyperprolactinemia
- Anthropometry, pubertal stage, and dysmorphisms
- *Breasts:* Synthetic estrogens effect—strong pigmentation of areolas and nipples
- External genitalia for ambiguities and cryptorchidism
- *Testis:* Size, nodularity, asymmetry, and consistency
- *Abdomen:* For adrenal masses

Investigations

- *Initial:*
  - Thyroid function tests
  - Testosterone
  - Estradiol
  - Human chorionic gonadotropin (HCG)
  - Luteinizing hormone (LH)
  - Prolactin
- *Selected cases:*
  - Karyotyping
  - Dehydroepiandrosterone sulfate (DHEAS)
  - Liver function tests (LFT)
  - Renal function tests (RFT)

An approach to the management of gynecomastia is given in **Flowchart 1**.

FLOWCHART 1: Approach to gynecomastia.

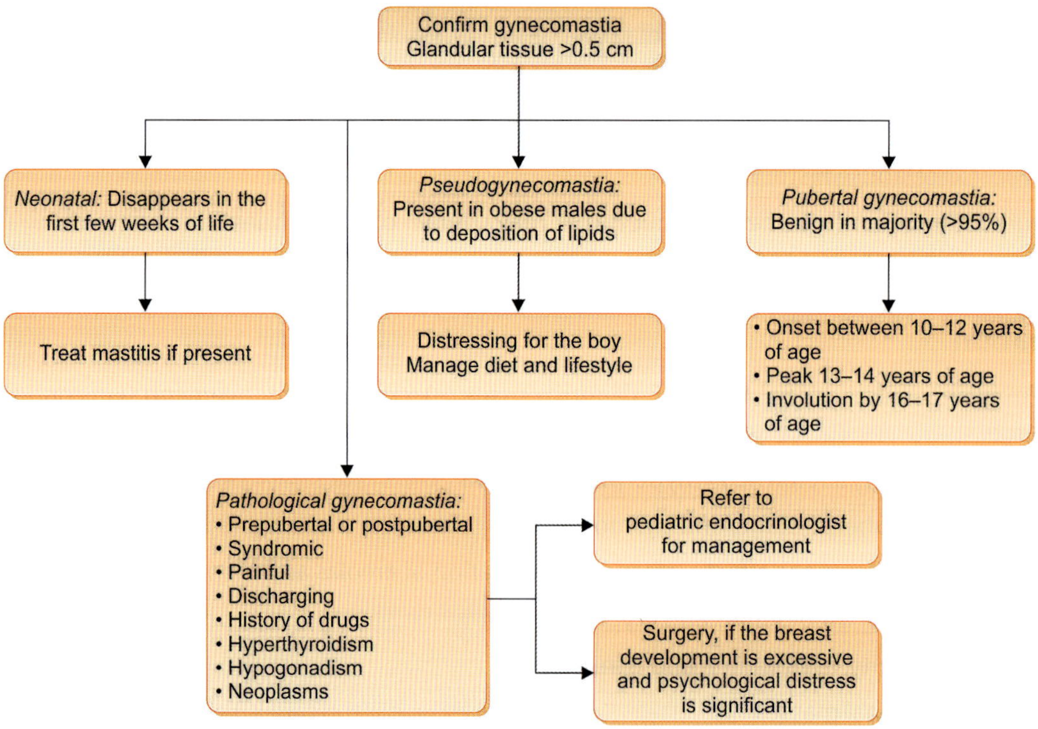

Suggested Reading

- Ali O, Donohue PA. Gynecomastia. In: Kleigman R M, St Geme JW, Blum NJ, Shah SS, Tasker RC, Wilson KM, Behrman R (Eds). Nelson Textbook of Pediatrics, 21st edition. Philadelphia: Elseiver; 2016. pp. 2742-3.
- Bhatt K. Pubertal Gynecomastia. In: Shah NS, Rao S (Eds). IAP Specialty Series on Pediatric Endocrinology. New Delhi. Jaypee Brothers Medical Publishers (P) Ltd; 2013.
- Pediatric Endocrinology Associates. (2024). Gynecomastia. [online] Available from https://pediatricendocrinologynj.com/gynecomastia/ [Last accessed April, 2024].
- Soliman AT, De Sanctis V, Yassin M. Management of Adolescent Gynecomastia: An Update. Acta Biomed. 2017; 88(2):204-13.

Acute Scrotum

47

Section Editor: **Gnanamurthy Narasimha**
Section Co-Editor: **Nagalatha Chidananda**
Authors: **Soundharya S, Ramesh Santhana Krishnan**

Definition

- The acute scrotum is defined as scrotal pain, swelling, and redness of acute onset.
- Acute scrotum in childhood is an important condition. It requires early evaluation and management to prevent the loss of testis.

Causes

It includes the following causes:

- *Torsion:*
  - Testicular torsion
  - Hydatid torsion
- *Infection:*
  - Epididymitis
  - Orchitis
- *Trauma:*
  - Hematoma
  - Hematocele
  - Testicular rupture
- *Systemic disease:*
  - Henoch–Schönlein purpura
  - Lymphoma/leukemia
- *Other causes:*
  - Incarcerated inguinal hernia
  - Scrotal edema
  - Scrotal emphysema
  - Appendicitis
  - Testicular tumor
  - Insect bite

History

- *Pain in the scrotum:* Sudden onset of excruciating pain
- *Vomiting* may be associated with torsion, but not always so.
- *Swelling and redness:* Nonspecific
- History of trauma
- *Urinary tract infection (UTI)* favors the diagnosis of epididymo-orchitis.

Examination

- *Pain in the scrotum:* Sudden onset of excruciating pain
- Swelling and redness of scrotum
- Tenderness
- *Prehn's sign:* Lifting the testis reduces the pain in epididymo-orchitis (negative Prehn's sign) whereas makes no difference in a testicular torsion (Positive Prehn's sign).
- *Cremasteric reflex*: Scratching the inner thigh causes an elevation in the testis. This may be absent in testicular torsion.

  **It is important to remember that these classically described signs may be difficult to demonstrate in a practical setting in a child with acute scrotal pain.*

- *Blue dot sign:* Pathognomonic for torsion of appendix of testis; small bluish discoloration in the upper pole on transillumination

Diagnostic Studies

- *Ultrasound with color doppler:* This detects reduced or absent perfusion *within the testis* compared to the opposite testis, suggesting ischemia.
- *Radionuclide imaging:* "Halo" of clear area in the midst of dense uptake; high sensitivity and specificity—90%
- *Blood investigations/bone marrow:* Only if systemic causes are suspected

Management Algorithm

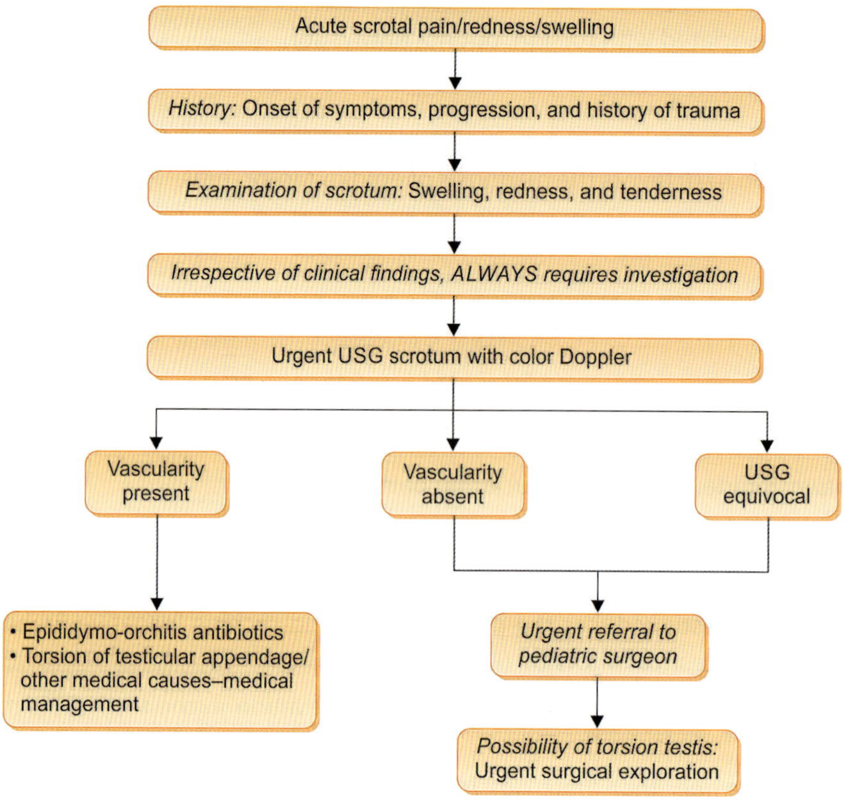

(USG: Ultrasonography)

Note: It is always safer to err on the side of overdiagnosis of torsion testis and involve a surgeon at the earliest to prevent any loss of testis.

The above dictum is acute scrotum is torsion unless proved otherwise.

Suggested Reading

- Gatti JM, Patrick Murphy J. Current management of the acute scrotum. Semin Pediatr Surg. 2007;16(1):58-63.
- Hutson JM. Undescended testis, torsion, and varicocele. In: Coran AG, Caldamone A, Adzick NS, Krummel TM, Laberge M, Shamberger R (Eds.). Pediatric surgery, 7th edition. Amsterdam, Netherlands: Elsevier; 2012. pp. 1003-19.
- Kapp A, Troxler D, Prüfer F, Holland-Cunz S, Frech M, Gros SJ. Testicular torsion in the absence of severe pain: Considerations for the pediatric surgeon. Children (Basel). 2021;8(6):429.
- Maheshwari PN, Arora AM. Let's not clinically miss testicular torsion in patients presenting with lower abdominal pain and vomiting. J Indian Assoc Pediatr Surg. 2021;26(1):68.
- Smith N. The acute scrotum in children. Surgery (Oxford). 2019;37(4):221-4.

Hypothyroidism

48

Section Editor: **Kripasindhu Chatterjee**
Section Co-Editors: **Atanu Bhadra, Ashim Kumar Ghosh**
Author: **Vani HN**

Introduction

- Hypothyroidism is the most common disorder of thyroid function in children.
- It is due to an insufficient thyroid hormone production.
- The causes could be either congenital or acquired.
- The fault could be in the thyroid gland (primary) or in pituitary or hypothalamus (central/secondary) or it may be due to peripheral causes like defects in transport/metabolism/action at the target site.

Etiology

Congenital	*Acquired*
• Dysgenesis – Aplasia – Hypoplasia – Ectopic • Dyshormonogenesis – Dual oxidases (Duox) – Peroxidase – Thyroglobulin • *Central causes:* Hypothalamus and pituitary development defects (genetic)—HESX1, PROP1, POUF1, and LHX3	• Autoimmune • *Drugs:* Amiodarone and lithium • Iodine deficiency • Head and neck causes: – Tumor – Surgery – Chemotherapy – Radiation

Red Flag Signs

Congenital

- Jaundice (beyond 2 weeks of life)
- Dry/ichthyosis skin
- Lethargy and skin mottling
- Hoarse cry
- Poor sucking
- Constipation
- Delayed development
- Umbilical hernia
- Periorbital swelling
- Macroglossia
- Large fontanelle
- Developmental delay

Majority of the newborns will be asymptomatic, hence newborn screening should be mandatory.

Acquired

- Weight gain
- Cold intolerance
- Dry skin
- Short stature (reduced height velocity)
- Hoarse voice
- Poor scholastic performance
- Delayed puberty
- Neck swelling (goiter)
- Periorbital puffiness
- Refractory anemia
- Menstrual disturbance
- Calf muscle hypertrophy (Kocher–Debré–Semelaigne)
- Rarely early puberty (Van Wyk–Grumbach)

Diagnostic Approach

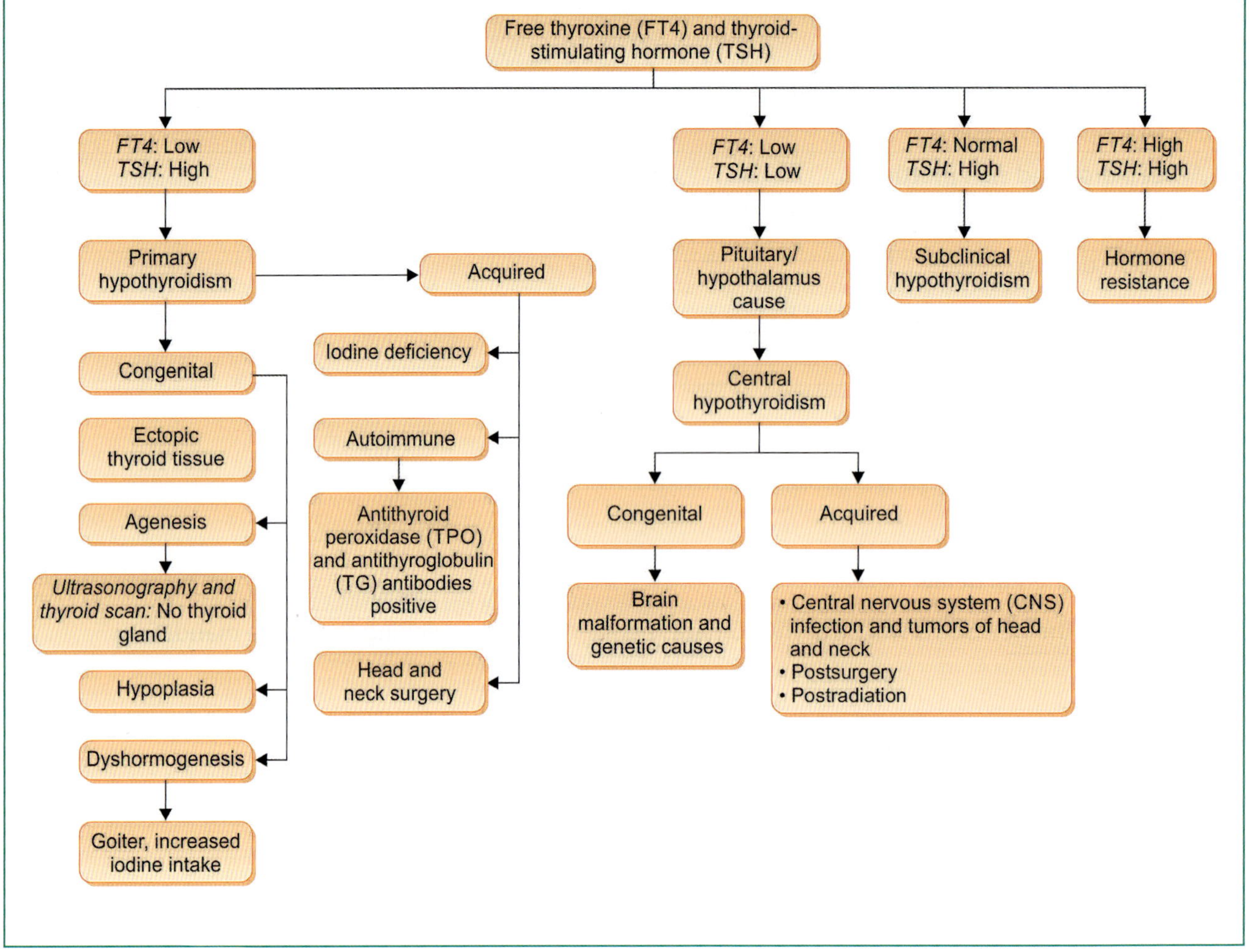

Suggested Reading

- Bekkering GE, Agoritsas T, Lytvyn L, Heen AF, Feller M, Moutzouri E, et al. Thyroid hormones treatment for subclinical hypothyroidism: A clinical practice guideline. BMJ. 2019;365:l2006
- Rivkees S, Bauer AJ. Thyroid disorders in children and adolescents. In: Sperling MA, Majzoub JA, Menon RK, Stratakis Ca (Eds). Sperling Pediatric Endocrinology, 5th edition. Philadelphia: Saunders; 2021. pp. 395-416.
- Sudhanshu S, Riaz I, Sharma R, Desai MP, Parikh R, Bhatia V. Newborn screening guidelines for congenital hypothyroidism in India: Recommendations of the Indian Society for Pediatric and Adolescent Endocrinology (ISPAE)—Part II: Imaging, Treatment and Follow-up. Indian J Pediatr. 2018;85(6):448-53.
- Van Trotsenburg P, Stoupa A, Léger J, Rohrer T, Peters C, Fugazzola L, et al. Congenital Hypothyroidism: A 2020–2021 Consensus Guidelines Update—An ENDO-European Reference Network Initiative Endorsed by the European Society for Pediatric Endocrinology and the European Society for Endocrinology. Thyroid. 2021;31(3):387-419.

Watery Eyes

49

***Section Editor:* Sumitha Nayak**
***Section Co-Editor:* Priya Shivalli**
***Author:* Ganesh Kulkarni**

Introduction

Watery eyes is a common pediatric symptom, which is also known as epiphora/lacrimation.

The cause is not always being an emotional upset. It may be due to:

- *Overproduction of tears (lacrimal fluid):* Lacrimation
- *Underdrainage of tears:* Epiphora

Anatomy of the gland: Lacrimal glands—one for each eye—are located on the outer edge of the upper eye, beneath the eyelid, and are the production house for a salty fluid that lubricates the eye with each blink. The moisture from tears helps prevent damage to the cornea, the outer covering of the eyeball, which can become inflamed or irritated if it is dry.

The congenital nasolacrimal duct obstruction at the valve of Hasner is the most common cause of epiphora in children.

Although the tears are meant to be protective, excessive lacrimation leads to watery eyes.

Etiology

Watery eyes could be benign, not needing any treatment.

It can be due to various underlying conditions. Some of the most common causes of epiphora include:

- *Congenital variety:* Congenital dacryocele/dacryocystitis/nasolacrimal duct obstruction
- Allergies
- Blepharitis
- Dry eyes
- Infections like conjunctivitis or sinusitis
- Styes

- Chalazions
- Entropion
- Eye injuries can also cause epiphora
- Environmental irritants like smoke or air pollution
- Scratched corneas (corneal abrasions)
- Dirt, debris, chemicals, or any foreign object that irritates the eye for long

Types

- *Gustatory epiphora:* It is referred to as crocodile tears. It occurs due to aberrant nerve regeneration.
- *Reflex epiphora:* It is a reactive mechanism of tear production due to irritation/injury to the corneal surface.
- *Obstructive epiphora:* It is caused due to blockage in any part of the lacrimal gland or ductular system.
- *Hypersecretive epiphora:* This is very rare. It occurs due to the excessive production of tears by the lacrimal glands.

Pointers

Pointers include:

- Eye pain
- Red/pink eye
- Heavy and wet eye
- Itchiness
- Cloudy/unclear vision

Red Flag Signs

- Pain around eyes
- A foreign body sensation
- Unilateral or bilateral watering of eyes beyond 9–10 months in infants—Chronic dacryocystitis
- Red eye—foreign body or trauma
- Cloudy/unclear vision—corneal abrasion

Diagnostics

These tests will help arrive at the diagnosis:

- Assessment of lid laxity
- Evaluate tear break-up time
- Dye disappearance test
- Probing and drainage

Approach

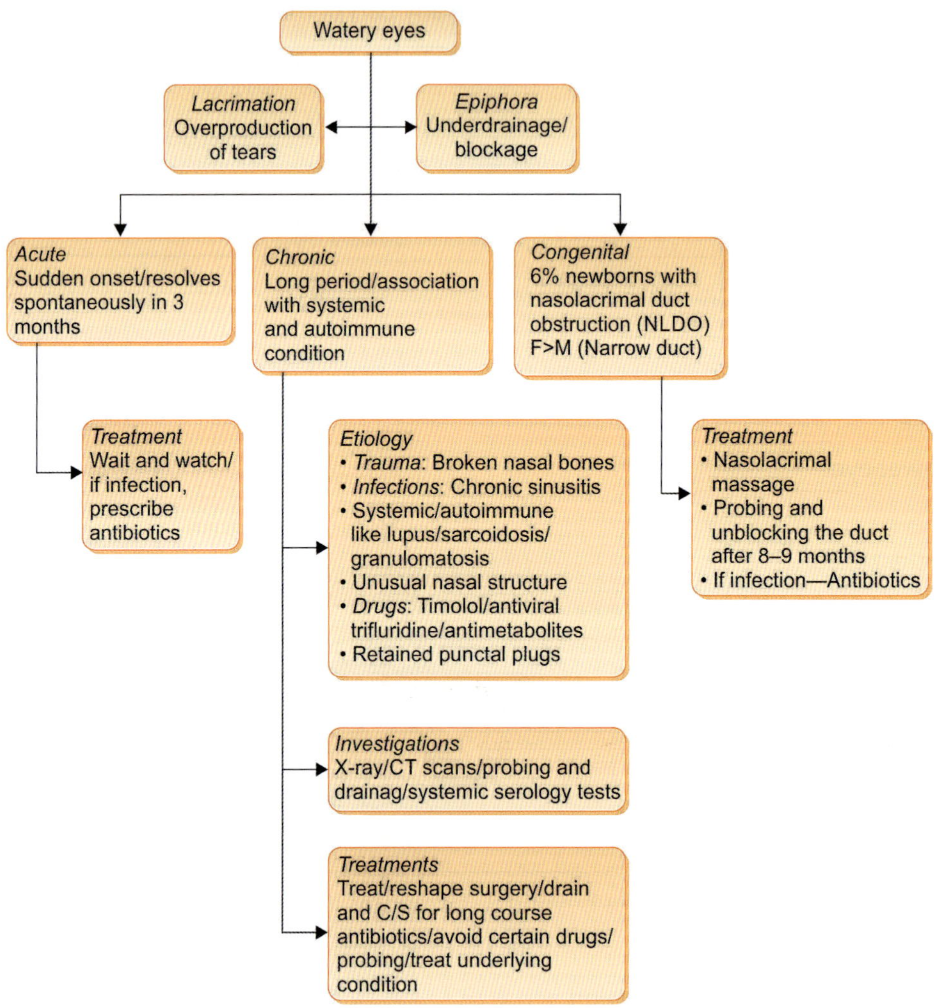

Suggested Reading

- Cleveland Clinic. (2024). Watery Eyes. [online] Available from https://my.clevelandclinic.org/health/symptoms/17944-watery-eyes. Accessed 12/16/2022.
- Merck Manual. (2023) Tearing. [online] Available from https://www.merckmanuals.com/professional/eye-disorders/symptoms-of-ophthalmologic-disorders/tearing?query=epiphora. [Last accessed April, 2024].
- Patel J, Levin A, Patel BC. Epiphora. In: StatPearls [Internet]. Treasure Island (FL): StatPearls Publishing; 2024. [online] Available from: https://www.ncbi.nlm.nih.gov/books/NBK557449/

Acute Eye Pain

50

***Section Editor:* Sumitha Nayak**
***Section Co-Editor:* Priya Shivalli**
***Authors:* Sahana Devadas, Sumitha Nayak**

Introduction

Ocular pain is a common complaint which must not be ignored. The children and their parents should seek immediate medical attention. Younger children may be unable to express pain and may manifest with continuous crying.

Etiology

Most often, eye pain occurs due to local causes in the eye. These include:

- Ocular foreign body
- Ocular trauma
- Conjunctival infections
- Dry eye
- Allergic diseases
  - Blepharitis—infections of the eyelid margins
  - Ocular infections—bacterial, viral
- Refractory errors
  - Episcleritis, scleritis, uveitis
  - Functional eye pain
  - Idiopathic eye pain

Approach to a Child with Eye Pain

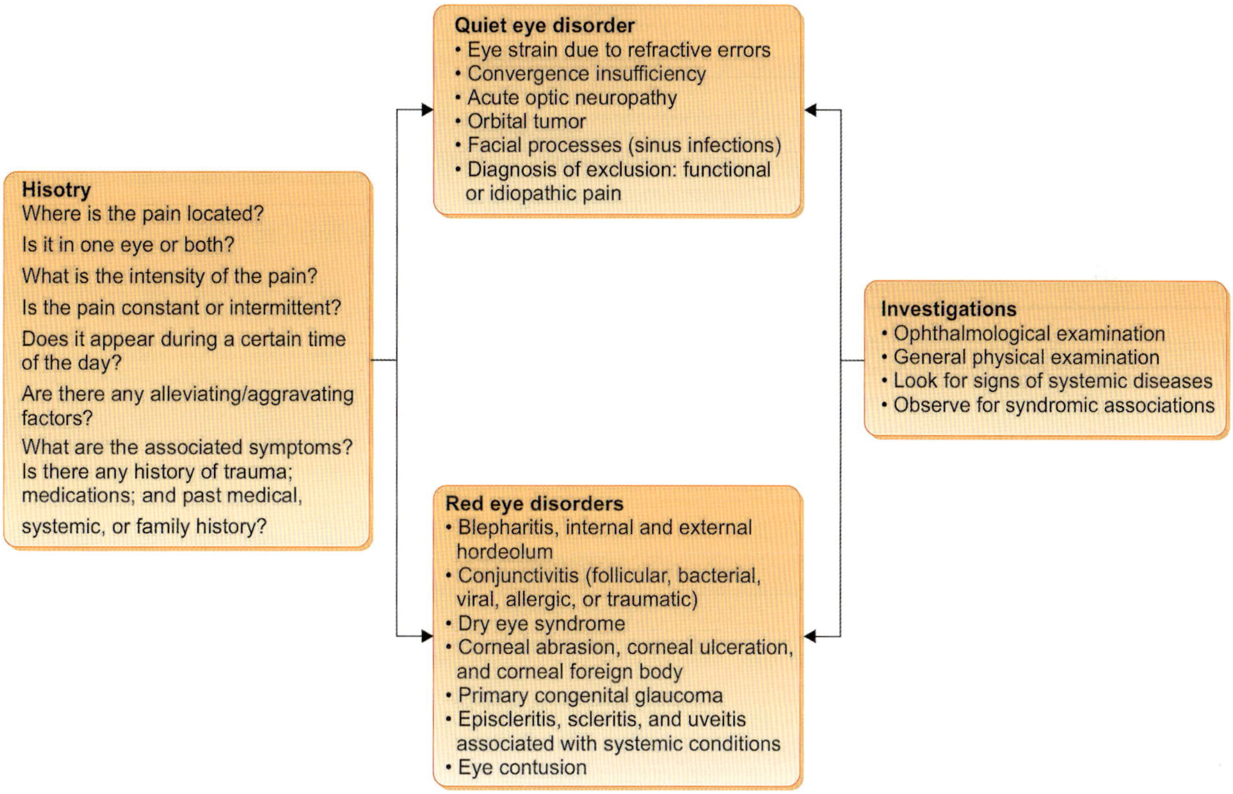

- Most commonly, eye pain is due to foreign body or blunt trauma to the eye.
- Specific ocular examinations could include vision testing as per age and other investigations if the cause has not been correctly identified.
- *Investigations to be done based on the findings obtained from the history and physical examination:*
  - All patients with eye pain should undergo a vision test for vision loss
  - Snellen's chart
  - Kinetic red test
  - Test for visual field defect
  - Visual acuity—up to 20% have visual loss
  - Slit-lamp examination

Diagnostic Pointers

Diagnostic pointers are given in **Tables 1 and 2**.

TABLE 1: History and its possible causes.

HISTORY	POSSIBLE CAUSES
Contact lens use	Corneal abrasion, keratitis, conjunctivitis
Decreased vision	Optic neuritis, keratitis, scleritis, uveitis, angle-closure glaucoma, and cellulitis
Foreign body sensation	Corneal abrasion, dry eye syndrome, keratitis, and retained foreign body
Headache	Acute angle closure glaucoma, scleritis, cluster headache, and migraine
Photophobia	Keratitis, uveitis, corneal abrasion, and migraines
Stabbing or boring eye pain	Scleritis and cluster headache

TABLE 2: Physical examination and its possible causes.

PHYSICAL EXAMINATION	POSSIBLE CAUSES
Conjunctival injection	Conjunctivitis, keratitis, uveitis, and scleritis
Eyelid swelling	Hordeolum, orbital cellulitis, and preseptal cellulitis
Increased intraocular pressure	Acute angle closure glaucoma
Pain with extraocular movement	Acute angle closure glaucoma, scleritis, optic neuritis, and orbital cellulitis
Positive penlight test	Keratitis, uveitis
Positive swinging flashlight test	Optic neuritis

Red Flag Signs

- Allergic eye disease is usually seen in young children, with a chief complaint of eye rubbing.
- Moderate or severe pain with discharge and photophobia: Corneal involvement/severe allergic disease
- Acute-onset pain with localized circumcorneal congestion—anterior segment etiology
- Diffuse congestion—posterior segment etiology
- Intolerance to bright light while watching screens and discharge

Algorithm for Eye Pain

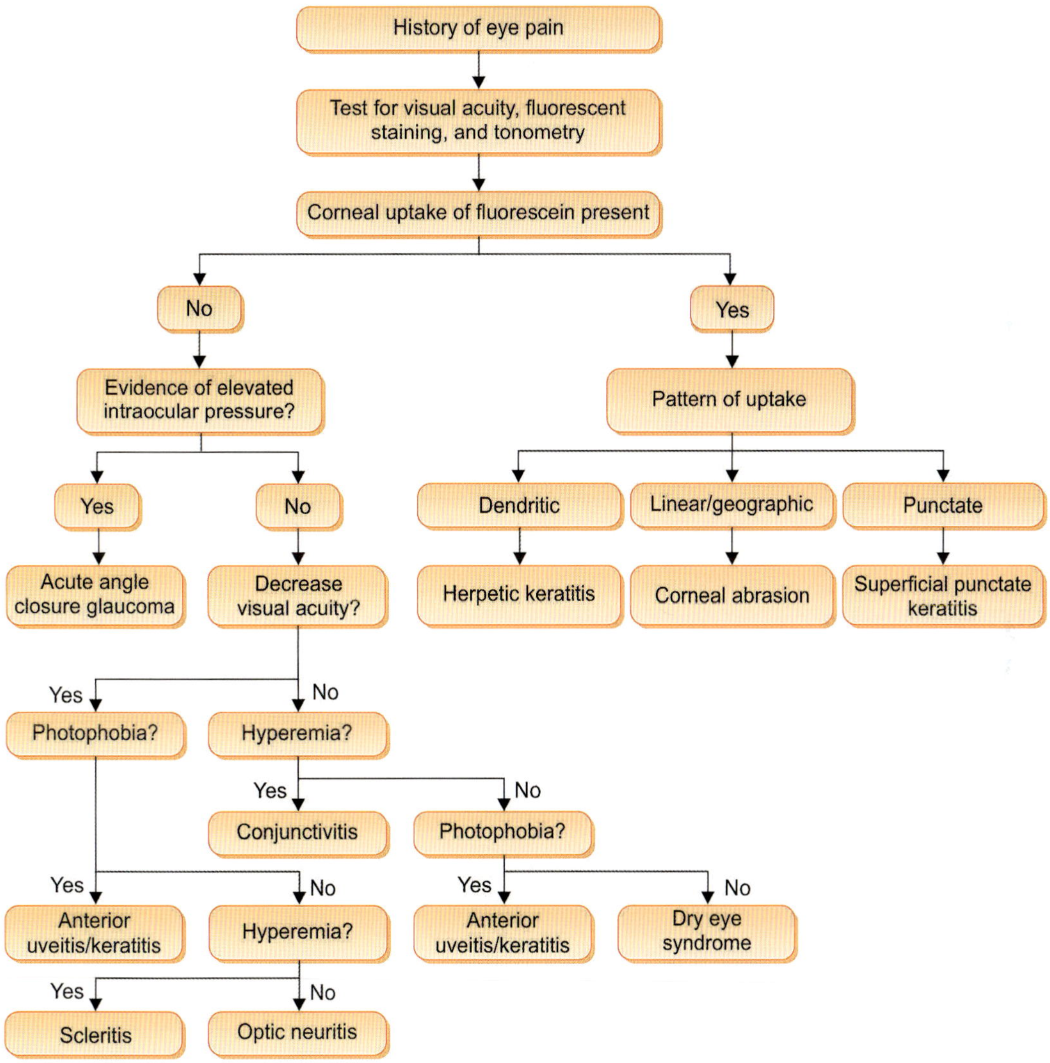

Suggested Reading

- Aguilera ZP, Chen PL. Eye Pain in Children. Pediatr Rev. 2016;37(10):418-25.
- Grönlund MA, Aring E, Landgren M, Hellström A. Visual function and ocular features in children and adolescents with attention deficit hyperactivity disorder, with and without treatment with stimulants. Eye (London, England). 2007;21(4):494-502.
- Indian Academy of Pediatrics (IAP). Standard Treatment Guidelines 2022. [online] Available from https://iapindia.org/pdf/Ch-101-Allergic-Conjunctivitis.pdf [Last accessed April, 2024].
- Murthy SI, Das S, Deshpande P, Kaushik S, Dave TV, Agashe P, et al. Differential diagnosis of acute ocular pain: Teleophthalmology during COVID-19 pandemic - A perspective. Indian J Ophthalmol. 2020;68(7):1371-9.

Limping Child

51

Section Editor: **Kripasindhu Chatterjee**
Section Co-Editors: **Atanu Bhadra, Ashim Kumar Ghosh**
Author: **Kalpana Datta Chatterjee**

Introduction

A limp is any deviation from the normal gait pattern. An abnormal gain in a child is a cause of concern for parents and pediatricians.

Patterns of *abnormal gait:*

- *Antalgic gait:*
  - Short stepping
  - Reduce stance time on affected side.
  - Spine pain
  - Slow stiff gradual movement to avoid jarring
- *Short-limb gait:*
  - Limb length discrepancy (LLD) >5%
  - Toe walk/shoulder drops on the same side
  - Compensatory knee bend on the contralateral side
- *Trendelenburg gait:*
  - Weak abductors, abnormal fulcrum
  - Pelvis drops on the opposite side
  - Compensatory leaning on the affected side
- Waddling gait
- *Duck-like gait* with bilateral hip involvement/neurologic disease

Causes of Limp

Common causes of limp in different ages are given in **Boxes 1 to 3**.

BOX 1: Causes of limp in toddlers (1–3 years).

PAINLESS LIMP	PAINFUL LIMP
• Developmental dysplasia of the hip • Neuromuscular disorder • Cerebral palsy	• Septic arthritis and osteomyelitis • Transient synovitis • Intervertebral diskitis • Occult trauma ("toddler's fracture") • Malignancy

BOX 2: Causes of limp in a child (3–10 years).

PAINLESS LIMP	PAINFUL LIMP
• Developmental dysplasia of hip • Legg–Calve–Perthes disease • Polio • Cerebral palsy • Muscular dystrophy (Duchene)	• Septic arthritis • Osteomyelitis • Myositis • Transient synovitis • Trauma • Rheumatological disorders • Juvenile idiopathic arthritis (JIA) • Intervertebral diskitis

BOX 3: Causes of limp in an adolescent (11–15 years).

PAINLESS LIMP	PAINFUL LIMP
• Slipped capital femoral epiphysis (chronic, stable) • Developmental dysplasia of hip (acetabular dysplasia) • Lower extremity length inequality • Neuromuscular disorder	• Septic arthritis • Osteomyelitis • Myositis • Trauma • Rheumatological disorder • Slipped capital femoral epiphysis (acute, unstable)

Clinical Assessment

History

A detailed history should be taken from the child and the parents.

Specific characteristics of the pain should be noted using the **OPQRST** pattern:

- ***Onset:*** When was the onset of pain? Was it gradual or acute? What are the inciting factors or history of trauma?
- ***Provocation:*** What makes the pain better or worse? Are anti-inflammatory medications helpful?
- ***Quality:*** Is it burning, dull, "achy"?
- ***Radiation:*** Does the pain radiate?
- ***Severity:*** Does it limit the child' s activity?
- ***Timing:*** How long do painful episodes last? Do episodes occur during sleep?

Associated symptoms: Fever, weight loss, night sweats, anorexia, and general malaise may indicate the etiology.

Previous medical and surgical history, recent travel, immunizations, and developmental history must be asked for.

Physical Examination

To identify the type of limp, localize the site of pathology.

Preferably observe the child barefoot and undressed for better assessment of stance and gait. Abdomen, pelvis, back, and extremities should also be inspected and palpated. Focal examination should be done if infection or trauma is suspected.

Laboratory Studies

- Routine investigations—complete blood count (CBC), C-reactive protein (CRP) and erythrocyte sedimentation rate (ESR)
- Synovial fluid analysis—septic arthritis/transient synovitis
- Blood culture—infective suspicion
- Immunologic laboratory studies—rheumatological origin

Radiographic Assessment

- Plain radiographs—anteroposterior and lateral views of the involved area with one joint above and below
- Ultrasonography
- CT scan
- MRI/MR angiography

Red Flags

- Fever and rigors
- Night pain, night sweats, lymphadenopathy, hepato/splenomegaly and weight loss
- Back pain and abnormal neurology
- Pallor, bruising and sickle cell disease
- Limp >4 weeks
- Failure to thrive
- Recurrent infections
- Age >10 years of age
- Obesity in children >8 years of age

Approach to a Child with Limp

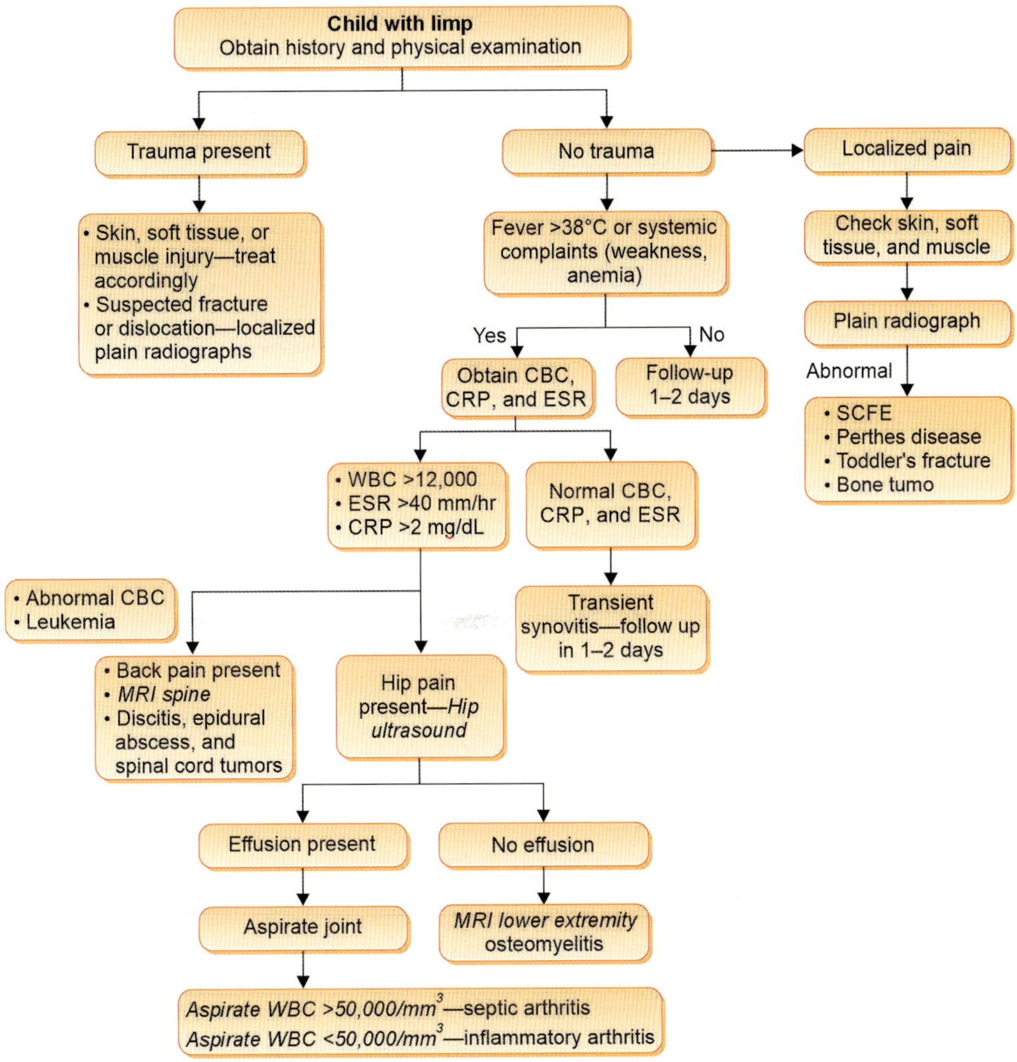

(CBC: complete blood count; CRP: C-reactive protein; ESR: erythrocyte sedimentation rate; SCFE: slipped capital femoral epiphysis; WBC: white blood cell)

Suggested Reading

- Barkin RM, Barkin SZ, Barkin AZ. The limping child. J Emerg Med. 2000;18(3):331-9.
- Chambers HG, Sutherland DH. A practical guide to gait analysis. J Am Acad Orthop Surg. 2002;10(3):222-31.
- Delaney RA, Lenehan B, O'Sullivan L, et al. The limping child: an algorithm to outrule musculoskeletal sepsis. Ir J Med Sci. 2007;176 (3):181-7.
- Flynn JM, Widmann RF. The limping child: evaluation and diagnosis. J Am Acad Orthop Surg. 2001;9(2):89-98.
- Sawyer JR, Kapoor M. The limping child: a systematic approach to diagnosis. Am Fam Physician. 2009;79(3):215-24.

Abdominal Mass

52

Section Editor: **B Rajsekhar**
Section Co-Editor: **Suchitra Pusapati**
Author: **Aathira Ravindranath**

Introduction

Children can present with an abdominal mass due to a number of underlying conditions including infection, inflammation, malignancy, or congenital reasons.

Approach

- The first step is to determine the site of origin of the mass which can originate from the parietal wall or intra-abdominal space. The intra-abdominal masses can originate from intraperitoneal or retroperitoneal sites **(Flowchart 1)**.
- Assess the organ of origin **(Table 1)**.
- Ascertain the possible etiology—infection, inflammation, malignancy, congenital.

FLOWCHART 1: Approach to mass abdomen.

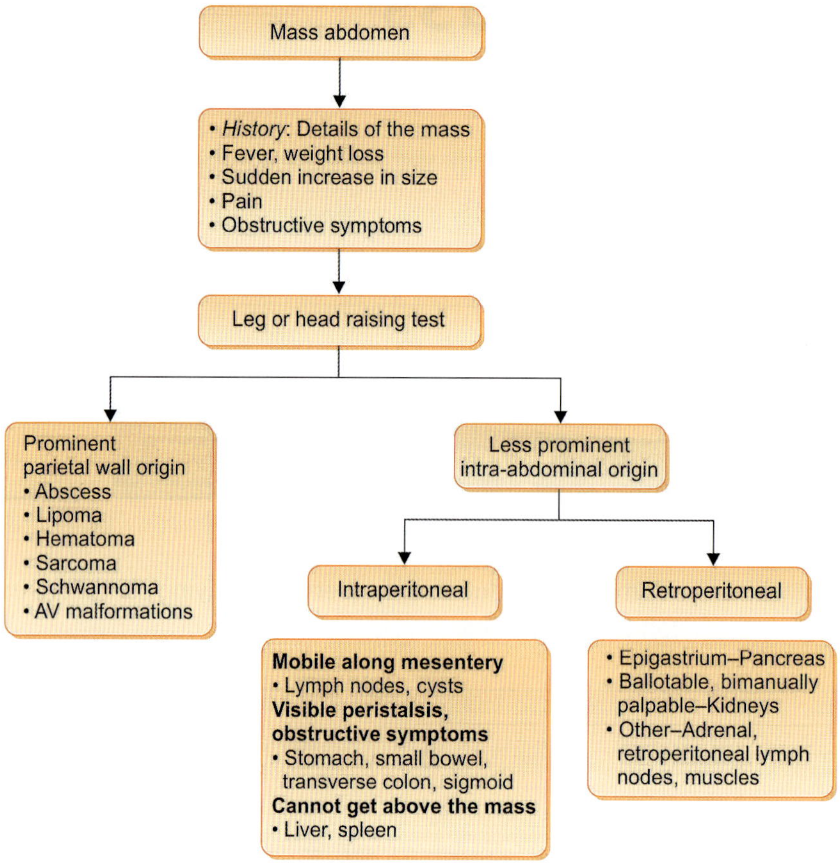

TABLE 1: Organ of origin in different quadrants.

Epigastrium	*Right hypochondrium*	*Left hypochondrium*	*Periumbilical*	*Right lumbar*	*Left lumbar*	*Hypogastrium*	*Right iliac*	*Left iliac*
Pancreatic mass	Liver	Spleen	Small bowel	Kidney	Kidney	Urinary bladder	Appendix	Recto-sigmoid
Gastric mass	Gallbladder	Kidney	Lymph nodes	Adrenal	Adrenal	Adnexa	Meckel's diverticulum	
Duodenal	Bile duct	Adrenal	Retroperitoneal muscles	Retroperitoneal muscles, lymph nodes	Retroperitoneal muscles, lymph nodes		Ileocecal region	
Lymph nodes	Hepatic flexure	Splenic flexure		Ascending colon	Descending colon			
Transverse colon								

History

- Age of the child
- Time when the mass was noticed
- Site of initial appearance of the mass
- Rate of increase in size—malignancies or intralesional bleed can increase the size rapidly
- Associated pain
- Constitutional symptoms
- Bowel habits, urinary symptoms

Red Flags

- Fever
- Weight loss
- Sudden increase in size of mass
- Severe pain
- Sudden pallor
- Symptoms of obstruction—vomiting, obstipation
- Jaundice
- Hematemesis or melena
- History of trauma

Investigations

- Investigations are based on the clinical suspicion.
- **Routine blood workup:** Hemogram, renal functions, liver function tests, electrolytes, and further tests may be planned based on the suspected etiology and organ of origin. For example, neuroblastoma—urinary metanephrine, normetanephrine, vasoactive intestinal peptide (VIP) in case of VIPoma, alpha-fetoprotein in case of hepatoblastoma.
- **Abdominal X-ray erect:** Air–fluid levels in case of obstruction.
- **Ultrasonogram:** To determine whether the lesion is solid or cystic and provide the first clue about the organ of origin.
- Cross sectional imaging like computed tomography with intravenous contrast or magnetic resonance imaging will determine the organ of origin and possible etiology.
- Image-guided biopsy may be needed based on the suspected etiology.

Suggested Reading

- Bilal M, Voin V, Topale N, Iwanaga J, Loukas M, Tubbs RS. The Clinical anatomy of the physical examination of the abdomen: A comprehensive review. Clin Anat. 2017;30:352-6.
- Ferguson CM. Inspection, Auscultation, Palpation, and Percussion of the Abdomen. In: Walker HK, Hall WD, Hurst JW (Eds). Clinical Methods: The History, Physical, and Laboratory Examinations, 3rd edition. Boston: Butterworths; 1990. (Chapter 93).

Hypertonia

53

Section Editor: Kripasindhu Chatterjee
Section Co-Editors: Atanu Bhadra, Ashim Kumar Ghosh
Author: Bela Verma

Introduction

Hypertonia or increased muscle tone is one aspect of an underlying problem of movement and posture.

Definition

Hypertonia—abnormally increased resistance to externally imposed movement around a joint. There are three subtypes of neurologically mediated hypertonia:

1. *Spasticity:* With one or both of the following signs:
   - Resistance to externally imposed movement increases with increasing speed of stretch and varies with the direction of joint movement
   - Resistance to externally imposed movement rises rapidly above a threshold speed or joint angle
2. *Dystonia*—movement disorder with involuntary sustained or intermittent muscle contractions causes twisting and repetitive movements, abnormal postures, or both
3. *Rigidity*—hypertonia with ALL of the following:
   - Resistance to externally imposed joint movement at very low speeds of movement, does not depend on imposed speed, and does not exhibit a speed or angle threshold
   - Simultaneous co-contraction of agonists and antagonists with an immediate resistance to a reversal of the direction of movement about a joint
   - The limb does not tend to return toward a particular fixed posture or extreme joint angle
   - Voluntary activity in distant muscle groups does not lead to involuntary movements about the rigid joints, although rigidity may worsen.

Mixed tone—when two subtypes of hypertonia are present.

Etiology

- Classification according to anatomical site:

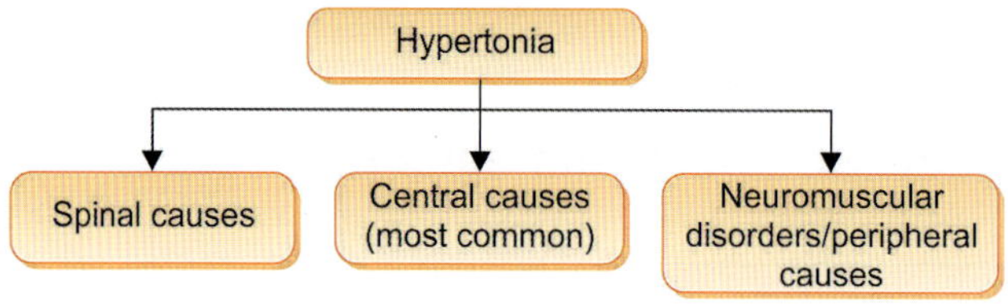

- Risk factors:

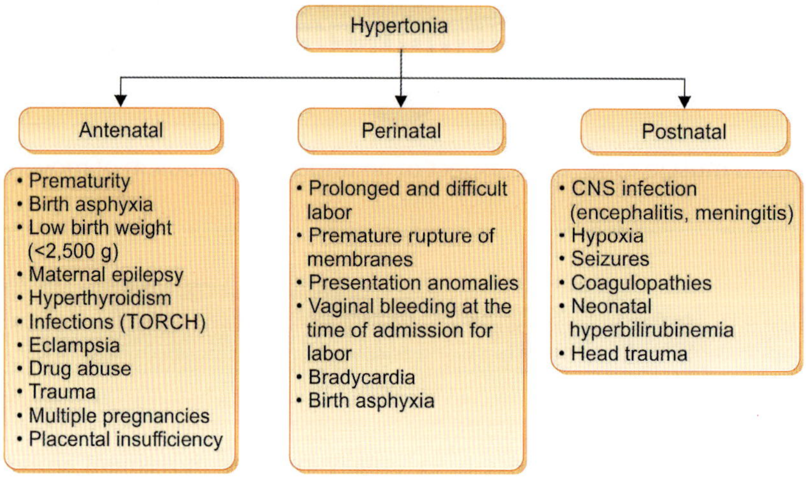

(CNS: central nervous system; TORCH: toxoplasmosis, others, rubella, cytomegalovirus, herpes simplex)

- According to time of presentation:

Neonatal hypertonia presenting on day 1 of life:

- Meningitis/meningoencephalitis
- Cerebral abscess
- Acute intracranial hemorrhage
- Ischemic stroke/cerebral sinus venous thrombosis
- Tonic seizures
- Hydrocephalus
- Congenital intracranial tumors
- Antenatal brain injury—antenatal hypoxia, fetal intracranial hemorrhage, vascular phenomena, and trauma

Neonatal hypertonia presenting after day 1 of life:

Central causes:

- Hypoxic ischemic encephalopathy (HIE)
- Spinal trauma/hemorrhage/cervical myelopathy
- Bilirubin encephalopathy
- Metabolic abnormalities (organic acidurias)
- Mitochondrial disorders
- TORCH infections

Peripheral causes:

- Neonatal tetanus
- Schwartz–Jampel syndrome types 1B and 2
- Hereditary hypertonia/Isaac syndrome

Red Flag Signs

SIGN	SUGGESTIVE OF
Shrill cry, and opisthotonus	Kernicterus
Irritability, fever, and signs of sepsis	Meningitis/meningoencephalitis
Bulging fontanelle, and sunset sign	Hydrocephalus
Encephalopathy, and signs of multiorgan dysfunction	Metabolic disturbance

Persistent hypertonia from birth is unusual and needs further evaluation.

Approach to Hypertonia

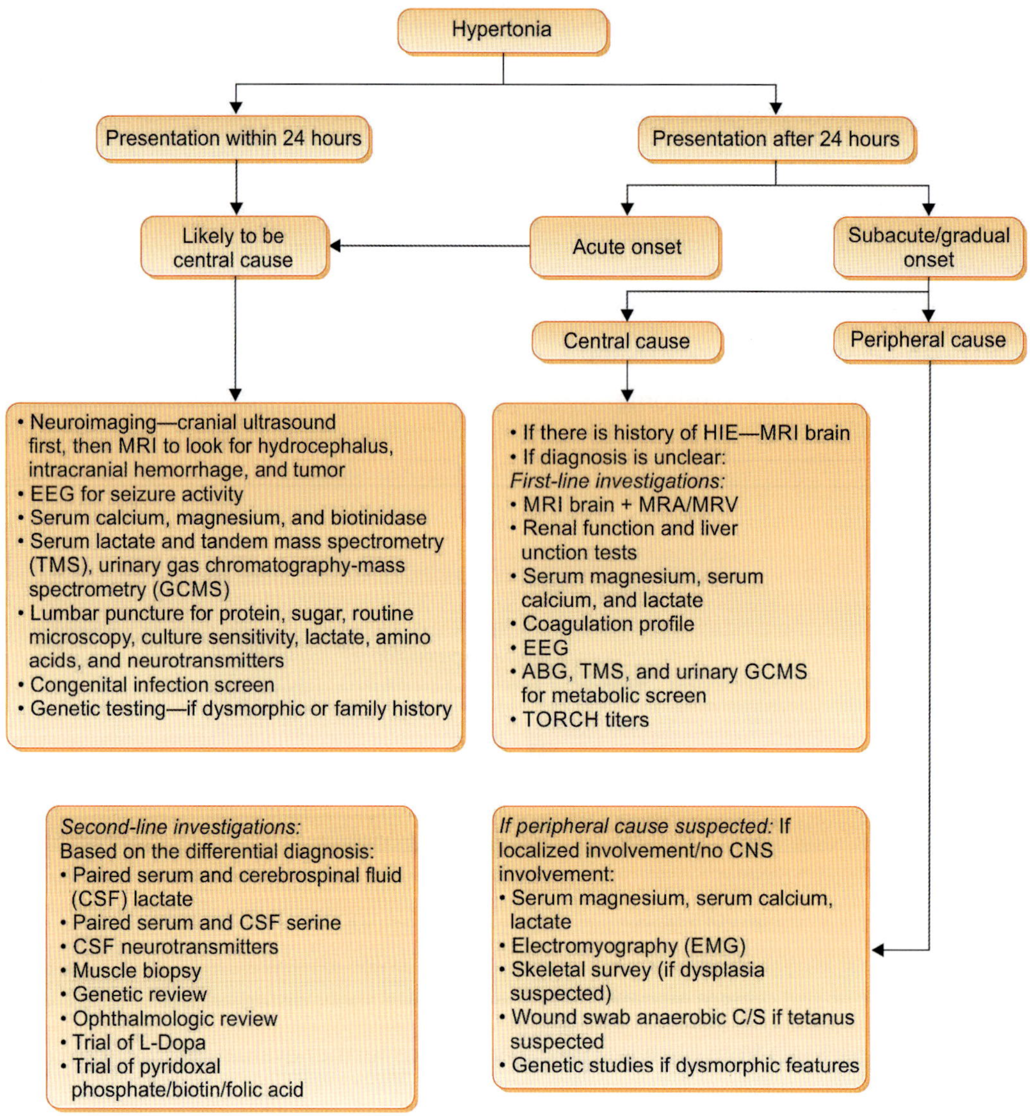

Suggested Reading

- Dy R, Roge D. Medical Updates in Management of Hypertonia. Phys Med Rehabil Clin N Am. 2020;31(1):57-68.
- Hart AR, Sharma R, Rittey CD, Mordekar SR. Neonatal hypertonia - a diagnostic challenge. Dev Med Child Neurol. 2015;57(7):600-10.
- Jethwa A, Mink J, Macarthur C, Knights S, Fehlings T, Fehlings D. Development of the Hypertonia Assessment Tool (HAT): a discriminative tool for hypertonia in children. Dev Med Child Neurol. 2010;52(5):e83-7.
- Lumsden DE, Cadwgan J. Fifteen-minute consultation: A clinical approach to the management of the child with hypertonia. Arch Dis Child Educ Pract Ed. 2020;105(5):276-81.
- Sanger TD, Delgado MR, Gaebler-Spira D, Hallett M, Mink JW; Task Force on Childhood Motor Disorders. Classification and definition of disorders causing hypertonia in childhood. Pediatrics. 2003;111(1):e89-97.

Hypotonia in Infants

54

Section Editor: **Kripasindhu Chatterjee**
Section Co-Editors: **Atanu Bhadra, Ashim Kumar Ghosh**
Authors: **Jaydeb Ray, Pradip Paria**

Introduction

- Hypotonia indicates a decreased muscle tone or physiologic resistance to movement of a muscle through its range of motion. It differs from weakness, which indicates a decrease in muscle power.
- Hypotonia may be apparent or subtle in presentation. It may be due to central (upper motor neuron) or peripheral (lower motor neuron) nervous system involvement. Central hypotonia is more common (70–80%).

Etiology

- *Central:*
  - Cerebral malformation
  - Hypoxic–ischemic encephalopathy
  - Intracranial hemorrhage
  - Congenital infection, e.g., TORCH
  - Endocrine—hypothyroidism
  - Inborn errors of metabolism, e.g., Pompe's disease, carnitine deficiency and mucopolysaccharidosis
  - Chromosomal/syndromes (with facial dysmorphism): Trisomy 21, Prader–Willi syndrome
  - Spinal cord injury—birth trauma

- *Peripheral:*
  - *Anterior horn cell:* Spinal muscular atrophy (SMA) type 1
  - *Peripheral nerve:* Charcot–Marie–Tooth (CMT) disease
  - *Neuromuscular junction:* Myasthenia gravis
  - *Muscles:* Congenital myopathies, muscular dystrophy, myotonic dystrophy

Red Flag Signs

- Diffuse encephalopathy
- Developmental regression
- Progressive hypotonia
- Seizure
- Metabolic crisis
- Respiratory failure

Approach

History

A history of polyhydramnios and fetal akinesia

Complicated delivery with birth trauma/perinatal depression. A family history of consanguinity, affected parents, siblings—in cases of congenital myotonic dystrophy, SMA, or metabolic disorders

Physical Examination

Dysmorphism in the case of Down syndrome, trisomies 13 and 18, peroxisomal disorder, or congenital disorder of glycosylation

Central nervous system (CNS) involvement—as abnormal head circumferences, encephalopathy, seizures, and respiratory and feeding abnormalities

Extraneural involvement—multiorgan dysfunction, organomegaly, and heart failure suggest systemic disorders. Respiratory (congenital myopathy, SMA), cardiovascular (cardiomyopathy, arrhythmias in muscular dystrophy) system involvement, associated hypogonadism, contracture, or joint laxity of joints in peripheral nervous system involvement (PNS)

Neurological Examination

It helps to decide whether cerebral or neuromuscular causes are involved.

Central hypotonia—poor axial but preserved appendicular/limb tone. Dysmorphism usually suggests a genetic cause. Peripheral hypotonia—frog-like posture, decreased antigravity movements of the limbs, and absent deep tendon reflexes **(Table 1)**

Persisting hypotonia can be assessed by picking up the baby when holding him/her under the arms. A hypotonic baby tends to slip through the fingers (vertical suspension). A hypotonic infant hangs like a rag doll when kept in the prone position (horizontal suspension). Is 1 a marked head lag when the infant is pulled forward by the arms from the supine position (pull to seat sign).

TABLE 1: Differences between central and peripheral hypotonia.

	CENTRAL	PERIPHERAL			
		ANTERIOR HORN CELL	NERVE	NEUROMUSCULAR JUNCTION	MUSCLE
Alertness	Reduced alertness	Alert	Alert	Alert	Alert
Seizure	+/– seizure	Absent	Absent	Absent	Absent
Strength	Normal	Generalized weakness	Weakness (distal > proximal)	Weakness + Involvement of facial/bulbar/eye muscles	Weakness (proximal > distal), may involve the face, extraocular muscles
DTRs	Normal/ increased, clonus +	Decreased/ absent	Decreased/ absent	Normal DTRs	Decreased DTRs
Fasciculations	Absent	Fasciculations +	+/– fasciculations	No fasciculations	No fasciculation
Associated features	+/– dysmorphism	–	–	+/– arthrogryposis	+/– contractures

(DTR: deep tendon reflexes)

Diagnosis

Prioritize the differentiation of neuraxial localization, i.e., CNS or PNS involvement. If the hypotonia is due to CNS involvement, neuroimaging (CT/MRI brain), electroencephalography (EEG), tandem mass spectrometry (TMS)/gas chromatography-mass spectrometry (GCMS), and ammonia/lactate estimation are the primary investigations. In PNS, the most useful initial test is creatine kinase (CK), thyroid profile, and nerve conduction study (NCS) with electromyography (EMG).

Approach to a Hypotonic Infant

Approach to a hypotonic infant is shown in **Flowchart 1**.

FLOWCHART 1: Diagnostic approach in hypotonia.

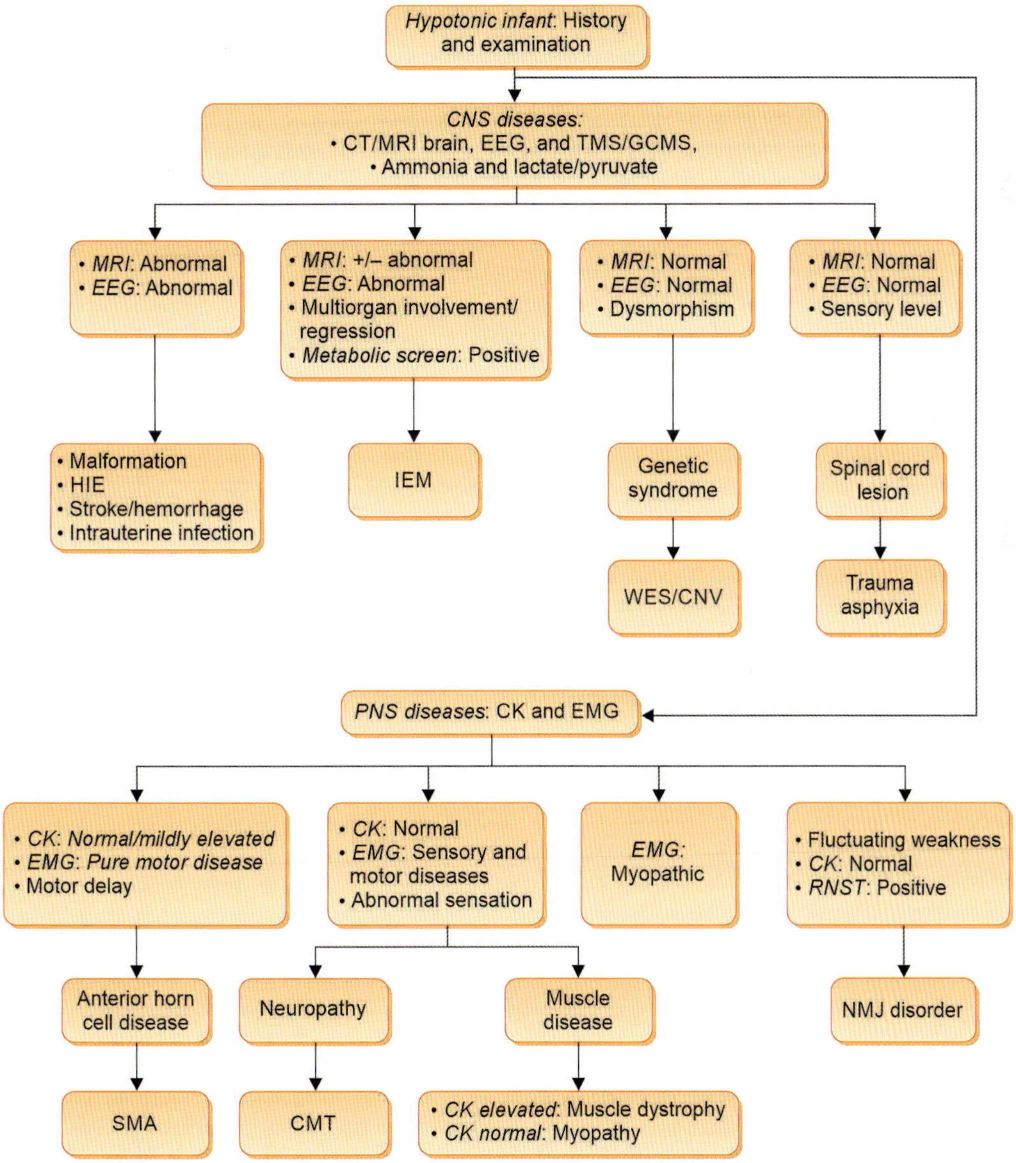

(CK: creatine kinase; CMT: Charcot—Marie–Tooth; CNS: central nervous system; CNV: copy number variation; EMG: electromyography; GCMS: gas chromatography-mass spectrometry; IEM: inborn error of metabolism; HIE: hypoxic ischemic encephalopathy; NMJ: neuromuscular junction; RNST: repetitive nerve stimulation test; SMA: spinal muscular atrophy; TMS: tandem mass spectrometry; WES: whole-exome sequencing)

Suggested Reading

- Bodensteiner JB. The evaluation of the hypotonic infant. Semin Pediatr Neurol. 2008;15(1):10-20.
- Johnston H. The floppy weak infant revisited. Brain Develop. 2003;25(3):155-8.
- Paro-Panjan D, Neubauer D. Congenital hypotonia: Is there an algorithm? J Child Neurol. 2004;19(6):439-42.
- Richer LP, Shevell MI, Miller SP. Diagnostic profile of neonatal hypotonia: An 11-year study. Pediatr Neurol. 2001;25(1):32-7.
- Sparks SE. Neonatal hypotonia. Clin Perinatol. 2015;42(2):363-71.

Jaundice

55

Section Editor: B Rajsekhar
Section Co-Editor: Suchitra Pusapati
Authors: GV Basavaraja, Sheetal Sajjan

Introduction

- Jaundice is yellowish discoloration of skin and sclera due to elevated serum bilirubin. Total serum bilirubin >1 mg/dL is considered abnormal beyond the neonatal period.
- *Conjugated hyperbilirubinemia:* Direct bilirubin >1 mg/dL with total bilirubin <5 mg/dL or the direct bilirubin is over 20% of the total bilirubin if total bilirubin is >5 mg/dL.
- Neonatal cholestasis has not been covered in this chapter.

Etiology

Hyperbilirubinemia beyond infancy is usually unconjugated. It is classified into three groups of causes as given in **Table 1**.

TABLE 1: Three groups of causes of hyperbilirubinemia.

JAUNDICE SECONDARY TO INCREASED PRODUCTION OF BILIRUBIN	JAUNDICE SECONDARY TO IMPAIRED BILIRUBIN UPTAKE IN THE LIVER	JAUNDICE SECONDARY TO IMPAIRED BILIRUBIN CONJUGATION
• Inherited red blood cell disorders like thalassemia, sickle cell disease, G6PD deficiency, and hereditary spherocytosis. • Infections—malaria, leptospirosis, and sepsis • Autoimmune hemolytic anemia • Microangiopathic hemolytic anemia • Drug-induced hemolytic anemia—cephalosporins, cotrimoxazole, NSAIDs, cyclosporine, and tacrolimus	• Cardiac failure • Portosystemic shunts	• Inherited disorders—Crigler–Najjar syndrome, and Gilbert syndrome • Acquired liver diseases like chronic hepatitis, chronic liver disease, and Wilson disease • Hyperthyroidism

(G6PD: glucose-6-phosphate dehydrogenase; NSAIDs: nonsteroidal anti-inflammatory drugs)

Conjugated hyperbilirubinemia. It is common in neonates and infants. Causes of conjugated hyperbilirubinemia in older children and adolescents are given in **Box 1**.

BOX 1: Causes of conjugated hyperbilirubinemia in older children and adolescents.

Obstructive causes
• Choledochal cyst • Stone/tumor/parasitic infection in the biliary tract
Hepatocellular causes
• *Infections:* Sepsis (endotoxemia, enterocolitis), hepatitis A, B, C, E, nontypeable hepatitis, HIV • *Metabolic causes:* Wilson disease, Dubin–Johnson syndrome, rotor syndrome, mitochondrial disorders, cystic fibrosis, hemochromatosis • *Endocrine disorders:* Hypothyroidism • *Autoimmune causes:* Autoimmune hepatitis, primary sclerosing cholangitis, and primary biliary cirrhosis • Disorders of intrahepatic bile ducts: Alagille syndrome, PFIC, and congenital hepatic fibrosis • Drugs, toxins, and total parenteral nutrition • *Miscellaneous:* Vascular anomalies, Budd–Chiari syndrome, cardiac insufficiency & hypoperfusion, and trisomy 21

(PFIC: progressive familial intrahepatic cholestasis)

Red Flag Signs

- Marked abdominal pain and tenderness
- Altered mental status
- Gastrointestinal bleeding (occult/gross)
- Features of coagulopathy: Ecchymoses, petechiae, and purpura
- Significant weight loss
- Signs of sepsis
- Rising serum bilirubin with decreasing alanine transaminase/aspartate transaminase (ALT/AST)

Approach to a Child with Jaundice

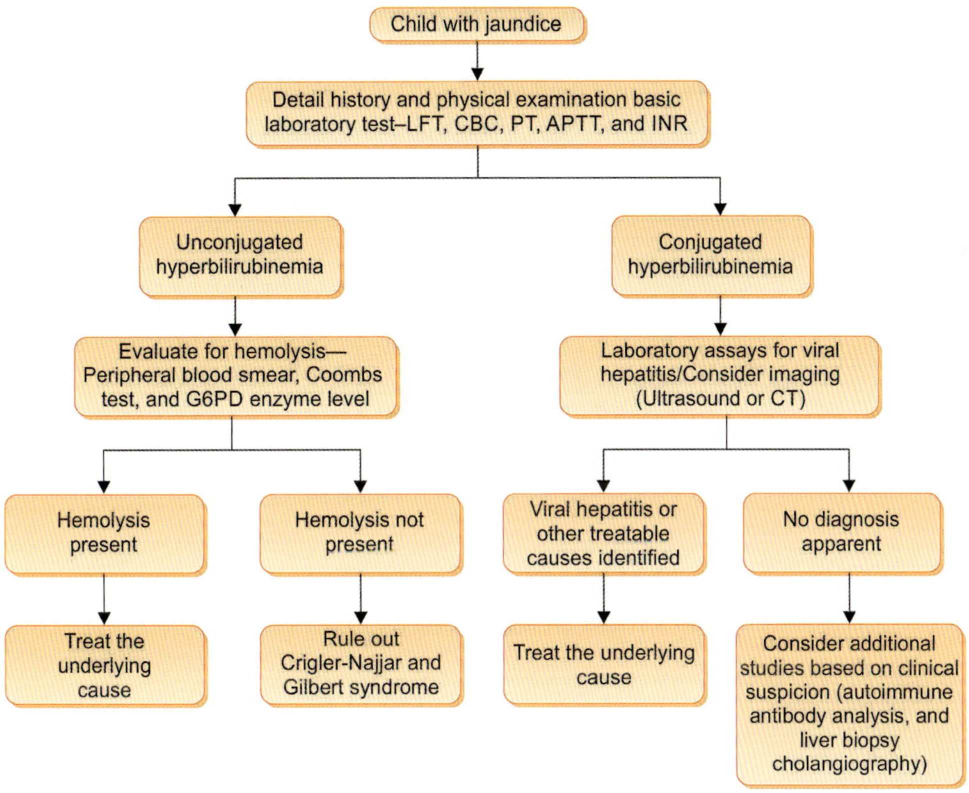

(APTT: activated partial thromboplastin time; CBC: complete blood count; G6PD: glucose-6-phosphate dehydrogenase; INR: international normalized ratio; LFT: liver function test; PT: prothrombin time)

Suggested Reading

- Muniyappa P, Kelley D. Hyperbilirubinemia in pediatrics: Evaluation and care. Curr Probl Pediatr Adolesc Health Care. 2020;50(8):100842.
- Siew SM, Kelly DA. Evaluation of jaundice in children beyond the neonatal period. Paediatr Child Health. 2016;26(10):451-8.
- Telega GW. Jaundice. In: Kliegman RM, Toth H, Bordini BJ, Basel D (Eds). Nelson Pediatric Symptom-Based Diagnosis: Common Diseases and Their Mimics, 2nd edition. Philadelphia: Elsevier; 2022. pp. 255-74.

Proptosis

56

***Section Editor:* Sumitha Nayak**
***Section Co-Editor:* Priya Shivalli**
***Authors:* Madhu S Pujar, Sumitha Nayak**

Introduction

- Proptosis or exophthalmos is defined as protrusion of eyeballs beyond the orbit margins of the eyes, when the patient is looking straight ahead.
- A 2 mm or greater asymmetry between the protrusion of the two eyes is considered as abnormal.

Symptoms and Signs

- Proptosis may be due to defects in the orbit or in the surrounding structures.
- It is manifested by displacement of the globe, associated with local pain, redness, and swelling. It is often accompanied by decreased vision, double vision, optic disc swelling, and impaired ocular movements. Early diagnosis and management are imperative to preventing permanent loss of vision and other complications.

Classification

Proptosis is based on laterality—could be unilateral or bilateral. The causes of each are described in **Box 1**.

BOX 1: Causes of proptosis.

UNILATERAL PROPTOSIS	BILATERAL PROPTOSIS
• Orbital cellulitis	• Associated with thyroid disease
• Developmental anomalies	• Orbital myositis
• Inflammations	• Thrombosis of cavernous sinus
• Anomalies of the vasculature	• Metastasis from neuroblastoma
• Neoplastic growths	
• Metabolic disease	

Differential Diagnosis

Differential diagnosis by age at presentation is given in **Table 1**.

TABLE 1: Differential diagnosis by age at presentation.

1–5 YEARS	5–10 YEARS	>10 YEARS
Dermoid cysts	Pseudotumor cerebri	Pseudotumor cerebri
Metastatic neuroblastoma	Orbital extension of retinoblastoma	Meningioma
Rhabdomyosarcoma	Lymphoma	Tumor of lacrimal glands
Epithelial cyst	Leukemia	Leukemia
Optic nerve glioma	Dermoid cysts	Lymphoma
Sphenoid wing meningioma	Hemangioma	Dermoid cysts
		Hemangioma

Approach

- Detailed history must include the time since onset and any trauma to the eye.
- *Associated pain:* Quality and severity, progression, unilateral or bilateral
- *Vision:* Any changes, diplopia whiter mono-ocular or binocular, horizontal or vertical diplopia
- A detailed history of past events must be elicited, including history of past illness, drug usage, etc.
- Physical examination of the involved eye:
  - Visual acuity, pupils, and intraocular pressure
  - Eye lid—palpebral fissure, and elevator function
  - Observe—any pulsations, globe displacement, and periorbital changes
  - Any bruits heard?
  - Examine anterior segment—conjunctiva status—chemosis, injection, dilated, or tortuous vessels
  - Corneal status

Approach to a Child with Proptosis

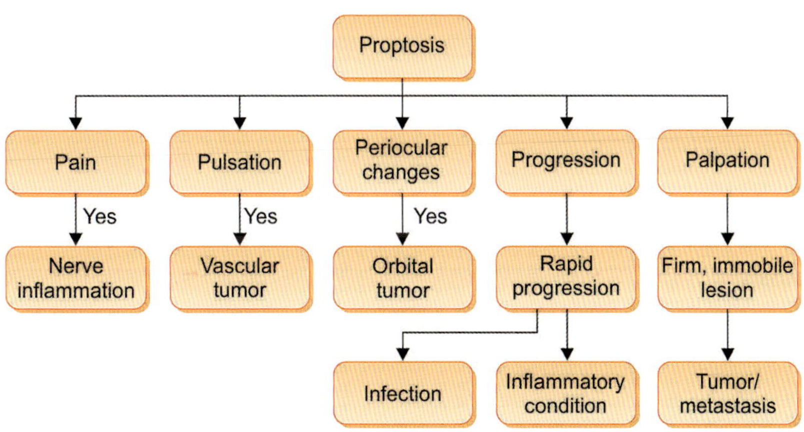

Investigations

- Ophthalmic examination—assess the visual acuity, field of vision
- Ocular pressure
- Examination of anterior and posterior chambers of the eye
- Imaging of the eye—CT and MRI help in clinching the diagnosis

In a nutshell, remember the Ps in History and examination:

- Pain
- Progression
- Palpation
- Pulsation
- Periorbital changes

Red Flag Signs

- Eye pain and redness
- Headache
- Loss of vision
- Diplopia
- Fever
- Pulsating proptosis
- Neonatal proptosis

Suggested Reading

- Dallow LR, Pratt GS, Green PJ. Approach to Orbital disorders and Frequency of Disease occurrence. In, Albert MD, Jakobiec AF (Eds). Principle and Practice of Ophthalmology, 2nd edition. Philadelphia: W B Saunders; 2000. pp. 3057-67.
- Ganessan K, Bakhshi S. Proptosis in children: Approach. Indian J Med Pediatr Onc. 2004;25(Suppl):33-4.
- Kanski J, Bowling B (Eds). Orbit. In: Kanski's Clinical Ophthalmology: A Systematic Approach, 8th edition. Amsterdam: Elsevier; 2016. pp. 82-7.
- Stefanyszyn MA, Robinson DH, Robert BP. Disorders of orbit. In: Nelson LB (Ed). Harley's Paediatric Ophthalmology, 4th edition. Philadelphia: WB Saunders; 1998. pp. 371-96.
- Topilow NJ, Tran AQ, Koo EB, Alabiad CR. Etiologies of proptosis: A review. Intern Med Rev (Wash DC), 2020;6(3). DOI10.18103/imr.v613.852

Sleep Disturbances

57

***Section Editor:* Kripasindhu Chatterjee**
***Section Co-Editors:* Atanu Bhadra, Ashim Kumar Ghosh**
***Authors:* Supratim Datta, Ashim Kumar Ghosh**

Introduction

- The average sleep required for good health in children is 8–10 hours per night.
- Sleep issues can have deleterious effects on school performance and in social relationships.

Results of Sleep Deprivation

Common sleep disorders include the following:

- *Insomnia*: It affects about 20–30% of children.
- Symptoms include difficulty in falling asleep, staying asleep, or both.
- It is divided into three categories:
    1. *Behavioral insomnia*: It is common up to 5 years of age. It is associated with resistance to sleep, taking a long time to fall asleep, and frequent night-time wakings.
    2. *Conditioned insomnia*: It is more common in older children and adolescents. It is associated with feelings of anxiety related to bedtime and sleep.
    3. *Transient sleep disturbances:* These involve temporary disruptions in a child's normal routine like traveling, illness, and stressful life events.
- *Obstructive sleep apnea:* It occurs when soft tissues in the throat block the air passage during sleep. Common causes are enlarged tonsils, obesity, and birth defects. It affects 1–5% of children.
- *Snoring in children:* It affects 10–17% of children. It is relatively common and does not always indicate a larger issue.

- *Sleepwalking and bedwetting:* Sleepwalking/somnambulism involves walking or engaging in other complex behaviors while asleep. Bedwetting/nocturnal enuresis is involuntary urination during asleep.

Both of these are more common in children than adults. Approximately 5% of children exhibit signs of sleepwalking and 15% of children experience bedwetting and both resolve with age.

- *Night terrors:* It is a type of parasomnia where the sleeper suddenly awakens feeling frightened and panicked, with no recollection of the event. It occurs in non-rapid eye movement (NREM) stage of sleep in 30% of children. A familial predisposition may occur.
- *Nightmares:* These occur during rapid eye movement (REM) stage of sleep associated with dreaming. Nightmares are associated with stress/major life events.
- *Restless leg syndrome or Willis–Ekbom disease:* It is a movement disorder that can significantly disturb sleep. The main symptom is a painless but overwhelming urge to move the legs. It may be due to iron deficiency or may be genetic. It is underdiagnosed in children.
- *Excessive daytime sleepiness:* It is associated with reduced alertness, increased sleepiness, and falling asleep during the day. It occurs in 10–20% children. It is commonly associated with a number of sleep-related and ill-health conditions.
- *Bruxism:* Bruxism, or repetitive teeth grinding, can occur during the day or night. If occurring at night, it can disrupt sleep. It may lead to painful symptoms—headaches, tooth damage, and jaw muscle injury. It may be associated with stress. It tends to lessen with age and can be recurrent.

Red Flag Signs

- Snoring
- Breathing pauses during breathing
- Trouble falling asleep
- Problems with sleeping through the night
- Trouble staying awake during daytime

Approach

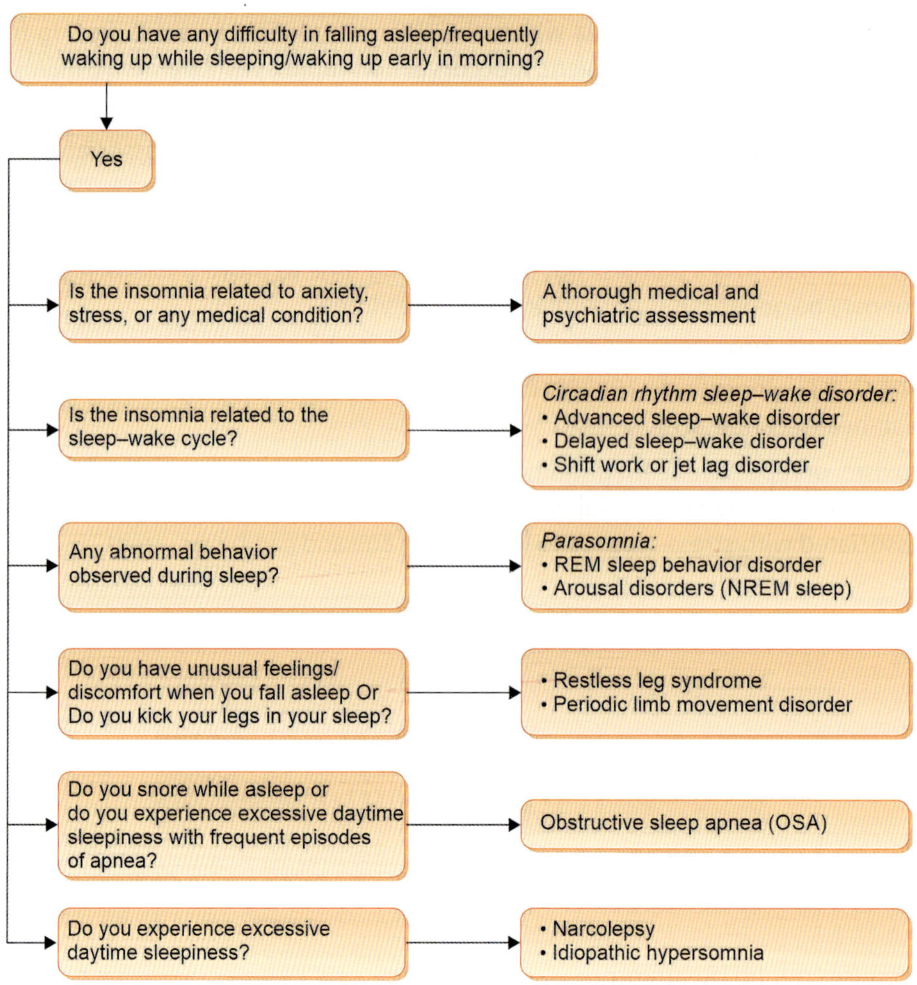
Do you have any difficulty in falling asleep/frequently waking up while sleeping/waking up early in morning?
Yes
Is the insomnia related to anxiety, stress, or any medical condition?
A thorough medical and psychiatric assessment
Is the insomnia related to the sleep–wake cycle?
Circadian rhythm sleep–wake disorder:
• Advanced sleep–wake disorder
• Delayed sleep–wake disorder
• Shift work or jet lag disorder
Any abnormal behavior observed during sleep?
Parasomnia:
• REM sleep behavior disorder
• Arousal disorders (NREM sleep)
Do you have unusual feelings/ discomfort when you fall asleep Or Do you kick your legs in your sleep?
• Restless leg syndrome
• Periodic limb movement disorder
Do you snore while asleep or do you experience excessive daytime sleepiness with frequent episodes of apnea?
Obstructive sleep apnea (OSA)
Do you experience excessive daytime sleepiness?
• Narcolepsy
• Idiopathic hypersomnia

Suggested Reading

- Mansur A, Castillo PR, Rocha Cabrero F, Rizwan A. Bokhari S. Restless Legs Syndrome. [Updated 2023 Feb 27]. In: StatPearls [Internet]. Treasure Island (FL): StatPearls Publishing; 2023 Jan-. [online] Available from https://www.ncbi.nlm.nih.gov/books/NBK430878/ [Last accessed May, 2024].
- Patel AK, Reddy V, Shumway KR, Araujo F. Physiology, Sleep Stages. [Updated 2022 Sep 7]. In: StatPearls [Internet]. Treasure Island (FL): StatPearls Publishing; 2023 Jan-. [online] Available from https://www.ncbi.nlm.nih.gov/books/NBK526132/ [Last accessed May, 2024].
- Schwab RJ. (2022). Insomnia and excessive daytime sleepiness (EDS). Merck Manual Consumer Version. [online] Available from https://www.merckmanuals.com/home/brain,-spinal-cord,-and-nerve-disorders/sleep-disorders/insomnia-and-excessive-daytime-sleepiness-eds [Last accessed May, 2024].
- Stallman HM, Kohler M. Prevalence of Sleepwalking: A Systematic Review and Meta-Analysis. PLoS One. 2016; 11(11):e0164769.
- Summer J, Vyas N. (2023). Sleep disorders in children. [online] Available from https://www.sleepfoundation.org/children-and-sleep/sleep-disorders-in-children [Last accessed May, 2024].
- Wieckiewicz M, Paradowska-Stolarz A, Wieckiewicz W. Psychosocial aspects of bruxism: The most paramount factor influencing teeth grinding. BioMed Res Int. 2014;2014:1-7.

Edema

58

Section Editor: **Nehal Patel**
Section Co-Editor: **Jay T Dhirwani**
Authors: **Kinnari Vala, Vaibhav Shah, Shaad Abqari**

Introduction

- Edema indicates an abnormal swelling of tissues, due to excess fluid accumulation in the extracellular fluid (ECF) compartment, due to sodium and water retention by the kidneys.
- It can be generalized or localized. Localized fluid accumulations in pleural or peritoneal cavities are pleural effusion and ascites.

Etiopathogenesis

Major causes of edema in children are given in **Table 1**.

TABLE 1: Major causes of edema in children as per pathogenesis.

PRIMARY RENAL SODIUM RETENTION	SECONDARY RENAL SODIUM RETENTION
Acute kidney injury (AKI)	Nephrotic syndrome (NS)
Glomerular disease	Cardiac failure
Chronic kidney disease (CKD)	Cirrhosis
	Nutritional deficiencies
	Hormonal factors
	Drug-induced edema

Red Flags

- Associated redness
- Breathlessness
- Diaphoresis and extreme irritability
- Feeding difficulty
- Respiratory distress and grunting in young infants

Etiopathological Approach

In a child with a history of some chronic organ involvement, the new-onset edema/worsening of edema could point to the worsening of the previous disease. Always ask for past history of illness **(Table 2)**.

TABLE 2: Systemic approach for edema in a child.

ORGAN/ SYSTEM INVOLVED	CAUSES	IMPORTANT HISTORY	PHYSICAL EXAMINATION	LABORATORY INVESTIGATIONS
Kidney	NS, AKI, glomerular disease, systemic vasculitis, CKD	Acute/chronic, may start with periorbital involvement, along with oliguria, anuria, history of hematuria, history suggestive of symptoms and signs of uremia, poor growth in CKD	Periorbital edema, hypertension, acidotic breathing, symptoms of pulmonary edema may occur in acute glomerulonephritis, stunting, and wasting in CKD	• Urine routine examination may show proteinuria and hematuria • Low serum albumin levels in NS, elevated creatinine, urea, low complement 3 levels, high ASO, hyperkalemia, metabolic acidosis, hyperphosphatemia, anemia
Heart	• Heart failure • Structurally normal heart—cardiomyopathies, myocarditis, arrhythmias, drugs, vasculitis, ischemic, noncardiac—sepsis • Congenital heart defects—volume overload (shunts, regurgitant lesions) and pressure overload (AS, PS) conditions	Tachypnea, diaphoresis during feeding, poor feeding, reduced weight gain, lethargy, and irritability	• Tachycardia, tachypnea, rales or wheezes, gallop rhythm, hepatomegaly, and edema (lower extremities) • Peripheral edema is generally less common in children with heart failure than in adult	• CXR, ECG, and ECHO • Biomarkers (BNP, NT-pro BNP), metabolic and genetic testing in selected cases. CMRI

Contd...

Contd...

ORGAN/ SYSTEM INVOLVED	CAUSES	IMPORTANT HISTORY	PHYSICAL EXAMINATION	LABORATORY INVESTIGATIONS
Gastrointestinal	• Protein malabsorption d/t celiac disease, exocrine pancreatic insufficiency, because of tropical sprue, and giardiasis • Protein-losing enteropathy d/t inflammatory bowel disease, intestinal tuberculosis, intestinal lymphangiectasia, immunodeficiency, and malignancy	Growth failure, chronic/recurrent diarrhea, blood/oil in stools, recurrent/ chronic vomiting/ abdominal pain, postprandial bloating, positive family history, recurrent skin/ respiratory infections, history of recurrent blood/albumin transfusions	Abdominal distension with wasting of peripheries, pallor, signs of fat malabsorption, perianal involvement, and skin lesions	Elevated tTG IgA, decreased fecal elastase, elevated fecal alpha-1-antitrypsin, stool giardia Ag positive, elevated fecal calprotectin, reduced immunoglobulins, HIV ELISA positive, primary immunodeficiency workup positive, MR/CT enterography showing changes of IBD/ITB, UGI ± LGI scopy with biopsies, and HPE examination of duodenal/small bowel/ colonic biopsies help in diagnosis of celiac Dx/ IBD/ITB/PID/PIL
Endocrinological causes	Hypothyroidism, SIADH, mineralocorticoids excess	History of medications, appetite, diet history, and voiding volume chart	Weight gain, mild edema, dry skin, mask-like face, and hypertension	Thyroid function tests, electrolytes, sugar levels, and urine routine examination
Nutritional	Kwashiorkor	Socioeconomic history, family history, h/o tuberculosis, and diet history	Other features s/o malnutrition, pallor, skin, and hair changes	Complete anthropometry, developmental examination, anemia, hypoalbuminemia, etc.
Drug-induced	Steroids, NSAIDs, penicillin, few antihypertensives, and vasodilators	History of ingestion of drug accidentally or excess dose taken	Features suggestive of drug toxicity may be present	–
Other	Excessive parenteral administration of sodium and water in hospitalized children	Intravenous infusions (one can ask number of bottles in a specified period)	Edema in variable severity	May check sodium level, and creatinine

(AKI: acute kidney injury; AS: aortic stenosis; ASO: antistreptolysin O; BNP: brain natriuretic peptide; CKD: chronic kidney disease; CMRI: cardiac magnetic resonance imaging; CXR: chest X-ray; Dx: disease; ECG: electrocardiography; ECHO: echocardiography; ELISA: enzyme-linked immunosorbent assay; HPE: histopathology; IBD: inflammatory bowel diseases; ITB: intestinal tuberculosis; LGI: lower gastrointestinal; NS: nephrotic syndrome; NSAIDs: nonsteroidal anti-inflammatory drugs; PID: pelvic inflammatory disease; PIL: primary intestinal lymphoma; PS: pulmonary stenosis; SIADH: syndrome of inappropriate antidiuretic hormone; UGI: upper gastrointestinal)

Bedside Approach to a Child Presented with Edema

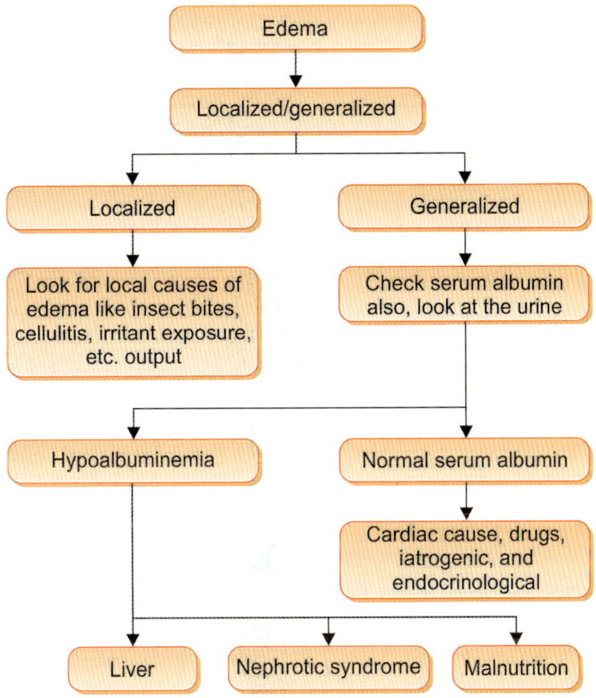

- Urine output may be decreased in nephrotic syndrome, acute kidney injury, and cardiac failure, due to medications.
- Any etiology leading to long-standing intravascular hypovolemia can cause pre- to intrinsic—acute kidney injury, with diminished urine output and edema

Suggested Reading

- Ahmed H, VanderPluym C. Medical management of pediatric heart failure. Cardiovasc Diagn Ther. 2021;11(1): 323-35.
- Das BB. Current state of pediatric heart failure. Children. 2018;5(7):88.
- Jayaprasad N. Heart Failure in Children. Heart Views. 2016;17(3):92-9.
- Meena J, Bagga A. Current Perspectives in Management of Edema in Nephrotic Syndrome. Indian J Pediatr. 87:633-40.
- Valentini RP. (2019). Pathophysiology and etiology of edema in children. UpToDate. [online] Available from https://medilib.ir/UpToDate [Last accessed May, 2024].

Strabismus

59

Section Editor: **Sumitha Nayak**
Section Co-Editor: **Priya Shivalli**
Authors: **Krishna Mohan, Manjusha K**

Introduction

- Strabismus is the misalignment of eyes, with one eye on target and the other eye deviated from the target.
- It is also referred to as "squint", "crossed eyes", and "wall eyes".

Risk Factors

- Down syndrome, cerebral palsy, Apert and Crouzon syndrome, premature infants with low birth weight, and positive family history.
- It can occur at any age and is usually noticed before 6 years with a peak onset around 3 years.

Classification

- *Pseudostrabismus or apparent squint:* Pseudoesotropia (due to prominent epicanthal fold) and pseudoexotropia (in hypertelorism)
- *Latent squint (heterophoria):*
  - Physiological causes—esophoria (hyperopes) and exophoria (myopes)
  - Anatomical causes—orbital asymmetry, abnormal interpupillary distance, mild weakness of extraocular muscles
- *Manifest squint (heterotropia):*
  - *Concomitant strabismus:* Same deviation in all fields of gaze, no restriction of eye movement or muscle paresis. Onset at first 6 months of life. Maybe infantile/congenital esotropia, intermittent esotropia, or accommodative esotropia **(Fig. 1)**
  - *Incomitant strabismus:* Deviation is different in different fields of gaze due to limited eye movement. Could be due to neurogenic causes like 3, 4, or 6 nerve palsy. Myogenic causes are associated with muscle disturbances. Myasthenia gravis may also be a cause **(Fig. 2)**.

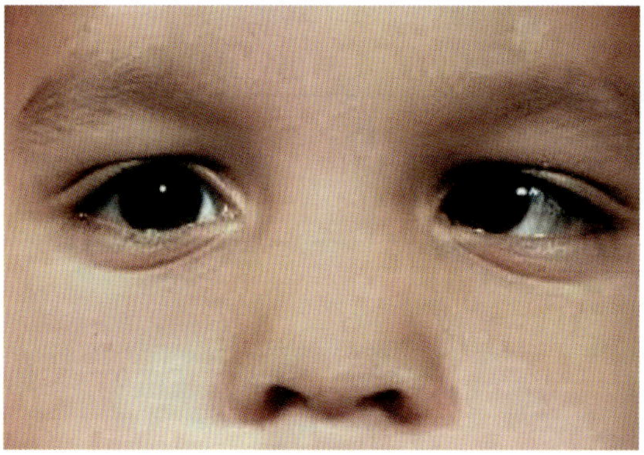

FIG. 1: Concomitant strabismus.

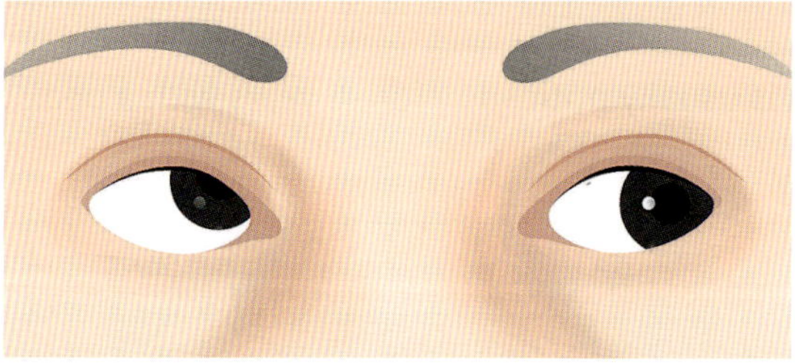

FIG. 2: Incomitant strabismus.

Red Flags

- Acquired strabismus
- Diplopia
- Limited eye movements
- Ptosis or other neurologic signs
- Poor vision or abnormal red reflex

Evaluation

Evaluation includes good history taking, ocular/physical examination, and appropriate investigations

- *Visual acuity:*
  - *Infants:* "CSM" (Central, Steady, and Maintained) method is a simple technique to observe fixation and the followability (observe the corneal reflex while moving a torch from side to side)
  - *Preverbal children:* Preferential looking tests, e.g., Cardiff picture cards
  - *Children:* Snellen charts, illiterate e-chart, Sheridan–Gardiner charts
- *Stereo acuity:*
  - Measures the visual sense of depth and fusion of images by the brain.
  - *Compensatory head posture (CHP):* Motor adaptation to attain binocular single vision
- *AC/A (accommodative convergence/accommodation) ratio:* Amount of convergence in prism diopters per diopter change in accommodation
- *Measurement of deviation:* Hirschberg test, Krimsky test, cover test–uncover test, alternate cover test, prism cover test, Maddox wing, Maddox rod test
- *Ocular motility:*
  - Extraocular movements involve the assessment of smooth pursuit movements followed by saccades.
  - We look for versions, ductions, vergence, near point of convergence, near point of accommodation, and fusional amplitudes
- *Binocular single-vision testing:* Worth four-dot test, diplopia charting
- Refraction
- *Forced duction test:* Assess limitation of movement
- Fundoscopy
- *Neuroimaging:* Hydrocephalus, optic nerve glioma, medulloblastoma, or craniopharyngioma

Complications

- Amblyopia
- Reduced stereopsis
- Asthenopia
- Diplopia
- Nystagmus
- Abnormal head and neck posture
- Impaired social and mental growth

Approach

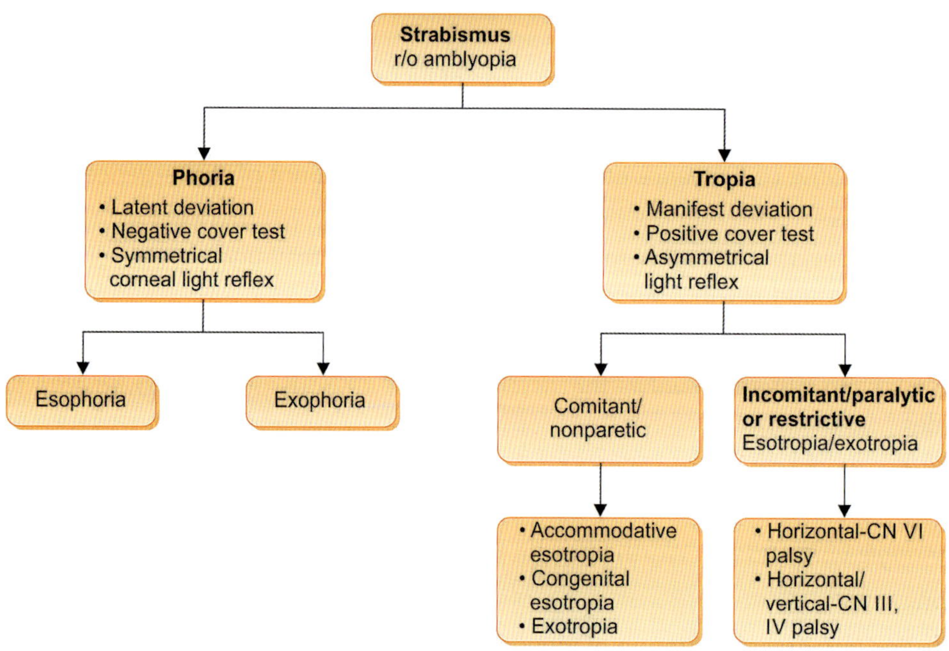

Suggested Reading

- Bateman JB, Isenberg SJ. Emery and Rimoin's Principles and Practice of Medical Genetics, 6th edition. Philadelphia: Elsevier; 2013.
- Brodsky MC. Pediatric Neuro-Ophthalmology. Springer: New York; 2016.
- Kanukollu VM, Sood G. Strabismus. Treasure Island (FL): StatPearls Publishing; 2024 Jan.
- Wright KW. Pediatric Ophthalmology for Primary Care. Illinois: American Academy of Pediatrics; 2007.
- Zhang XJ, Lau YH, Wang YM, Kam KW, Ip P, Yip WW, et al. Prevalence of strabismus and its risk factors among school aged children: The Hong Kong Children Eye Study. Sci Rep. 2021;11:13820.

Epistaxis

60

Section Editor: **Rupesh Masand**
Section Co-Editor: **Hema Gupta Mittal**
Author: **Ravi Bhatia**

Introduction

- Epistaxis is also referred to as "nose bleeds".
- It may be an isolated occurrence or may occur repeatedly.
- Though there is no consensus on the definition of recurrent epistaxis in children, some studies have defined it as five or more episodes in a year.
- The most common age of presentation is between 3 and 8 years of age. The incidence of epistaxis declines after the age of puberty.
- Indian data show that approximately 0.5% of all emergency room visits are due to epistaxis. About 30% of children aged 2–5 years, 56% of children aged 6–10 years, and 64% of children aged 11–15 years develop epistaxis during their lifetime.

Anatomy

The most common site of bleeding is from the Kiesselbach plexus, located at the anteroinferior area of the nasal septum where vessels from internal carotid and external carotid arteries converge.

Classification

Epistaxis could be primary or secondary.

- *Primary (most common):* Idiopathic
- *Secondary:* These may be local or systemic
  - *Local cause:*
    - *Nose picking (most common cause):* In hot or cold weather, when the ambient humidity is low, the nasal septal mucosa becomes dry and friable. It is predisposed to bleeding, even with minor trauma as may occur with nose picking, rubbing, blowing, or sneezing. Increased atmospheric pollutant concentrations (of airborne particulate matter and atmospheric ozone) may also irritate the nasal respiratory epithelium.
    - Rhinitis
    - Foreign body in nasal cavity
    - Upper respiratory tract infection
    - Nasal polyp
    - Juvenile nasal angiofibroma
  - *Systemic*:
    - *Infections:* Dengue fever
    - *Noninfectious:* Hypertension, leukemia, idiopathic thrombocytopenic purpura, Von Willebrand disease
  - Drugs like aspirin, nonsteroidal anti-inflammatory drugs (NSAIDs)

Red Flags

Though mostly self-limiting, sometimes its presentation may be sinister. Watch out for the following:

- Pallor
- Sick-looking child
- Child having prolonged fever
- Febrile child in a dengue-endemic area
- Adolescent female with a history of menorrhagia
- Recurrent nasal bleeds
- Severe/life-threatening bleed/hemodynamically unstable patient

Investigations

Epistaxis is a clinical diagnosis and does not require any investigations. However, patients with red flag signs may require some investigations:

- Complete blood count (CBC) with peripheral blood film
- Serology for dengue and other secondary diseases as per clinical pointers
- Coagulation profile (Von Willebrand disease)

Approach

- A detailed history must be taken to establish cause and severity of epistaxis specifically for:
  - Recurrent or frequent episodes of epistaxis
  - Easy bruising
  - Past history of bleeding after surgical challenges (e.g., dental extractions, tonsillectomy, circumcision), trauma, etc.
  - Family history of bleeding, menorrhagia, recurrent epistaxis
  - Medications, e.g., NSAIDs, nasal sprays
- Do a thorough general physical examination looking for clues of any trauma to the head neck area and bleeding disorder. Also examine:
  - Airway—assess for airway compromise (e.g., in cases of facial trauma)
  - Breathing
  - Circulation
- Assess site of bleeding, if feasible

Algorithm: Approach to a Child with Epistaxis

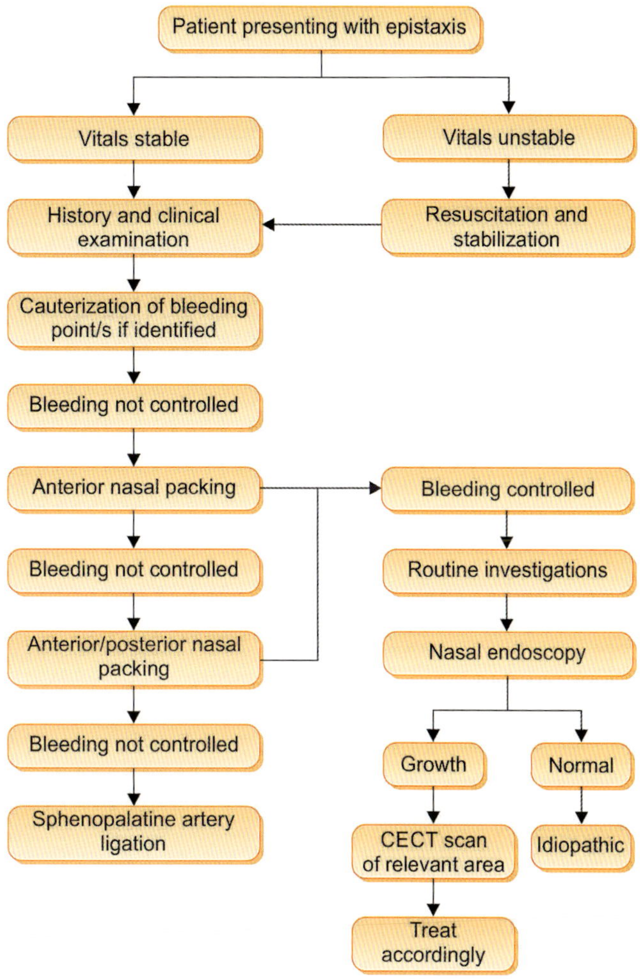

Suggested Reading

- Gupta S, Borgohain AG, Rao S. Epistaxis in children. Standard Treatment Guidelines 2022. Under the Auspices of the IAP Action Plan 2022. [online] Available from https://iapindia.org/pdf/ch-069-epistaxis-in-children.pdf [Last accessed May, 2024].
- Haddad Jr J, Keesecker S. Epistaxis. In: Kliegman RM, Stanton BF, St. Geme JW, Schor NF (Eds). Nelson Textbook of Pediatrics, 20th edition, Vol. 2. Philadelphia, PA: Elsevier; 2016. pp. 2009-10.

Halitosis

61

Section Editor: **Rupesh Masand**
Section Co-Editor: **Hema Gupta Mittal**
Author: **Ravi Bhatia**

Introduction

- Halitosis originates from the Latin word "halitus" which means "bad breath". It refers to the foul odorous breath emitted from the mouth due to either oral or nonoral causes.
- Studies across the world have put a prevalence of halitosis between 5 and 40%.

Classification

According to International Society for Breath Odor Research, halitosis is classified into three main categories:

1. *Genuine halitosis:* Here, the breath malodor can be verified objectively and it has an intensity beyond the socially acceptable levels.
2. *Pseudohalitosis:* When the bad odor has not been documented objectively but still the patient insists on its presence
3. *Halitophobia:* It is the belief of existence of malodor by a patient even after successful treatment of either genuine halitosis or pseudohalitosis.

Cause

Breakdown of epithelial cells, food debris, salivary or serum proteins, mainly by gram-negative species and proteolytic obligate anaerobes present in the oral cavity, results in production of volatile sulfur compounds, aromatic compounds and amines, short-medium-chain fatty acids or organic acids, alcohols, aliphatic compounds, aldehydes, and ketones which account for the bad odor.

Etiology

- *Oral (90% cases)*:
  - Poor oral hygiene
  - Periodontal diseases
  - Coated tongue
  - Dental caries
  - Food lodgment
  - Gingivitis
  - Oral malignancy
- *Extraoral (10% cases)*:
  - Foreign body (nose/lung)
  - Rhinosinusitis
  - Adenoid hypertrophy
  - Tonsillitis
  - *Gastrointestinal:* Pharyngeal pouch, Zenker diverticulum, gastroesophageal reflux disease, pyloric stenosis, acute liver failure
  - Bronchiectasis
  - Leukemia
  - Diabetic ketoacidosis
  - End-stage renal failure
  - Intake of raw garlic, onions, tobacco products, betel, alcohol, and solvent drug abuse

Approach

- Diagnosis is mostly clinical; often the parents or the class teacher are among the first ones to detect halitosis in children.
- *Take a detailed history:* Any history of tender or bleeding gums, pain during chewing, toothache, nasal discharge and stuffiness, snoring, mouth breathing, headache, any dental procedures, choking following food intake, chronic productive cough, polyuria, polydipsia, polyphagia associated with growth failure and/or altered sensorium, intake of specific odorous food substances.

Investigations

- Organoleptic assessment measures the strength of target odors and the value is expressed and compared to a predefined scale. This is considered the gold standard for diagnosing and assessing halitosis. It involves the measurement of the unpleasant odors by smelling the air exhaled from the nose and mouth and then calculation of organoleptic score by a trained examiner.
- Volatile sulfur compounds (VSC) monitoring involves detection of hydrogen sulfide and mercaptans by gas chromatography.
- Microbiological tests involve detection of bacteria in plaque, tongue coating taken from a patient having halitosis, by appropriate culture methods.
- Relevant investigations like CBC, peripheral blood smear, random blood sugar, blood urea, serum creatinine, liver function tests, ABG, Chest X-ray, HRCT thorax, upper GI endoscopy, 24-hour impedance monitoring to rule out systemic causes as suspected by history and physical examination.

Algorithm

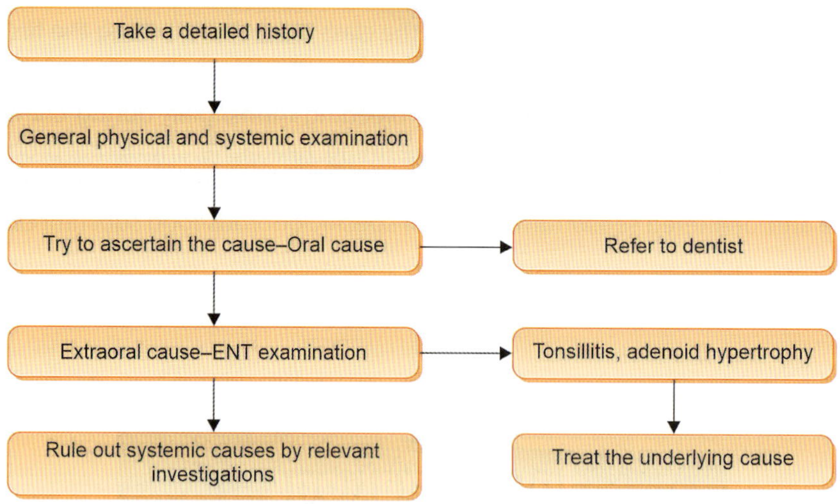

Suggested Reading

- Ayilikci BU, Colak H. Halitosis: From diagnosis to management. J Natural Sci Biol Med. 2013;4(1):14-23.
- Rosing CK, Loesche W. Halitosis: an overview of epidemiology, etiology and clinical management. Braz Oral Res. 2011;25(5):466-71.

Nystagmus

62

Section Editor: **Sumitha Nayak**
Section Co-Editor: **Priya Shivalli**
Author: **Shreekrishna GN**

Introduction

- Nystagmus is the rhythmic oscillations of one or both eyes.
- It may be due to an abnormality in any one of the three basic mechanisms that regulate position and movement of the eyes: Fixation, conjugate gaze, or vestibular mechanism.

Etiology

- Nystagmus can be congenital or acquired.
- It may be benign in origin, or associated with abnormal visual development, or associated with an underlying neurological disorder.

Classification

- *Physiological:*
  - Oculokinetic nystagmus—people looking out of a window in a moving train
  - Peripheral—abnormalities in the vestibular system
  - Central—abnormalities in the central vestibular system or cerebellum
  - Retinal—inability to fixate
- To decide whether central or peripheral:
  - If it persists or fatigues
  - Whether it is associated with vertigo
  - Whether it improves with visual fixation

	SUSTAINED	FATIGUE	VERTIGO	FIXATION
Central	+	–	–	–
Peripheral	–	+	+	+

Whether symmetrical movement at the same speed in both directions—pendular nystagmus

Fast phase in one direction and slow phase in the other—jerk nystagmus

Red Flag Signs

- Later onset of the nystagmus
- Constant oscillopsia (older children)
- Dysconjugate/gaze evoked/seesaw/convergence–retraction nystagmus
- Horizontal nystagmus becoming vertical in vertical gaze
- Vertical or torsional nystagmus (after exclusion of retinal pathology, e.g., achromatopsia)
- Any associated neurological signs/symptoms in a systemically unwell child

Approach

History

Time of onset	• Spasmus nutans occurs in the age group of 3–15 months and disappears by age 3–4 years • Sensory defect nystagmus begins in the first 3 months of life if vision loss is present at birth
Family history	• Congenital motor nystagmus has a strong hereditary component • Commonly sex-linked dominant form • Autosomal transmission is uncommon
Head positioning	With time, the child adopts abnormal head positioning if there was a null position associated with the nystagmus
Presence of photophobia	Albinism and oculocutaneous albinism can lead to nystagmus presenting as sensory defect nystagmus

Examination Findings

Visual acuity	• Congenital motor nystagmus associated with relatively good visual acuity 20/40 to 20/70 • Sensory defect nystagmus is associated with poor vision
Color vision	• Achromatopsia (red monochromatism), present at birth, is complete color blindness • The first signs are presence of sensory defect nystagmus and light sensitivity with squinting in bright light • An electroretinogram may show an abnormal photopic signal with maintenance of a normal scotopic signal
Slit-lamp examination	A slit-lamp examination will differentiate ocular albinism, optic nerve hypoplasia, and congenital cataracts, all of which will manifest as sensory defect nystagmus
Neuroimaging—CT scan and MRI	• Imaging is necessary to rule out organic and neurologic causes of nystagmus • Required in: – Decreased vision and abnormal optic nerve – All acquired nystagmus – Atypical congenital waveforms – Spasmus nutans

Algorithm

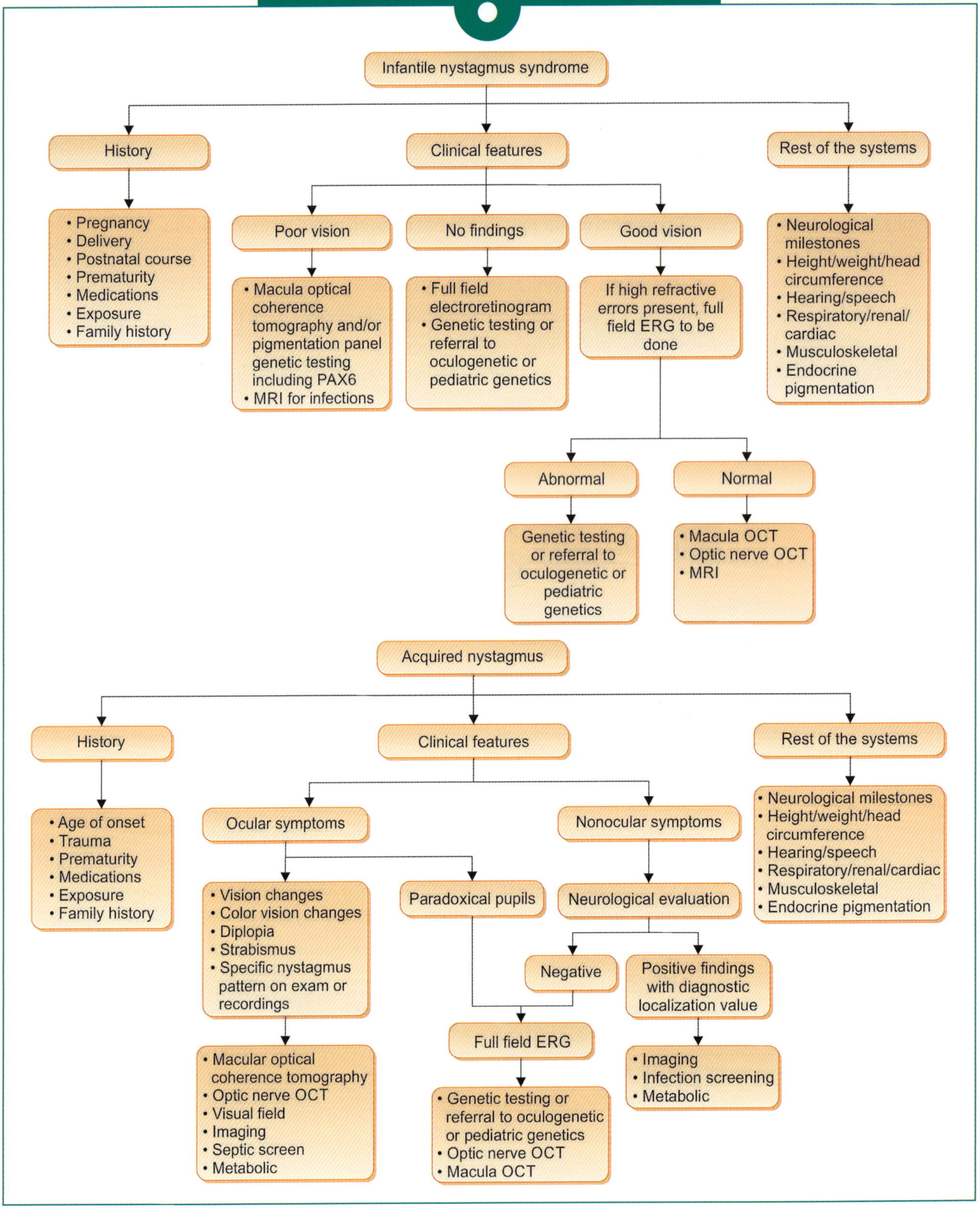
Infantile nystagmus syndrome
History
Clinical features
Rest of the systems
• Pregnancy
• Delivery
• Postnatal course
• Prematurity
• Medications
• Exposure
• Family history
Poor vision
No findings
Good vision
• Macula optical coherence tomography and/or pigmentation panel genetic testing including PAX6
• MRI for infections
• Full field electroretinogram
• Genetic testing or referral to oculogenetic or pediatric genetics
If high refractive errors present, full field ERG to be done
Abnormal
Normal
Genetic testing or referral to oculogenetic or pediatric genetics
• Macula OCT
• Optic nerve OCT
• MRI
• Neurological milestones
• Height/weight/head circumference
• Hearing/speech
• Respiratory/renal/ cardiac
• Musculoskeletal
• Endocrine pigmentation
Acquired nystagmus
History
Clinical features
Rest of the systems
• Age of onset
• Trauma
• Prematurity
• Medications
• Exposure
• Family history
Ocular symptoms
Nonocular symptoms
• Vision changes
• Color vision changes
• Diplopia
• Strabismus
• Specific nystagmus pattern on exam or recordings
Paradoxical pupils
Neurological evaluation
Negative
Positive findings with diagnostic localization value
Full field ERG
• Macular optical coherence tomography
• Optic nerve OCT
• Visual field
• Imaging
• Septic screen
• Metabolic
• Genetic testing or referral to oculogenetic or pediatric genetics
• Optic nerve OCT
• Macula OCT
• Imaging
• Infection screening
• Metabolic
• Neurological milestones
• Height/weight/head circumference
• Hearing/speech
• Respiratory/renal/cardiac
• Musculoskeletal
• Endocrine pigmentation

Suggested Reading

- American Academy of Ophthalmology. (2020). Clinical Guidelines: Childhood Nystagmus Workup [Internet]. [online] Available from https://www.aao.org/education/disease-review/clinical-guidelines-childhood-nystagmus-workup [Last accessed May, 2024].
- American Academy of Ophthalmology. (2018). Nystagmus in Infancy and Childhood [Internet]. [online] Available from https://www.aao.org/education/disease-review/nystagmus-in-infancy-childhood [Last accessed May, 2024].
- Self JE, Dunn MJ, Erichsen JT, Gottlob I, Griffiths HJ, Harris C, et al. Management of nystagmus in children: a review of the literature and current practice in UK specialist services. Eye [Internet]. 2020;34(9):1515-34.

Urticaria

63

Section Editor: **Gnanamurthy Narasimha**
Section Co-Editor: **Nagalatha Chidananda**
Author: **Sowmya A Nagarajan**

Introduction

Affecting approximately 15–25% of the global population at some point in their lives, urticaria can occur as an acute or a chronic condition. Its pathogenesis is complex, involving various immune and nonimmune mechanisms.

Etiology

- *Allergic urticaria:* IgE-mediated hypersensitivity reactions (drugs, food, insect bites)
- *Nonallergic urticaria:*
  - Autoimmune urticaria (autoimmune diseases like lupus, rheumatoid arthritis)
  - Physical urticarias (cold, heat, pressure)
  - Infective urticarias (viral, bacterial infections)
  - Urticarial vasculitis
  - Hereditary angioedema
  - Mast cell disorders (mastocytosis)
  - Erythema multiforme
  - Cutaneous vasculitis

Classification

ACUTE URTICARIA	CHRONIC URTICARIA	
Urticaria lasts for <6 weeks	Urticaria lasts for >6 weeks	
Causes	Chronic spontaneous urticaria	Chronic inducible urticaria
• Infection • Food • Contact • Physical agents	Idiopathic, autoimmune; rarely infections, cancer, hypothyroidism, hyperthyroidism, rheumatic diseases	Triggers including cold, heat, pressure, ultraviolet and visible light, vibration, water, sweating, contact allergens

Approach to Diagnosis

- Comprehensive patient history including possible triggers, drugs taken, foods eaten, pollen exposure, animal contact, etc.
- Detailed skin examination, including the presence of angioedema. Evaluation for systemic signs of vasculitis/other associated findings
- *Laboratory investigations:*
  - Complete blood counts
  - Erythrocyte sedimentation rate (ESR) and C-reactive protein (CRP)
  - Serum tryptase levels (to assess mast cell disorders)
  - Autoimmune antibodies screening, including antinuclear antibody (ANA), rheumatoid factor (RF)
- *Dermatological tests:*
  - Skin prick test for suspected allergens
  - Cold stimulation and ice cube test for cold urticaria
- *Skin biopsy and histopathology:*
  - Indicated in cases of urticarial vasculitis or suspected mastocytosis

Red Flags

- Swelling of the face, lips, or eyes
- Fever and systemic symptoms
- *Respiratory distress and wheezing:* Could indicate anaphylaxis
- *Joint pain and swelling:* Point to underlying systemic disease, like rheumatoid arthritis/lupus
- *Persistent or recurrent episodes:* Over 6 weeks/recurs frequently; further investigation is required to rule out autoimmune or underlying systemic diseases.
- *Failure to thrive and growth retardation:* Evaluate for any underlying condition.

Clinical Pointers

CAUSE	CLINICAL FEATURES
Allergens	Itchy red welts on the skin with or without angioedema (e.g., food, insect bite)
Nonallergic triggers	• Hives • Infections • Physical triggers like pressure, cold, heat • Symptoms worsen with exposure to a specific trigger
Autoimmune or systemic diseases	• Itchy red welts on the skin • Joint pain and swelling • Fever, fatigue, weight loss
Idiopathic chronic urticaria	• Recurrent episodes • Symptoms lasting over 6 weeks

Approach

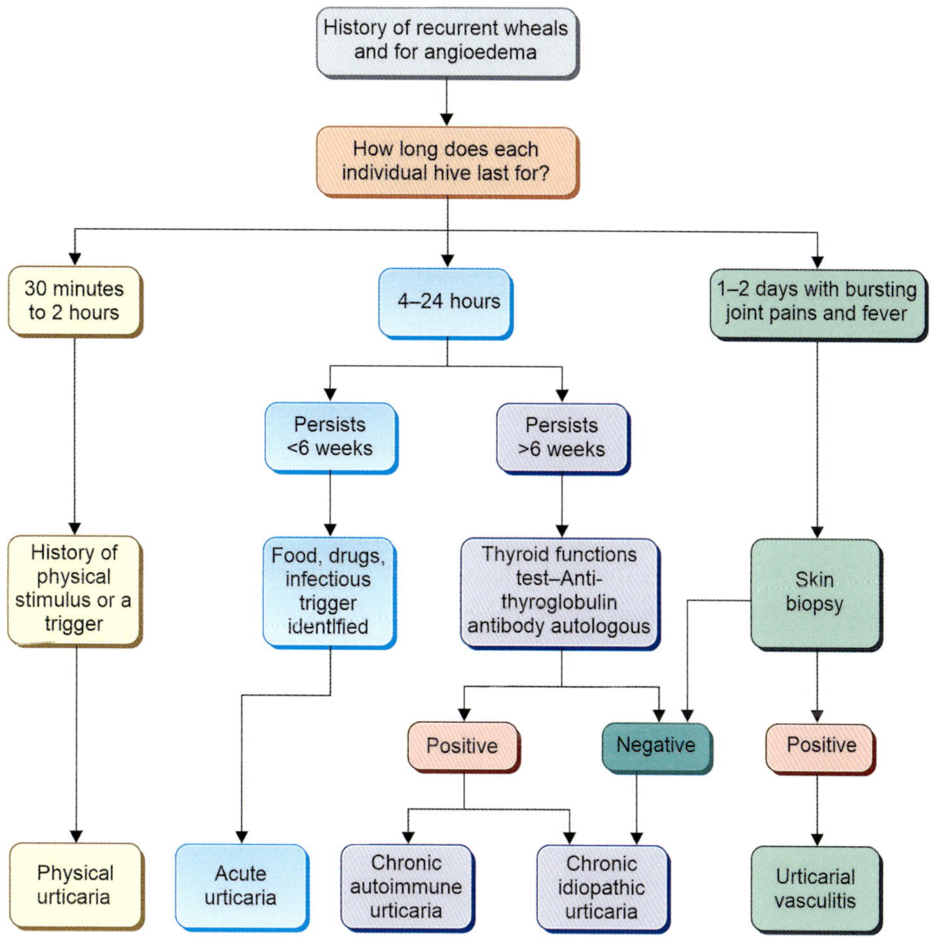
History of recurrent wheals and for angioedema
How long does each individual hive last for?
30 minutes to 2 hours
4–24 hours
1–2 days with bursting joint pains and fever
Persists <6 weeks
Persists >6 weeks
History of physical stimulus or a trigger
Food, drugs, infectious trigger identified
Thyroid functions test–Anti-thyroglobulin antibody autologous
Skin biopsy
Positive
Negative
Positive
Physical urticaria
Acute urticaria
Chronic autoimmune urticaria
Chronic idiopathic urticaria
Urticarial vasculitis

Suggested Reading

- Champion RH, Roberts SO, Carpenter RG, Roger JH Br. Urticaria and angio-oedema. A review of 554 patients. Br J Dermatol. 1969;81:588-97.
- Greaves M. Chronic urticaria. J Allergy Clin Immunol. 2000;105:664-72.
- Kaplan AP. Chronic urticaria: pathogenesis and treatment. J Allergy Clin Immunol. 2004;114:465-74.
- Kulthanan K, Jiamton S, Thumpimukvatana N, Pinkaew S. Chronic idiopathic urticaria: prevalence and clinical course. J Dermatol. 2007;34:294-301.
- Maurer M, Zuberbier T, Metz M. The Classification, Pathogenesis, Diagnostic Workup, and Management of Urticaria: An Update. Handb Exp Pharmacol. 2022;268:117-33.
- Saini SS, Kaplan AP. Chronic Spontaneous Urticaria: The Devil's Itch. J Allergy Clin Immunol Pract. 2018;6(4): 1097-106.
- Szymanski K, Schaefer P. Urticaria and Angioedema. Prim Care. 2023;50(2):237-52.
- Tidman MJ. Managing urticaria in primary care. Practitioner. 2015;259:25-8.
- Toubi E, Kessel A, Avshovich N, Bamberger E, Sabo E, Nusem D, et al. Clinical and laboratory parameters in predicting chronic urticaria duration: a prospective study of 139 patients. Allergy. 2004;59:869-73.
- van der Valk PG, Moret G, Kiemeney LA. The natural history of chronic urticaria and angioedema in patients visiting a tertiary referral centre. Br J Dermatol. 2002;146:110-3.
- Zuberbier T, Aberer W, Asero R, Bindslev-Jensen C, Brzoza Z, Canonica GW, et al. The EAACI/GA(2) LEN/EDF/WAO Guideline for the definition, classification, diagnosis, and management of urticaria: the 2013 revision and update. Allergy. 2014;69:868-87.

Ptosis

64

Section Editor: Sumitha Nayak
Section Co-Editor: Priya Shivalli
Author: Uday A Pai

Introduction

- Ptosis of the eyelid refers to drooping of the upper eyelid. It is significant when it obstructs vision and causes disablement.
- It may be due to a congenital or acquired abnormality of the muscles that elevate the eyelid.
- Ptosis may be the presenting sign or symptom of a serious neurologic disease.

Classification

Ptosis is classified into congenital or acquired.

Types of Acquired Ptosis

- *Neurogenic:* This is due to defective innervation of the levator muscle of upper eyelid. For example, 3rd nerve palsy, Horner syndrome, Marcus Gunn jaw-winking syndrome, multiple sclerosis
- *Myogenic:* Levator muscle myopathy or defect at neuromuscular junction. For example, myasthenia gravis, ocular myopathy, simple congenital, blepharophimosis syndrome
- *Mechanical:* Impairment of levator function due to the mass effect of some abnormal external mass/ structure such as neoplasm, chalazion, contact lens in the upper fornix, scarring, etc.
- *Aponeurotic* or *involutional ptosis:* Due to a defective levator aponeurosis by aging, trauma, or postoperative complication
- *Traumatic:* Any kind of direct/indirect trauma to the eyelid leading to levator transection, cicatrization, eyelid laceration, or orbital rooftop fracture with ischemia

Clinical Evaluation

- The upper lid margin covers >2 mm of the cornea, making palpebral fissure narrower than normal.
- Observation of both eyes and the general evaluation of the patient.
- Backward tilting of head, wrinkled skin of the forehead, and elevated eyebrows present with compensatory changes.
- Examine for any scar, swelling, or abnormal structure near eyelids.
- It may also present with eyeball deviation/shrinking/bulging.

Look for the following signs:

- Absent upper lid crease—congenital ptosis
- Pupillary function, i.e., anisocoria in Horner syndrome (miosis) and CN III palsy (mydriasis)
- Ocular motility—assess 3rd cranial nerve paresis
- Jaw-winking sign—Marcus Gunn jaw-winking syndrome
- Bell's phenomenon and tear film:
    - Bell's phenomenon is a protective mechanism and preoperative assessment in every case of ptosis surgery. Normal Bell's phenomenon consists of an upward and outward movement of the eyes associated with eyelid closure.
    - Ptosis surgery induces changes in Meibomian gland (MG) and tear film and effect on astigmatism and aberrations.
- Phenylephrine test to assess Müller's muscle functions. Topical phenylephrine (alpha-adrenergic sympathomimetic) is administered in the superior fornix, and eyelid elevation in response shows ideal candidacy for this surgery.

Physical Assessment

- *Levator muscle function:* Place the thumb firmly against the patient's eyebrow, with eyes in downward gaze. Then the patient looks upward, and the amount of excursion is measured with a scale.

  Grades:
    - Normal (15 mm)
    - Excellent (>12 mm)
    - Good (9–11 mm)
    - Fair (5–9 mm)
    - Poor (<4 mm)

- *Margin-reflex distance (MRD):* Patient fixates on torchlight held by the examiner, and the distance between its corneal reflection and the upper lid margin is measured. A value of 4–5 mm is normal MRD.

  Palpebral fissure height: Normally, the upper lid margin covers 2 mm and lower lid margin covers 1 mm of the cornea. Measure distance between them. Normal is 7–10 mm in males and 8–12 mm in females. Compare with the contralateral side. Calculate the difference. This quantifies the unilateral ptosis as mild (1–2 mm), moderate (3–4 mm), or severe (>4 mm).
- *Margin crease distance:* This is the distance between the lid margin and skinfold of upper lid measured in downward gaze. Normal values: 7–8 mm (males); 8–10 mm (females). It is above normal in aponeurotic ptosis and absent/vague in congenital ptosis.

Pseudoptosis—False Perception of the Ptosis

- Contralateral retracted lid
- Downward deviated ipsilateral eyeball followed by the upper lid
- Overhanging skin over the upper lid
- Brow ptosis
- Upper lid swelling, i.e., preseptal cellulitis, orbital cellulitis, chalazion
- Volume deficit as seen in microphthalmos, phthisis bulbi, enophthalmos, etc.

Diagnosis

- Slit-lamp examination
- Visual field testing
- Ocular motility (eye movement) test
- Tensilon test (uses the drug Tensilon, also known as edrophonium, to diagnose myasthenia gravis)

Additional Investigations

- *Iliff test:* Early detection in *infancy* to check levator muscle function.
- On everting the upper eyelid when the child looks down, if the eyelid reverts on its own, it indicates a good levator function.
- Patients with ptosis should be investigated clinically by an ophthalmologist and neurologist, for blood tests, X-rays, and CT/MRI scans of the brain, orbit, and thorax.

Algorithms

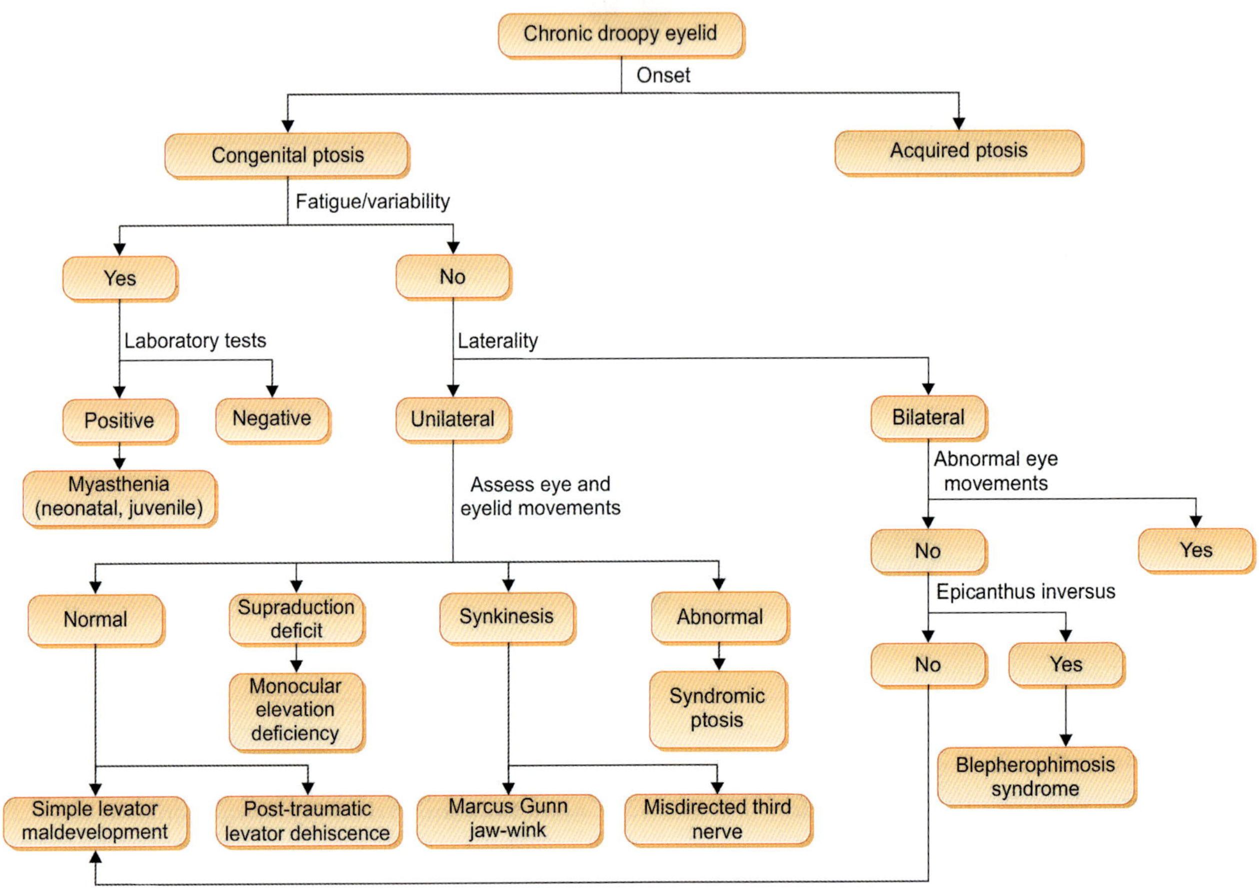

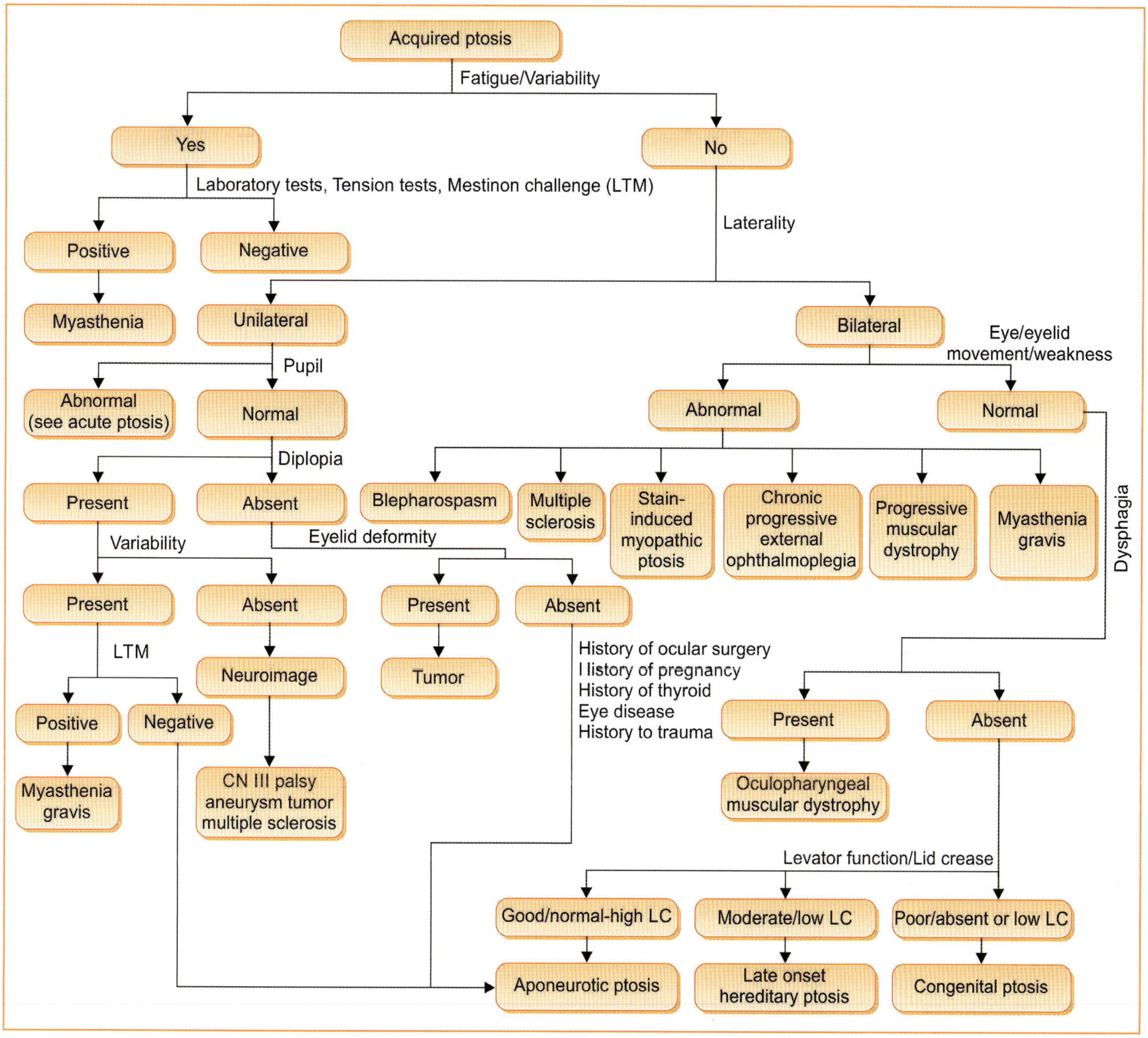

Suggested Reading

- American Academy for Pediatric Ophthalmology and Strabismus. Ptosis (https://aapos.org/glossary/ptosis). Updated 03/2023. Accessed 8/9/2023.
- American Academy of Ophthalmology. What is Ptosis (https://www.aao.org/eye-health/diseases/what-is-ptosis)? Reviewed/Edited 9/9/2022. Accessed 8/9/2023.
- National Library of Medicine (U.S.). Eyelid drooping (https://medlineplus.gov/ency/article/001018.htm). Accessed 8/9/2023.
- Shahzad B, Siccardi MA. Ptosis (https://www.ncbi.nlm.nih.gov/books/NBK546705/). 2023 Feb 19. In: StatPearls [Internet]. Treasure Island (FL): StatPearls Publishing; 2023 Jan-. Accessed 8/9/2023.

Hypertension in Children and Adolescents

65

Section Editor: **Nehal Patel**
Section Co-Editor: **Jay T Dhirwani**
Authors: **Fagun Shah, Suprita Kalra**

Introduction

- Hypertension (HTN) is not uncommon in childhood and adolescence.
- The pooled prevalence in pediatrics per worldwide systematic analysis was reported as 4%.

Definition

Normal Blood Pressure

- *For children aged 1–13 years:* Both systolic BP (SBP) and diastolic BP (DBP) < 90th percentile for age, sex, and height
- *For children >13 years:* <120/80 mm Hg

CHILDREN 1–13 YEARS OF AGE		CHILDREN >13 YEARS OF AGE
Normal BP	<90th percentile of SBP and DBP	<120/80 mm Hg
Elevated BP	SBP and/or DBP ≥ 90th percentile to <95th percentile or 120/80 mm Hg to <95th percentile (whichever is lower)	120/<80 to 129/<80 mm Hg
Stage I HTN	SBP and/or DBP ≥ 95th percentile to <95th percentile + 12 mm Hg, or 130/80 to 139/89 mm Hg (whichever is lower)	130/80 to 139/89 mm Hg
Stage II HTN	SBP and/or DBP ≥95th percentile + 12 mm Hg or ≥140/90 mm Hg (whichever is lower)	≥140/90 mm Hg

(DBP: diastolic blood pressure; HTN: hypertension; SBP: systolic blood pressure)

Etiology and Classification

1. *Primary hypertension (HTN):* No identifiable cause
2. *Secondary HTN is more common in younger ages:* Underlying identifiable cause
   - *Renal*: *Forms 90% of secondary cause of hypertension*. Includes parenchymal diseases (glomerulonephritis, congenital abnormalities of kidneys and urinary tract), renovascular
   - *Cardiac:* Coarctation of aorta
   - *Endocrinal:* Cushing's disease, Addison's disease, pheochromocytoma, etc.
   - *Monogenic:* Liddle's syndrome, apparent mineralocorticoid excess, congenital adrenal hyperplasia, etc.
   - *Miscellaneous:* Drugs and toxins, genetic syndromes, pulmonary developmental disorders

- *Etiology and classification:*
  - *White-coat HTN:* Isolated office HTN with office BP readings ≥95th percentile but normal BP outside hospitals
  - *Masked HTN:* Normal BP in hospital settings, but HTN on ambulatory BP monitoring. Important risk factor for left ventricular hypertrophy (LVH) and cardiovascular disease

Whom to Screen?

- Prematures (<32 weeks), intrauterine growth restriction (IUGR), small for gestational age (SGA)
- Prolonged neonatal intensive care unit/pediatric intensive care unit (NICU/PICU) stay, history of umbilical catheterization
- Recurrent urinary tract infection (UTI), hematuria/proteinuria
- Congenital renal and urinary tract abnormalities
- Family history of congenital renal disease
- Malignancy/other systemic illnesses associated with hypertension (e.g., neurofibromatosis, tuberous sclerosis complex, sickle cell disease)
- Drugs known to cause hypertension (e.g., caffeine, nonsteroidal anti-inflammatory drugs, glucocorticoids)
- Evidence of elevated intracranial pressure
- Obesity
- Types 1 and 2 diabetes
- Coarctation/aortic stenosis

Screening Frequency

- *Without risk factors:* Above 3 years during annual health checkups
- *With risk factors:* All children irrespective of age should be screened for HTN during every health care visit

Evaluation of Hypertension

Diagnostic Pointers

- Prepubertal age, thin patients, absence of family history and other comorbid conditions causing risk of cardiovascular disease (CVD) points toward secondary HTN
- Recurrent UTI
- Glomerulonephritis
- CAKUT (congenital anomalies of the kidneys and urinary tracts)
- Ambiguous genitalia
- History of drugs causing HTN

Laboratory Evaluation

- Basic investigations include:
  - Complete blood count (CBC)
  - Renal function test (RFT), serum electrolytes
  - Urinalysis
  - Lipid profile
  - Glycated hemoglobin (Hb1AC) for obese children
  - Kidney ultrasound
  - Echocardiography
- Further evaluation if suspected secondary cause of HTN

Red Flags

- *Hypertensive emergency:* Acute severe rise in BP with life-threatening symptoms and/or evidence of target organ damage
- *Hypertensive urgency:* Acute severe rise in BP without life-threatening symptoms and evidence of acute end-organ damage
- BP normally >30 mm Hg above 95th centile for age, sex, and height

Approach

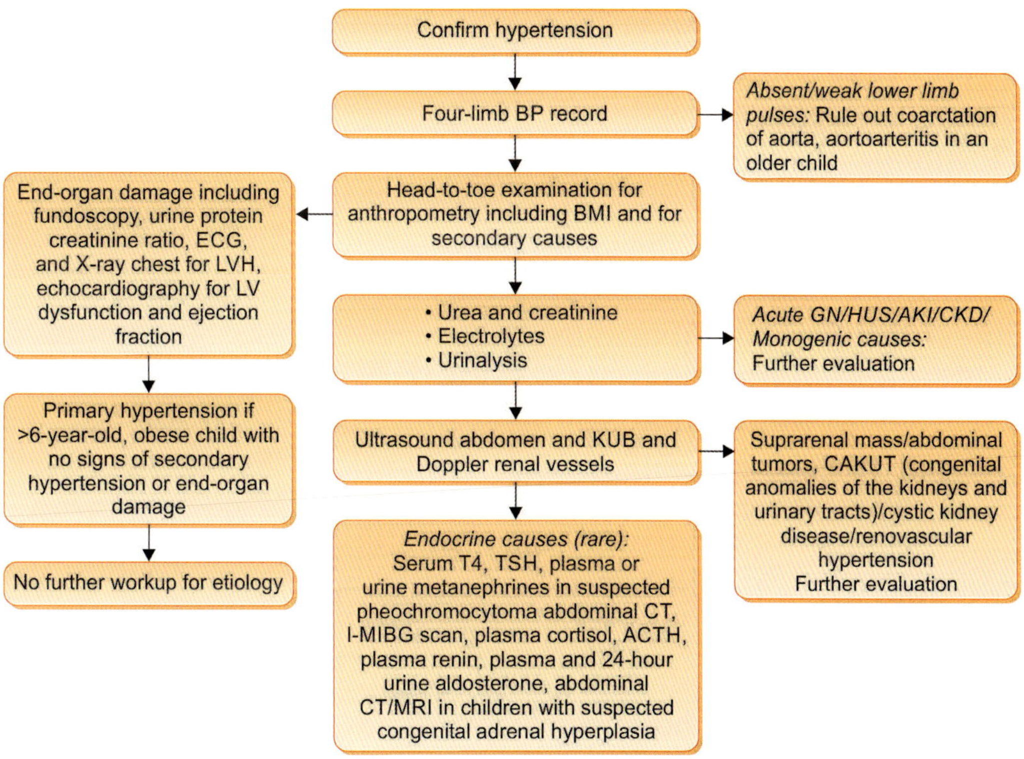

(ACTH: adrenocorticotropic hormone; AKI: acute kidney injury; CKD: chronic kidney disease; GN: glomerulonephritis; HUS: hemolytic uremic syndrome; T4: thyroxine; TSH: thyroid-stimulating hormone)

Suggested Reading

- Falkner B, Gidding SS, Baker-Smith CM, Brady TM, Flynn JT, Malle LM, et al; American Heart Association Council on Hypertension; Council on Lifelong Congenital Heart Disease and Heart Health in the Young; Council on Kidney in Cardiovascular Disease; Council on Lifestyle and Cardiometabolic Health; and Council on Cardiovascular and Stroke Nursing. Pediatric Primary Hypertension: An Under recognized Condition: A Scientific Statement From the American Heart Association. Hypertension. 2023;80(6):e101-11.
- Flynn JT, Kaelber DC, Baker-Smith CM, Blowey D, Carroll AE, Daniels SR, et al; Subcommittee on Screening and Management of High Blood Pressure in Children. Clinical Practice Guideline for Screening and Management of High Blood Pressure in Children and Adolescents. Pediatrics. 2017;140(3):e20171904.

Ear Discharge

66

Section Editor: **Rupesh Masand**
Section Co-Editor: **Hema Gupta Mittal**
Authors: **Mohammad Asif, Bhavya Verma**

Introduction

- Ear discharge refers to the drainage of aqueous substances from the ear which may be serous, serosanguineous, or purulent.
- Associated symptoms include earache, fever, pruritus, vertigo, tinnitus, and hearing loss.
- It may originate from the ear canal, middle ear, or cranial vault.

Etiology

Based on the duration of discharge:

- Acute discharge: Discharge <6 weeks
  - Acute otitis media (AOM) with perforated tympanic membrane
  - Recurrent AOM with adenoids
  - Chronic suppurative otitis media with/without cholesteatoma
  - Otitis externa (OE)
  - Cerebrospinal fluid (CSF) leak caused by head trauma
  - Posttympanostomy tube drainage
- Chronic discharge: Discharge >6 weeks
  - Foreign body (FB)
  - Cholesteatoma
  - Chronic purulent otitis media
  - Necrotizing OE
  - External and middle ear neoplasms
  - Granulomatosis with polyangiitis

Common Bacterial Pathogens

These include *Pseudomonas aeruginosa*, *Staphylococcus aureus*, *Proteus* species, *Streptococcus pneumoniae*, *Haemophilus influenzae*, *Moraxella catarrhalis*, etc.

Red Flag Signs

- Recent major head trauma
- Facial palsy
- Vertigo and tinnitus
- Sudden-onset hearing loss
- Fever and pain
- Spreading cellulitis
- Suspected mastoiditis
- Any neurologic symptoms (difficulty in swallowing/speech)

Diagnostic Pointers

- *Features of drainage:* Onset, duration, color, and consistency of otorrhea, quality and duration of discharge **(Table 1)**

DURATION OF DISCHARGE	
Acute onset: ASOM	*Recurrent:* CSOM
Purulent with acute onset: ASOM with perforation of tympanic membrane	Persistent otitis externa

TABLE 1: Quality of discharge and diseases.

QUALITY OF DISCHARGE	DISEASES
Thin, white debris-filled discharge	Bacterial otitis externa
Mucoid discharge	Tympanic membrane (TM) perforation, contact dermatitis
Clear or thin bloody discharge	Cerebrospinal fluid (CSF) otorrhea
Purulent discharge	Acute suppurative otitis media (ASOM), foreign body (FB), middle ear or severe external canal infections
Blood-tinged discharge	Trauma, FB, granuloma, or carcinoma
Foul-smelling discharge	Cholesteatoma, neoplasm

- *Fever:* It suggests acute middle ear infection/necrotizing external otitis **(Flowcharts 1 and 2)**.
- *Pain:* On manipulation of the tragus/gentle traction on the auricle: *Classic sign of bacterial otitis externa*
- *Pruritus:* Prominent in OE, otomycosis, allergic dermatitis, and FB
- *Swimming:* Important history in acute otitis externa.
- *Foreign body:* It leads to persistent otorrhea. Common FB include paper, insects, pebble, foam/cotton wool.
- *Trauma:* Any obvious head trauma or signs of basilar skull fracture (e.g., raccoon eyes, battle sign) should raise suspicion for CSF otorrhea. Minor external trauma like cleaning with cotton swabs/fingers may lead to bacterial OE **(Flowchart 1)**.
- *Medication usage:* Topical medications (e.g., neomycin, benzocaine, propylene glycol) may trigger a contact dermatitis of external auditory canal. Other allergens include new cosmetics, ointments, and certain outdoor plants (e.g., poison ivy) **(Flowchart 3)**.
- *Previous treatments:* A persistently draining ear despite antibiotic treatment may indicate chronic suppurative otitis, otomycosis, noninfectious causes of otorrhea **(Flowchart 2)**.

Physical Examination

- Examination of the ear:
  - Auricle, pinna, mastoid, postauricular area, pre/postauricular lymph nodes
  - Otoscopy of the external canal, tympanic membrane, and middle ear
  - Tympanic membrane for signs of middle ear infection (injection, dullness, and bulging), perforation, bullae, evidence of trauma, etc.
  - In patients without obvious tympanic membrane perforation or bulging, assessment of tympanic membrane by pneumatic otoscopy.

- Keratinous debris and retraction pocket formation may suggest chronic suppurative otitis media with cholesteatoma.
- Thin white debris filled discharge suggest bacterial otitis externa.

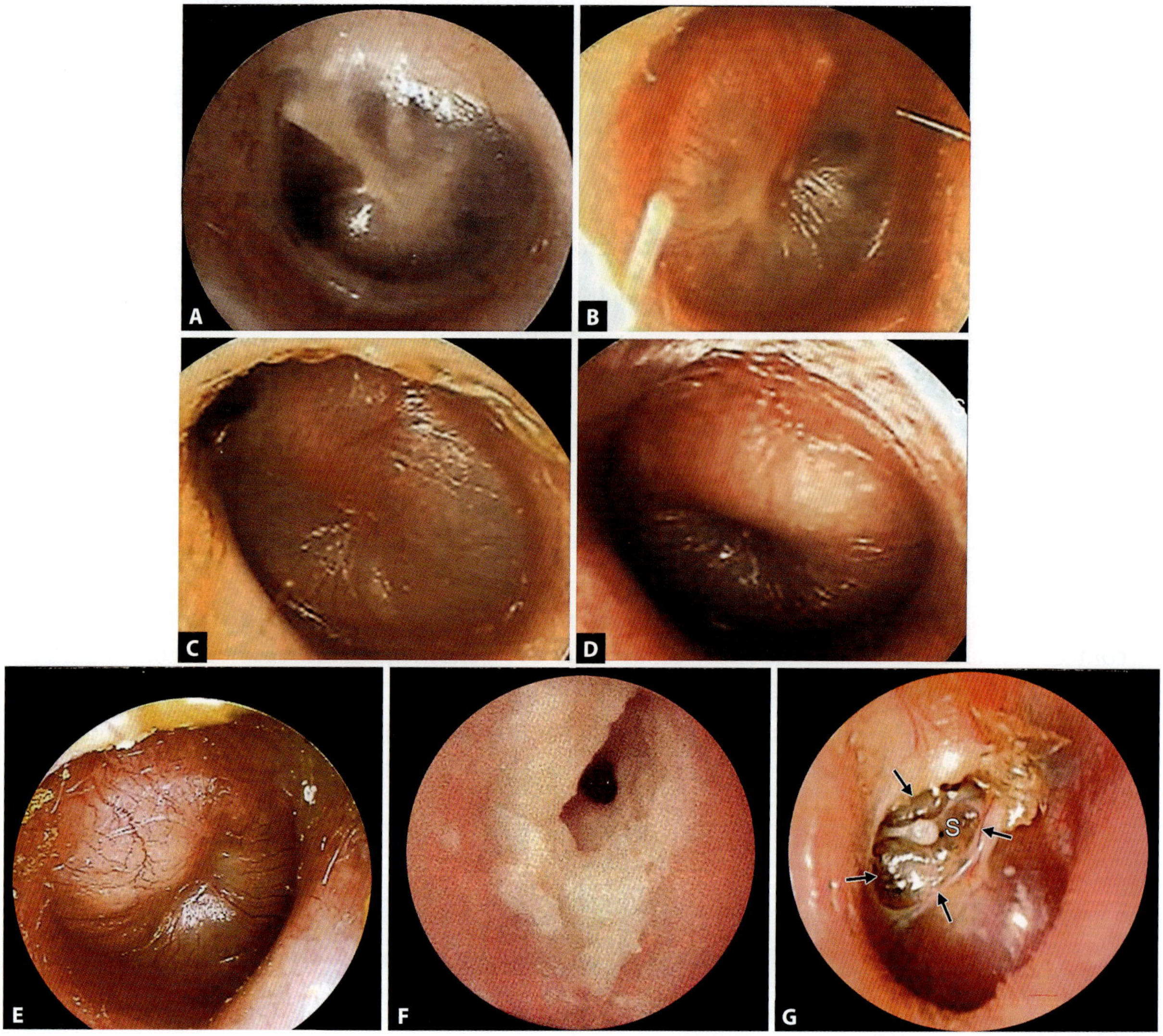

(A) Normal tympanic membrane; (B) Mild bulging; (C) Moderate bulging; (D) Severe bulging; (E) Tympanic membrane in acute otitis media; (F) Otitis externa; (G) Cholesteatoma (S: head of stapes)

- **Hearing assessment:** Rinnes test, Weber's test and audiometry tests.
- **Neurologic assessment:** In children with facial nerve palsy, vertigo, tinnitus, sudden onset hearing loss and difficulty in swallowing and speech.
- **Laboratory investigations:** History and physical examination are sufficient to diagnose and manage most causes but in few cases we may do.
  - *Culture of ear drainage:* The most common organism reported is *Pseudomonas aeruginosa*. Culture of ear drainage may be done in suspected necrotizing otitis externa and otitis media with chronic drainage, where previous treatment has failed.
  - *Testing for cerebrospinal fluid otorrhea:* When in doubt about the presence of a CSF leak. Beta trace protein or beta-2-transferrin provide accurate testing for the presence of CSF but are not widely available.
  - *Imaging:* It is indicated in basilar skull fracture with CSF leakage, spontaneous CSF leakage, necrotizing OE, cholesteatoma, external auditory canal mass, chronic polyps etc.
  - *Tissue biopsy:* May be indicated in chronic external auditory mass.

Algorithm

FLOWCHART 1: Approach to otorrhea in children.

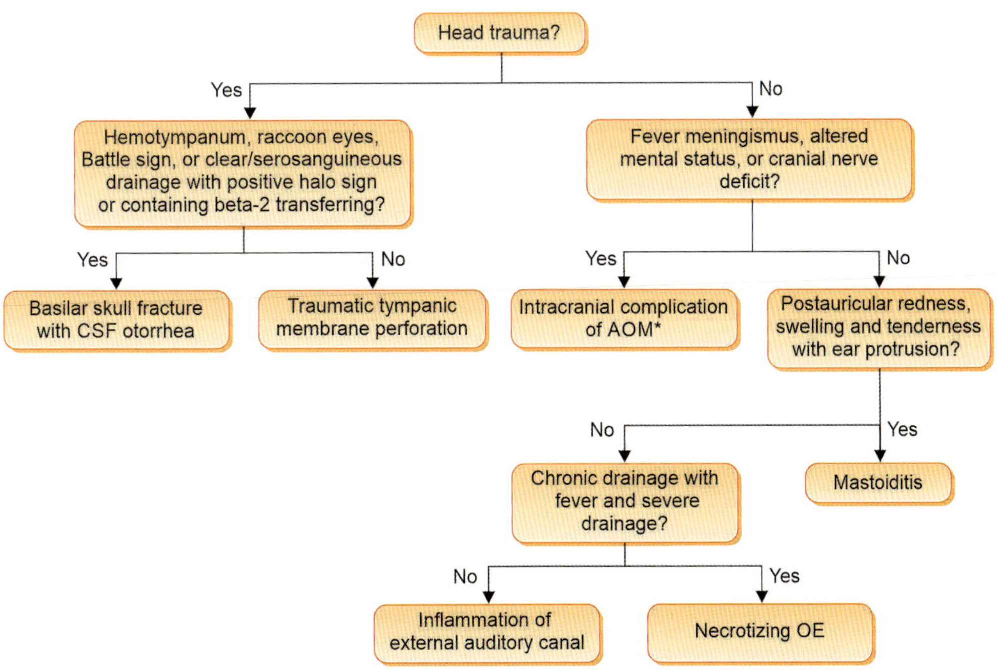

(AOM: acute otitis media; CSF: cerebrospinal fluid; OE: otitis externa)

*Meningitis, Brain abscess, Epidural abscess, Subdural empyema, Lateral or Cavernous sinus, Thrombosis, Carotid, Artery thrombosis

FLOWCHART 2: Otorrhea without external auditory canal inflammation.

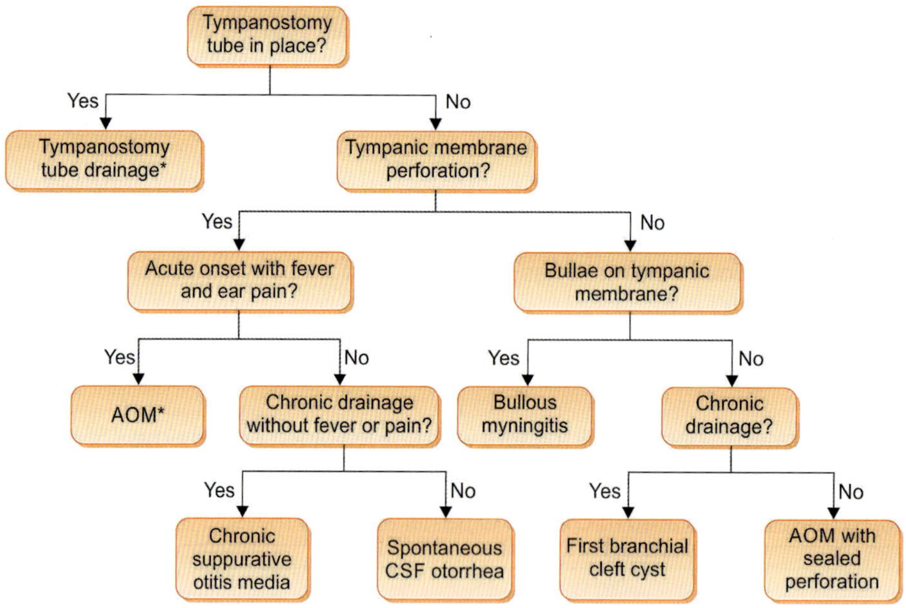

(AOM: acute otitis media; CSF: cerebrospinal fluid)

*10 to 30 % children with tympanostomy tube associated with ear discharge, i.e., foul smelling, mucoid and mixed with blood

FLOWCHART 3: Otorrhea with external auditory canal inflammation.

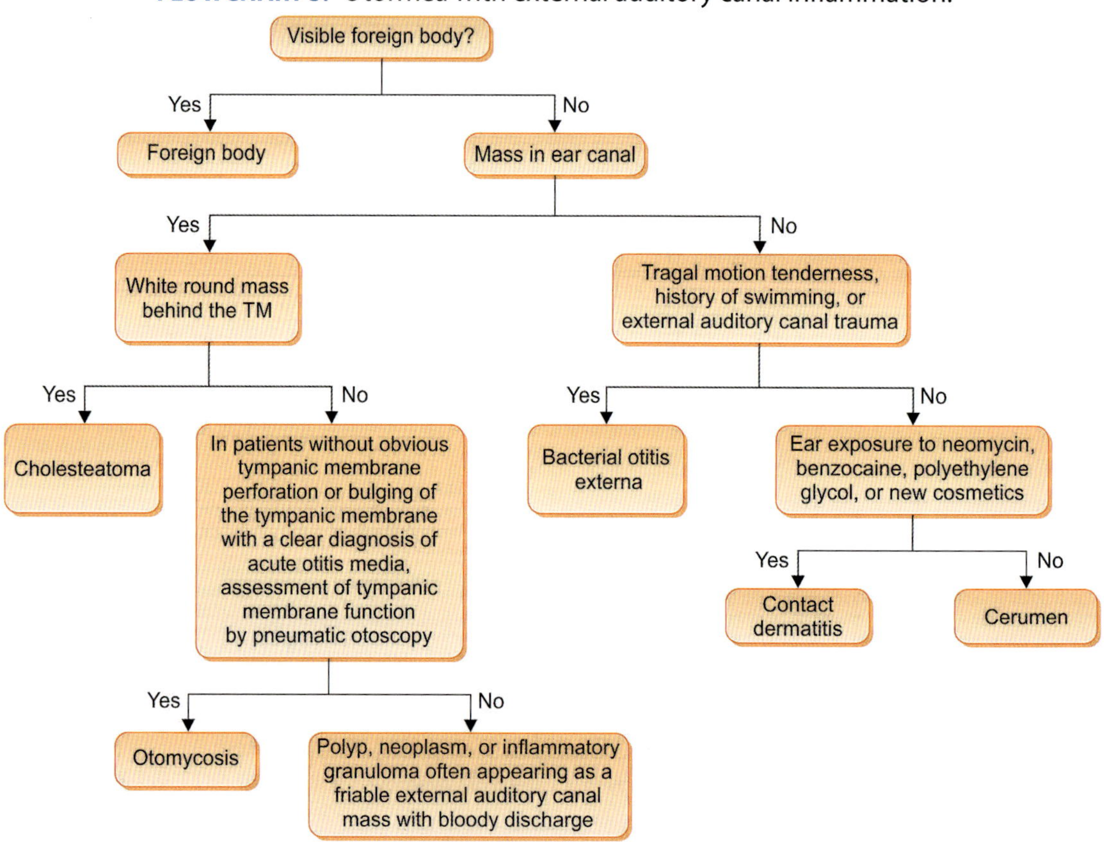

Suggested Reading

- Bardanis J, Batzakakis D, Mamatas M. Types and causes of otorrhea. Auris Nasus Larynx. 2003;30(3):253-7.
- Rowlands G. The child with ear discharge. Paediatr Child Health. 30(1):P39-42.
- Schoem SR, Darrow DH. Pediatric Otorhinolaryngology. Illinois: American Academy of Pediatrics.
- Strother CG, Sadow K. (2023). Evaluation of otorrhea (ear discharge) in children. UpToDate. [online] Available from https://www.uptodate.com/contents/evaluation-of-otorrhea-ear-discharge-in-children [Last accessed May, 2024].
- Watkinson JC, Clarke RW. Scott Brown's Textbook of Otorhinolaryngology Head and Neck Surgery, Pediatrics: The Ear Skull Base, 8th edition, volume 2. Boca Raton, FL: Chapman and Hall/CRC; 2018.

Difficulty in Breathing (Dyspnea)

67

Section Editor: **Rupesh Masand**
Section Co-Editor: **Hema Gupta Mittal**
Author: **Pawan Kalyan Pinnamaneni**

Introduction

Commonly known as dyspnea, it is characterized by a feeling of labored and uncomfortable respiration. It can arise from various factors, like heightened exertion of the respiratory muscles, activation of neuroreceptors in the respiratory tract, or stimulation of chemoreceptors—both peripheral and central.

Etiology

- *Congenital anomalies:* Structural anomalies in the airways or lungs, such as choanal atresia, macroglossia, laryngomalacia, tracheobronchomalacia, tracheo-esophageal fistula, congenital lobar emphysema
- *Respiratory infections:* Common cold, tonsillopharyngitis, bronchiolitis, croup, pneumonia
- Bronchial asthma
- *Foreign body aspiration:* Inhalation or swallowing of small objects, causing airway blockage and breathing difficulties
- *Cardiovascular:* Congenital heart disease (acyanotic/cyanotic/obstructive), rheumatic heart disease, myocarditis, cardiomyopathy, pericarditis, pericardial effusion, arrhythmias
- *Miscellaneous:* Anemia, diabetic ketoacidosis, central nervous system (CNS) depression
- Duchenne muscular dystrophy, anxiety or panic attacks, chest trauma, costochondritis

Red Flag Signs

VISIBLE CHEST RETRACTIONS ABSENT BREATH SOUNDS ON AUSCULTATION INABILITY TO SPEAK IN FULL SENTENCES DUE TO SHORTNESS OF BREATHS CYANOSIS	CONFUSION, LETHARGY, EXTREM FATIGUS SIGNS OF CHOKING OEDEMA/ ANASARCA OLIGURIA
Absent breath sounds on auscultation	Signs of choking
Inability to speak in full sentences due to shortness of breath	Confusion, lethargy, or extreme fatigue
Cyanosis	Edema/anasarca/oliguria

Relevant Investigations

- *Pulse oximetry:* To assess respiratory function
- *Complete blood count (CBC):* For infection/anemia
- *Chest X-ray:* Identifies lung structural abnormalities or infections
- Skin prick tests or IgE estimation to identify potential allergens
- *Pulmonary function tests:* Assess lung function and potential underlying asthma
- *ECG, Echo-2D:* Heart structure, function, rules out congenital heart defects
- *Arterial blood gas:* Acidosis/alkalosis
- Blood sugar estimation/ketonuria
- Serum electrolytes, blood urea, serum creatinine

Diagnostic Pointers

- *Detailed history:* Inquire about the presenting symptoms, duration, triggers, family history, and associated symptoms.
- Response to oxygen inhalation in the form of increasing oxygen saturation points toward a possible respiratory cause of dyspnea.
- *Physical examination:* General appearance, special sitting position to facilitate breathing, breathing pattern, lung sounds, and signs of respiratory distress (e.g., nasal flaring, use of accessory muscles). Cardiac examination for gallop rhythm, murmurs, etc.
- *Observation of symptoms:* Document any cough, stridor, wheezing, changes in breathing patterns.
- *Response to medications:* Evaluate response to bronchodilators, which can be helpful in diagnosing and managing asthma or reactive airway disease.

Approach

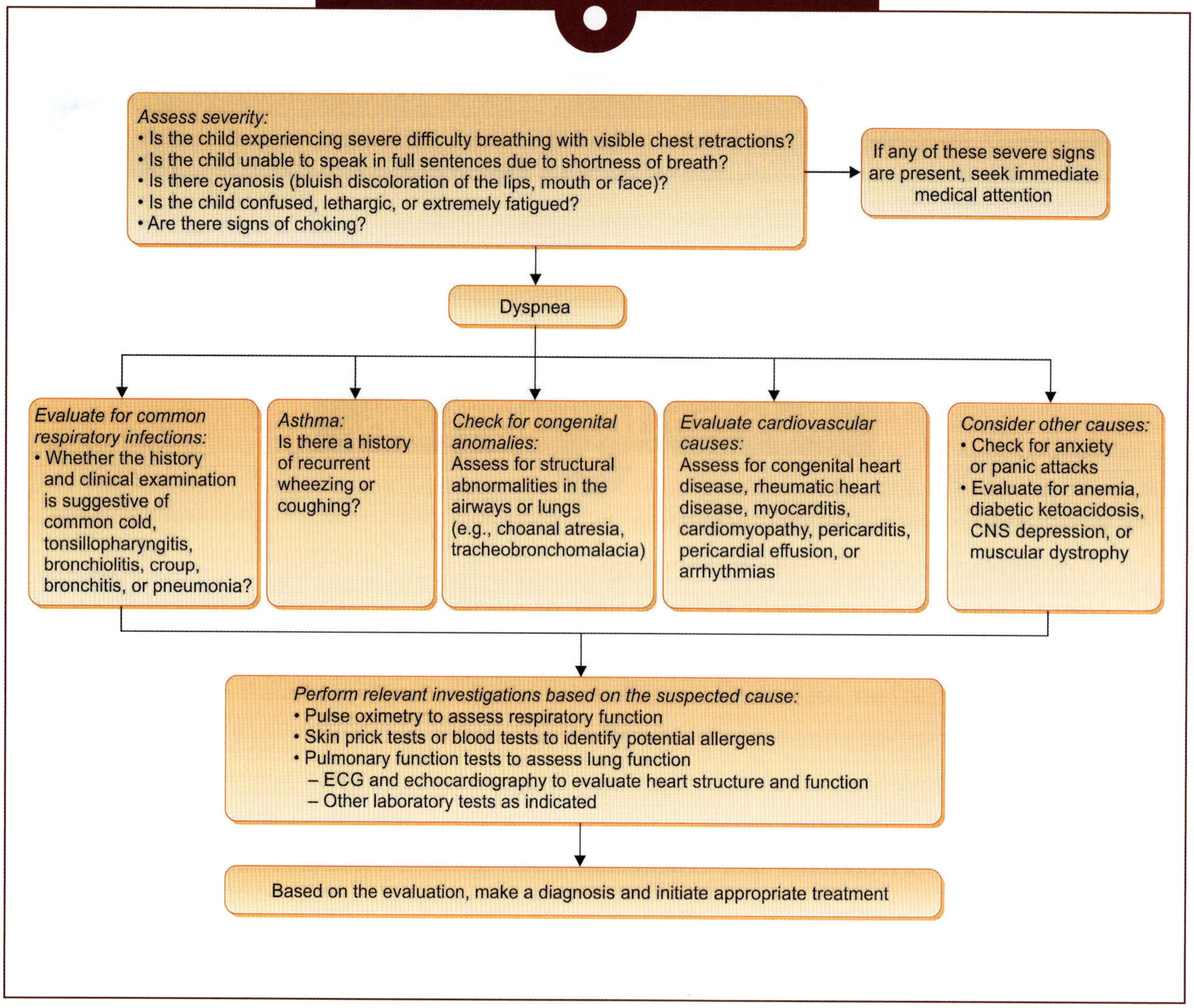
Assess severity:
• Is the child experiencing severe difficulty breathing with visible chest retractions?
• Is the child unable to speak in full sentences due to shortness of breath?
• Is there cyanosis (bluish discoloration of the lips, mouth or face)?
• Is the child confused, lethargic, or extremely fatigued?
• Are there signs of choking?
If any of these severe signs are present, seek immediate medical attention
Dyspnea
Evaluate for common respiratory infections:
• Whether the history and clinical examination is suggestive of common cold, tonsillopharyngitis, bronchiolitis, croup, bronchitis, or pneumonia?
Asthma:
Is there a history of recurrent wheezing or coughing?
Check for congenital anomalies:
Assess for structural abnormalities in the airways or lungs (e.g., choanal atresia, tracheobronchomalacia)
Evaluate cardiovascular causes:
Assess for congenital heart disease, rheumatic heart disease, myocarditis, cardiomyopathy, pericarditis, pericardial effusion, or arrhythmias
Consider other causes:
• Check for anxiety or panic attacks
• Evaluate for anemia, diabetic ketoacidosis, CNS depression, or muscular dystrophy
Perform relevant investigations based on the suspected cause:
• Pulse oximetry to assess respiratory function
• Skin prick tests or blood tests to identify potential allergens
• Pulmonary function tests to assess lung function
– ECG and echocardiography to evaluate heart structure and function
– Other laboratory tests as indicated
Based on the evaluation, make a diagnosis and initiate appropriate treatment

Suggested Reading

- Brogan TV, Thiagarajan RR. Dyspnea in children. Pediatr Clin. 2019;66(3):539-56.
- Kotecha S, Bansal S. Approach to dyspnea in children. Indian J Pediatr. 2017;84(2):128-36.
- Nair A, Kirthi V. Dyspnea in Children. In: StatPearls [Internet]. StatPearls Publishing; 2021.
- Patil S, Caples SM. Respiratory compromise: A pediatric perspective. Respir Care. 2010;55(6):776-87.
- Weese-Mayer DE, Morrow AS. Dyspnea in Children. In: StatPearls [Internet]. StatPearls Publishing; 2020.

Chest Pain

68

Section Editor: **Rupesh Masand**
Section Co-Editor: **Hema Gupta Mittal**
Authors: **Sonia Bhatt, Payal Mittal**

Introduction

Chest pain is a common complaint for emergency and outpatient department (OPD) visits. According to literature, the most common causes of chest pain in children are musculoskeletal (33%) and psychogenic (28.4%).

Etiology

Chest pain includes both cardiac and non-cardiac causes.

Causes of chest pain are given in **Table 1**.

TABLE 1: Causes of chest pain.

CATEGORY	CLINICAL DISORDERS
Idiopathic	
Musculoskeletal	Costochondritis, Tietze's syndrome, precordial catch
Respiratory	Bronchial asthma, pleuritic processes (pneumonia/pneumothorax/pulmonary embolus)
Psychogenic	Anxiety, hyperventilation/disordered, breathing
Gastrointestinal	Acid reflux, esophagitis, gastric ulceration
Miscellaneous	Herpes zoster, sickle cell crisis, tumors (chest wall/mediastinal)
Cardiac	Pericarditis, arrhythmia, myocardial ischemia (e.g., aortic stenosis, hypertrophic obstructive cardiomyopathy, coronary artery disease), mitral valve prolapse, myocarditis

Approach to a child with Chest Pain

Complete history and physical examination: It gives clues to possible diagnosis.

Diagnostic Pointers

Features associated with cardiac etiology of chest pain are given in **Table 2**.

TABLE 2: Cardiac etiology of chest pain and associated features.

FEATURES	PROBABLE ETIOLOGY
Associated with exercise	Left heart obstruction or myocardial ischemia
Radiation to the jaw and left arm	Coronary ischemia
Radiation to left shoulder tip	Pericarditis
Associated with palpitation	Pathological arrhythmia
Associated with syncope	Left heart obstruction or arrhythmia

Features associated with non-cardiac etiology of chest pain are given in **Table 3**.

TABLE 3: Non-cardiac etiology of chest pain and associated features.

FEATURES	PROBABLE ETIOLOGY
Well-localized, superficial tenderness worse on movement	Musculoskeletal
Associated with chest tightness and cough	Respiratory
Presented as retrosternal/epigastric pain, sharp or burning in nature. Associated with eating and posture	Gastrointestinal
Anxiety and hyperventilation, history of stressors, recurrent	Psychogenic

Red Flag Signs

- Chest pain associated with exercise and exertion
- Significant palpitations with chest pain
- Syncopal attacks during exercise
- Significant family history of arrhythmia, sudden death, or genetic disorders
- History of cocaine/amphetamine use (in adolescents)

Investigations

If suspected organic causes:

- *ECG:* Rate, rhythm, hypertrophy determination (using normal values for age), signs of pericarditis, ischemia
- *Chest X-ray:* History of acute severe pain, pain when walking, cough, fever, history of trauma, or abnormal examination findings
- *Blood tests: Complete blood count* (CBC), erythrocyte sedimentation rate (ESR), C-reactive protein (CRP), blood cultures
- *Echocardiogram (echo):* It can help to diagnose the following:
    - Pericardial effusions
    - Cardiomyopathy
    - Ventricular dysfunction
    - Left-sided obstructive lesions
    - Aortic root measurements and assessment for dissection
    - Heart valve function
    - Coronary arteries (origins and appearance)
    - Pulmonary hypertension
    - Assessment of intracardiac cardiac devices

Further Investigations

- In case of history of palpitations, a *24-hour ambulatory ECG* helps to capture episodes of arrhythmia and identify atrial/ventricular arrhythmia/heart block.
- *Exercise stress test* (for exertional chest pain)

Approach

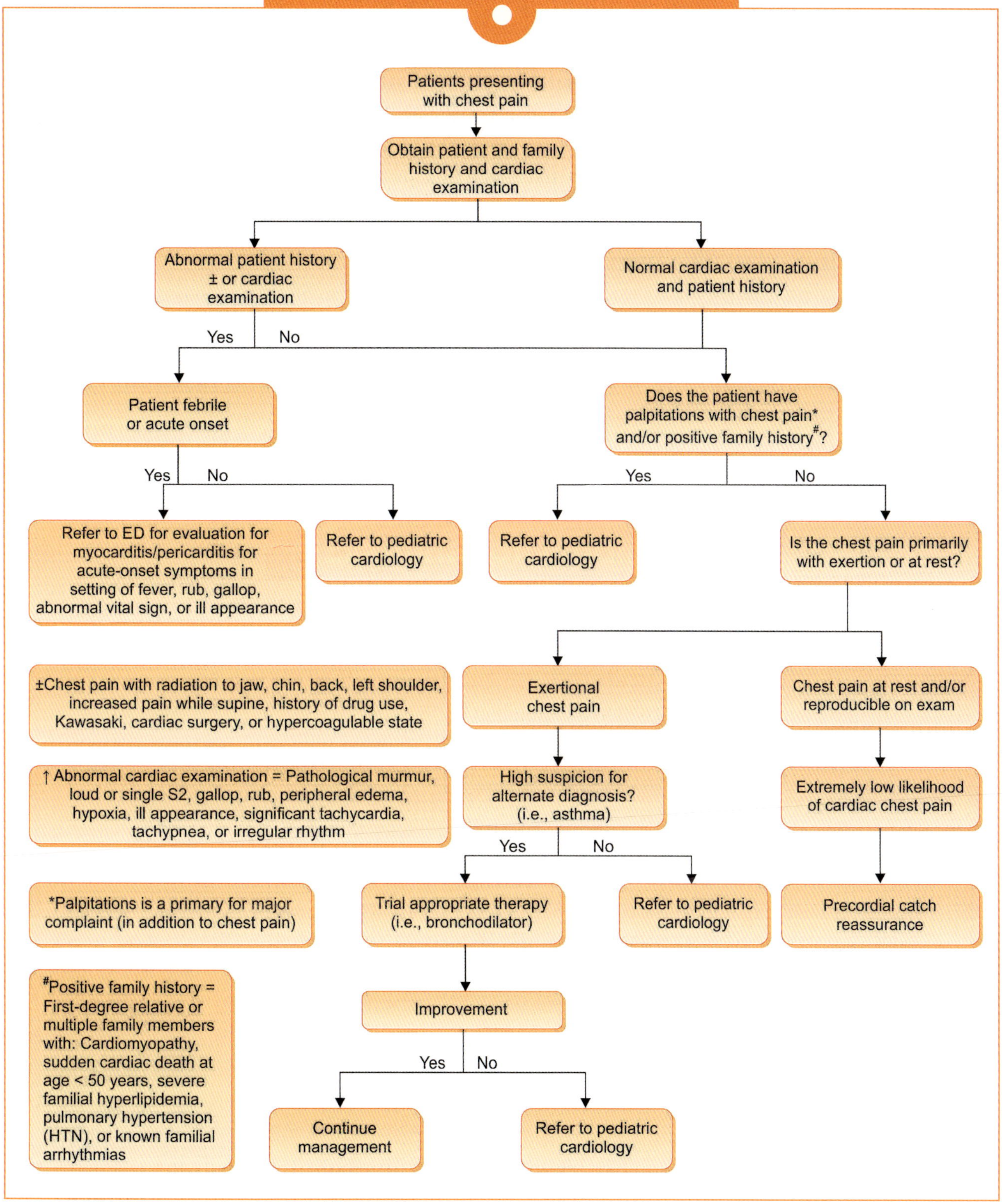
Patients presenting with chest pain
Obtain patient and family history and cardiac examination
Abnormal patient history ± or cardiac examination
Normal cardiac examination and patient history
Yes
No
Patient febrile or acute onset
Does the patient have palpitations with chest pain* and/or positive family history#?
Yes
No
Yes
No
Refer to ED for evaluation for myocarditis/pericarditis for acute-onset symptoms in setting of fever, rub, gallop, abnormal vital sign, or ill appearance
Refer to pediatric cardiology
Refer to pediatric cardiology
Is the chest pain primarily with exertion or at rest?
±Chest pain with radiation to jaw, chin, back, left shoulder, increased pain while supine, history of drug use, Kawasaki, cardiac surgery, or hypercoagulable state
Exertional chest pain
Chest pain at rest and/or reproducible on exam
↑ Abnormal cardiac examination = Pathological murmur, loud or single S2, gallop, rub, peripheral edema, hypoxia, ill appearance, significant tachycardia, tachypnea, or irregular rhythm
High suspicion for alternate diagnosis? (i.e., asthma)
Extremely low likelihood of cardiac chest pain
Yes
No
*Palpitations is a primary for major complaint (in addition to chest pain)
Trial appropriate therapy (i.e., bronchodilator)
Refer to pediatric cardiology
Precordial catch reassurance
#Positive family history = First-degree relative or multiple family members with: Cardiomyopathy, sudden cardiac death at age < 50 years, severe familial hyperlipidemia, pulmonary hypertension (HTN), or known familial arrhythmias
Improvement
Yes
No
Continue management
Refer to pediatric cardiology

Suggested Reading

- Andrew WB, Julian F. How to evaluate a child with chest pain. Curr Paediatr. 2004;14:64-70.
- Aygun E, Aygun ST, Uysal T, Aygun F, Dursun H, Irdem A. Aetiological evaluation of chest pain in childhood and dolescence. Cardiol Young. 2020;30:617-23.
- Collins SA, Griksaitis MJ, Legg JP. 15-minute consultation: a structured approach to the assessment of chest pain in a child. Arch Dis Child Educ Pract Ed. 2014;99(4):122-6.
- Deshpande SS, Vidya G, Bendre NS, Ghate MR. Children with Medically Unexplained Pain Symptoms: Categorization and Effective Management. Indian J Psychol Med. 2011;33:163-6.
- Kane DA, Fulton DR, Saleeb S, Zhou J, Lock JE, Geggel RL. Needles in hay: chest pain as the presenting symptom in children with serious underlying cardiac pathology. Congenit Heart Dis. 2010;5(4):366-73.

Dysmenorrhea

69

Section Editor: **Kripasindhu Chatterjee**
Section Co-Editors: **Atanu Bhadra, Ashim Kumar Ghosh**
Author: **Pavithra Nagaraj**

Introduction

- Dysmenorrhea is a Greek word meaning "painful monthly bleeding". This is the most common cause of pelvic pain in young girls, with a prevalence of around 80% in Indian adolescents. It is associated with significant emotional, psychological, and functional health problems resulting in school absenteeism and impaired quality of life.
- No adolescent should leave the clinic without understanding that dysmenorrhea is potentially harmful and that no girl "needs to put up with it".

Etiology

- *Primary dysmenorrhea:* When adolescents attain ovulatory cycles, i.e., within 6–12 months of menarche with no underlying cause.
- *Secondary dysmenorrhea:* Painful menstrual cycle secondary to a pelvic pathology/any other medical condition, inside or outside the uterus.

BOX 1: Causes of secondary dysmenorrhea.

- Endometriosis
- Adenomyosis
- *Infections:* Genital Koch's, STD, pelvic inflammatory disease (PID)
- Congenital obstructive mullerian malformations, cervical stenosis
- Ovarian cysts
- Fibroid uterus (endometriomas)
- Uterine polyps

(STD: sexually transmitted disease)

Associated Symptoms

- Gastrointestinal symptoms like nausea, vomiting, diarrhea, bloating
- Irritability, headache, muscle cramps
- Poor sleep quality
- School absenteeism

Red Flags

- High body mass index
- Early menarche
- Family history of dysmenorrhea
- Depression/anxiety
- Smoking
- Nulliparity

Algorithm for Approach

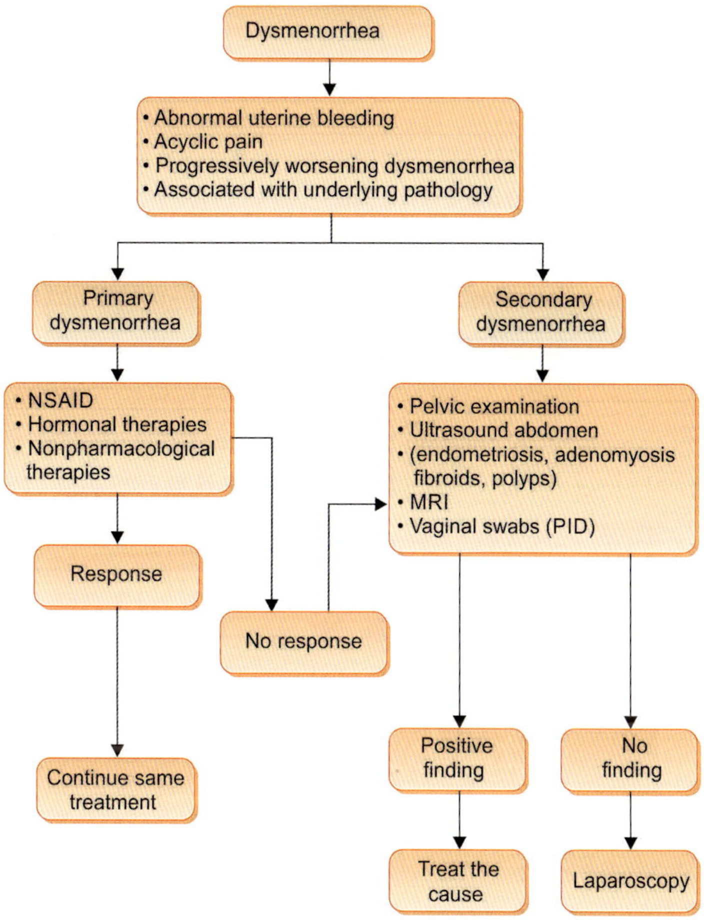

(NSAID: nonsteroidal anti-inflammatory drug; PID: pelvic inflammatory disease)

Suggested Reading

- Chauhan G, Kodnani A. A study of prevalence and impact of dysmenorrhea and its associated symptoms among adolescent girls residing in slum areas of Vadodara City, Gujarat. Int J Med Sci Public Health. 2016;5(3):510.
- Gantt PA, McDonough PG. Adolescent dysmenorrhea. Pediatr Clin North Am. 1981;28(2):389-95.
- Harel Z. Dysmenorrhea in adolescents. Ann N Y Acad Sci. 2008;1135:185-95.
- Sharghi M, Mansurkhani SM, Larky DA, Kooti W, Niksefat M, Firoozbakht M, et al. An update and systematic review on the treatment of primary dysmenorrhea. JBRA Assist Reprod. 2019;23(1):51-7.

Joint Pain

70

Section Editor: Janani Shankar
Section Co-Editor: Arathi Srinivasan
Authors: R Venkateswari, Shama Sowdagar

Introduction

Joint pain is a common complaint in children. It can be a manifestation of a benign condition or a serious condition like malignancy. A thorough history and clinical examination will help in arriving at the diagnosis.

Etiology

Etiology of joint pain is given in **Box 1**.

BOX 1: Etiology of joint pain.

- *Infection:* Septic arthritis, osteomyelitis, adjacent soft-tissue infections
- Reactive and postinfectious arthritis
- Trauma
- *Hematologic disorders:* Leukemia, bleeding diathesis, hemoglobinopathies
- Rheumatic diseases
- Epiphyseal disorders
- Juvenile idiopathic arthritis (JIA)
- Metabolic bone diseases
- Bone tumors
- Growing pain

Pointers

Duration:

- Acute onset, short duration—infectious/traumatic
- Chronic pain—with juvenile idiopathic arthritis (JIA)

Single/multiple joint involvement:

- Monoarticular joint pain: Bacterial infection, trauma

Pain characteristics:

- Early morning joint stiffness/pain that worsens after a period of inactivity: JIA
- Pain that worsens with activity: Trauma
- Nocturnal pain with frequent night awakening: Malignancy like leukemia or bone tumors
- Nocturnal pain can also be seen in benign conditions like growing pain. With growing pains, the child is well throughout the day; the pain is more in the lower limbs and gets relieved with massaging.
- Migratory joint pain: Acute rheumatic fever

Joint swelling: With signs of inflammation like warmth, redness, and restriction of movements; suggests an infectious/inflammatory cause

Fever:

- High grade with single joint involvement: Bacterial infection
- With respiratory or gastrointestinal symptoms preceding the onset of joint pain: Reactive arthritis
- Fever may be a manifestation of malignancy and inflammatory conditions like JIA, systemic lupus erythematosus (SLE), vasculitis, etc.
- A specific pattern of fever like quotidian fever: Systemic-onset JIA

Trauma: It can be the actual cause of joint pain. Sometimes, minor trauma might lead to unmasking of an unrelated condition.

Gait abnormality: History of limp due to pain/abnormality in gait to be asked

Associated symptoms: History of fever, skin rash, weight loss, abdominal pain, and redness of eyes can point to underlying etiology.

Known medical condition: Underlying bleeding diathesis like hemophilia, hemoglobinopathies like sickle cell anemia, connective tissue diseases like dermatomyositis, and inflammatory bowel disease can present with joint pain.

Red Flag Symptoms

- Nocturnal pain
- Pain severe enough to interfere with weight bearing
- Presence of systemic symptoms like fever and weight loss
- Pallor, bleeds

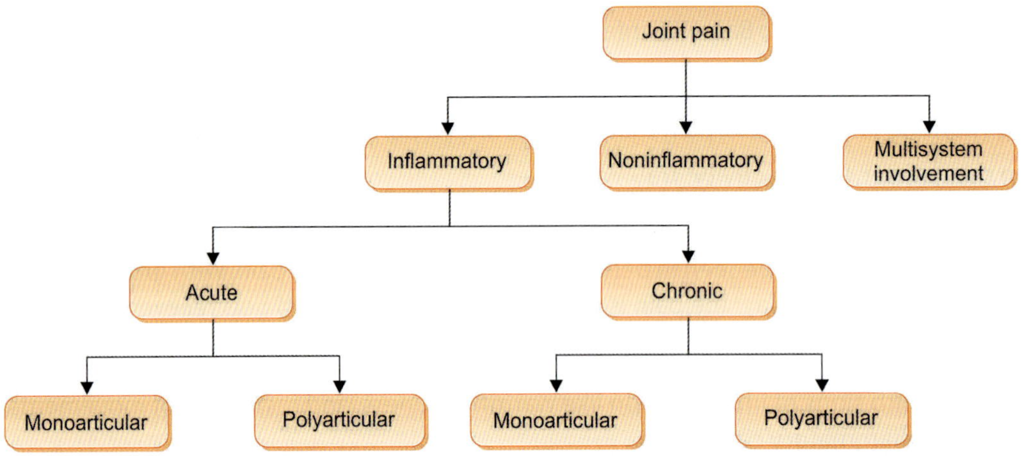

- *Noninflammatory:* Growing pain, joint hypermobility, vitamin D deficiency, osteochondrosis, dysplasia
- *Acute:* Infections, reactive arthritis, fracture, vasculitis, bone tumor, osteochondrosis, slipped capital femoral epiphysis (SCFE), trauma, hemarthrosis, acute leukemia, sickle cell
- *Chronic (>6 weeks):* JIA, connective tissue diseases, tuberculosis (TB)

Physical Examination

- General appearance: Well or sick looking
- Anthropometry, temperature, and BP
- Look for pallor, bleeds, lymphadenopathy, organomegaly
- Examination of skin, oral cavity, eyes
- pGALS (pediatric gait, arms, legs, and spine) assessment
- Focused examination of the affected joint and examination of other joints: Presence of warmth, erythema, range of movements, joint effusion, synovial thickening, muscle atrophy, limb length discrepancy
- Evaluation of muscle strength, look for joint hypermobility

Investigations

- *Complete blood count:* Provides clue to infectious and inflammatory pathology
- *Acute phase reactants:* C-reactive protein (CRP), erythrocyte sedimentation rate (ESR): Provide clue to infectious and inflammatory pathology
- *Liver and renal function test:* Should be done in those with systemic symptoms
- *Creatine phosphokinase (CPK):* To be done in those with muscle involvement
- Joint aspiration and analysis of synovial fluid for cell count, protein, glucose, Gram stain, culture, and polymerase chain reaction (PCR). In a child with suspected septic or reactive arthritis, aspiration and analysis of joint fluid will help in confirming the diagnosis.
- *Imaging studies:*
  - *X-ray:* A plain radiograph has limitations in sensitivity. Imaging of the contralateral unaffected joint is useful for comparison.
  - *USG of the joint:* Look for effusion, synovial changes
  - *MRI:* More valuable information than other modalities in children with bone and joint infection, bone tumors, and other inflammatory conditions
  - *CT:* Reserved for evaluating structural bone conditions
- *Specific tests:* Antistreptolysin O (ASO) titer, throat swab culture, antinuclear antibody (ANA), rheumatoid arthritis (RA) factor, immunoglobulin profile, human leukocyte antigen (HLA) B27

Algorithm

Approach to joint pain is shown in **Flowchart 1**.

FLOWCHART 1: Approach to joint pain.

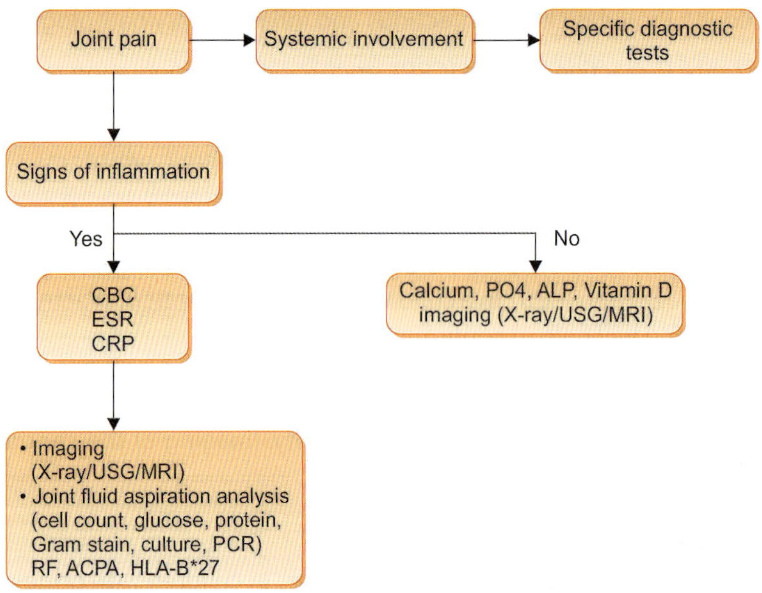

(ACPA: anti-citrullinated peptide antibody; ALP: alkaline phosphatase; CBC: complete blood count; CRP: C-reactive protein; ESR: erythrocyte sedimentation rate; HLA: human leukocyte antigen; PCR: polymerase chain reaction; PO4: phosphate; RF: rheumatoid factor)

Suggested Reading

- Sawhney S. Approach to a child with joint pains. In: Sawhney S, Aggarwal A (Eds). Pediatric Rheumatology. Singapore: Springer. pp. 159-72.
- Yukiko Kimura, Taunton R Southwood (2023). Evaluation of the child with joint pain and/or swelling. UpToDate. Retrieved May 2024, from https://www.uptodate.com/contents/evaluation-of-the-child-with-joint pain-and/or-swelling.

Acute-onset Cough

71

Section Editor: **Rupesh Masand**
Section Co-Editor: **Hema Gupta Mittal**
Author: **Somu Sivabalan**

Introduction

- Cough is the sound of forced expulsion of air against a closed glottis. It can happen voluntarily or involuntarily.
- This is a defensive reflex that protects the airway from aspiration of foreign materials, by enhancing clearance of secretions and particulates from the airways.

Types

- *Acute:* Cough that persists for <3–4 weeks
- *Chronic:* Daily cough of at least 4 weeks' duration. It is usually associated with an underlying/serious disorder.

Etiology

- Cough may be a manifestation of a respiratory disease.
- As respiratory bronchioles and alveoli lack cough receptors, their affection does not cause cough.
- Cough receptors are distributed along the respiratory system and nonrespiratory sites. It may be a secondary manifestation of cardiac, upper gastrointestinal, or neurological disease.
- Occasionally, somatic cough syndrome (previously called psychogenic/habit cough).

- Acute life-threatening cough may be due to aspiration syndrome including foreign bodies/sudden critical airway collapse due to a spectrum of severe airway malacias (laryngotracheobronchomalacia).

Pointers to Etiology

- Allergic shiners, Dennie–Morgan line, transverse crease on nose secondary to allergic salute
- Adenoid facies, chronic open mouth breathing—adenoid hypertrophy
- Harrison sulcus, increased anteroposterior diameter of the chest wall—chronic pathology

BOX 1: Disorders presenting with acute cough.

Disorders
Postinfectious cough syndrome [respiratory syncytial virus (RSV), parainfluenza virus, Mycoplasma, Chlamydia, and pertussis)
Aspiration syndrome: • *Intrinsic:* Gastroesophageal reflux disease (GERD), laryngopharyngeal reflux (LPR), aerodigestive communications: Tracheoesophageal fistula (TEF) and clefts • *Extrinsic:* Foreign body
Asthma
Upper airway cough syndrome (UACS) • Nonallergic rhinitis • Allergic rhinitis • Vasomotor rhinitis • Chronic bacterial sinusitis
Persistent moist cough: Protracted bacterial bronchitis (PBB)
Pertussis: Paroxysmal cough

TABLE 1: Localization of respiratory sounds/noises.

RESPIRATORY SOUNDS/NOISES	LOCALIZATION
Snuffle/snort	Nasal passage/nasopharynx
Snore	Oronasopharynx
Rattle	Either or both extra- and intrathoracic airways
Stridor associated with: • Normal voice, normal cough • Hoarse voice, barky cough • Normal voice, loud brassy, honky cough	• Extrathoracic airway • Supraglottic • Glottic • Subglottic
Wheeze	Intrathoracic airway
Grunt	Alveolar/lung parenchyma

Red Flags

- Daily moist/productive cough
- Feeding difficulties, choking, drooling
- Chest pain, chronic/exertion dyspnea
- Hemoptysis
- Persistent voice change
- Failure to thrive (FTT)
- *Abnormal auscultatory findings in the chest:* Added sounds or variation in sound quality
- Digital clubbing
- Hypoxia (SaO_2 <92%)
- Dropping SaO_2 >3 from baseline at rest, activity, or sleep
- Cyanosis

Approach to Acute-onset Cough (Flowchart 1)

- *Step 1:* Is it a significant cough?
  - Since birth
  - With acute life-threatening event (ALTE)
  - >2 weeks of progressive nature
  - <2 weeks disturbing the day-to-day activity and/or sleep
  - Beyond 4 weeks
  - With distress, hypoxia, chest pain, or hemoptysis
  - With persisting voice change or feeding/swallowing difficulties
- *Step 2:* Cough with other respiratory symptoms
- *Step 3:* Cough with multisystem involvement
- *Step 4:* Cough with red flags

Features of Cough

- *Character of the cough:* Is it moist or dry?
- *Diurnal variation:*
  - When is it more during day time or during night?
  - *Early morning cough:* Lower airway
  - Is it present when awake and also during sleep?
- *Changing posture:* Upper airway cough syndrome (UACS) commonly known as postnasal drip induces cough when child is in supine position on bed.
- *Paroxysmal:* Pertussis, GERD, LPR
- *With voice change:* Laryngeal

TABLE 2: Disorders bearing predisposition to develop respiratory disease.

DISORDERS	RESPIRATORY DISEASE
Orocraniofacial anomaly: Down syndrome, mucopolysaccharidosis, Pierre–Robin sequence	Upper airway obstruction
Kyphosis, scoliosis, pectus carinatum, absent ribs	Restrictive lung disease
Neuromuscular/neurodevelopmental	Ineffective cough, aspiration/stagnation, with collapse or infection
Rheumatological, vasculitis	Interstitial lung disease
Immunodeficiency	Severe, persistent, unusual, and recurrent respiratory infections

FLOWCHART 1: Approach to acute-onset cough

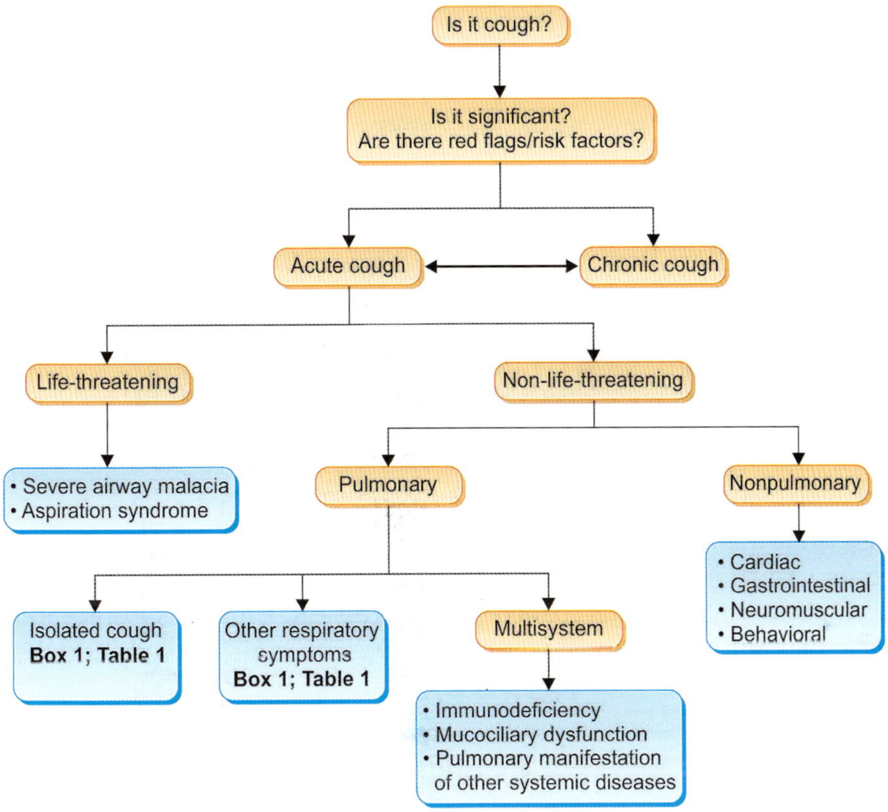

Suggested Reading

- Amdekar Y, Chokhani R, Palaniraman R. Management of Cough in Office Practice. Indian Academy of Pediatrics (IAP). Standard Treatment Guidelines 2022. [online] Available from https://iapindia.org/pdf/Ch-150-Management-of-Cough-inOffSTANDARD%20 TREATMENT%20GUIDELINES%202022ice-Practice.pdf [Last accessed May, 2024].
- Chang AB, Landau LI, Van Asperen PP, Glasgow NJ, Robertson CF, Marchant JM, et al.; Thoracic Society of Australia and New Zealand. Cough in children: definitions and clinical evaluation. Med J Aust. 2006;184(8):398-403.
- Desai PP, Thomas PK, Abhyankar N, Vora A, Jaggi V, Jog P, et al. INDIan Consensus on the mAnagemenT of cOugh at pRimary care setting (INDICATOR). J Assoc Physicians India. 2023;71(6):11-2.
- Kasi AS, Kamerman-Kretzmer RJ. Cough. Pediatr Rev. 2019;40(4):157-67.

Bleeding Child

72

Section Editor: **Janani Shankar**
Section Co-Editor: **Arathi Srinivasan**
Author: **Ajeitha Loganathan**

Introduction

- Bleeding in children is an unusual manifestation and a cause of alarm.
- The causes may range from a congenital abnormality in the bleeding or clotting mechanisms or acquired causes associated with other systemic disorders like immune thrombocytopenia (ITP), vitamin K deficiency, disseminated intravascular coagulation (DIC), aplastic anemia, leukemia, and inherited causes including hemophilia and von Willebrand disease (VWD).

Etiology

Etiology of bleeding in children is given in **Table 1**.

TABLE 1: Etiology of bleeding in children.

ETIOLOGY	EXAMPLES	TYPE OF BLEED
Systemic illnesses	Sepsis, DIC, aplastic anemia, leukemia	Multiple sites, concurrent bleed
Local cause	Trauma, surgery, tumor	Single site, recurrent bleed
Underlying bleeding disorder	Discussed below	Recurrent bleeds—different sites with no/trivial trauma

(DIC: disseminated intravascular coagulation)

Bleeding Disorders

Bleeding disorders could be disorders of primary or secondary hemostasis **(Table 2)**.

TABLE 2: Bleeding disorders.

CLINICAL FEATURES	PRIMARY HEMOSTASIS (PLATELET DISORDERS, VWD, VESSEL WALL DISEASE)	SECONDARY HEMOSTASIS (CLOTTING FACTOR DEFICIENCY)
Site	Skin/mucous membrane	Soft tissue, muscle, joints
Petechiae	Common	Absent/rare
Hemarthroses, soft-tissue hematoma	Rare	Common
Bleeding after surgery	Immediate	Delayed

(VWD: von Willebrand disease)

Causes

Causes of bleeding in children are given in **Box 1**.

BOX 1: Causes of bleeding in children.

PLATELET DISORDERS	COAGULATION DISORDERS
Thrombocytopenia: • *Decreased platelet survival* – Immune mediated - Immune thrombocytopenia (ITP) - Drug induced – Thrombotic microangiopathy - Disseminated intravascular coagulation (DIC) - Hemolytic uremic syndrome (HUS) - Thrombotic thrombocytopenic purpura (TTP) – Wiskott–Aldrich syndrome (WAS) • *Decreased platelet production* – Malignancies (leukemia, lymphoma) – Sepsis – Marrow failure • *Platelet sequestration* – Hypersplenism – Giant hemangiomas (Kasabach–Merritt syndrome) • *Disorders of platelet function* – Congenital - Glanzmann's thrombasthenia - Bernard–Soulier syndrome – Acquired - *Drug induced:* Aspirin	• *Congenital* – Hemophilia – Other factor deficiencies – von Willebrand disease (VWD) • *Acquired* – DIC – Vitamin K deficiency – Liver disease – Warfarin – Renal disease – Cyanotic congenital heart disease

Age, Pattern, and Gender-based Etiology

Etiology based on age, pattern, and gender is given in **Table 3**.

TABLE 3: Age, pattern, and gender-based etiology.

FEATURE	DISORDER
Infant while weight bearing—joint bleeds	Clotting factor deficiency (e.g., hemophilia)
Boy with mucocutaneous bleeding, eczema	WAS (X linked)
Infant, newborn, prolonged PT, aPTT	Vitamin K deficiency bleeding
Well child, mucosal bleeding, low platelets	ITP
Bleeding from intact skin, many sites, normal coagulation profile	Hematohidrosis

(aPTT: activated partial thromboplastin time; ITP: immune thrombocytopenia; PT: prothrombin time; WAS: Wiskott–Aldrich syndrome)

Approach

- History taking
- Clinical examination
  - *Systemic features:* Lymphadenopathy, hepatosplenomegaly, pallor (leukemia)
  - Petechiae versus purpura versus ecchymoses, e.g., palpable purpura in lower limbs (IgA vasculitis)
  - *Unusual bruises:* Battered baby syndrome
  - *Icterus:* Liver disease
  - *Fever/toxemia:* Sepsis, DIC
  - Compartment syndrome
  - Hemodynamic status
  - *Joint laxity:* Collagen vascular disease
  - Skin

- *Congenital anomalies:* Hand and thumb anomalies [Fanconi anemia, thrombocytopenia-absent radius (TAR) syndrome]
- *Hemangioma:* DIC
- Fundoscopy is vital.

❍ Evaluation

Evaluation is given in **Table 4**.

TABLE 4: Tests for evaluation.

TEST	LOOK FOR	DIAGNOSIS
Complete blood counts	• Anemia • Leucopenia/leukocytosis • Thrombocytopenia	• Aplastic anemia, hemolysis, massive blood loss, leukemia • Leukemia, aplastic anemia, sepsis
Peripheral smear	• Platelet number and morphology • Schistocytes (microangiopathic hemolytic anemia)	• *Small platelets:* WAS • *Giant platelets:* ITP, Bernard–Soulier syndrome • HUS, TTP, DIC
Bleeding time and clotting time	Obsolete	
PT	Elevation (normal—approximately 10–11 seconds)	Deficiency of extrinsic (tissue factor, factor VII) or common pathway factors (II, V, X, and fibrinogen)
aPTT	Elevation (normal—approximately 26–35 seconds)	Deficiency of intrinsic (VIII, IX, XI, or XII), common pathway factors, presence of inhibitors (e.g., lupus anticoagulant/heparin)
Mixing studies	Normalization of clotting test (PT or aPTT) following a 1:1 dilution with normal pooled plasma	• Clotting factor deficiency • Persistent abnormal PT/aPTT with mixing—indicates inhibitors
Specific coagulation factor assays	Low	Specific factor deficiency
Fibrinogen	Low	• Congenital afibrinogenemia, hypofibrinogenemia • Consumption, e.g., DIC

(aPTT: activated partial thromboplastin time; DIC: disseminated intravascular coagulation; HUS: hemolytic uremic syndrome; ITP: immune thrombocytopenia; PT: prothrombin time; TTP: thrombotic thrombocytopenic purpura; WAS: Wiskott–Aldrich syndrome)

Approach to a Child with Bleeding Disorder

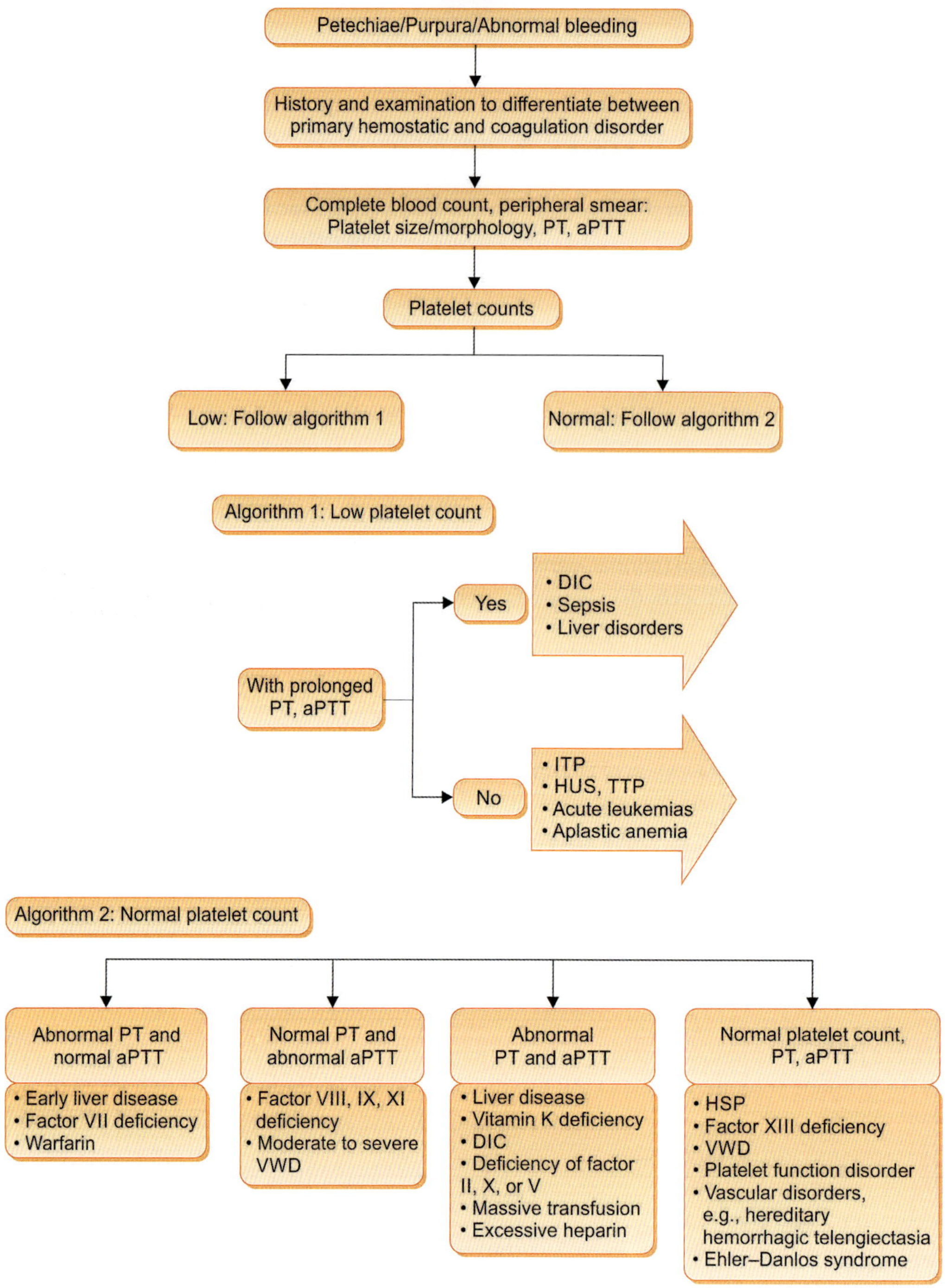

(aPTT: activated partial thromboplastin time; DIC: disseminated intravascular coagulation; PT: prothrombin time; HUS: hemolytic uremic syndrome; ITP: immune thrombocytopenia; TTP: thrombotic thrombocytopenic purpura VWD: von Willebrand disease)

Red Flags

- Severe pallor
- Altered mental status (intracranial bleed)
- Bleeding from multiple sites (DIC)
- Compartment syndrome
- Hemarthroses
- Bone pains (leukemia)
- Any transfusion requirement

Suggested Reading

- A l-Huniti A, Sharath kumar A, Manwani D. Approach to the pediatric patient with a bleeding disorder. In: Shaz BH, Hillyer CD, Gil MR (Eds). Transfusion Medicine and Hemostasis. Philadelphia: Elsevier; 2019. pp. 565-70.
- Allen GA, Glader B. Approach to the bleeding child. Pediatric Clin. 2002;49(6):1239-56.
- Bansal D, Oberoi S, Marwaha RK, Singhi SC. Approach to a child with bleeding in the emergency room. Indian J Pediatr. 2013;80:411-20.
- Blanchette VS, Breakey VR, Revel-Vilk S (Eds): SickKids Handbook of Pediatric Thrombosis and Hemostasis. Basel: Karger; 2013. pp. 14-22.

Amenorrhea

73

Section Editor: **Kripasindhu Chatterjee**
Section Co-Editors: **Atanu Bhadra, Ashim Kumar Ghosh**
Authors: **Eshita Bhowmik, Sweta Mandal**

Definition

- *Primary amenorrhea:* Absence of menarche by 15 years of age or a delay of >3 years from the onset of thelarche
- *Secondary amenorrhea:* A gap of 1 year from the last menstrual period; however, any gap >90 days from the last menstrual period in girls >1 year post menarche needs evaluation.

Etiology

- *Primary hypogonadism/hypergonadotropic hypogonadism:*
  - Turner syndrome
  - Primary ovarian failure/insufficiency: Genetic (*FMR, FOXL2* mutation), autoimmune
  - Surgery
  - Chemotherapy
  - Local irradiation
  - Oophoritis (mumps)
  - Galactosemia
  - Gonadal dysgenesis due to disorder of sex development (DSD)
- *Secondary hypogonadism/hypogonadotropic hypogonadism (HH):*
  - Constitutional delay in growth and puberty (CDGP)
  - Functional HH
  - Chronic illness
  - Athletic amenorrhea
  - Eating disorder

- *Isolated gonadotropic deficiency:* Congenital, Kallman syndrome, other genetic causes (*KISS1*, *TAC3*, *TAC3R*), syndromic (Prader–Willi syndrome, Bardet–Biedl syndrome)
- *Combined pituitary hormone deficiency:* Mutation in *PROP1*, *LHX3*
- *Tumor of hypothalamopituitary axis:* Craniopharyngioma, glioma
- Cranial irradiation
- Traumatic brain injury
- *Postinflammation:* Meningitis, encephalitis

- *Nonhypothalamic, nonovarian causes:*
  - Pregnancy
  - Obesity
  - Cushing syndrome
  - Untreated hypothyroidism
  - Hyperprolactinemia
- *Hyperandrogenism:* Polycystic ovarian disease
- *Abnormal genital structure:*
  - Uterine adhesion
  - Imperforate hymen
  - Mayer–Rokitansky–Küster–Hauser (MRKH) syndrome
  - Complete androgen insensitivity syndrome (CAIS) in genetic male

Red Flag Signs

- No breast development (Tanner stage 1) by 13 years of age
- No menarche after 3 years of onset of thelarche
- No menarche by age 15 years
- *Irregular menstrual cycle:* >90 days for any one cycle (>1 year post menarche), cycles <21 days/ >45 days (>1 year to <3 year postmenarche), cycle < 21 days/ >35 days (>3 year post menarche)
- Short stature, other stigmata of Turner syndrome
- Excessive weight loss/recent weight gain/obesity
- Feature of raised intracranial tension, visual field defect, headache, vomiting

Investigations

- Assessment of growth, plotting in growth chart with midparental height
- Tanner staging of breast and pubic hair, genital examination to rule out DSD. 46XY undervisilised boy with 17-alpha-hydroxylase deficiency
- *Karyotyping:* 46XY. Complete androgen insensitivity syndrome presents with complete breast development, amenorrhea, and absent pubic hair.
- 46XX girl with nonclassic congenital adrenal hyperplasia (NCCAH)/nonsalt-wasting type of CAH presents with menstrual abnormality features of virilization and clitoromegaly.

Other Investigations

- *Visual field, fundus examination:* Rule out central midline tumor
- Formal smell testing for anosmic variety of Kallman syndrome
- Dysmorphic features like webbed neck, cubitus vulgus, hyperconvex nails with short stature—Turner syndrome
- *Bone age assessment:* Delayed bone age in a short child with delayed puberty with a growth rate consistent with bone age with family history of delayed onset of puberty is a strong indicator of CDGP
- *Hormone assays:* Hyperandrogenism, with raised testosterone, free androgen index, dehydroepiandrosterone sulfate (DHEAS), and hirsutism with oligoanovulation indicates polycystic ovarian syndrome (PCOS).
- *Pelvic USG:* DSD, MRKH syndrome
- *MRI brain:* Suspected intracranial space-occupying lesion (SOL)/Kallman syndrome

Approach

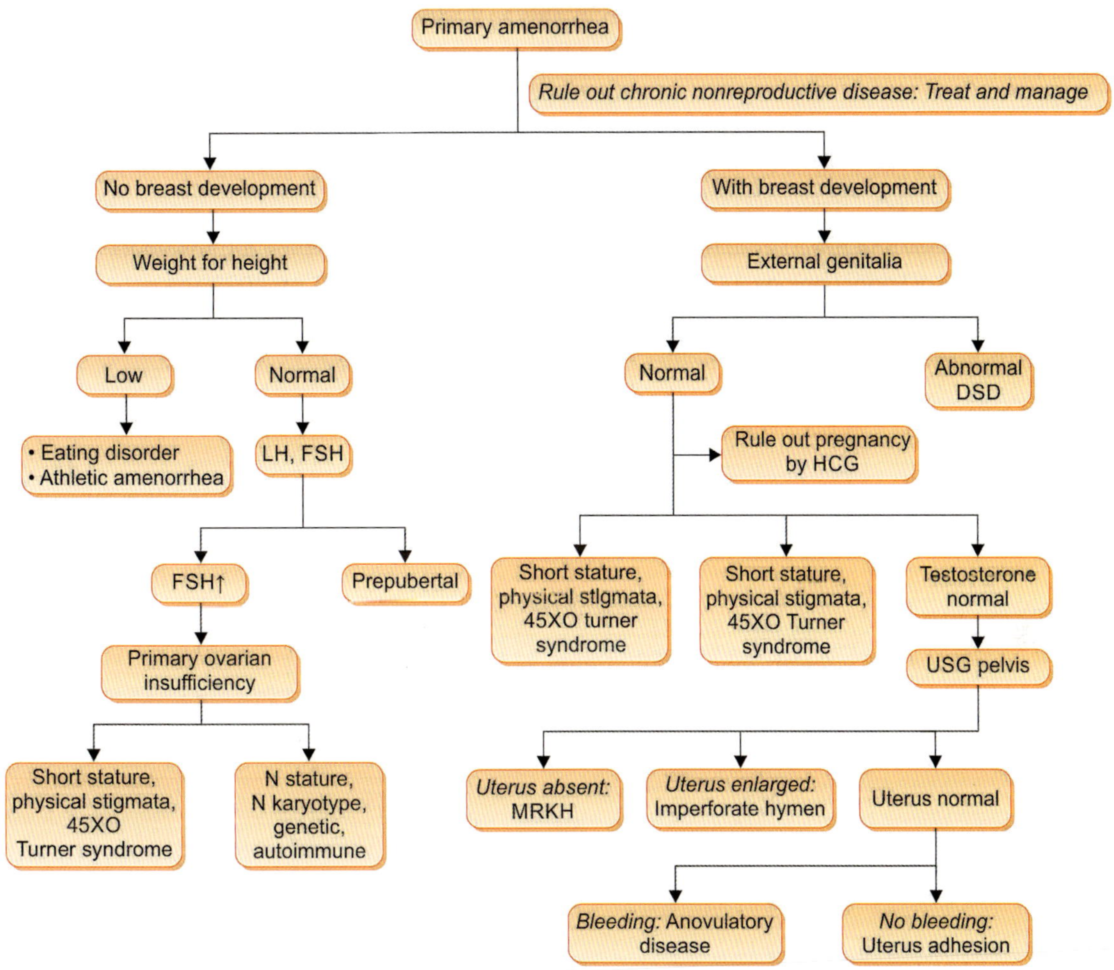

(DSD: disorder of sex development; FSH: follicle-stimulating hormone; HCG: human chorionic gonadotropin; LH: luteinizing hormone; MRKH: Mayer–Rokitansky–Küster–Hauser)

Suggested Reading

- ACOG Committee Opinion No. 651: Menstruation in girls and adolescents: using the menstrual cycle as a vital sign. Obstet Gynecol. 2015;126(6):e143-6.
- Peña AS, Witchel SF, Hoeger KM, Oberfield SE, Vogiatzi MG, Misso M, et al. Adolescent polycystic ovary syndrome according to the international evidence-based guideline. BMC Med. 2020;18(1):72.
- Rosenfield RL, Cooke DW, Radovick S. Puberty in the female and its disorders. In: Sperling Pediatric Endocrinology, 5th edition. Philadelphia: Elsevier; 2021. pp. 528-626.
- Styne DM. Physiology and disorders of puberty. In: Melmed S, Auchus RJ, Goldfine AB, Koenig RJ, Rosen CJ (Eds). Williams Textbook of Endocrinology, 14th edition. Philadelphia: Elsevier; 2020. pp. 1023-164.
- Zacharin M, Banerjee I. Delayed puberty. In: Desai MP, Menon PSN, Bhatia V, Seth A (Eds). Pediatric Endocrine Disorders, 4th edition. Hyderabad: Universities Press (India) Private Limited; 2022. pp. 139-52.

Dysphagia

74

Section Editor: **Rupesh Masand**
Section Co-Editor: **Hema Gupta Mittal**
Author: **Neminathan**

Definition

Dysphagia is disruption in swallow sequence owing to the affection of the upper gastrointestinal (GI) tract from the lip to the lower esophageal sphincter.

Classification

- *Oropharyngeal:* Difficulty in initiating the swallowing
- *Esophageal:* Difficulty in food passage down the esophagus

Clinical Presentation

- Dysphagia—always an acute/chronic symptom of underlying disorders.
  - *Oropharyngeal dysphagia:* Changes in speech, choking, food spillage, food sticking in mouth/throat, nasal regurgitation, uncoordinated oral movements
  - *Esophageal dysphagia:* Chest/epigastric pain, food bolus, food sticking in throat/retrosternum, heartburn, vomiting
- Dysphagia may be associated with primary affection of other systems like:
  - Dysmorphism (Down syndrome, Pierre–Robin sequence), intellectual disability, improper posture control, seizure disorder, recurrent aspiration, stridor, immobility
  - Cyanosis, increased suck–swallow–rest cycle, stridor, noisy breathing, recurrent aspiration of feeds [congenital heart disease (CHD), double aortic arch]
  - Failure to thrive, recurrent wheeze, infections attributed to respiratory illness like pulmonary dysplasia

Etiology

Etiology of dysphagia is given in **Table 1**.

TABLE 1: Etiology of dysphagia.

OROPHARYNGEAL	ESOPHAGEAL	OTHERS
• Anatomical disruption of head and neck structures • Nasopharyngeal/tongue base masses • Vocal cord paralysis • Laryngeal cleft • Cervical abscess	*Congenital:* • Tracheoesophageal fistula • Esophageal atresia • Hiatus hernia • Congenital webs/rings of upper esophagus • Diverticula • Esophageal duplication cyst • Obstruction by vascular anomalies—aberrant right subclavian/Aortic aneurysm *Acquired:* • Reflux esophagitis • Gastroesophageal reflux disease (GERD) • Peptic stricture • Caustic esophagitis • Foreign body • Achalasia • Eosinophilic esophagitis • Systemic sclerosis • Crohn's disease	*Neuromuscular/Neurological:* • Developmental disorders • Cerebral palsy • Degenerative disorders • Traumatic brain injury *Behavioral:* • Feed avoidance • Temper tantrums

Red Flags

SYMPTOMS	SIGNS
• Poor weight gain, poor suck, weak cry, floppy muscle • Shortness of breath/aspiration • With/without fever, increase fatiguability • Choking/globus sensation	• Failure to thrive • Aspiration pneumonia • Foreign body

Investigations

- Fluoroscopic/video fluoroscopic evaluation of swallowing (gold standard
- Upper GI endoscopy
- Chest X-ray
- CT/MRI of neck, thorax (structural abnormalities, chronic side effects of radiation therapy—dysphagia/ aspiration-related structures where MRI is better than CT)
- pH multichannel intraluminal impedance [gold standard—gastroesophageal reflux disease (GERD)]
- High-resolution esophageal manometry (motility disorder)

A multidisciplinary approach is advisable in systemic involvement.

Approach to Dysphagia

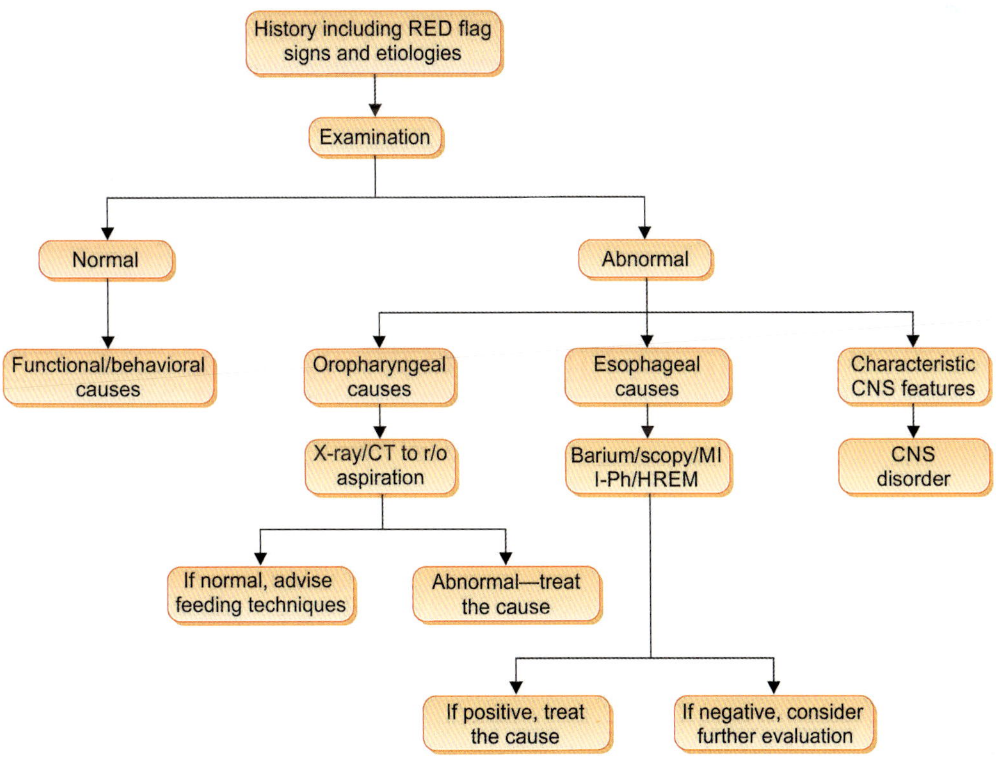

(CNS: central nervous system; HREM: high-resolution esophageal manometry)

Suggested Reading

- Dodrill P, Gosa MM. Pediatric dysphagia: Physiology, assessment, and management. Ann Nutr Metab. 2015;66 (Suppl 5):24-31.
- Krishnamurthy R, Balasubramanium RK, Kamath N, Bhat KG. A Delphi survey based construction and validation of test for oropharyngeal dysphagia in Indian neonates. Int J Pediatr Otorhinolaryngol. 2021;140:110306.
- Lanzoni G, Sembenini C, Gastaldo S, Leonardi L, Bentivoglio VP, Faggian G, et al. Esophageal dysphagia in children. Front Pediatr. 2022;10:885308.
- Lawlor CM, Choi S. Diagnosis and management of pediatric dysphagia: A review. JAMA Otolaryngol Head Neck Surg. 2020;146(2):183-91.

Hoarseness of Voice

75

Section Editor: **Rupesh Masand**
Section Co-Editor: **Hema Gupta Mittal**
Authors: **Partha Pratim Borah, Chiranjeet Narayan Dev**

Definition

- Hoarseness is a symptom of vocal cord dysfunction.
- It presents as a breathy, harsh, coarse, strained, or raspy voice.
- In children, hoarseness can be used to describe both the quality of the voice and the quality of the cry.

Etiology

Hoarseness is classified as follows:

- *Congenital*: Infants presenting with an unusual cry or respiratory distress should be evaluated for congenital abnormalities like laryngeal webs or hemangiomas. Those with cardiac anomalies have a higher incidence of congenital laryngeal anomalies.
- *Paralysis of the vocal cord:* May be unilateral/bilateral vocal cord paralysis

  Unilateral paralysis presents with symptoms of chronic aspiration and weak/absent cry
- *Bilateral paralysis:* Vocal cords assume a midline position, protecting the airway from aspiration and permitting a normal cry
- *Acquired:* Allergic/infectious laryngitis, laryngitis due to gastroesophageal reflux
- *Pathophysiology:* The smaller airways of children are more susceptible to inflammation and edema of the subglottic airway. Laryngitis occurs with viral respiratory infections, secondary to acute vocal strain, submucosal vocal cord inflammation, or hemorrhage. Laryngotracheobronchitis/croup is more common in children <5 years of age and commonly viral in origin.

Laryngopharyngeal reflux (LPR) is defined as reflux of gastric or duodenal juices beyond the esophagus into the larynx, oropharynx, or nasopharynx.

Gastroesophageal reflux disease and LPR disease are common causes of pediatric hoarseness.

Metabolic/endocrinal causes due to disruption of normal enzymatic activity, causing abnormal infiltration/faulty muscle and nerve function. In Urbach–Wiethe disease/mucopolysaccharidosis, dysphonia occurs due to laryngeal involvement.

In hypothyroidism, generalized hypotonia and myxedematous infiltrations in the vocal folds

Recurrent respiratory papillomatosis is more common in a first-born child, young primigravid mothers, and low socioeconomic groups.

- *Functional:* Personality disorders, adjustment problems/anxiety, psychological trauma, disturbed parent–child relationship, attention deficit hyperactive disorder (ADHD)

  Chronic usage of metered dose inhalers containing budesonide without the aid of spacer device can also lead to laryngitis and oral thrush.

Red Flags

- Heartburn
- Apnea
- Persistent cough
- Stridor
- Respiratory distress with progression
- Hemoptysis
- Dysphagia, odynophagia
- Cervical lymphadenopathy
- Fever, night sweats, and unexplained weight loss

If any of these are present and the hoarseness is persistent beyond 3 weeks, an urgent referral to an otorhinolaryngologist should be made.

Investigations

- *Thorough* clinical assessment and endoscopic examination
- The laryngoscopic examination for the diagnosis of the laryngeal lesions and correct treatment
- Endoscopy with transnasal flexible scope for identifying the morphodynamic alterations
- Stroboscopy—only in the older age group of children
- Laryngeal ultrasound—to assess the subglottic diameter, laryngeal stenosis, subglottic hemangiomas, and vocal fold paralysis
- Computed tomography (CT) and magnetic resonance imaging are usually advised for any neoplastic assessment in the larynx.

Algorithm: Approach to Hoarseness of Voice

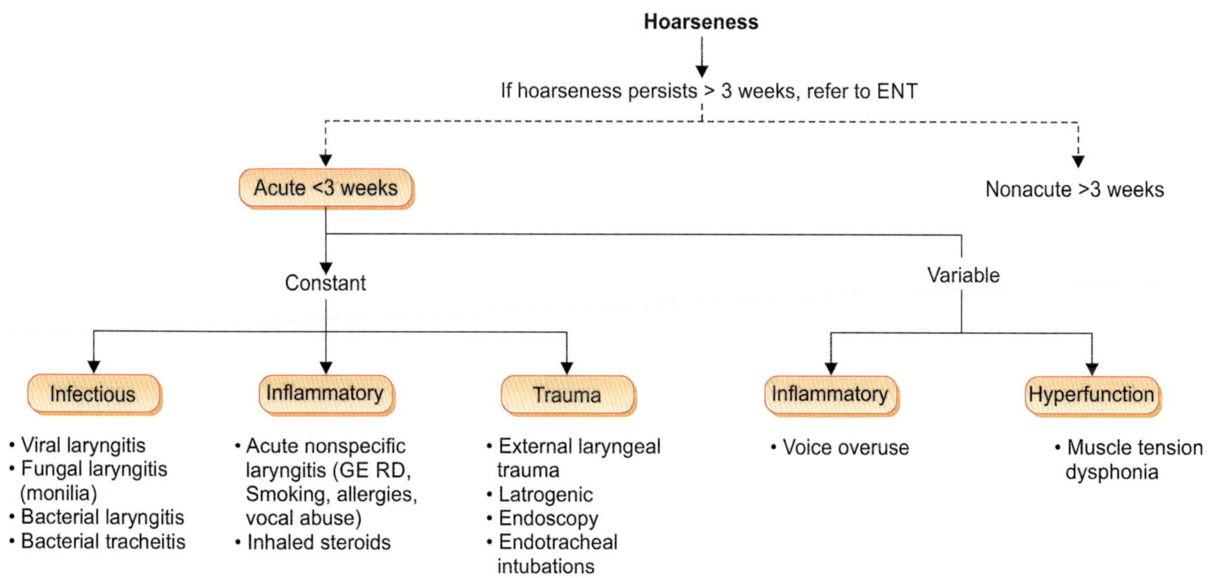

(ENT: ear, nose, throat; GERD: gastroesophageal reflux disease)

Suggested Reading

- Elbanna MM, Elmaghraby RM. Predisposing factors of childhood dysphonia in primary school children. Egypt J Otolaryngol. 2021;37:105.
- Swain SK, Nayak B, Sahoo L, Munjal S, Sahu MS. Pediatric dysphonia - A review. Indian J Child Health. 2019;6(1):1-5.
- Tavares ELM, Brasolotto A, Santana MF, Padovan CA, Martins RHG. Epidemiological study of dysphonia in 4-12 year-old children. Braz J Otorhinolaryngol. 2011;77(6):736-46.
- Worthen M, Chandran S. Hoarseness in children. Int J Head Neck Surg. 2016;7 (2):130-5.

Irritability and Fussiness 76

Section Editor: **Sumitha Nayak**
Section Co-Editor: **Priya Shivalli**
Authors: **Prasant Kumar Saboth, Shikha Garg**

Introduction

- Irritability/fussiness is an externalizing behavioral response to any internal or external stressor/stimuli.
- In infants and younger children, it may be a response to some physical/environmental stressor. Often, it is a means of communication of distress. In older children and adolescents' excessive irritability may indicate a deficit in emotional regulation in response to stressors.
- The onset and severity of irritability, associated physical features, and child's developmental trajectory are important factors to be considered while assessing irritable children.
- Occasional anger outbursts in older children and adolescents may be developmentally appropriate responses to frustrating situations. Chronic irritability is more concerning and needs closer examination. This could be a strong predictor of future mental health issues in children and adolescents.

Etiology

- *Acute onset (<2 weeks)*
  - Infections—localized (e.g., ear infections), systemic
    - Trauma/head injury/CNS infections
    - Gastroesophageal reflux
    - Constipation/colic
    - Diaper dermatitis in younger children
    - Hernia—obstructed/irreducible
    - Nasal obstruction/upper respiratory infection (URI)
    - Sleep disturbances due to any reason
    - Cyanotic spells/arrythmias

- *Persistent (>2 weeks)*
- *Infants*
  - Nutrition-related protein-energy malnutrition (PEM)/severe acute malnutrition (SAM)
  - Failure to thrive—nutritional/metabolic disorders, etc.
  - Gastrointestinal (GI) problems: Gastroesophageal reflux/colic/cow milk protein allergy/constipation
  - Central nervous system (CNS) conditions: Encephalopathy/seizures/evolving tonal abnormalities
  - Dental problems
  - Sleep disorders
  - Diaper dermatitis
  - Chronic disorders, e.g., atopic dermatitis/allergy
  - Sensory issues: Vision/hearing impairment
  - Poor mother–infant bonding
- *Preschoolers:* Developmentally normal
  - Infections—localized (e.g., ear infections) or systemic—CNS infections
  - Trauma/head injury
  - GI issues—gastroesophageal reflux disorder/constipation
  - Sleep disturbances due to any reason
  - Neurological causes—encephalopathy/seizures
  - Metabolic disorders
  - Chronic disorders, e.g., atopic dermatitis/allergy
  - Temperament issues—temper tantrums
  - Psychological issues—arrival of a sibling/parental disharmony, etc.
- *Preschoolers with developmental delay:* Chronic medical causes plus
  - Autism
  - Attention-deficit hyperactivity disorder (ADHD)
  - Sensory processing disorders
  - Sensory issues: Vision/hearing impairment
  - Social communication disorders
- *School-going children:*
  - Various chronic medical conditions as mentioned above
  - Family-related
    - Stress
      - Conflicts with/among parents
      - High parental expectations
      - Sibling rivalry

- School factors
  - Change of school
    - Bullying
    - Authoritarian teachers
    - Maladjustment in school
- Individual factors
  - High expectations
    - Body image issues
      - ADHD
      - Anxiety disorders
      - Depression
      - Cyberbullying
      - Adverse childhood experiences/post-traumatic stress disorder (PTSD)
      - *Abuse:* Physical/sexual/substance
      - Mood disorders

Red Flags

SYMPTOMS	SIGNS
• Continuous cry for >2 hours	• Temperature >101°F
• Cyanotic spells	• Tachypnea
• Fast breathing	• SpO_2-<92% in room air
• Self injury behavior (Hand banging)	• Visible peristalsis
• High grade fever	• Rashes/bite marks
• Skin rashes	• Meningeal signs present
• Sleep disorders	• BP >95th percentile
• Suicidal attempt/tendencies	

Approach to Irritability and Fussiness in Children

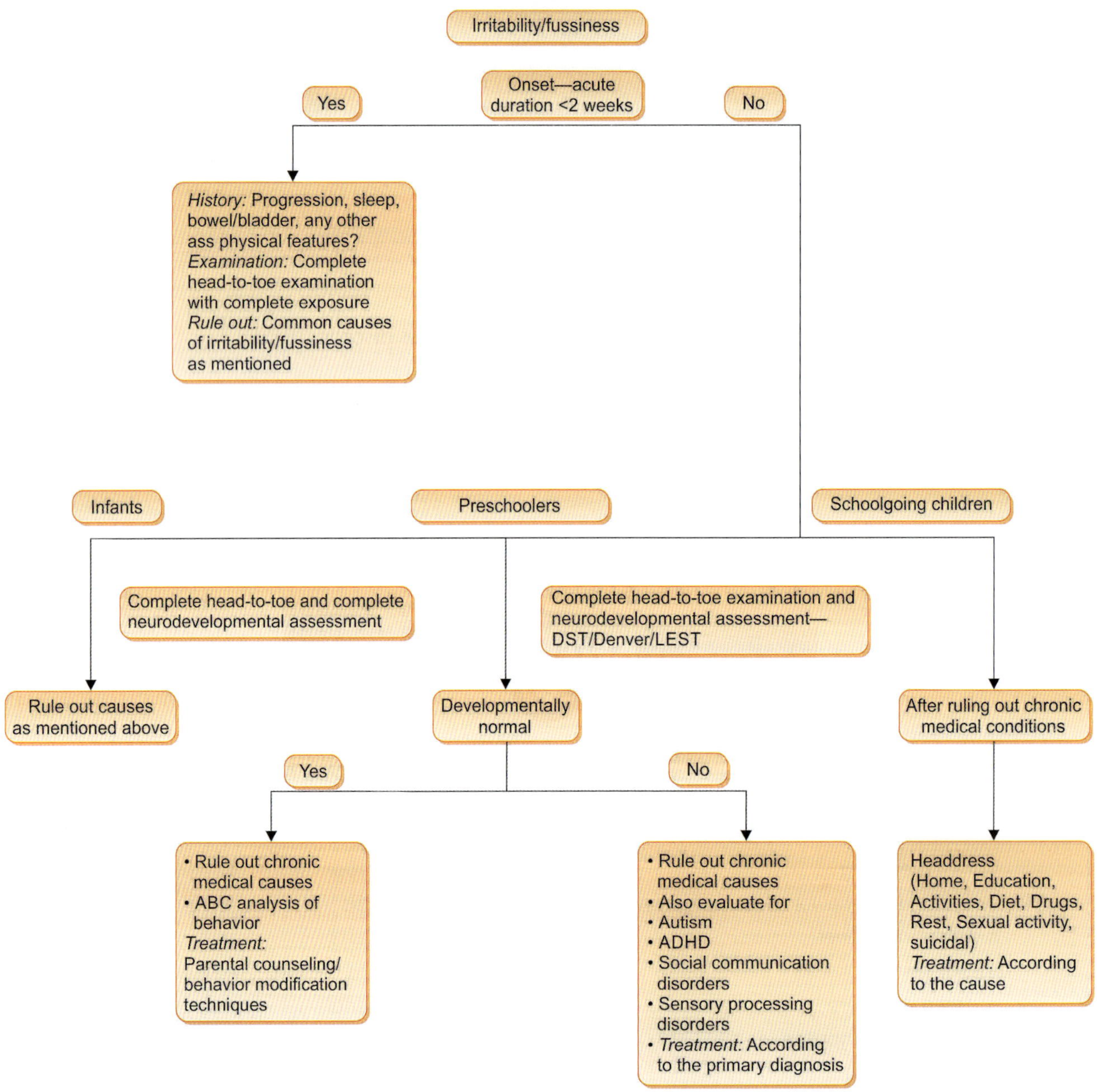

(ABC: antecedent-behavior-consequence; ADHD: attention-deficit/hyperactivity disorder; DST: development screening test; LEST: language evaluation scale trivandrum)

Suggested Reading

- Fourneret P, Desombre H. [The Severe Chronic Irritability Concept: A clinical dimension to consider in child and adolescent]. Encephale. 2017;43(2):187-91.
- Hameed U, Dellasega CA. Irritability in Pediatric Patients: Normal or Not? Prim Care Companion CNS Disord. 2016;18(2):10.4088/PCC.15br01893.
- Krieger FV, Leibenluft E, Stringaris A, Polanczyk GV. Irritability in children and adolescents: Past concepts, current debates, and future opportunities. Revista Brasileira de Psiquiatria. 2013;35(Suppl 1):S32-9.

Persistent Nasal Discharge/Nasal Obstruction

77

Section Editor: **Rupesh Masand**
Section Co-Editor: **Hema Gupta Mittal**
Author: **Dipti Pujari**

Introduction

- Persistent nasal discharge and nasal obstruction are common presenting symptoms in a pediatric clinic.
- They may occur together as symptoms of "allergic rhinitis" (AR). As the pollen allergy season continues to get longer and more intense due to global warming, the prevalence of AR in India is also increasing, affecting 13% of 6–7-year-old children and almost 22% of adolescents.

Etiology

Some of the causes of persistent nasal discharge/blockage are as follows:

- *AR:*
  - *Indoor pollens:* House dust mites, pets, cockroaches, molds
  - *Outdoor pollens:* Tree/grass/weed pollens, molds
- Classified depending on symptom—duration and severity as follows:
  a. Mild intermittent
  b. Mild persistent
  c. Moderate-severe intermittent
  d. Moderate-severe persistent

- *Infective rhinitis* (discharge/blockage lasts almost till the duration of the infection)
  - Viral
  - Bacterial
  - Fungal
- *Nonallergic vasomotor rhinitis:* By triggers like:
  - Strong smells
  - Sudden weather changes
  - Certain medications
  - Exercise
- *Rhinitis medicamentosa:* From overuse of topical nasal decongestants:
  - Phenylephrine
  - Oxymetazoline
- *Atrophic rhinitis:*
  - Congenital
  - Estrogen imbalance
  - Lack of iron or vitamins A or D
  - Secondary to autoimmune diseases
  - After radiation therapy
- *Cerebrospinal fluid (CSF) leak:* History of base of the skull trauma but rarely could be nontraumatic CSF rhinorrhea

SYMPTOMS	THINK OF
Unilateral nasal obstruction with/without rhinorrhea	Sinonasal tumor/FB
Persistent unilateral blood-stained discharge	Carcinomas/prolonged presence of foreign body
Persistent clear watery leak	CSF leak/acute FB insertion
Fever, pain, or foul smell in the nose with congestion or runny nose in an immunocompromised host	Fungal sinusitis
Obstruction and persistent nasal discharge since very early infancy	Hemangiomas

(CSF: cerebrospinal fluid; FB: foreign body)

Red Flags

- Unilateral nasal obstruction with/without rhinorrhea (sinonasal tumor)
- Persistent unilateral blood-stained discharge (Carcinoma)
- Persistent clear watery leak (CSF leak)
- Fever, pain or foul smell in the nose with congestion or runny nose in an immunocompromised host (Fungal sinusitis)
- Obstruction and persistent nasal discharge present since very early infancy (hemangiomas)

Investigations

- Thorough *history and examination*
- *Skin prick test or serum-specific IgE* for indoor and outdoor aeroallergens (strongly guided by the history only):
  - Early morning sneeze—house dust mite sensitization
  - Sneezing and rhinorrhea while playing outside in the park—grass/tree/weed pollen allergies
- *Nasal eosinophil count:* >10 eosinophils/high-power field may point to nasal allergy.
- *CT scan of paranasal sinuses:* To evaluate polyps, turbinate hypertrophy, nasal septal deviation, obstruction of osteomeatal complex
- *Peak nasal inspiratory flow rate (PNIFR):* Simple tool to measure nasal obstruction in the outpatient department (OPD). Normal flow is 100–300 L/min. Less than 100 L/min is symptomatic of nasal obstruction.

Algorithm for the Diagnosis of Allergic Rhinitis

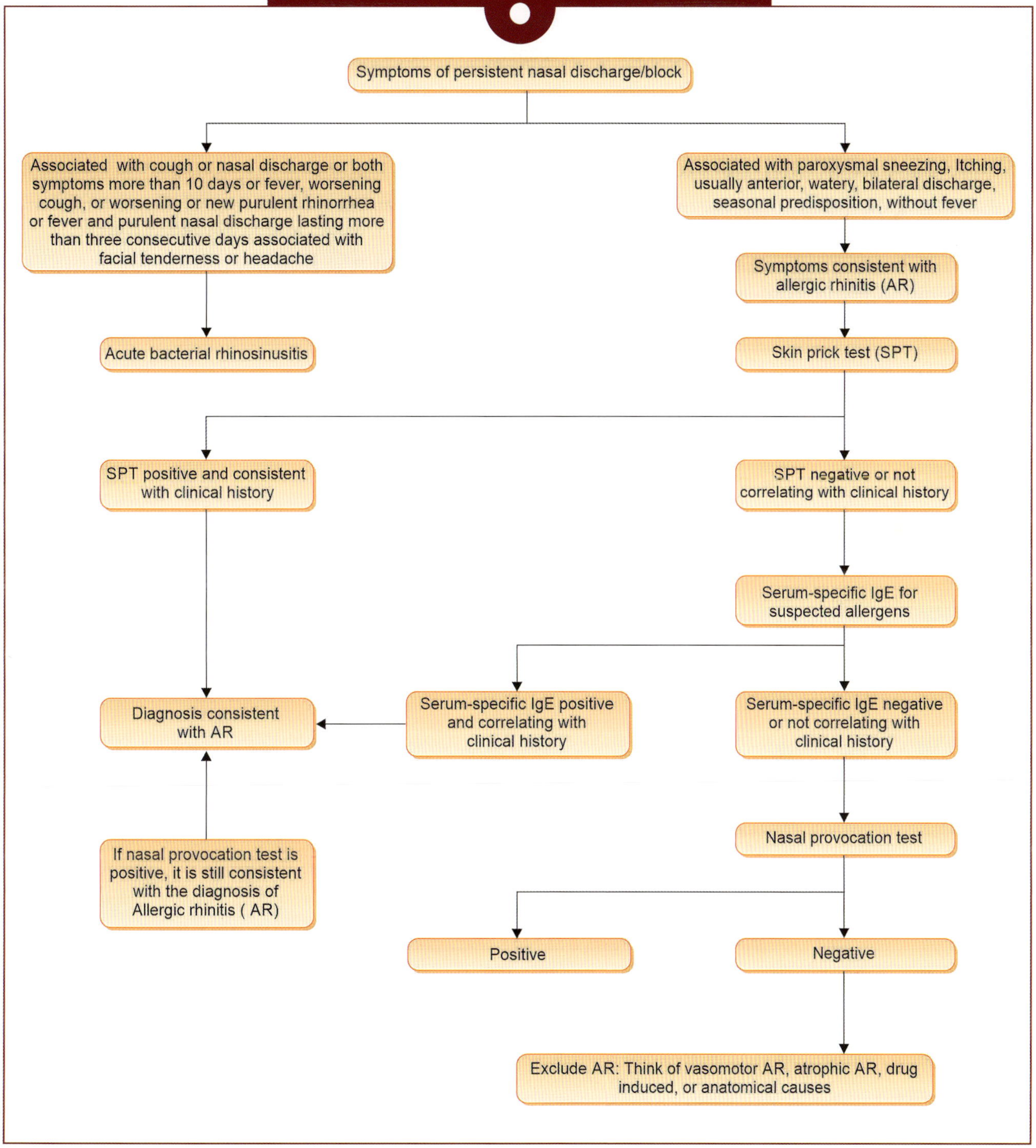

Suggested Reading

- Australasian Society for Clinical Immunology and Allergy. (2022). Allergic rhinitis clinical update. [online] Available from https://www.allergy.org.au/images/stories/pospapers/ar/ASCIA_HP_Allergic_Rhinitis_2022.pdf [Last accessed May, 2024].
- Bousquet J, Toumi T, Sousa-Pinto B, Anto JM, Bedbrook A, Czarlewski W, et al. The Allergic Rhinitis and Its Impact on Asthma (ARIA) Approach of Value-Added Medicines: As-Needed Treatment in Allergic Rhinitis. J Allergy Clin Immunol Pract. 2022;10(11):2878-88.
- Dykewicz MS, Wallace DV, Baroody F, Bernstein J, Craig T, Finegold I, et al. Treatment of seasonal allergic rhinitis: an evidence-based focused 2017 guideline update. Ann Allergy Asthma Immunol. 2017;119(6):489-511.e41.
- Paramesh H, Nagaraju K, Sukumaran TU, Agarkhedkar S, Bhakta S, Tilak R, et al. Airway Diseases Education and Expertise (ADEX) in Pediatrics: Adaptation for Clinical Practice in India. Indian Pediatr. 2016;53(2):154-8.

Poor Scholastic Performance

78

Section Editor: **Sumitha Nayak**
Section Co-Editor: **Priya Shivalli**
Author: **Lalitha Wadhwa**

Introduction

- Poor scholastic performance is referred to as specific developmental disorders of scholastic skills (SDDSS).
- This is an abnormality in cognitive processing. This is largely attributed to biological dysfunction.
- SDDSS comprises groups of disorders manifested by specific and significant impairments of scholastic skills.
- The occurrence of SDDSS is more common in boys than in girls.

Etiology

Etiology of SDDSS is given in **Table 1**.

TABLE 1: Etiology of SDDSS.

TYPE	DISORDER
• Medical problems	• Hearing and visual impairment
• Emotional disorders	• Repeated failures
• Psychiatric disorders	• Fear of bullying
• Neurological disorders	• Substance abuse
• Environmental factors	• Malnutrition

Presentation

- SDDSS frequently occurs in conjunction with other clinical syndromes such as attention-deficit hyperactivity disorder (ADHD), conduct disorder, and specific developmental disorder of motor function or speech and language.
- The normal patterns of skill acquisition are disturbed from early stages of development, e.g., poor scholastic achievement, language delay, severe spelling disorder, reading disorder.

Diagnostic Pointers

- There must be a clinically significant degree of impairment in the specified scholastic skill.
- The impairment must be specific.
- The impairment must be developmental.
- There must be no external factors.
- It must not be due to corrected visual/hearing impairment.

Red Flags

- Delayed achievement of early milestones should raise the suspicion of associated scholastic impairment.
- Delayed milestones act as pointers. Some of these include the following:

No visual fixation by	2 months
No localization by	6 months
No sitting with support	9–10 months
No standing alone by	16 months
No walking alone by	18 months
No single words by	18 months
No imaginative play by	3 years

- A multipronged management is required. The team should comprise pediatricians, ophthalmologists, otorhinolaryngologists, pediatric neurologists, child psychiatrists, child psychologists, and counselors.
- Some standard tests like WISC (Wechsler Intelligence Scale for Children) or the SBIS (Stanford Binet Intelligence Scale) may be undertaken for determining the child's IQ.

Approach to a Child with Poor Scholastic Performance

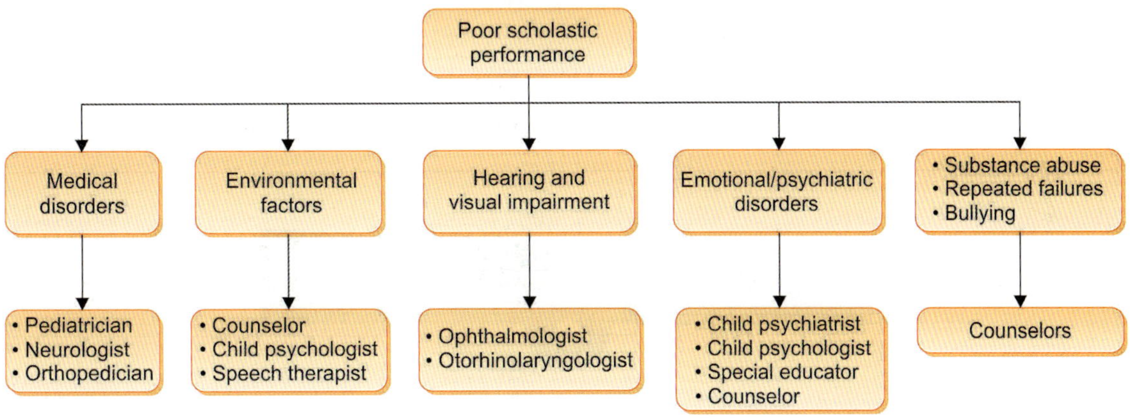

Suggested Reading

- American Psychiatric Association. Diagnostic and Statistical Manual of Mental Disorders, 5th edition. Washington, DC: American Psychiatric Association; 2013. [online] Available from: https://doi.org/10.1176/appi.books.9780890425596 [Last accessed May, 2024].
- Karande S, Kulkarni M. Poor school performance. Indian J Pediatr. 2005;72:961-7.
- Narayan J, Madhavan T, Mukhopadhyaya S. A study of children with poor scholastic performance. Indian J Psychol Med. 1990;13(2):173-85.
- World Health Organization. The ICD-10 Classification of Mental and Behavioural Disorders. Geneva: World Health Organization; 1992. [online] Available from https://www.who.int/publications/i/item/9241544228 [Last accessed May, 2024].

Self-harm

79

Section Editor: Sumitha Nayak
Section Co-Editor: Priya Shivalli
Author: Manini Moudgal

Introduction

Self-harm is also known as self-mutilation, self-abuse, and nonsuicidal self-injury (NSSI).

Definition

- According to Diagnostic and Statistical Manual of Mental Disorders, Fifth Edition (DSM-V), self-harm is when an individual engages in intentional self-inflicted damage to the surface of his or her body, on 5 or more days in the past 1 year, with the expectation that the injury will lead to only mild or moderate physical harm.
- Most often, it is a coping mechanism for an emotionally distressing situation.
- *Long-standing and repeated episodes of NSSI are a strong risk factor for future suicidal behavior.*
- Nonsuicidal self-injury (NSSI) is uncommon in children. It tends to peak in midadolescence (13–16 years) and falls by 18 years of age.

Common Types

Common types of NSSI are cutting, scratching, branding, picking and pulling skin and hair, burning, biting, head banging, hitting self, and excessive body piercing and tattooing.

Risk Factors and Comorbidities

- *Gender difference:* More in females per some studies, whereas some found no difference. Girls tend to cut more and boys hit.
- *Adverse early childhood experiences:* Sexual abuse, parental neglect, and bullying
- *Social media:* Excessive exposure to NSSI content
- *Neurobiological factors:* Abnormalities in the hypothalamic–pituitary–adrenal axis
- *Psychiatric illnesses:* Borderline personality disorder, depression, attention deficit hyperactivity disorder (ADHD), anxiety, substance abuse, schizophrenia
- *Coexisting syndromes:* Autism, Gilles de la Tourette syndrome, Lesch–Nyhan syndrome, severe mental retardation

In case of any suspected comorbidity, the patient has to be investigated accordingly.

Red Flags

HISTORY	SIGNS AND SYMPTOMS
Stress at school: Exams, peer and parental pressure, bullying	Cuts in various stages of healing, especially over wrists, arms, thighs, and abdomen
Stress at home: Domestic abuse, violence	Bruises of varying stages over forehead
Life events: Death, relationship failures, moving	Always dressed in long sleeves, refusing a complete physical exam
Addictions: Substances, media, electronics	Unusual hair loss pattern
Body image issues: Anorexia, bulimia	Collecting sharp objects
Low self-esteem, extreme sadness	
Struggles with sexual orientation	

Approach to Self-harm

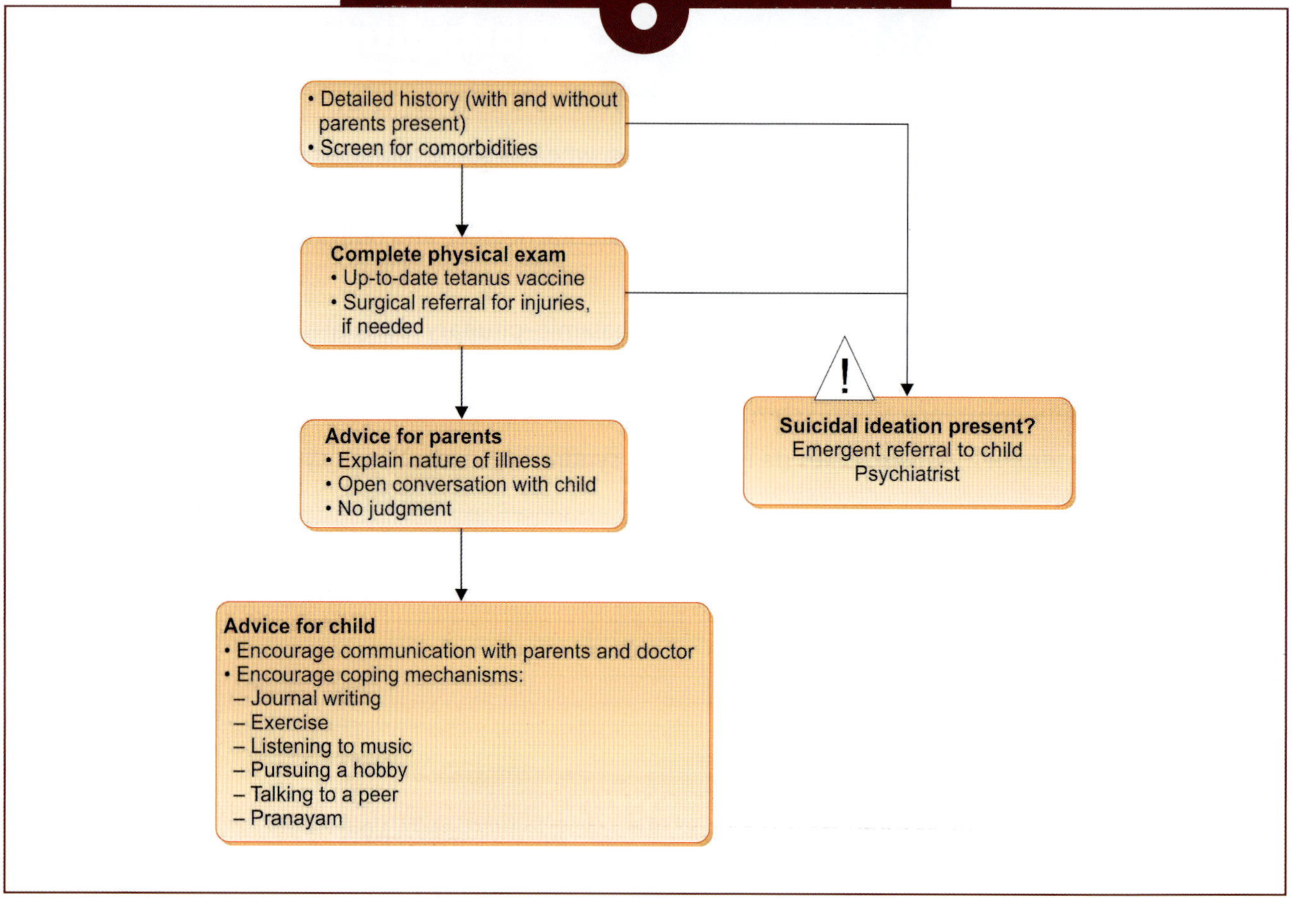

Suggested Reading

- American Psychiatric Association. Diagnostic and Statistical Manual of Mental Disorders, 5th edition. Arlington: American Psychiatric Publishing; 2013.
- Bhola P, Munivenkatappa M, Rajappa V, Phillip M. Predictors of non-suicidal and suicidal self-injurious behaviours, among adolescents and young adults in urban India. Asian J Psychiatry. 2017:29:123-8.
- Krishnakumar P, Geeta MG, Riyaz A. Deliberate self-harm in children. Indian Pediatr. 2010;48:367-71.
- Patra BN, Sen MS, Sagar R, Bhargava R. Deliberate self-harm in adolescents: A review of literature. Ind Psychiatry J. 2023;32(1):9-14.
- Review and update on non-suicidal self-injury: who, how and why. Vega D, Sintes A, Fernández M, Punti J, Soler J, Santamarina P, et al. Actas Esp Psiquiatr . 2018 Jul;46(4):146-55.
- UNICEF. What is self-harm? [online] Available from https://www.unicef.org/parenting/mental-health/what-is-self-harm [Last accessed May, 2024].

Weight Loss

80

Section Editor: **Kripasindhu Chatterjee**
Section Co-Editors: **Atanu Bhadra, Ashim Kumar Ghosh**
Authors: **Swapan Kumar Ray, Rajyashree Chamaria**

Introduction

- Weight loss in children is a concerning issue, often requiring a thorough evaluation to identify the underlying causes.
- Presentations may be acute or progressive and may be intentional or unintentional.
- Unintentional weight loss is of major concern.

Clinically significant weight depending on age:

- *Newborns:* >12%—normal neonates lose 7–10% of birth weight in the first few postnatal days.
- *Children:* >5% from baseline
- *Adolescents:* >5% and/or body mass index (BMI) percentile (BMI ≤17.5 kg/m^2)

Etiology

Below 6 months of age:

- *Commonly:*
  - Acute infection
  - Problems with feeding
  - Milk protein allergy
  - Malnutrition or failure to thrive
  - Gastroesophageal reflux disease
  - Pyloric stenosis
  - Child neglect
  - Surgical causes like intestinal volvulus, etc.

Dehydration associated with any etiology can be severe.

Older Infants, Children, and Adolescents

- *Acute:*
  - Infections
  - Excessive losses from vomiting and diarrhea
  - Gastroesophageal reflux disease
  - Excessive activity
  - Surgery
  - Difficulty in establishing breast feeding in infants
  - Inappropriate dilution of formula in infants
  - Psychological stress
- *Chronic:*
  - *Gastrointestinal disorders:* Conditions like celiac disease, Crohn's disease, or chronic pancreatitis
  - *Endocrine disorders:* Thyroid dysfunction or diabetes
  - Cystic fibrosis
  - *Eating disorders:* Anorexia nervosa, bulimia, and avoidant/restrictive food intake disorder (ARFID) are chronic conditions characterized by disordered eating behaviors and require specialized treatment.
  - *Malignancies:* Pediatric cancers, such as leukemia or lymphoma
  - Inflammatory bowel disease
  - Malabsorption
  - Chronic infections like tuberculosis or HIV
  - Psychiatric affective disorders, especially depression
  - Congenital heart disease
  - Child abuse
  - Craniofacial abnormalities

Red Flags

- Rapid weight loss
- Failure to thrive
- Changes in appetite
- *Gastrointestinal (GI) symptoms:* Persistent vomiting, diarrhea, or abdominal pain
- Unexplained fever
- Chronic fatigue

Approach

History

- Detailed history including diet, birth history, urinations and bowel movements/day, vomiting, diarrhea, fatigue, details of breast feeding/if formula fed dilution
- For adolescents, consider HEEADSSS (home, education/employment, eating, activities, drugs, sexuality, suicide/depression, and safety), menstrual history for girls, and body image issues.

Investigations (Guided by Clinical Suspicion)

- Complete blood count, peripheral smear
- Erythrocyte sedimentation rate (ESR), C-reactive protein
- Comprehensive metabolic panel
- IgA tissue transglutaminase (TTG)
- Mantoux test, HIV test
- Thyroid function test
- Stool test (ova, fat content, and calprotectin)
- Urinalysis
- *Imaging:* X-rays, ultrasounds, or CT scans may be needed.
- Upper GI endoscopy or colonoscopy to visualize the gastrointestinal tract (GIT) and biopsy
- *Psychological assessments:* In eating disorder or emotional distress

Acute Weight Loss in Children and Adolescents

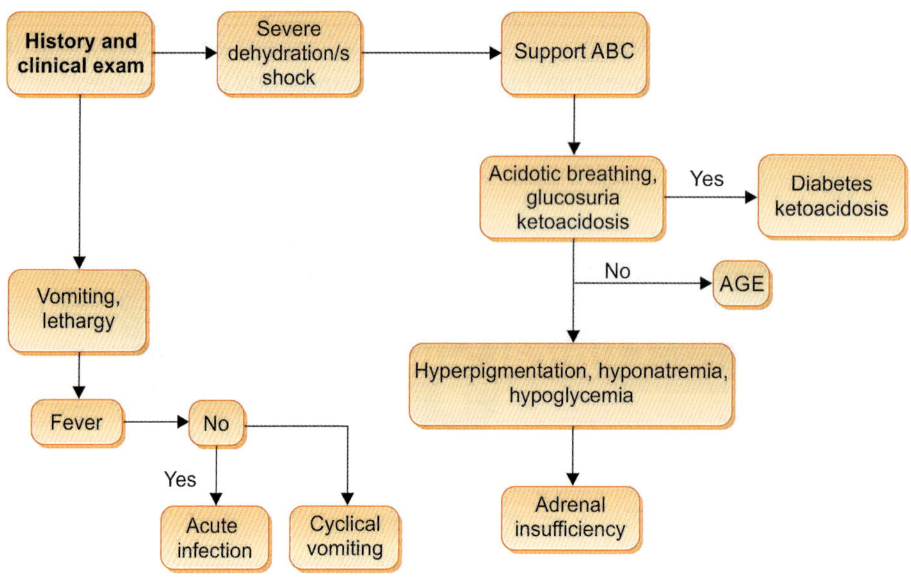

(AGE: acute gastro enteritis; ABC: airway, breathing, circulation)

Chronic Weight Loss in Children and Adolescents

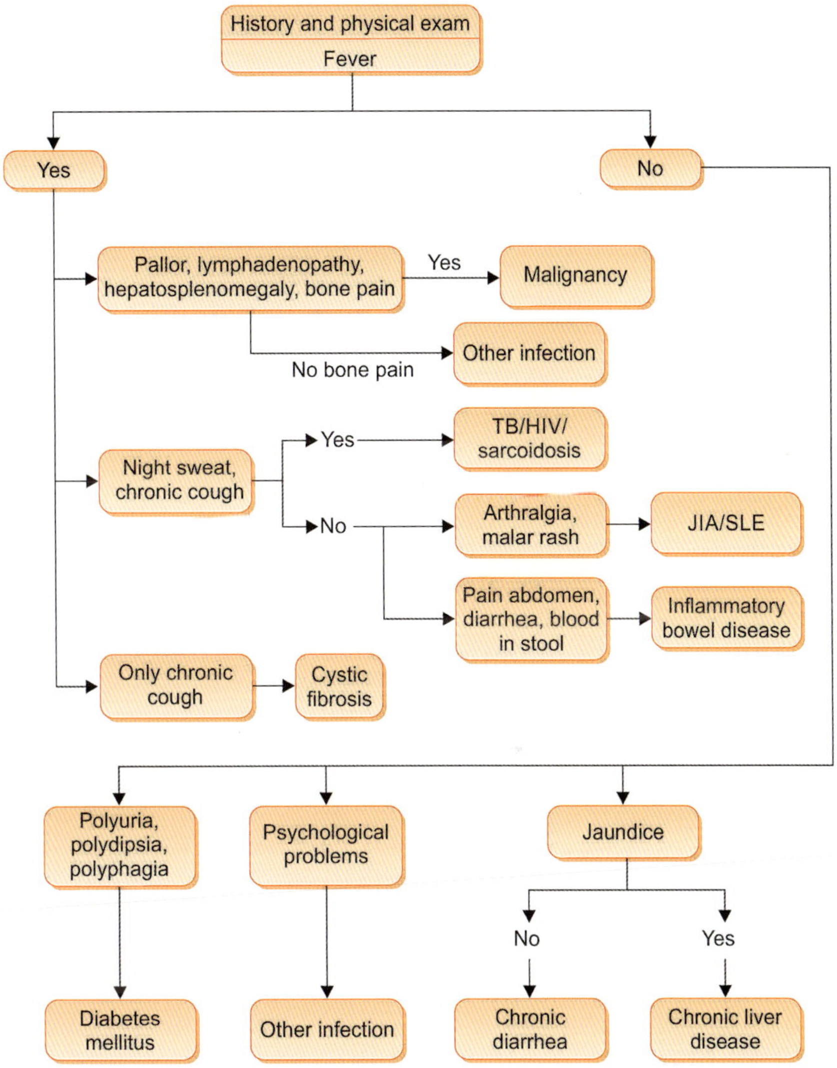

(HIV: human immunodeficiency virus; JIA: juvenile idiopathic arthritis; SLE: systemic lupus erythematosus; TB: tuberculosis)

Weight Loss in Infants below 6 Months

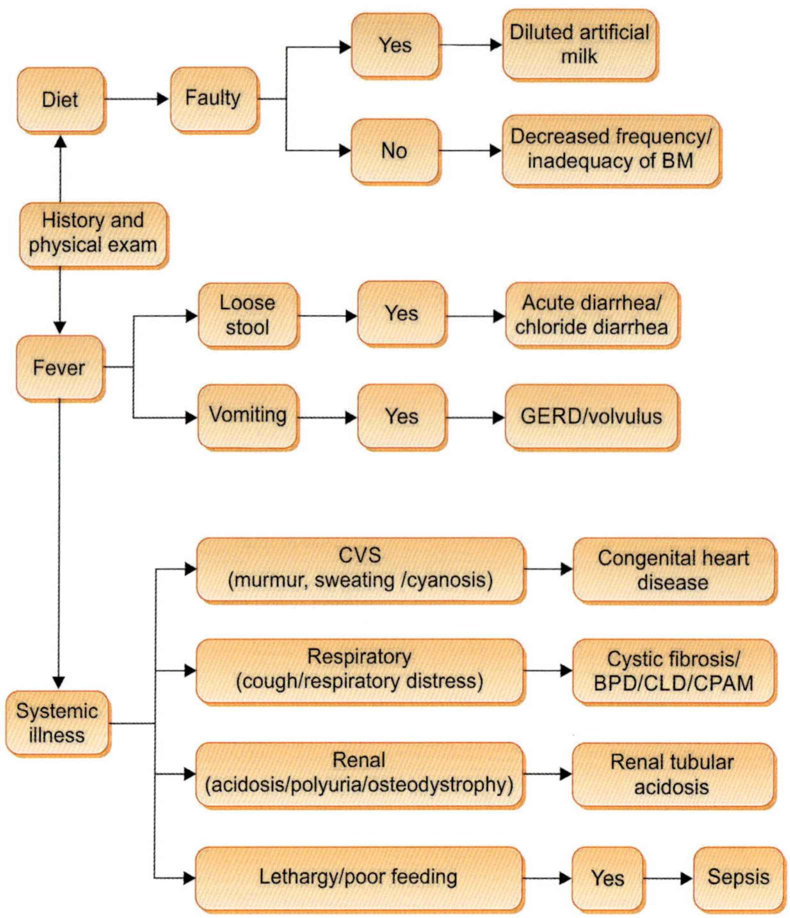

(BM: breast milk; BPD: bronchopulmonary dysplasia; CLD: chronic lung disease; CPAM: congenital pulmonary airway malformation; CVS : cardio vascular system; GERD: gastroesophageal reflux disease)

Suggested Reading

- Alibhai SM, Greenwood C, Payette H. An approach to the management of unintentional weight loss in elderly people. CMAJ. 2005;172:773-80.
- Bouras EP, Lange SM, Scolapio JS. Rational approach to patients with unintentional weight loss. Mayo Clin Proc. 2001;76:923.
- Gaddey HL, Holder K. Unintentional weight loss in older adults. Am Fam Physician. 2014;89:718.
- Gupta R, Evans AT. Approach to the patient with unintentional weight loss, UpToDate. [online] Available from https://www.uptodate.com/contents/approach-to-the-patient-with-unintentional-weight-loss. [Last accessed May, 2024].
- McMinn J, Steel C, Bowman A. Investigation and management of unintentional weight loss in older adults. BMJ. 2011;342:d1732.
- Meltzer AA, Everhart JE. Unintentional weight loss in the United States. Am J Epidemiol. 1995;142:1039.
- Moriguti JC, Moriguti EK, Ferriolli E, de Castilho Cação J, Junior NL, Marchini JS. Involuntary weight loss in elderly individuals: assessment and treatment. Sao Paulo Med J. 2001;119:72.
- Sahyoun NR, Serdula MK, Galuska DA, Zhang XL, Pamuk ER. The epidemiology of recent involuntary weight loss in the United States population. J Nutr Health Aging. 2004;8:510.
- Wannamethee SG, Shaper AG, Lennon L. Reasons for intentional weight loss, unintentional weight loss, and mortality in older men. Arch Intern Med. 2005;165:1035.
- Wong CJ. Involuntary weight loss. Med Clin North Am. 2014;98:625.

Abdominal Distension

81

Section Editor: **B Rajsekhar**
Section Co-Editor: **Suchitra Pusapati**
Author: **Arti Pawaria**

Introduction

- Abdominal distension is defined as an increase in the abdominal girth/prominence of the abdominal wall.
- A detailed history, clinical assessment, early diagnosis, and intervention can significantly improve outcomes.

Etiology

The etiological categorization of abdominal distension based on the underlying mechanism causing the distension is crucial for tailored investigative workup and treatment strategies.

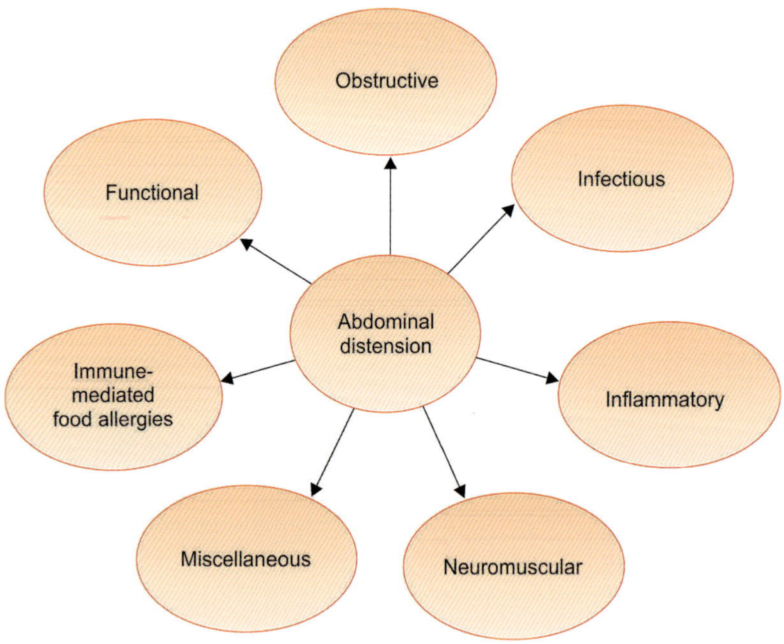

- *Obstructive causes:*
  - Intestinal atresia/stenosis
  - Malrotation and volvulus
  - Intussusception
- *Infectious causes:*
  - *Necrotizing enterocolitis:* Mostly seen in premature infants
  - Gastroenteritis
  - Abdominal tuberculosis
- *Inflammatory causes:*
  - *Inflammatory bowel disease (IBD):* Crohn's disease, ulcerative colitis
  - Appendicitis
  - Meckel's diverticulitis
  - Pancreatitis
  - Peritonitis
- *Functional causes:*
  - *Functional gastrointestinal disorders (e.g., irritable bowel syndrome):* Disorders of gut–brain interaction
  - Overeating or aerophagia (swallowing air)
  - Constipation
- *Neuromuscular causes:*
  - Hirschsprung's disease
  - *Gastroparesis:* Hypomotility of gut–IBS, postenteritis gastroparesis
  - Chronic intestinal pseudo-obstruction
- *Allergic or immune-mediated food allergies:*
  - Celiac disease
  - Lactose intolerance
  - *Other food allergies:* Bovine milk protein allergy, multiple food protein allergy
- *Miscellaneous causes:*
  - Ascites—transudative/exudative
  - *Tumors or cysts:* Benign or malignant growths causing distension

Red Flags

- Persistent vomiting
- Significant weight loss
- Chronic diarrhea
- Blood in stools
- Jaundice
- Weight loss/failure to thrive
- Ascites
- Associated fever
- Evidence of intestinal obstruction
- Lethargy, temperature instability, feeding intolerance, vomiting, and bloody stools, especially in cases of necrotizing enterocolitis (NEC)

Investigations

Investigations are done after a comprehensive history and physical examination:

- Complete blood count (thrombocytosis—iron deficiency anemia, IBD)
- Inflammatory markers [erythrocyte sedimentation rate (ESR), C-reactive protein (CRP)]
- Liver function tests [hypoalbuminemia—malabsorption, gastrointestinal (GI) loss from ulcerations, transaminitis—celiac hepatitis]
- *Stool studies:* Occult blood, *Clostridium difficile* toxin and antigen, opportunistic infection, fecal calprotectin
- *X-ray abdomen:* Free air under diaphragm, pattern of bowel dilatation (small bowel vs. large bowel), fixed bowel loops, double bubble sign, etc.
- Pneumatosis intestinalis on X-ray abdomen serves as a hallmark diagnostic sign, alongside portal venous gas. In advanced cases, pneumoperitoneum indicates intestinal perforation
- Abdominal ultrasound, specific tests based on suspected diagnosis such as endoscopy or colonoscopy for IBD, and imaging like CT or MRI for suspected abdominal tuberculosis
- Barium meal follow-through, barium enema

Algorithm on Approach to Abdominal Distension in Children

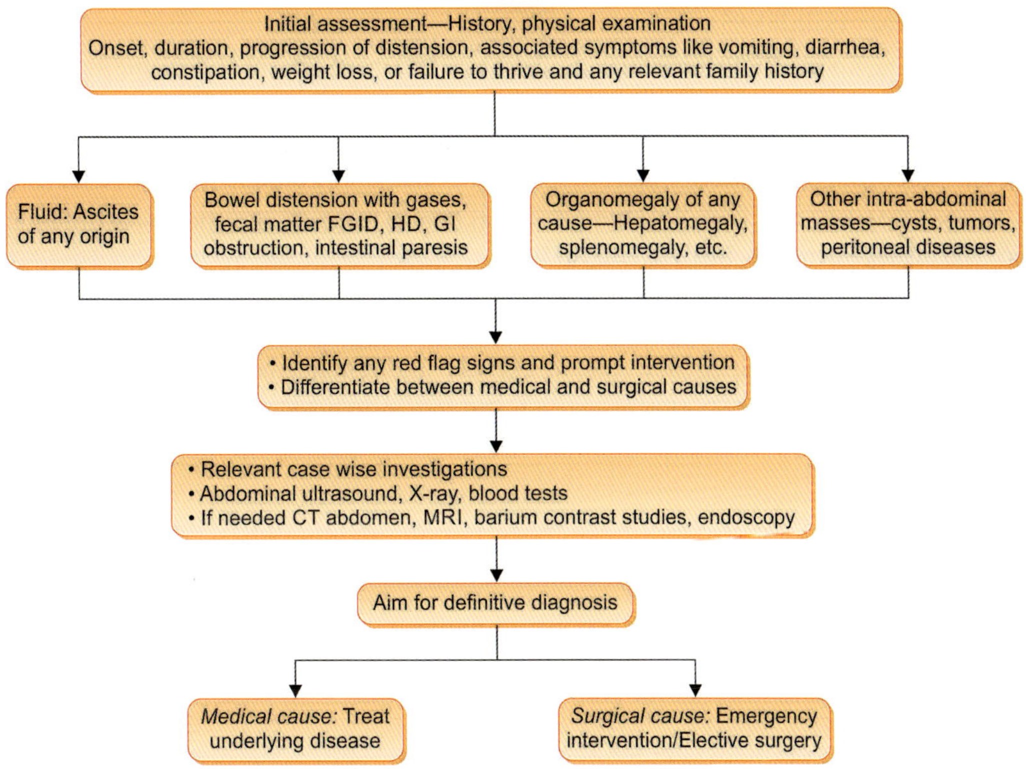

(FGID: functional gastrointestinal disorder; GI: gastrointestinal; HD: Hirschsprung's disease)

Suggested Reading

- Bavdekar A, Thakur A. Ascites in children. Indian J Pediatr. 2016;83(11):1334-40.
- Cai X, Liebe HL, Golubkova A, Leiva T, Hunter CJ. A review of the diagnosis and treatment of necrotizing enterocolitis. Curr Pediatr Rev. 2023;19(3):285-95.
- Giefer MJ, Murray KF, Colletti RB. Pathophysiology, diagnosis, and management of pediatric ascites. JPGN. 2011; 52(5):503-13.
- Makharia G, Srivastava S, Das P, Goswami P, Singh U, Tripathi M, et al. Clinical, endoscopic, and histological differentiations between Crohn's disease and intestinal tuberculosis. Am J Gastroenterol. 2010;105(3):642-51.
- Mari A, Backer FA, Mahamid M, Amara H, Carter D, Boltin D, et al. Bloating and abdominal distension: Clinical approach and management: Adv Ther. 2019;36:1075-84.
- Poddar U, Yachha SK, Srivastava A, Kumari N. Pediatric inflammatory bowel disease: Is it really uncommon in Asian children? J Gastroenterol Hepatol. 2020;4:860-6.
- Turner D, Ruemmele FM, Orlanski-Meyer E, Griffiths AM, de Carpi JM, Bronsky J, et al. Management of pediatric ulcerative colitis: Joint ECCO and ESPGHAN evidence-based consensus guidelines. JPGN. 2012;55(3):292-310.

Cervical Swellings

82

Section Editor: **Rupesh Masand**
Section Co-Editor: **Hema Gupta Mittal**
Authors: **Dhiraj Mohan Gupta, Showkat Hussain Tali**

Introduction

Cervical swellings are mostly benign reactive lymph nodes originating from common viral infections. However, unusual pathologies such as embryologic anomalies, vascular lesions, or neoplasms may also present similarly.

Classification

Cervical swelling is based on position (midline or lateral), time of appearance (congenital or acquired), and duration (acute and chronic), as mentioned below.

Pointers on History and Examination

Pointers on history and examination are given in **Table 1**.

TABLE 1: History taking and examination.

Age at onset	Tender/nontender, rubbery/nonrubbery
Duration	Solid/cystic/fluctuating
Position: Supraclavicular, submandibular, submental, posterior triangle	Mobile/fixed
Single/multiple	Overlying skin free/fixed with indurations
Secondary to other etiologies—tick-borne diseases, etc.	
Relation to swallowing/protrusion of tongue/any relation to neck movement	Associated sinus/fistula

Comprehensive Head and Neck Examination

Look for insect bites, evidence of trauma, and dermatological conditions. Examine oral cavity and assess cranial nerves.

Characteristics of Various Cervical Swellings

Characteristics of various cervical swellings are given in **Tables 2 and 3**.

TABLE 2: Congenital midline cervical swellings.

DISEASE	AGE OF PRESENTATION	OCCURRENCE	SIGN/SYMPTOM	INVESTIGATION
Thyroglossal cyst/sinus	School age	• Most common congenital anomaly • Infrahyoid location more common than suprahyoid	Elevates on protrusion of tongue/swallowing	• USG • CT scan • MRI sinogram
Aberrant/ ectopic thyroid	School age, puberty, pregnancy, and menopause	70% present as hypothyroidism	Dysphagia, dysphonia upper respiratory tract obstruction/sleep apnea syndrome	Technetium-99M scintigraphy
Thyroid swelling	Any age	As hypothyroidism—goiter	Elevates on swallowing and deglutition, neck swelling, hoarseness of voice	• USG • Technetium-99M scintigraphy
• Dermoid cyst • Epidermoid cyst	• 40% at birth • 60% <5 years	Epithelial lining with/without skin appendages	Neck swelling	• USG • CT scan
• Ranula • Plunging ranula	Congenita/ acquired	• Obstruction of sublingual gland • Can extend into the neck through mylohyoid	• Benign cystic, mobile, nonblanching, nontender • Blue colored	• Imaging • USG • CT scan • MRI
Cervical cleft	Congenital lesion	Impaired fusion of branchial arches	• Erythematous rash • Projectile elevated mass on upper portion • On lower portion—may be sinus/tract	• USG • CT scan

Congenital Midline and Lateral Cervical Swellings

TABLE 3: Congenital midline and lateral swellings.

DISEASE	AGE OF PRESENTATION	SPECIFICITY	SIGN/SYMPTOM	INVESTIGATION
Congenital hemangioma	At birth	Never involutes	Lesions are raised usually pink to blue color	Prenatal USG scanning
Infantile hemangioma	At birth—as a bruise mark	• *Proliferation:* At 2–4 weeks • *Rapid proliferation:* At 4–6 months • *Regression:* At 1 year of age	Presents as flat violaceous lesion mistaken for bruises	• USG • CT scan
Port-wine stain	At birth	• Capillary malformation • Does not proliferate	Light pink/dark discoloration of the skin	• USG • CT scan
Cystic hygroma or lymphangioma	• 50% present at birth • 90% by age of 2 years	Lymphatic malformation	Violaceous, rubbery, dough-like consistency swelling, borders not well defined	• Transillumination test • USG

Congenital Lateral Cervical Swellings

Anomalies of congenital lateral cervical swellings are given in **Table 4**.

TABLE 4: Congenital lateral cervical swellings.

DISEASE	AGE OF PRESENTATION	SPECIFICITY	SIGN/SYMPTOM	INVESTIGATION
Branchial cleft cyst or sinus	Infancy/young children	• Second most common congenital lesions of head and neck • Second branchial cleft involvement most common	As cyst/discharging sinus	• CT with fistulogram • MRI with contrast
Torticollis or fibromatosis or wry neck	Infancy	Congenital/acquired	Head typically tilted laterally toward the ipsilateral affected muscle; chin rotated contralateral to the contracture	• USG • CT scan
Thymic cysts	• 2–15 years • Common in males	Uncommon 1–3% of all anterior mediastinal masses	Painless unilocular cyst mass	• USG • CT scan • MRI with contrast

Contd...

Contd...

DISEASE	AGE OF PRESENTATION	SPECIFICITY	SIGN/SYMPTOM	INVESTIGATION
Laryngocele	Childhood to adulthood	Herniation of laryngeal saccule—externally or internally	Cystic lesion	Direct laryngoscopy/ fiberoptic/CT with contrast

Acquired lymphadenopathy due to acute infections (<2 weeks) is given in **Table 5**.

TABLE 5: Acquired lymphadenopathy due to acute infections (<2 weeks).

DISEASE	AGE OF PRESENTATION	SPECIFICITY	ANATOMICAL PRESENTATION	SIGN/ SYMPTOM	INVESTIGATION
Viral—EB virus, cytomegalovirus, influenza, measles, mumps, Coxsackie	Younger ages	Nonspecific	Mostly lateral	Nontender, discrete with variable signs, secondary to URTI/ postexanthem	• Nonspecific tests • FNAC
Bacterial—*Staphylococcus aureus* and *Streptococcus pyogenes*	<5 years of age	Post-URTI, otitis media, skin or scalp lesions	Laterally, anterior, and posterior triangles	Malaise, fever, sore throat dysphagia, dysphonia	• CBC • Throat swab • Culture • Serological tests

(CBC: complete blood count; EB: Epstein–Barr; FNAC: fine needle aspiration cytology; URTI: upper respiratory tract infection)

Acquired lymphadenopathy due to chronic infections (>2 weeks) is given in **Table 6**.

TABLE 6: Acquired lymphadenopathy due to chronic infections (>2 weeks).

DISEASE	AGE OF PRESENTATION	SPECIFICITY	ANATOMICAL PRESENTATION	SIGN/ SYMPTOM	INVESTIGATION
Atypical *Mycobacterium*	Toddler and school age	Consumption of unpasteurized milk	Posterior triangle	• Painless fluctuant lymph nodes • Bluish skin over it, necrosis later	• PPD test • CBNAAT • FNAC • X-ray
Mycobacterium tuberculosis	Any age	• Fever >2 weeks • Unremitting cough • History of contact	• Generalized lymphadenopathy • Cervical and occipital lymph nodes	• Fever • Cough • Loss of weight	• CBNAAT • Gastric lavage and sputum • X-ray

Contd...

Contd…

DISEASE	AGE OF PRESENTATION	SPECIFICITY	ANATOMICAL PRESENTATION	SIGN/ SYMPTOM	INVESTIGATION
HIV	Any age		Generalized lymphadenopathy	• PUO • Recurrent pneumonia • Oral rash • Diarrhea • Opportunistic infections	• Bone marrow cytology, • HIV serology • FNAC

(CBNAAT: cartridge-based nucleic acid amplification test; FNAC: fine-needle aspiration cytology; HIV: human immunodeficiency virus; PPD: purified protein derivative; PUO: pyrexia of unknown origin)

Neoplastic Neck Masses

Neoplastic neck masses are given in **Tables 7 and 8**.

TABLE 7: Benign neck masses.

DISEASE	AGE OF PRESENTATION	ANATOMICAL PRESENTATION	SIGN/SYMPTOM	INVESTIGATION
Pilomatrixoma	5–10 years	Posterior triangle and suboccipital lymph node	Superficial rock hard mobile neck masses; bluish hue	Clinically diagnosed

TABLE 8: Malignant neck masses.

DISEASE	AGE OF PRESENTATION	SPECIFICITY	ANATOMICAL PRESENTATION	SIGN/SYMPTOM	INVESTIGATION
Hodgkin lymphoma	Older children	RS cells	Lymph node in posterior triangle	Nontender lymph node supradiaphragmatic, profound weight loss, high fever, drenching night sweats	• CT staging • FNAC • Bone marrow biopsy
Non-Hodgkin lymphoma	<10 years	RS cells absent	Generalized occipital posterior triangle	Unexplained weight loss, fever, night sweat, abdominal pain	• CT staging • FNAC • Bone marrow biopsy

Contd…

Contd...

DISEASE	AGE OF PRESENTATION	SPECIFICITY	ANATOMICAL PRESENTATION	SIGN/SYMPTOM	INVESTIGATION
Neuro-blastoma	<5 years; in 1st month of life	Most common tumor in <5 years; older children present with abdominal mass	Lateral side of neck	• Airway obstruction and dysphagia • Horner syndrome • Cranial neuropathy	• CT • MRI
Rhabdomyo-sarcoma	<10 years	Highly malignant tumor of soft tissues	Lump in neck, groin, and armpit	Painful lump, headache, dysuria, bone pains, constant cough	• CT • MRI
Immuno-deficiency disorders	Infants to <5 years	Recurrent opportunistic infections	Scattered discrete nodes tender/nontender	• Pyrexia of unknown origin • Pneumonia • Diarrhea • Skin infections	• Blood culture • CD4, CD8 counts • Serological tests

(FNAC: fine-needle aspiration cytology; RS: Reed–Sternberg)

Red Flags

SYMPTOMS	SIGNS
• Persistent lymphadenopathy >6 weeks	• A lymph node that is firm, hard, or larger than >2 cm
• Rapidly increasing lymphadenopathy >2 cm	• Generalized lymphadenopathy
• Past history of malignancy	• A lump >2 cm
• Pain following fall/trauma	• A supraclavicular mass
• Sudden unexplained weight loss	• Severe pallor/petechiae/bone tenderness
• Prolonged fever	• Organomegaly
• Difficulty in breathing/feeding	• Discharging sinus

Investigations

Imaging

- *Ultrasonography (USG):* Size and extent of masses, consistency, cystic/solid; does not delineate the deeper lesions
- *Color Doppler USG* demonstrates the vascularization of mass and displaced normal surrounding vessels/intraregional flow
- *PET/CT neck:* Morphologic characterization, staging, precise visualization of fine bone structures, calcifications, and deep soft-tissue compartments
- *MRI:* Superior contrast resolution in evaluating masses in complex areas including head and neck
- *MRI with gadolinium or Doppler USG:* Gold standard for diagnosis of vascular lesions; also measures flow
- *MRI with fistulogram:* Helps to determine the extent and direction of the fistula/sinus

Histopathological Examination

- *Fine-needle aspiration cytology (FNAC):* Simple, quick minimal invasive, inexpensive and OPD-based procedure; determines the etiology
- *Excision biopsy:* Definitive diagnosis of cervical lesions, especially if the FNAC is unable to pick up the characteristic lesions and clinical suspicion is high

Cervical Swellings: A Summary

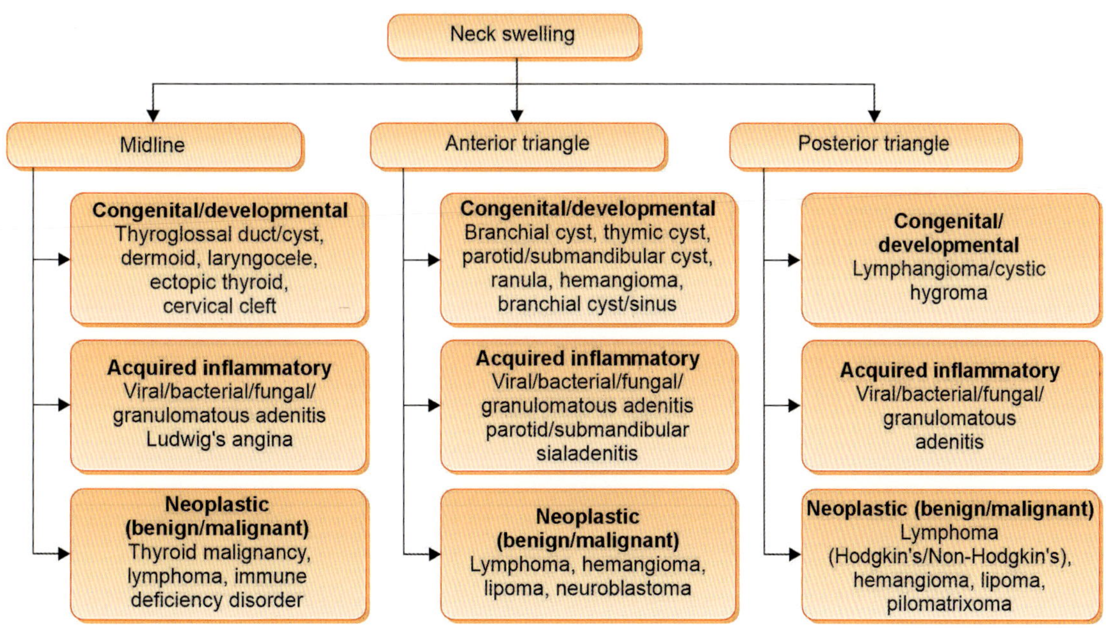

Algorithm for Diagnosis of Cervical Swelling in Children

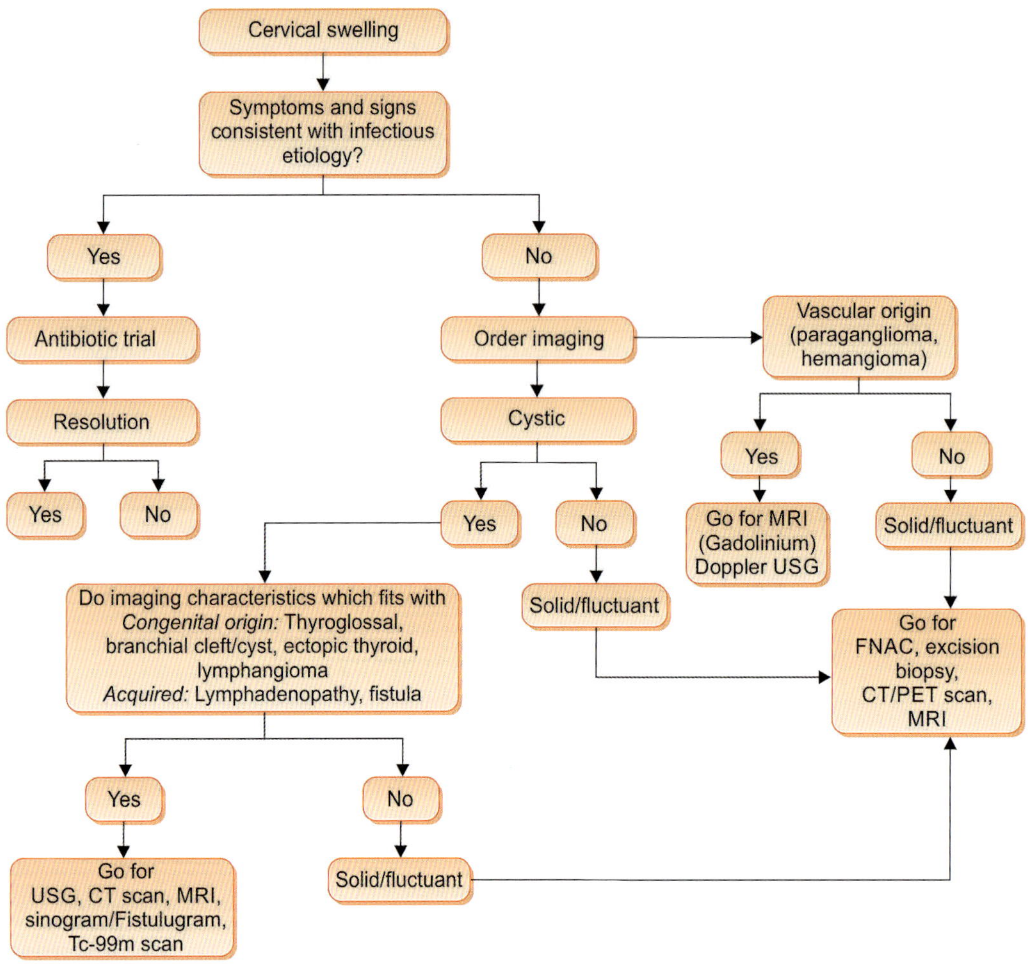

Suggested Reading

- Danielson-Cohen A, Linn SS, Huges A. Head and neck pilomatrixoma in children. Arch Otolaryngol Head Neck Surg. 2001;127(12):1481-3.
- Harish K. Neck dissections: radical to conservative. World J Surg Oncol. 2005;3:21.
- Jackson D. Evaluation and management of pediatric neck masses. Phys Assist Clinics. 2018;3(2):245-69.
- Krakovitz PR, Zdanski CJ, Parikh SR. Head and neck surgery. In: Parikh SR (Ed). Pediatric Otolaryngology Head and Neck Surgery: Clinical Reference Guide, 1st edition. San Diego, CA: Plural Publishing; 2014. pp. 422-613.
- Mittal MK, Malik A, Sureka B. Cystic Masses of neck: a pictorial review. Indian J Radiol Imaging. 2012;22(4):334-3.

Chronic Cough

83

Section Editor: **Rupesh Masand**
Section Co-Editor: **Hema Gupta Mittal**
Author: **Kana Ram Jat**

Introduction

Cough is one of the most common symptoms, yet there is lack of consensus on the definition of chronic cough.

Classification

Classification of cough is based on:

- *Duration of cough:* Acute cough (<2 weeks), subacute/protracted cough (2–4 weeks), chronic cough (>4 weeks)
- *Cough characteristics:* Dry/productive/wet/particularly recognized cough, e.g., paroxysmal cough, barking cough

Etiology in Decreasing Order of Frequency

Etiology in decreasing order of frequency is given in **Table 1**.

TABLE 1: Etiology in decreasing order of frequency.

INFANTS (<12 MONTHS)	1–5 YEARS	ABOVE 5 YEARS
Protracted URTI	Protracted URTI	Protracted URTI
GER	Bronchial asthma	Bronchial asthma
Chlamydia infection	Rhinosinusitis	Rhinosinusitis
Airway malacia	Inhaled irritants (passive smoke, air pollution)	Inhaled irritants
CHD	GER	Pulmonary tuberculosis
Inhaled irritants (passive smoke, air pollution)	Foreign body aspiration	Chronic suppurative lung disease (CF, PCD, etc.)
Recurrent wheezing	Chronic suppurative lung disease (CF, PCD, etc.)	Habit cough

(CF: cystic fibrosis; CHD: congenital heart disease; GER: gastroesophageal reflux; PCD: primary ciliary dyskinesia; URTI: upper respiratory tract infection)

Red Flags

VERY EARLY ONSET OF COUGH	UNILATERAL FINDINGS ON EXAMINATION OR CHEST X-RAY
Persistent wet cough	Recurrent pneumonia
Failure to thrive	Developmental delay
Clubbing	Not responding to asthma treatment
Associated persistent fever	Multisystem involvement

Approach to Chronic Cough

- Detailed history and examination provide clues to focused investigation and specific management.
- Asthma is suspected if there are (1) signs/symptoms of airway obstruction (cough, wheezing, breathing difficulty), (2) recurrent symptoms; child well between episodes, (3) multiple triggers [upper respiratory tract infection (URTI), dust, smoke, laughing, crying, running, etc.), (4) reversibility (by history/spirometry), and (5) history of atopy/family history of atopy/asthma.
- Habit cough if: (1) cough is only during day time or worsens in the presence of care givers/healthcare providers; (2) there is presence of stressors like school examinations or scolding by teachers/parents; (3) no pathology is found after relevant sufficient workup; (4) there is secondary gain from cough (e.g., leaves from school, more attention of parents); and (5) child is not appearing sick/cough stops when the child is engaged in activity.

Investigations

Chest X-ray, tuberculin skin test (Mantoux test), hemogram, spirometry (>5 years of age) are recommended. If chest X-ray is abnormal, sputum (if present)/induced sputum/gastric lavage should be sent for GeneXpert.

Other Investigations

CECT chest, flexible bronchoscopy, echocardiography, workup for immunodeficiency, serology for mycoplasma/chlamydia infection, sweat chloride test for cystic fibrosis, barium studies for tracheo-esophageal fistula or gastroesophageal reflux (GER), tests for primary ciliary dyskinesia (PCD), etc.

Pointers in History

Pointers in history are given in **Table 2**.

TABLE 2: Pointers in history.

SPECIFIC CLUES IN HISTORY	SUGGESTED POSSIBILITY/IES
Character of cough	
Barking/brassy cough	LTB, airway malacia, habit cough
Paroxysmal cough	Pertussis, cystic fibrosis, chlamydia/mycoplasma, viruses (adenovirus, RSV, parainfluenza), foreign body aspiration
Expectoration of casts	*Plastic bronchitis:* Asthma, postcardiac surgery
Acute-onset cough	Foreign body aspiration
Cough with wheezing	Asthma, foreign body aspiration
Cough with stridor	LTB, laryngeal lesions
Persistent wet cough	*Chronic suppurative lung disease:* Cystic fibrosis, PCD, postinfectious bronchiectasis
Timing of the cough	
Associated with feeding, choking	*Aspiration syndromes:* TEF, GER, laryngeal cleft, pharyngeal incoordination
Multiple triggers: Exercise, laughing, crying, allergens, etc.	Asthma
Night cough	Asthma GER, postnasal drip, congestive heart failure
Cough noticeable when people are around, subsides during sleep, stressors	Functional/psychogenic cough
Associated symptoms	
Large, bulky, foul smelling, oily stools with failure to thrive	Cystic fibrosis
Chest pain	Pleural effusion, asthma
Prolonged fever and weight loss	Tuberculosis, chronic suppurative lung disease
Progressive exertional dyspnea, dry cough	Interstitial lung disease, HP (if history of exposure to pigeon, other antigens)
Family history	
Allergic rhinitis or asthma	Asthma
Family history of TB	TB
Consanguinity, immunodeficiency or cystic fibrosis	Immunodeficiency or cystic fibrosis

(GER: gastroesophageal reflux; LTB: laryngotracheobronchitis; PCD: primary ciliary dyskinesia; RSV: respiratory syncytial virus; TB: tuberculosis; TEF: tracheoesophageal fistula)

Specific Examination Findings

Specific examination findings are given in **Table 3**.

TABLE 3: Specific examination findings.

SPECIFIC CLUES ON EXAMINATION	SUGGESTED POSSIBILITY/IES
Failure to thrive	Chronic suppurative lung disease, cystic fibrosis, TB
Clubbing	Chronic suppurative lung disease, cystic fibrosis, cyanotic CHD, ILD
Atopic dermatitis	Asthma
Allergic rhinitis markers (allergic shiner, Dennie's lines, allergic crease, allergic salute, mouth breathing)	Asthma
Nasal polyp	Asthma, cystic fibrosis, PCD
Harrison's sulcus	Any chronic lung disease, associated rickets
Increased AP diameter of chest	Asthma, cystic fibrosis
Polyphonic generalized wheezing	Asthma
Monophonic localized wheeze	Foreign body aspiration, intraluminal/extraluminal airway obstruction
Murmur	Heart disease
Stridor	Laryngeal or subglottic lesions

(AP: anteroposterior; CHD: congenital heart disease; GER: gastroesophageal reflux; ILD: interstitial lung disease; PCD: primary ciliary dyskinesia; TB: tuberculosis)

Approach

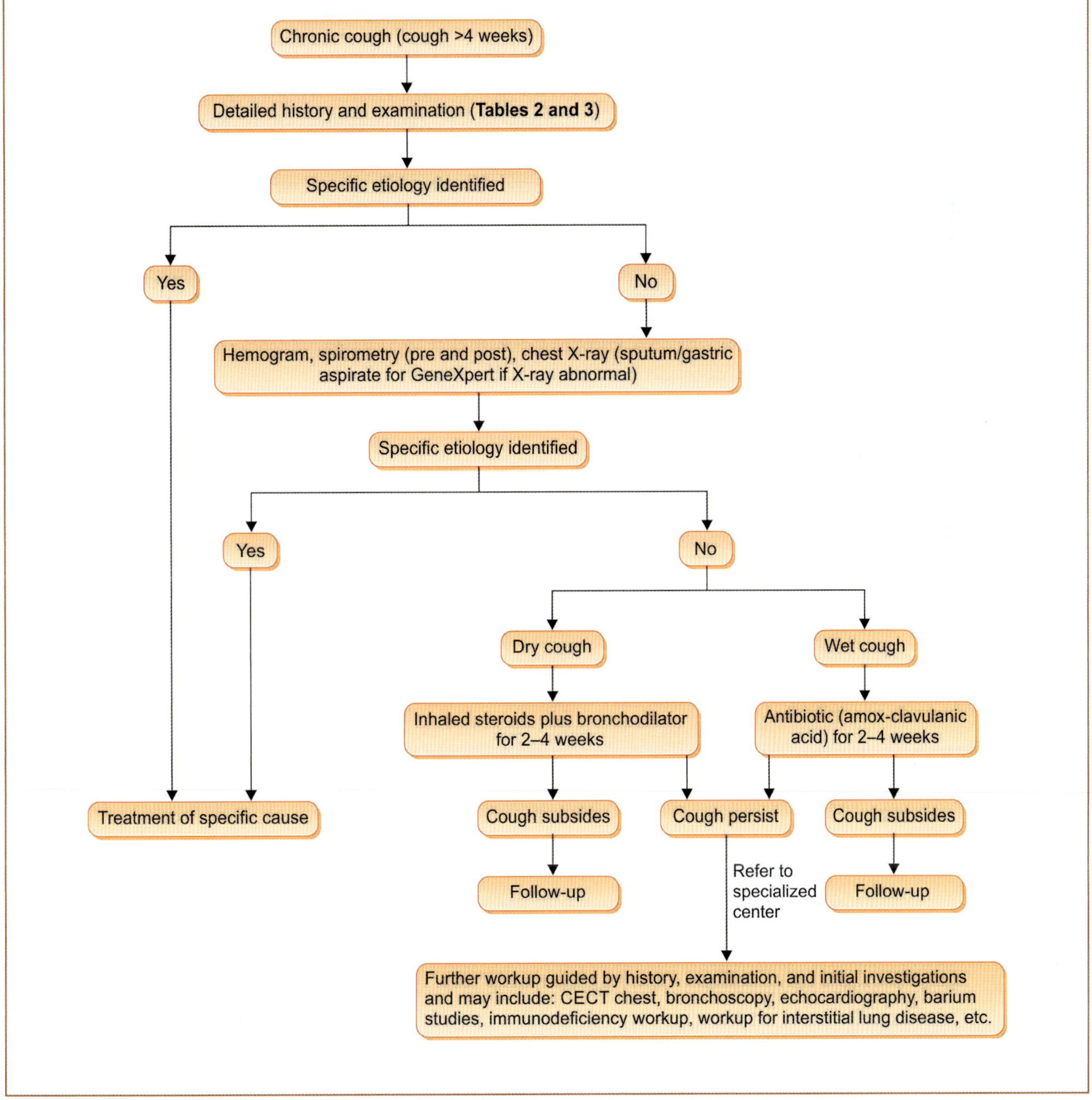
Chronic cough (cough >4 weeks)
Detailed history and examination (**Tables 2 and 3**)
Specific etiology identified
Yes
No
Hemogram, spirometry (pre and post), chest X-ray (sputum/gastric aspirate for GeneXpert if X-ray abnormal)
Specific etiology identified
Yes
No
Dry cough
Wet cough
Inhaled steroids plus bronchodilator for 2–4 weeks
Antibiotic (amox-clavulanic acid) for 2–4 weeks
Treatment of specific cause
Cough subsides
Cough persist
Cough subsides
Follow-up
Refer to specialized center
Follow-up
Further workup guided by history, examination, and initial investigations and may include: CECT chest, bronchoscopy, echocardiography, barium studies, immunodeficiency workup, workup for interstitial lung disease, etc.

Suggested Reading

- Carr BC. Efficacy, abuse, and toxicity of over-the-counter cough and cold medicines in the pediatric population. Curr Opin Pediatr. 2006;18:184-8.
- Chang AB, Oppenheimer JJ, Irwin RS; CHEST Expert Cough Panel. Managing chronic cough as a symptom in children and management algorithms. CHEST guideline and expert panel report. Chest. 2020;158:303-29.
- Kantar A, Marchant JM, Song WJ, Shields MD, Chatziparasidis G, Zacharasiewicz A, et al. History Taking as a Diagnostic Tool in Children With Chronic Cough. Front Pediatr. 2022;10:850912.
- Marchant JM, Chang AB, Kennedy E, King D, Perret JL, Schultz A, et al. Cough in Children and Adults: Diagnosis, Assessment and Management (CICADA). Summary of an updated position statement on chronic cough in Australia. Med J Aust. 2024;220(1):35-45.
- Marchant JM, Newcombe PA, Juniper EF, Sheffield JK, Stathis SL, Chang AB. What is the burden of chronic cough for families? Chest. 2008;134:303-9.
- Shields MD, Bush A, Everard ML, McKenzie SA, Primhak R. British thoracic society guidelines recommendations for the assessment and management of cough in children. Thorax. 2008;63:iii1-iii15.

Constipation

84

Section Editor: **B Rajsekhar**
Section Co-Editor: **Suchitra Pusapati**
Author: **Nagendra Kumar VR**

Introduction

- Constipation is common, especially in the under-5-year age group. It can have a significant psychological impact on the child and caretakers.
- Delay or difficulty in passing stools leading to significant distress should be considered as constipation
- Normal stool frequency in Indian children is around 7 times per week. The stool consistency corresponding to Bristol stool chart types 1 and 2 should be considered as constipation.
- Besides this, also consider other conditions like straining, painful defecation, fear of passing stools, standing defecation, and fecal soiling of undergarments.
- Details of Bristol stool chart are given in **Figure 1**.

Bristol stool chart

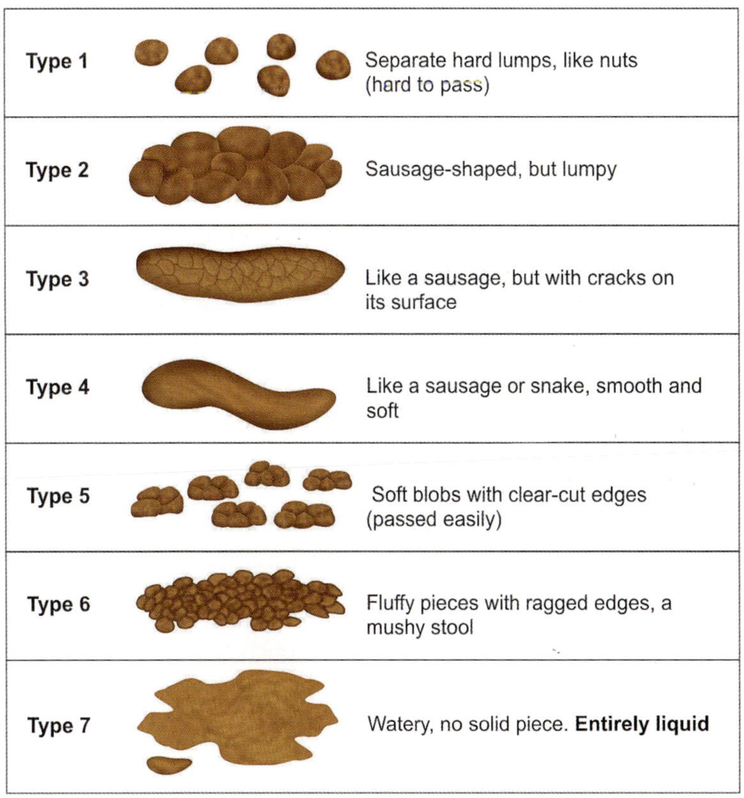

Etiology

- Constipation may be due to functional or organic causes.
- More than 95% of children have functional constipation. This is defined as the presence of two or more of the following criteria lasting over 1 month:
  1. Stool frequency ≤2 per week, history of hard and painful bowel movements, retention of stools, large-diameter stool obstructing the toilets, fecal incontinence, fecal mass on per abdomen or per rectum examination.
  2. Causes for functional constipation include improper diet, sedentary lifestyle, postponing defecation, unavailability of toilet, stressful events, intercurrent illness, toilet training, and drugs.

Causes

Organic causes of constipation are mentioned in **Table 1**.

TABLE 1: Organic causes of constipation.

SYSTEM	DISORDER
Abnormalities of colon and rectum	Ectopic anus, anal or colonic stenosis
Spinal cord anomalies	Meningomyelocele, sacral agenesis, tethered cord syndrome
Enteric nervous system and motility	Hirschsprung's disease, chronic intestinal obstruction, pelvic dyssynergia
Metabolic and allergy	Celiac disease, food protein allergy, cystic fibrosis
Endocrine	Hypothyroidism, diabetes mellitus
Central nervous system	Cerebral palsy, demyelinating disorders, developmental delay, seizure disorders
Drugs and poisons	Anticholinergic and antimotility, opiates, antiepileptics, lead poisoning

Red Flags

Table 2 describes red flag clinical features and related disorders.

TABLE 2: Red flag clinical features and related disorders.

RED FLAGS	DISORDER
Delayed passage of meconium and recurrent enterocolitis	Hirschsprung's disorder (beyond 48 hours)
Abdominal distension	Hirschsprung's disorder, chronic intestinal pseudo-obstruction, anal stenosis
Bilious vomiting and pain abdomen	Intestinal obstruction
Short stature, delayed development, poor scholastics, lethargy, obesity	Hypothyroidism
Thin-diameter hard stools	Anal stenosis
Global developmental delay, feeding issues, seizures, neurological deficits, failure to thrive	Cerebral palsy, neurodegenerative disorders, seizure disorders
Tuft of hair at back of the spine, abnormal neurological signs in lower limbs, gait abnormality	Tethered cord syndrome, spina bifida
Meconium ileus, recurrent respiratory tract infections, failure to thrive	Cystic fibrosis

Approach

- Complete history including duration of illness, type of stools, defecation position, straining, withholding behavior, toilet training, school timings, drugs, pain in the abdomen, and red flag symptoms should be taken.
- Thorough examination of growth, abdomen, lower back, perianal, and neurological areas should be done.
- Per rectal examination should be done in suspected anal stenosis/fecal impaction with/without fecal soiling.
- Investigations are not required unless red flag symptoms or signs are present.

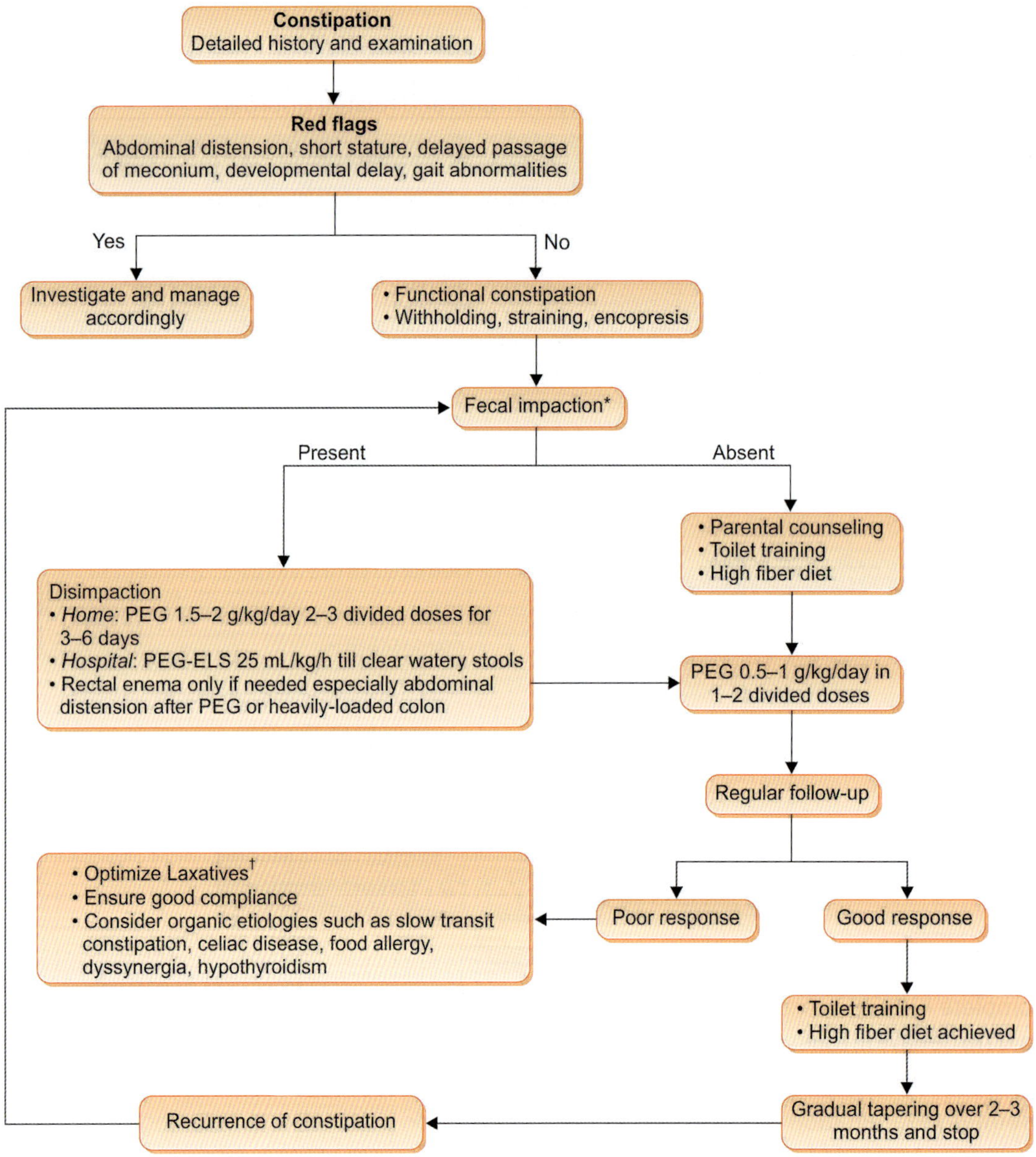

*Fecal impaction is diagnosed in the presence of a hard fecal mass in the lower abdomen or rectum

†Stimulant laxatives are not a part of the routine management and should be reserved for rescue therapy

Suggested Reading

- Poddar U. Approach to Constipation in Children. Indian Pediatr. 2016;53:319-27.
- Poddar U, Singh S, Pawaria A, Srivastava A, Yachha SK. Aetiological spectrum, clinical differentiation and efficacy of polyethylene glycol over lactulose in children with constipation: Experience of 316 cases. J Paediatr Child Health. 2019;55(2):162-7.
- Tabbers MM, DiLorenzo C, Berger MY, Faure C, Langendam MW, Nurko S, et al. Evaluation and treatment of functional constipation in infants and children: evidence-based recommendations from ESPGHAN and NASPGHAN. J Pediatr Gastroenterol Nutr. 2014;58:258-74.
- Yachha SK, Srivastava A, Mohan N, Bharadia L, Sarma MS, Indian Society of Pediatric Gastroenterology, et al. Management of Childhood Functional Constipation: Consensus Practice Guidelines of Indian Society of Pediatric Gastroenterology, Hepatology and Nutrition and Pediatric Gastroenterology Chapter of Indian Academy of Pediatrics. Indian Pediatr. 2018;55(10):885-92.

Delayed Puberty

85

Section Editor: **Kripasindhu Chatterjee**
Section Co-Editors: **Atanu Bhadra, Ashim Kumar Ghosh**
Authors: **Anurag Bajpai, Sayan Banerjee**

Introduction

- Delayed puberty is a common presentation in clinical practice.
- Differentiation between the physiological causes and the pathological ones presents a major challenge.

Criteria for Diagnosis

Criteria for diagnosis are given in **Table 1**.

TABLE 1: Criteria for diagnosis.

CRITERIA	FEMALES	MALES
Delayed puberty	• No breast development at 13 years • No menarche at 16 years	No testicular development at 14 years
Stalled puberty	• Secondary amenorrhea • No menarche after 4 years of thelarche	• Inadequate progression • Regression of testicular volume

Etiology

- *Hypogonadotropic hypogonadism (HH):*
  - Constitutional delay of growth and puberty (CDGP)—most common cause
  - Permanent HH
    - Isolated or syndromic HH (Prader–Willi, Bardet–Biedel)
    - Multiple pituitary hormone deficiency (MPHD)

- Congenital—malformations
- Acquired—mass lesions, infections, infiltrative disorders (histiocytosis), radiation
- *Functional HH:* Malnutrition, systemic illness
- Hyperprolactinemia
- *Hypergonadotropic hypogonadism:*
  - Gonadal dysgenesis
    - Turner syndrome (female)
    - Klinefelter syndrome (male)
  - Autoimmune ovarian insufficiency
  - Pelvic insult (radiation, cyclophosphamide)
  - Steroidogenic defects
    - XX—StAR, SCC, 17BHSD
    - XY—17-hydroxylase, 17BHSD, StAR
  - 5-alpha reductase deficiency (male)
  - Complete androgen insensitivity syndrome (CAIS)
  - Structural abnormalities (imperforate hymen, Mullerian agenesis)

Pointers to Constitutional Delay of Growth and Puberty

- Normal height and bone age
- Pubarche
- Stalled puberty

Red Flag Signs

- Stalled puberty, headache, rash, neurological insult
- Galactorrhea
- Tenderness, abdominal mass

Diagnostic Pointers

- *CDGP:* No pubertal development, delayed bone age (height normal for bone age), family history of delayed menarche (mother) and delayed shaving (father)
- *Permanent HH:* Anosmia, micropenis, pubarche, skeletal dysplasia, deafness
- *Syndromic HH:* Acromicria, almond-shaped eyes, polydactyl
- *Functional HH:* Sick child, with no pubertal development
- *Congenital MPHD:* Hypoglycemia, midline defects, vision abnormalities
- *Acquired MPHD:* Stalled puberty, secondary amenorrhea
- *Turner syndrome:* Webbing of neck, shield chest, short stature
- *Klinefelter syndrome:* Small and shotty testis, gynecomastia, tall stature
- *17-Hydroxylase deficiency:* Hypertension
- *Structural:* Normal breast and pubarche, amenorrhea
- *CAIS:* Amenorrhea, normal thelarche, no pubarche, inguinal gonads
- *5-Alpha reductase:* Atypical genitalia, virilization at puberty
- *Autoimmune:* Alopecia, vitiligo

Relevant Investigations

- *Screening investigations:* Comple blood count (CBC), liver function test (LFT), renal function test (RFT), tissue transglutaminase (TTG), random blood sugar (RBS)
- *Gonadotropins:* Luteinizing hormone (LH), follicle-stimulating hormone (FSH)
- *HH (LH < 0.1 mU/L):*
  - Gonadotropin hormone-releasing hormone (GnRH) stimulation—differentiates CDGP (LH >5 mU/L) from permanent HH (LH < 5 mU/L)
  - Permanent HH—prolactin, 8 AM cortisol, free thyroxine (FT4), thyroid-stimulating hormone (TSH), growth hormone (GH) stimulation test, MRI of the hypothalamic–pituitary region
- *Hypergonadotropic hypogonadism (FSH >15 mU/L):*
  - Karyotype, genetic studies (if karyotype normal)
  - Testosterone, dihydrotestosterone (DHT) levels—differentiate synthetic defects (both low), 5ARDII defect (high testosterone with low DHT), and CAIS (both high) in males

Approach to Delayed Puberty in Girls

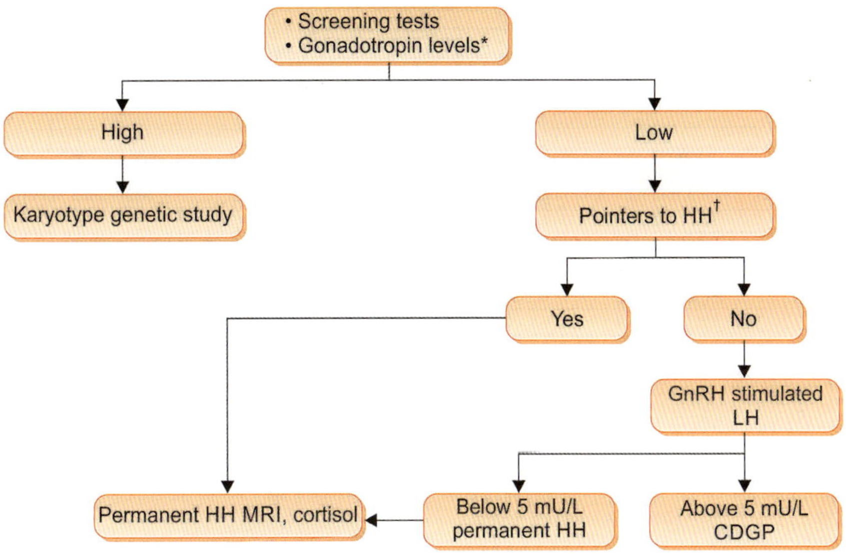

*CBC, ALT, creatinine, TTG, FT4, TSH, prolactin.

†Anosmia, synkinesia, CNS features.

(ALT: alanine transaminase; CBC: complete blood count; CDGP: constitutional delay of growth and puberty; CNS: central nervous system; FT4: free thyroxine; GnRH: gonadotropin hormone-releasing hormone; HH: hypogonadotropic hypogonadism; TSH: thyroid-stimulating hormone)

Source: Adapted with permission from Bajpai A, Dave C. (2023). Delayed Puberty. MedEClasses Online Course in Pediatric Endocrinology. [online] Available from learning.growsociety.in [Last accessed May, 2024].

Approach to Delayed Puberty in Boys

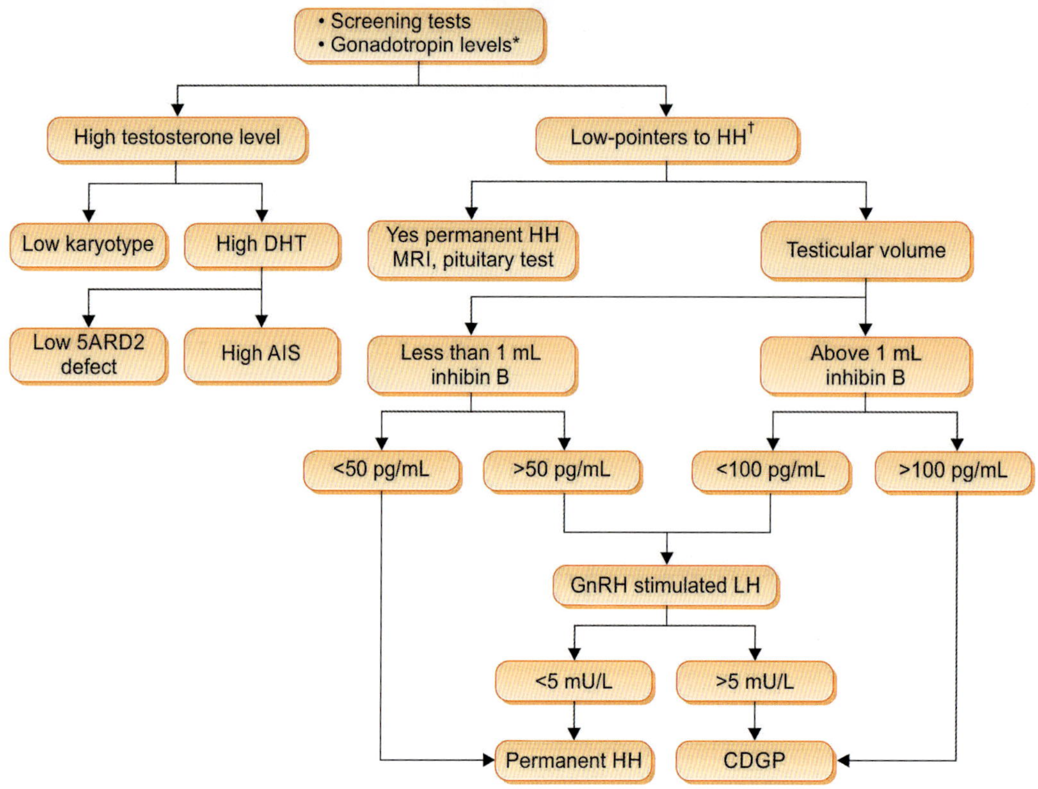

*CBC, ALT, creatinine, TTG, FT4, TSH.

†Micropenis, undescended testis, anosmia, synkinesia, CNS features.

(ALT: alanine transaminase; CBC: complete blood count; CDGP: constitutional delay of growth and puberty; CNS: central nervous system; FT4: free thyroxine; GnRH: gonadotropin hormone-releasing hormone; HH: hypogonadotropic hypogonadism; TSH: thyroid-stimulating hormone)

Source: Adapted with permission from Bajpai A, Dave C. (2023). Delayed Puberty. MedEClasses Online Course in Pediatric Endocrinology. [online] Available at from learning.growsociety.in [Last accessed May, 2024].

Suggested Reading

- Bajpai A. Delayed puberty. In: Shah N, Rao S (Eds). IAP Specialty Series on Pediatric Endocrinology, 2nd edition. New Delhi: Jaypee Digital; 2013. (Chapter 11).
- Harrington J, Palmert MR. An approach to the patient with delayed puberty. J Clin Endocrinol Metab. 2022;107(6): 1739-50.
- Kaplowitz PB. Delayed puberty. Pediatr Rev. 2010;31(5):189-95.
- Persani L, Bonomi M, Cools M, Dattani M, Dunkel L, Gravholt CH, et al. ENDO-ERN expert opinion on the differential diagnosis of pubertal delay. Endocrine. 2021;71:681-8.
- Young J, Xu C, Papadakis GE, Acierno JS, Maione L, Hietamäki J, et al. Clinical management of congenital hypogonadotropic hypogonadism. Endocr Rev. 2019;40(2):669-710.

Earache

86

Section Editor: **Rupesh Masand**
Section Co-Editor: **Hema Gupta Mittal**
Author: **Piyali Bhattacharya**

Introduction

Earache is a common complaint, especially among younger children in the primary/emergency care, peaking between the ages of 6 months and 2 years.

Types

- *Primary:* Pain originating inside the ear.
- *Secondary/referred:* Pain originating outside the ear.

Etiology

Primary Otalgia

- *Infections:*
  - *Acute otitis media with/without effusion: Common causes—Streptococcus pneumoniae, Hemophilus influenzae*, and *Moraxella catarrhalis* infection. Shorter eustachian tubes, which are compliant and horizontally placed, allow bacteria to easily traverse the middle ear cavity, causing swelling and inflammation.
  - *Otitis externa/"swimmer's" ear: Causes—Pseudomonas/Staphylococcus aureus* infection. It is seen in children going swimming during summer months. Due to poor hygiene, the skin lining the ear canal can become infected/irritated.
  - *Furunculosis: Cause—S. aureus.* Outer one-third cartilaginous portion of the external auditory canal is involved.

- *Perichondritis: Cause—S. aureus/Pseudomonas*. Infection of auricle/external auditory canal
- *Cellulitis*: *Streptococcus pyogenes* infection of the auricle
- *Herpes zoster:* Vesicles on the auricle and external auditory canal
- *Bullous myringitis: Causes*—Respiratory syncytial virus/influenza virus. Uncommonly due to *S. pneumoniae*, *H. influenzae*, and *M. catarrhalis*.

- *Trauma:* From falls, blows, self-induced by a sharp fingernail/sticks, clips, and safety pins, etc., used to scratch the ears/remove cerumen. Extreme heat or cold (frostbite), perforation of tympanic membrane due to slap injury/explosive blast
- *Impacted cerumen:* Hardened cerumen can cause increased pain, inflammation, and irritation.
- *Foreign body:* Playfully inserted small objects—beads, peas, crayons into ears. Can block/scratch the inner lining of the ear and cause earache
- *Barotrauma:* Lack of pressure equalization between the middle ear cavity and external environment during airplane descent causes severe earache.

Secondary/Referred Otalgia

- Aphthous ulcers, stomatitis, sinusitis, gingivitis, glossitis, toothache due to teething/dental caries/impacted teeth, mumps parotitis, temporomandibular joint dysfunction
- Bell's palsy
- Tonsillitis, pharyngitis, peritonsillar abscess, retropharyngeal abscess, postoperative phase of tonsillectomy
- Laryngitis, laryngeal or esophageal foreign body, esophagitis, gastroesophageal reflux
- Cervical lymphadenitis, arthritis, trauma of the cervical spine
- Migraine
- Psychogenic

Red Flags

- Unilateral episodic excruciating earache
- Dysphagia, dysphonia, odynophagia, or sore throat
- Cervical lymphadenopathy
- Unilateral hearing loss without obvious cause (e.g., cerumen)
- Persistent or unexplained otalgia without apparent cause and with normal examination
- Reddish swelling behind the ear
- Outer ear red, swollen, and painful
- Neck stiffness
- Immunosuppressed state

Investigations

Investigations may include:

- Otoscopy

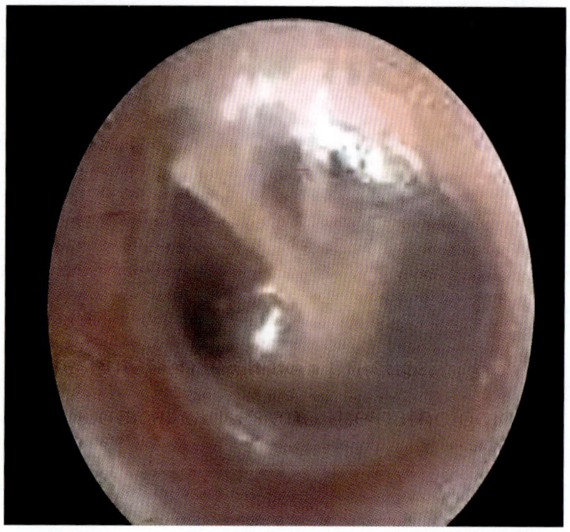

Normal tympanic membrane

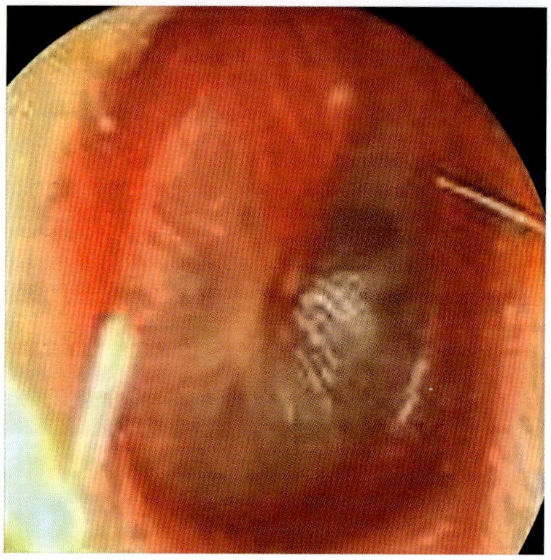

Bulging tympanic membrane

- Blood tests [complete blood count, erythrocyte sedimentation rate (ESR), C-reactive protein (CRP)]
- Aural discharge for culture and sensitivity
- Audiology—in case of recurrent infection/delayed speech development
- *Imaging (X-ray, CT scan):* X-ray cervical spine, paranasal sinuses, soft tissues of neck
- *Tympanometry:* Evaluation of middle ear functioning

Approach to Earache

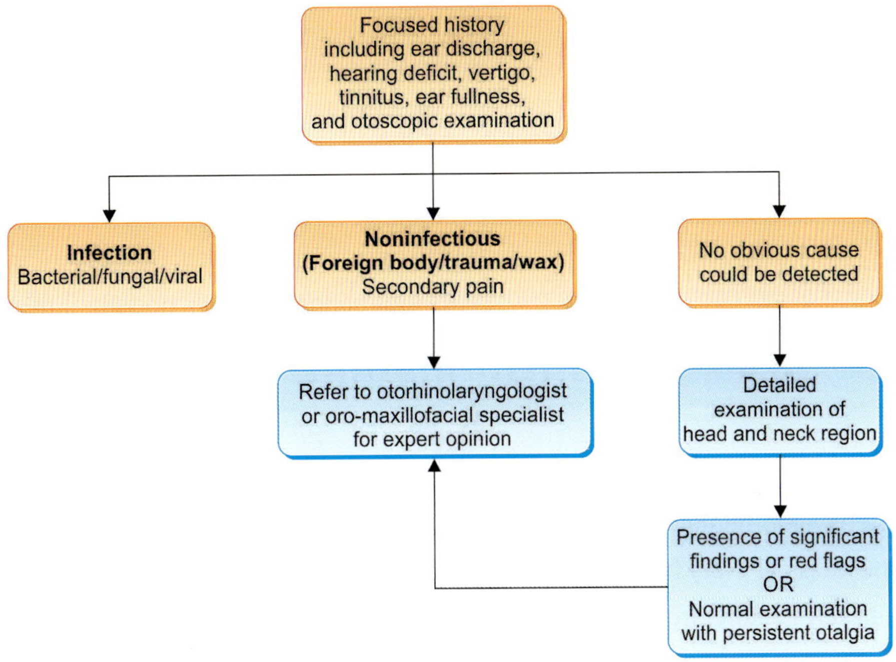

Suggested Reading

- Earwood JS, Rogers TS, Rathjen NA. Ear Pain: Diagnosing Common and Uncommon Causes. Am Fam Physician. 2018;97(1):20-7.
- Harrison E, Cronin M. Otalgia. Aust Fam Physician. 2016;45(7):493-7.
- Hwa TP, Brant JA. Evaluation and management of otalgia. Med Clin North Am. 2021;105(5):813-20.

Fecal Incontinence

87

Section Editor: **B Rajsekhar**
Section Co-Editor: **Suchitra Pusapati**
Authors: **Vishnu D Biradar, Siddhant Chavan**

Introduction

- Fecal incontinence (FI) is defined as the voluntary or involuntary defecation in an inappropriate place by children with a developmental age of 4 years or above.

  In children, the rates of FI vary from 1.6% to 4.4%.
- Boys are more likely to suffer from FI in comparison to girls.

Rome IV Criteria

- Recurrent uncontrolled passage of fecal material in an individual with a developmental age of at least 4 years
- Criterion fulfilled for the past 3 months

Etiology

Etiology of FI is given in **Box 1**.

BOX 1: Etiology of fecal incontinence (FI).

CONSTIPATION-RELATED FI	SPHINCTER-RELATED FI	NEUROGENIC FI
• Decreased fiber intake • Pelvic dyssynergia • High fatty meals	• Anorectal malformations • Hirschsprung's disease—postoperative status • Perianal abscesses/fistula • Anal sphincter trauma	• *Congenital:* – Myelomeningocele – Myelodysplasia – Spina bifida – Sacral agenesis – Arnold–Chiari syndrome • *Acquired:* – Spinal cord injury – Myelitis – Tumor(s) in the spinal cord

Investigations

- Detailed history, per abdominal and complete neurological examination
- Per rectal examination
  - To look for fecal impaction
  - To look for internal anal sphincter tone
  - To evaluate for squeeze pressure (external anal sphincter muscles)
  - Any perianal fistula
- Whole spine examination
  - To look for stigmata of spina bifida
  - Any swelling or other abnormality

Specific Tests

- Anorectal manometry
- Barium enema
- MRI whole spine ± Brain
- Endoanal ultrasound
- Colonic transit study

Referral to pediatric gastroenterologist, surgeon, or neurologist may be done based on the clinical diagnosis.

Red Flag Symptoms and Signs

Delayed passage of meconium, ribbon-like stools, significant abdominal distension	Hirschsprung disease
Fear of anal examination, scars in perianal region	Child sexual abuse
• Hair tuft/hemangioma/scars on spine • Abnormal anal and cremasteric reflex • Lower limb weakness • Delayed development	Neurological abnormalities
Blood in stools, failure to thrive	Other organic disorders

Approach to Fecal Incontinence in Children

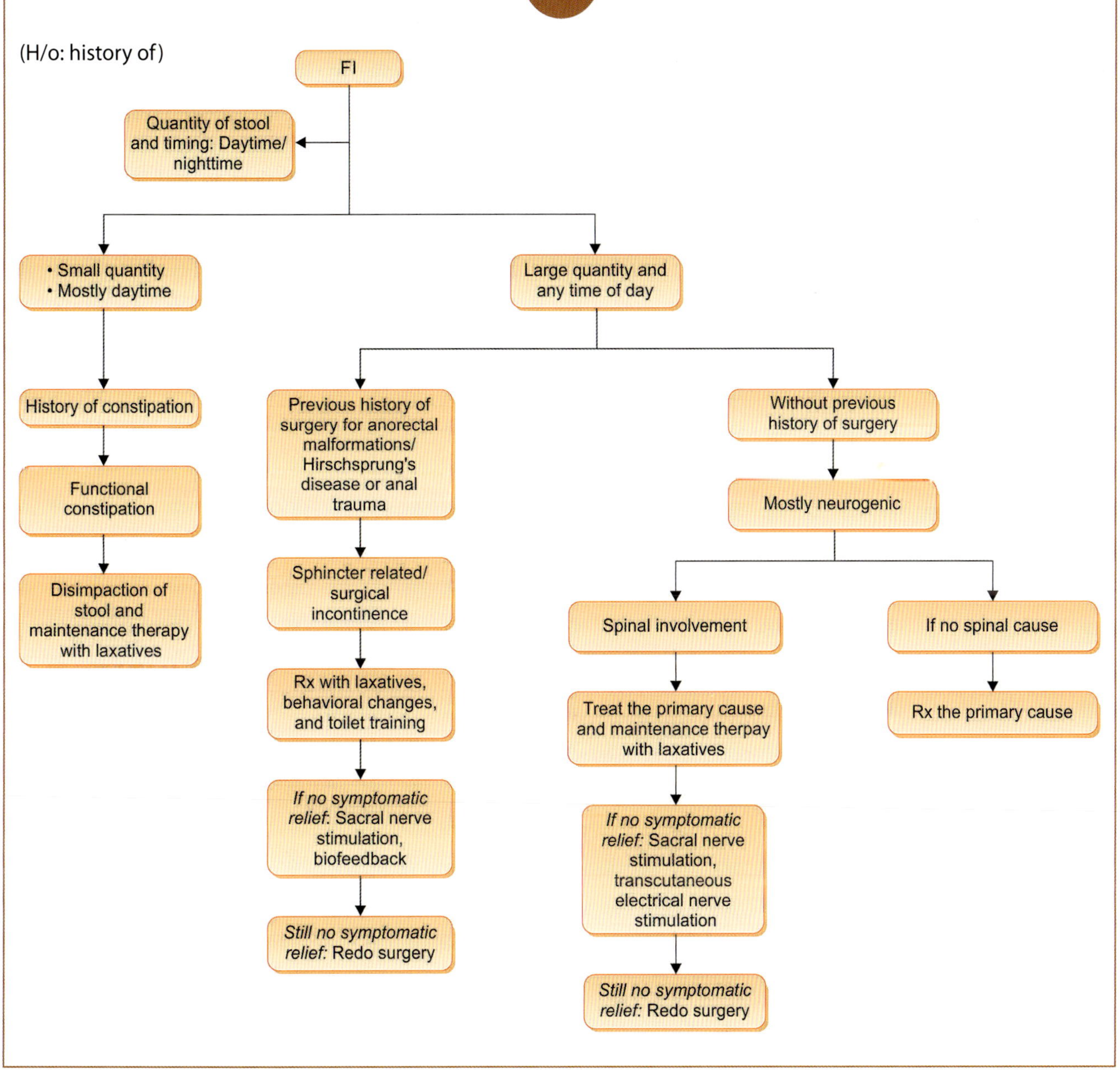

Suggested Reading

- Mansi S, Vaz K, Santucci NR, El-Chammas K, Graham K, Rosen NG, et al. Anal Sphincter Defect and Fecal Incontinence. JPGN Rep. 2022;3(4):e254.
- Rajindrajith S, Devanarayana NM, Thapar N, Benninga MA. Functional fecal incontinence in children: Epidemiology, pathophysiology, evaluation, and management. J Pediatr Gastroenterol Nutr. 2021;72(6):794-801.
- Shen Z-Y, Zhang J, Bai Y-Z, Zhang S-C. Diagnosis and management of fecal incontinence in children and adolescents. Front Pediatr. 2022;10:1034240.
- Tabbers MM, DiLorenzo C, Berger MY, Faure C, Langendam MW, Nurko S, et al. Evaluation and Treatment of Functional Constipation in Infants and Children: Evidence-Based Recommendations from ESPGHAN and NASPGHAN. JPGN. 2014;58:258-74.

Limb Pain

88

***Section Editor:* Janani Shankar**
***Section Co-Editor:* Arathi Srinivasan**
***Author:* Palash Das**

Introduction

- Children have a very active lifestyle and are prone to injuries and pain. The usual causes of limb pain in childhood are benign, self-limiting, and often trauma-related.
- The antecedent cause is usually evident in acute cases. In those with insidious-onset long-standing pain, a careful examination is required to find the underlying causes.
- Take the history using anagram SOCRATES (S—Site, O—Onset, C—Character, R—Radiation, A—Associated features, T—Timing, E—Exacerbating and Relieving factors, S—Severity)
- *Clinical examination:* p-GALS (pediatric gait, arms, legs, and spine) is a validated rapid method to examine the musculoskeletal system.
  - Observing from front and back—for rash/wasting/swelling
  - Gait on walking on heels/tiptoe
  - Holding hands straight/making fist/pinching thumb and index/touching tips of fingers with thumb
  - Squeezing of metacarpophalangeal joint by physician
  - Putting hands together—palm–palm and back–back
  - Reach up and touch the sky/putting hands behind neck/touching ear to shoulder
  - Putting three fingers in the mouth
  - Patellar tap/active and passive movement of knee and hip joint
  - Bend forward to touch toes

A detailed systemic examination to look for any of the following:

- *Pallor:* Consider leukemia/sickle cell anemia/metastatic tumors
- *Bleeding tendency:* Leukemia/hemophilia
- *Rash:* Palpable purpura—Henoch–Schonlein purpura (HSP), photosensitive rash (systemic lupus erythematosus)
- *Hepatosplenomegaly:* Leukemia

Etiology

Etiology of limb pain is given in **Box 1**.

BOX 1: Etiology of limb pain.

• *Trauma:* – Fracture – Sprains – Delayed-onset muscle soreness (after strenuous exercise)	• *Muscular:* – Viral myositis – Juvenile dermatomyositis	• *Vascular:* – Sickle cell pain crisis – Deep vein thrombosis
• *Infective:* – Osteomyelitis – Cellulitis	• *Joint:* – Juvenile idiopathic arthritis – Henoch–Schonlein purpura – Inflammatory bowel disease (IBD)-associated arthritis	• *Orthopedic conditions:* – Osteoid osteoma – Legg–Calve–Perthes disease – Osgood–Schlatter disease
• *Others:* – Benign nocturnal limb pain or growth pains – Spinal cord compression – Benign hypermobility syndrome	• *Malignancy:* – Leukemia – Metastatic tumors – Osteosarcoma/ chondrosarcoma	Nonaccidental injury

Red Flags

- Painful limping
- Severe pain as per pain scale
- *Systemic symptoms:* Fever, weight loss, night sweats, fatigue, or pallor
- Bleeding tendencies
- Movement restriction
- *Signs of inflammation:* Redness/tenderness/swelling
- Persistent pain as opposed to intermittent or pain that is progressively increasing in severity
- *Pain occurring in the morning/with activities:* Evaluate for inflammatory arthritis or trauma
- Nocturnal pain not relieved by analgesics

Relevant Investigations

- History/proper physical examination
- X-ray of the involved part, especially if fracture is suspected
- *MRI:* To detect joint pathologies/malignancies
- Complete blood count (CBC), C-reactive protein (CRP), erythrocyte sedimentation rate (ESR): Any patient with systemic symptoms of fever, pain in limbs, bleeding tendencies, etc.
- Antinuclear antibody (ANA)/double-stranded DNA (dsDNA)/urine analysis: If inflammatory pathology is suspected from history
- Vitamin D levels/creatine phosphokinase (CPK) levels/high-performance liquid chromatography (HPLC), etc., based on history and examination for identifying etiology

Approach to a Child with Limb Pain

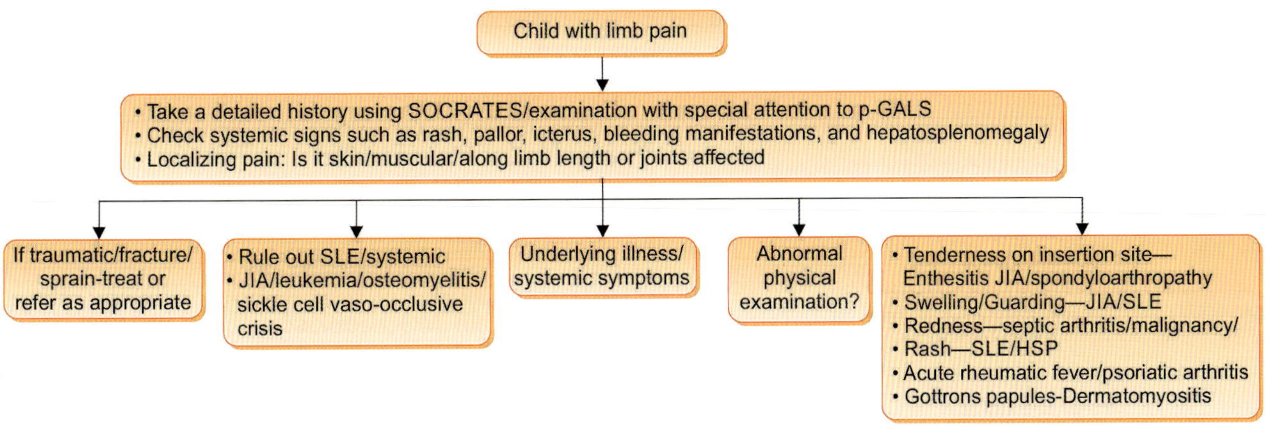

(HSP: Henoch–Schonlein purpura; JIA: juvenile idiopathic arthritis; SLE: systemic lupus erythematosus)

Suggested Reading

- Junnila JL, Cartwright VW. Chronic musculoskeletal pain in children: part I. Initial evaluation. Am Fam Physician. 2006;74(1):115-22.
- Naranje S, Kelly DM, Sawyer JR. A systematic approach to the evaluation of a limping child. Am Fam Physician. 2015;92(10):908-16.
- Tse SM, Laxer RM. Approach to acute limb pain in childhood. Pediatr Rev. 2006;27(5):170-80.

Stridor

89

Section Editor: **Rupesh Masand**
Section Co-Editor: **Hema Gupta Mittal**
Author: **Javeed Iqbal Bhat**

Introduction

- Stridor refers to a distinctive, high-pitched respiratory sound during inhalation, exhalation, or both. This symphony is due to turbulent airflow through partially obstructed airways at the level of the supraglottis, glottis, subglottis, or trachea.
- Stridor is a manifestation of many congenital and acquired abnormalities.

Etiology of Stridor in Children

Etiology of stridor in children is given in **Box 1**.

BOX 1: Etiology of stridor in children.

CONGENITAL STRIDOR	ACQUIRED STRIDOR
• Laryngomalacia • Tracheomalacia • Subglottic stenosis • Subglottic hemangioma • Vocal cord paralysis • Laryngeal web (vocal cord web) • Vascular rings • Vallecular cyst • Bronchogenic cyst • Laryngeal cleft • Other structural malformations affecting the upper airway	• Viral croup (laryngotracheitis) • Spasmodic croup • Bacterial tracheitis • Acute epiglottitis • Retropharyngeal abscess • Peritonsillar abscess • Vocal cord dysfunction • Foreign body aspiration • Anaphylaxis • Acquired vocal cord paralysis • Postventilation subglottic stenosis and upper airway tumors

Red Flags

- Increased work of breathing
- Cyanosis
- Difficulty swallowing or drooling
- Rapid onset stridor
- Altered mental status
- Stridor at rest
- Rapid progression of stridor

Evaluation

Assessment of patient's airway and respiratory effort must be performed and suitable intervention done as indicated. The following investigations aid in the evaluation of a stridulous child:

- Laboratory tests, complete blood count (CBC), differential counts to attempt to differentiate between viral and bacterial causes.
- Additional tests like imaging and bronchoscopy may be conducted.
- Imaging and endoscopy aid in outlining the lesions responsible for stridor.
- *Radiography:* Lateral film to assess retropharyngeal space size. A widened space may suggest a retropharyngeal abscess. In croup, a classic "steeple sign" on neck anteroposterior (AP) view indicates subglottic arch edema. The "thumb sign" seen on lateral soft-tissue radiograph of the neck suggests a diagnosis of acute infectious epiglottitis.
- *Computed tomography (CT) scan chest and neck:* To diagnose retropharyngeal cellulitis, enlarged lymph nodes, tumors, aberrant arteries, and vascular rings. It may help in the diagnosis of stenotic lesions and foreign bodies.
- Magnetic resonance imaging (MRI) is a valuable tool for diagnosing tracheal stenosis in pediatric patients.

Algorithmic Approach to Evaluation of a Child with Stridor

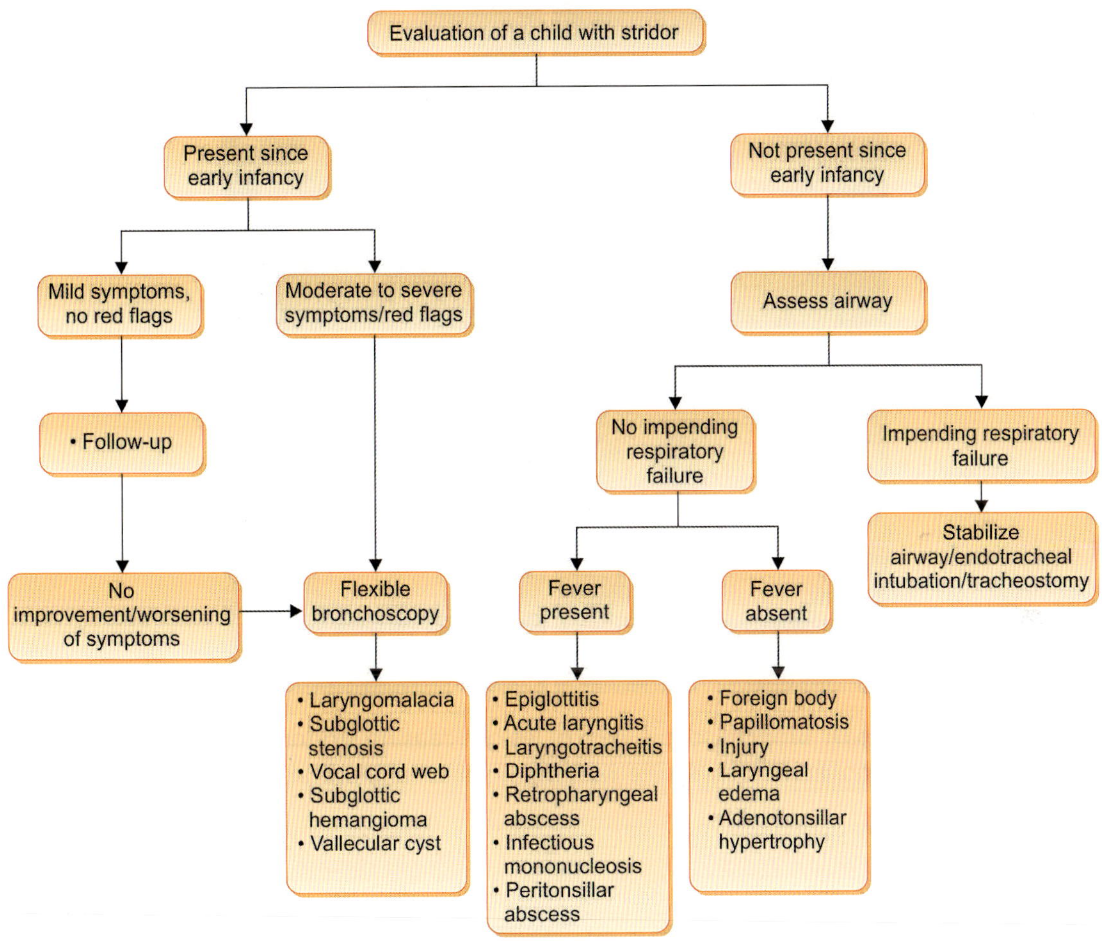

Nasopharyngoscopy, laryngoscopy, and bronchoscopy provide a definitive diagnosis of stridor causes in most of the children **(Figs. A to D)**. Multiple airway abnormalities may coexist, necessitating a comprehensive assessment of both upper and lower airways.

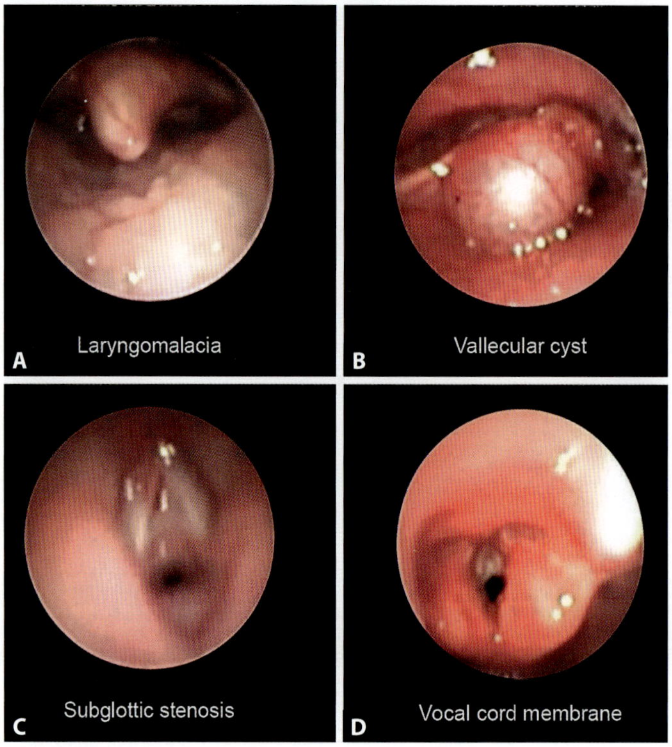

FIGS. A to D: Bronchoscopic view of lesions causing stridor in children.
Courtesy: Department of Pediatrics, Sher-e-Kashmir Institute of Medical Sciences, or Srinagar.

Suggested Reading

- Boudewyns A, Claes J, Van de Heyning P. Clinical practice: an approach to stridor in infants and children. Eur J Pediatr. 2010;169:135.
- Celmina M, Paule S. Stridor in children. Breathe (Sheff). 2018;14(3):e111-7.
- Quintero R, Fakhoury K. (2022). Assessment of stridor in children. [online] Available from www.uptodate.com/contents/assessment-of-stridor-in-children. [Last accessed May, 2024].
- Sicari V, Zabbo CP. Stridor in Children. [Updated 2023 Nov 12]. In: StatPearls [Internet]. Treasure Island (FL): StatPearls Publishing; 2023 Jan.

90

Vomiting

Section Editor: **B Rajsekhar**
Section Co-Editor: **Suchitra Pusapati**
Authors: **B Rajsekhar, Suchitra Pusapati**

Introduction

- Vomiting is defined as the involuntary, forceful retrograde ejection of the stomach contents via the mouth.
- Children often present with this symptom in the outpatient department. It can cause significant dehydration and may be a symptom of life-threatening illnesses.
- Vomiting must be differentiated from regurgitation which is effortless retrograde flow of duodenal/gastric contents, due to an incompetent/immature lower esophageal sphincter

Etiology

Based on the age of presentation

Infant
- Gastroenteritis
- Overfeeding
- Gastroesophageal reflux disease (GERD)
- Anatomical obstruction
- Meningitis, sepsis, and otitis media

Child
- Gastroenteritis
- Infections—sepsis and meningitis
- Gastritis
- Toxic ingestion/poisoning

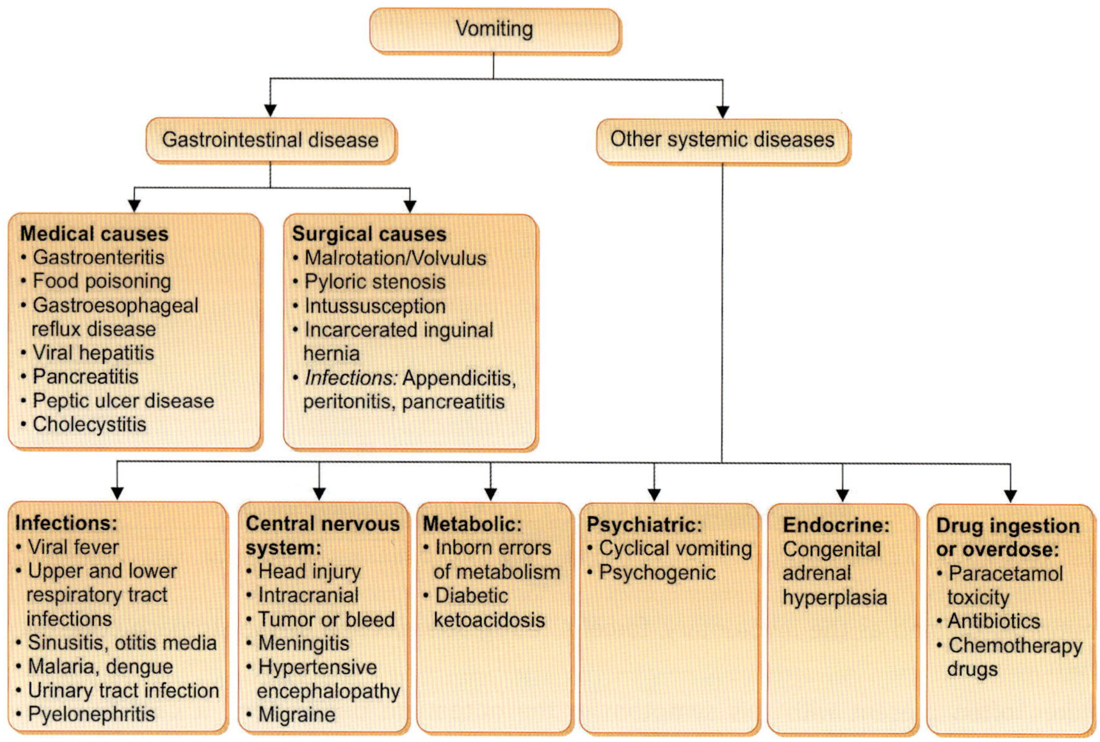

Note: List is not exhaustive and presentations can overlap.

Red Flags

SYMPTOM	POSSIBLE CAUSES
Hematemesis	Mallory–Weiss tear, erosive esophagitis, gastritis, peptic ulcer, and esophageal/gastric varices
Marked abdominal distension	Intestinal obstruction, appendicitis, sepsis
Dehydration, and shock	Acute gastroenteritis, sepsis, and inborn errors of metabolism
• Headache, irritable/drowsy, and seizures • Bulging fontanelle in neonate or young infant	Meningitis, encephalitis, space-occupying lesions, and nonaccidental injury in infant
History of head trauma	Intracranial bleeding
Bilious vomiting	Intestinal obstruction—atresia, volvulus, and intussusception
Projectile vomiting in an infant <12 weeks of age	Pyloric stenosis

Approach

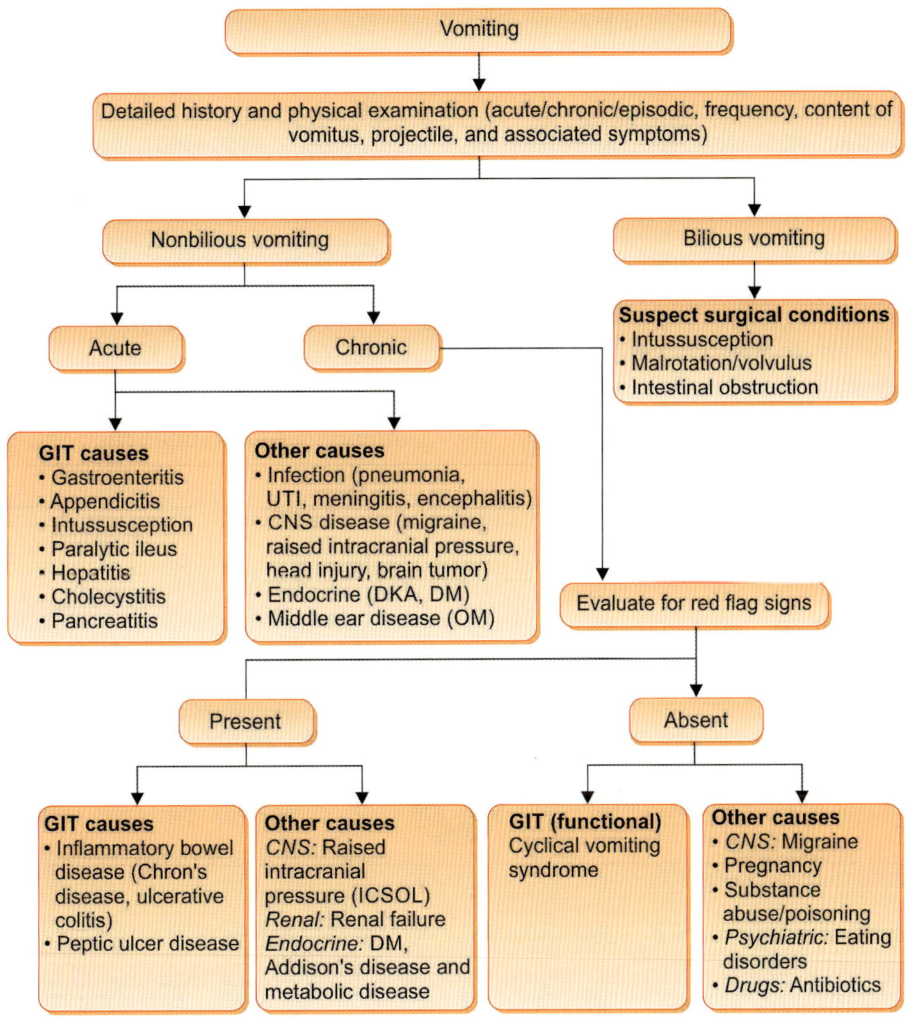

(CNS: central nervous system; ICSOL: intracranial space-occupying lesion; GIT: gastrointestinal tract; DKA: diabetic ketoacidosis; DM: diabetes mellitus; OM: otitis media; UTI: urinary tract infection)

Investigations

Most well children will not require any testing, but the following may be considered.

Indication	Investigations
Raised intracranial pressure, head trauma	CT brain
Intestinal obstruction or abdominal cause	Liver and renal function test, amylase, lipase, abdominal X-ray or ultrasound
Poisoning	Paracetamol levels, venous blood gas, ECG
Signs of infection	Complete blood count (CBC), C-reactive protein (CRP), blood culture, urine and stool microscopy & culture, viral serology, lumbar puncture, and chest X-ray
Metabolic causes	Blood glucose, urine ketones, arterial blood gas, ammonia, beta-human chorionic gonadotropin (HCG)

Referral to a pediatric surgeon, gastroenterologist, or neurologist may be done based on the clinical diagnosis

Suggested Reading

- Nelson WE. Nelson Textbook of Pediatrics. 21st edition. Amsterdam: Elsevier; 2021.
- Samprathi M, Jayashree M. Child with Vomiting. Indian J Pediatr. 2017;84(10):787-91.
- Kliegman RM, Toth H, Bordini BJ, Basel D. Nelson Pediatric Symptom-Based Diagnosis: Common Diseases and Their Mimics. Philadelphia, PA: Elsevier; 2022.

Bell's Palsy

91

Section Editor: **Kripasindhu Chatterjee**
Section Co-Editors: **Atanu Bhadra, Ashim Kumar Ghosh**
Author: **Asok Kumar Datta**

Introduction

- Bell's palsy is an acute neurological disorder caused due to lower motor neuron (LMN) type of lesion of the facial nerve (7th cranial nerve). It is characterized by sudden onset of weakness of unilateral facial muscles with/without loss of taste sensation of anterior one-third of tongue or hyperacusis, depending on the level of lesion.
- This commonly develops abruptly after about 2 weeks of a systemic viral infection.

Causes

Bell's Palsy is caused commonly due to compression of the facial nerve by inflammatory or immunological reactions with edema while passing through the bony facial canal. Other conditions like nucleus damage, cerebellopontine angle compression, ischemic, or trauma may also be causative.

Common Etiologies

- Herpes simplex virus type-1 infection
- Varicella zoster virus infection
- When associated with vesicles in auricle or external auditory canal—known as Ramsay Hunt syndrome

Less Common Causes

Viruses

- Epstein–Barr virus
- Cytomegalovirus
- Mumps
- Human Herpesvirus 6

- Human immunodeficiency virus (HIV)
- Intranasal inactivated influenza vaccine
- Influenza vaccination
- Hepatitis-B vaccination
- Nasal vaccine against HIV

Rare Causes

- Trauma
- Space-occupying lesion
- Mycoplasma infection
- Rickettsia infection
- Diabetes mellitus type 1—most often associated with concomitant viral infection
- Guillain–Barré syndrome
- Lyme disease
- Hypertension
- Melkersson–Rosenthal syndrome
- Narrowing of the bony canal
- Sarcoidosis
- Ribavirin
- Interferon alpha
- Peripheral facial nerve paralysis

Red Flags

- Gradual onset and gradual progress of paralysis beyond 3 weeks
- Recurrence
- Earache/otitis media
- Vesicles in the external meatus/soft palate
- Mastoid swelling and/or tenderness
- Involvement of other cranial nerves
- Parotid gland swelling
- Pain or paresthesia, limb paresis, and postural imbalance
- Lymphadenopathy, pallor, or bruising
- Hypertension
- Retinal changes associated with hypertension and/or diabetes

Clinical Manifestations

- Sudden onset, sometimes preceded by pain in the ear/sore throat
- Paralysis within 2–3 days after onset of ear pain
- Unable to close the eye of the affected side due to paralysis of orbicularis oculi muscle with dryness of the eye due to loss of secretion of lacrimal fluid caused by damage to the parasympathetic nerve, which is associated with the facial nerve
- Exposure keratitis may occur
- Unable to lift the eyebrows/frowning due to paralysis of frontalis and corrugator supercilli muscle
- Deviation of angle of the mouth toward the opposite side with dribbling of saliva, water and food, and loss of nasolabial fold on the same side
- Loss of taste sensation of the anterior two-third of the tongue of the same side if chorda tympani nerve is damaged
- Hyperacusis, if damage is caused to the nerve to stapedius
- A small percentage of patients exhibit dysfunction of other cranial nerves, including the glossopharyngeal and vestibulocochlear nerves
- Bilateral facial palsy, although uncommon, may result from congenital developmental anomalies, trauma, infectious or postinfectious granulomatous or neoplastic disorders.
- Bilateral hypoplasia or aplasia of the sixth and seventh cranial nerve in Moebius syndrome, Poland syndrome, rarely in collagen vascular diseases, and osteopetrosis
- Partial unilateral lower lip palsy in a neonate may result from involvement of the depressor anguli oris muscle, associated with cardiac, skeletal, and genitourinary abnormalities.

House–Brackmann Classification of Facial Function

GRADE	DESCRIPTION	GROSS FUNCTION	RESTING APPEARANCE	DYNAMIC APPEARANCE
1	Normal	Normal	Normal	Normal
2	Mild dysfunction	Slight weakness with efforts and may have mild synkinesis	Normal	Mild oral and forehead asymmetry and complete eye closure with minimal effort
3	Moderate dysfunction	Obvious asymmetry with movement, noticeable synkinesis, or contracture	Normal	Mild oral asymmetry; complete eye closure with effort, and slight forehead movement
4	Moderately severe dysfunction	Obvious asymmetry and disfiguring asymmetry	Normal	Asymmetric mouth, incomplete eye closure, and no forehead movement
5	Severe dysfunction	Barely perceptible movement	Asymmetric	Slight oral/nasal movement with effort and incomplete eye closure
6	Total paralysis	None	Asymmetric	No movement

Investigations

- High-resolution magnetic resonance imaging (MRI)—compression by lesions and to compare with the opposite site
- Ultrasound of the facial nerve for functional outcome
- Diffusion tensor tractography to enable a tridimensional display of facial nerve axons

Prognosis

- Most cases have favorable prognosis. Recovery begins within 2–4 weeks—maximum within 6 months (6–12 months). Recurrences are rare.
- Almost 85% patients fully recover.
- 10% cases have mild residual lesion.
- 5% cases are left with permanent severe disability.

Diagnostic Algorithm

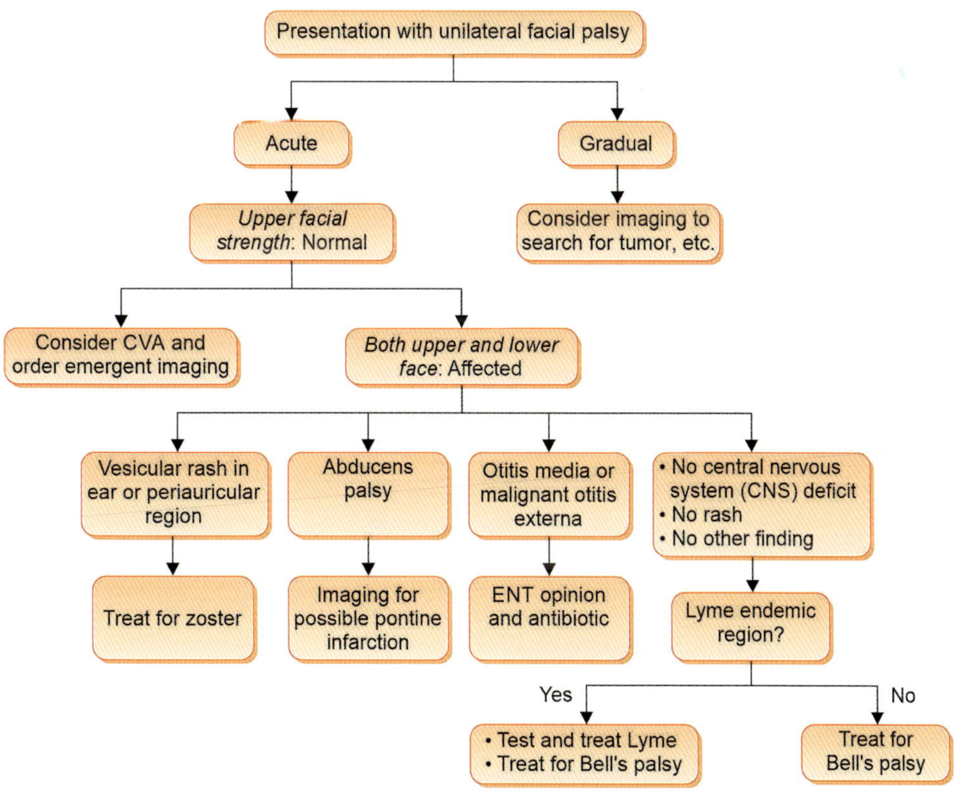

Suggested Reading

- Loscalzo J, Kasper DL, Longo DL, Fauci AS, Beal M, Houser S (Eds). Harrison's Principle of Internal Medicine, 20th edition. United States of America: McGraw-Hill Education; 2018. pp. 3169-70.
- Ryan MM. Bell's palsy. In: Kliegman RM, St. Geme III JW. Nelson Textbook of Pediatrics, 21st edition. Philadelphia, Pennsylvania: Elsevier; 2020. pp. 3339-40.
- Singh A, Deshmukh P. Bell's Palsy: A Review. Cureus. 2022;14(10):e30186.
- Swaiman KF, Ashwal S, Ferriero DM, Schor NF, Finkel RS, Gropman AL, Pearl PL, Shevell (Eds). Bell's Palsy. Swaiman's Pediatric Neurology, 5th edition. Amsterdam, Netherlands: Elsevier; 2011. pp. 1503-6.
- Zhang W, Xu L, Luo T, Wu F, Zhao B, Li X. The etiology of Bell's palsy: A review. J Neurol. 2020;267(7):1896-1905

Toe Walking

92

Section Editor: **Kripasindhu Chatterjee**
Section Co-Editors: **Atanu Bhadra, Ashim Kumar Ghosh**
Authors: **Jeevan Silwal, Ananda Kesavan TM**

Introduction

- Toe walking (TW) refers to a child walking with contact pattern on forefoot, rather than the heel strike.
- Idiopathic toe walking (ITW) is a pathological gait pattern in which children walk on their tip toes with no orthopedic/neurological reason after 2–3 years of age.
- A subset of children may have a genetic cause of the condition with a family history. The majority will resolve by the age of 5 years and those who continue beyond are described as persistent idiopathic toe walkers (ITWp).

Etiology

- *Neurological:* Cerebral palsy, spinal dysraphism, tethered cord syndrome, hereditary spastic paraplegia, and Chiari malformation
- *Neuromuscular:* Muscular dystrophy and hereditary motor sensory neuropathy
- *Musculoskeletal:* Congenital contracture of Achilles tendon or calf muscles, congenital clubfoot, leg length discrepancies (unilateral TW), and arthrogryposis
- *Developmental:* Autism spectrum disorder, attention-deficit/hyperactivity disorder (ADHD), and language and communication disorders
- ITW
- Genetic causes (rare)

Red Flags

- *Bowel and bladder symptoms:* Spinal pathology
- *Asymmetry:* Hemiplegic cerebral palsy and limb length discrepancy
- *Headache:* Chiari malformations
- *TW after a period of normal gait:* Neuromuscular etiology
- *Muscle atrophy and weakness:* Hereditary neuropathy
- *Calf pseudohypertrophy, Gowers's sign, proximal lower limb weakness:* Muscular dystrophy
- *Limited range of ankle joint:* May need early surgical intervention.

Approach

- *History:* Premature birth/perinatal complication, delayed motor milestones, bowel/bladder complaints, leg and/or back pain, course (progressive, episodic, or variable throughout the day), and family history.
- *Enquire:* Age of onset, episodic/continuous, whether normally walking in between, whether TW started after normal initial gait, frequent falls, etc.
- *General examination:* Examine foot, spine, general gait, dorsal midline skin lesions, and range of ankle motion.
- *Neurological examination:* Observe features of symmetry of TW, ataxia, muscular dystrophy features (Gowers's sign, calf hypertrophy, and proximal muscle weakness), mild hemiplegic gait, long tract signs (spasticity and brisk reflexes), and lower motor neuron (LMN) signs (pes cavus, muscle atrophy/weakness, sensory loss, and hyporeflexia)

  The approach to the management of a child with TW is given in **Flowchart 1**.

FLOWCHART 1: Approach to a child with toe walking.

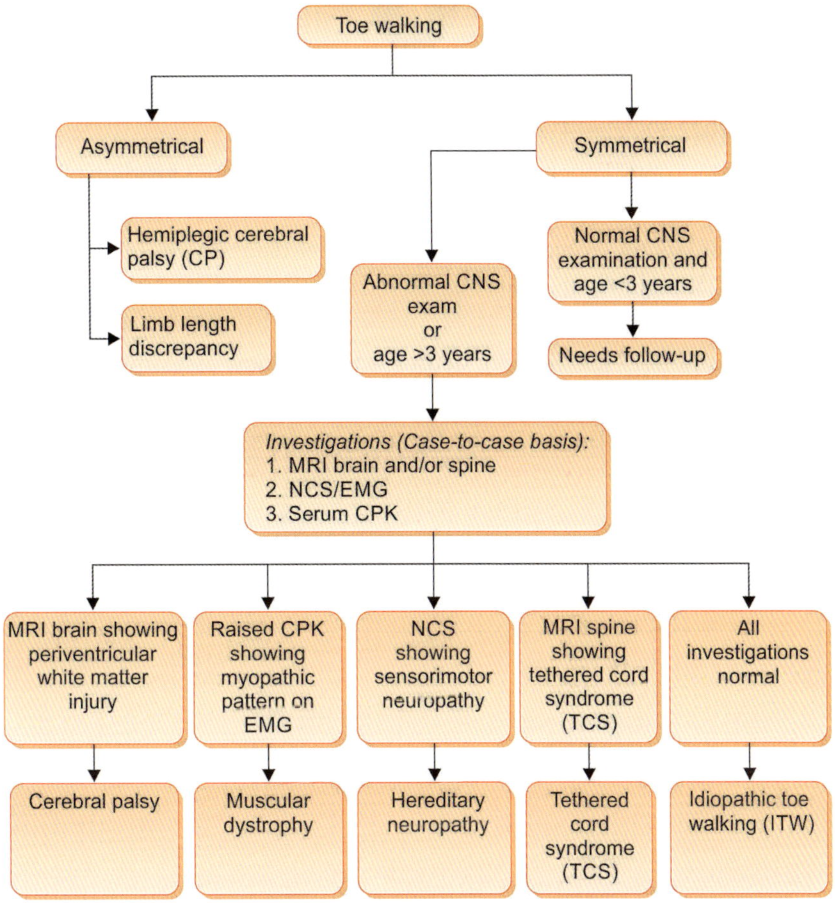

(CNS: central nervous system; CPK: creatine phosphokinase; EMG: electromyography; NCS: nerve conduction study)

Diagnosis and Investigation

- No standard testing recommendations exist for the diagnosis of ITW.
- Testing for other neurologic causes of TW is common on cases-to-case basis. For example, magnetic resonance imaging (MRI) brain and/or spine, nerve conduction studies (NCS), electromyography (EMG), serum creatine phosphokinase (CPK), radiograph (spine, ankle, and foot), and genetic tests (exome analysis)

Suggested Reading

- Bauer JP, Sienko S, Davids JR. Idiopathic toe walking: An update on natural history, diagnosis and treatment. J Am Acad Orthop Surg. 2022;30(22):e1419-e1430
- Caserta AJ, Pacey V, Fahey M, Gray K, Engelbert RH, Williams CM. Interventions for idiopathic toe walking. Cochrane Database Syst Rev. 2019;10(10):CD012363.
- Pomarino D, Martin S, PomarinoA, Pomarino P. The differential diagnosis of idiopathic toe walking. Medical Research Archives. 2017;5(9). [online] Available from https://esmed.org/MRA/mra/article/view/1504 [Last accessed June 2024].
- Ruzbarsky JJ, Scher D, Dodwell E. Toe walking: Causes, epidemiology, assessment, and treatment. Curr Opin Pediatr. 2016,28(1):40-6.
- Sala DA, Shulmann LH, Kennedy RF, Grant AD, Chu ML. Idiopathic toe-walking: A review. Dev Med Child Neurol. 1999;41(12):846-8.

Ataxia

93

Section Editor: **Kripasindhu Chatterjee**
Section Co-Editors: **Atanu Bhadra, Ashim Kumar Ghosh**
Author: **Debasis Panigrahi**

Introduction

- Ataxia refers to the failure of motor coordination leading to clumsiness, poor balance, irregularities in movements, inability to execute fine movements, or smooth sequence of movement.
- It is often benign and self-limited.

Etiology

Ataxia may occur due to dysfunction of cerebellum or failure of proprioceptive/vestibular afferents reaching the cerebellum.

Causes

- *Acute ataxia*
  - Postinfectious inflammatory conditions
  - Toxins
  - Tumors
  - Trauma

- *Acute and recurrent ataxia*
  - Migraine syndrome
  - Seizures
  - Inborn error of metabolism
  - Episodic ataxia type 1
  - Episodic ataxia type 2
- *Chronic*
  - Brain tumors
  - Hydrocephalus
  - Metabolic/Nutritional
  - Congenital malformations
  - Hereditary ataxias (ataxia telangiectasia, spinocerebellar ataxia, Friedreich's ataxia, etc.)
  - Basilar artery migraine
  - Seizure disorder

Red Flags

- Sudden onset/rapid progression
- Associated with headache, vomiting, confusion, and altered consciousness
- Neck stiffness
- Focal neurological deficit and cranial nerve involvement
- Abnormal eye movement like nystagmus
- Regression of milestones
- Family history of neurodegenerative disorder
- Associated tone abnormalities and abnormal reflexes

Investigations

Investigations are done depending on the suspected etiology:

- *Blood tests:* Specific tests can be considered based on etiology.
  - *Alpha-fetoprotein:* Ataxia telangiectasia
  - *Lipid profile:* Abetalipoproteinemia
  - *Serum and urinary copper:* Wilson's disease
  - *Lactate level:* Pyruvate dehydrogenase deficiency
  - *Cerebrospinal fluid (CSF) glucose:* Glucose transporter type-1 (GLUT1) deficiency, etc.
- *Magnetic resonance imaging (MRI) brain:* To assess the brain structure, particularly the cerebellum.
- Electromyography (EMG) and nerve conduction studies (NCS)
- *Genetic testing:* Can identify mutations associated with specific disorders.

Approach

Employ a multidisciplinary approach.

Underlying cause: Identify and treat the underlying cause **(Table 1)**.

TABLE 1: Treatable causes of inherited ataxia.

DISORDER	CLINICAL CLUES	TREATMENT
Ataxia with vitamin E deficiency	Ataxia, areflexia, and retinopathy	Vitamin E
Abetalipoproteinemia	Acanthocytosis, and retinitis pigmentosa	Vitamin E
Hartnup disease	Pellagra rash and intermittent ataxia	Niacin
Episodic ataxia 1 and 2	Episodic attacks of ataxia	Acetazolamide
Mitochondrial disorder	Encephalomyelopathy	Riboflavin and coenzyme Q10
Multiple carboxylase deficiency	Alopecia, rash, and variable organic acidemia	Biotin

The approach to diagnosis of ataxia in children is given in **Flowchart 1**.

FLOWCHART 1: Approach to diagnosis of ataxia in children.

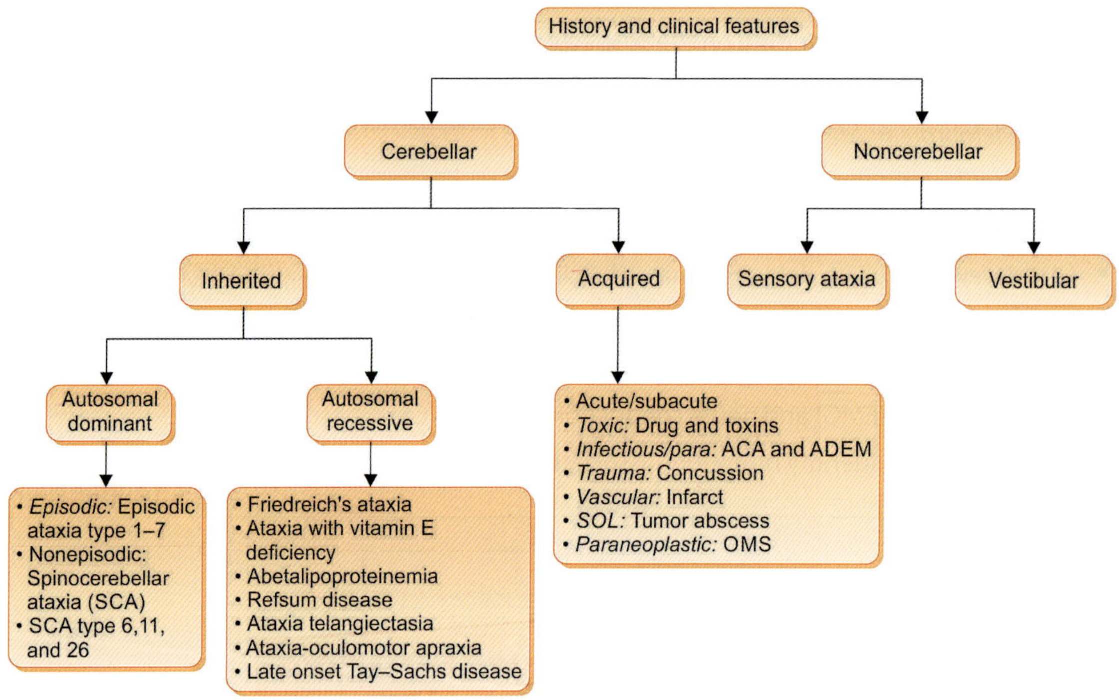

(ACA: acute cerebellar ataxia; ADEM: acute disseminated encephalomyelitis; OMS: opsoclonus–myoclonus syndrome)

Suggested Reading

- Lemma PC, Saravanan RV, Ravi LA. Approach to a child with ataxia. IJPP. 2016;18(2):109-21
- Overby P, Kapklein M, Jacobson RI. Acute ataxia in children. Pediatric Rev. 2019;40(7):332-43.
- Pavone P, Praticò AD, Pavone V, Lubrano R, Falsaperla R, Rizzo R, et al. Ataxia in children: Early recognition and clinical evaluation. Ital J Pediatr. 2017;43(1):6.
- Sharma P, Sonakar AK, Tyagi N, Suroliya V, Kumar M, Kutum R, et al.; GOMED-Ataxia study group. Genetics of ataxias in Indian population: A collative insight from a common genetic screening tool. Adv Genet (Hoboken). 2022;3(2):2100078.
- Swaiman KF, Ashwal S, Ferriero DM, Schor NF, Finkel RS, Gropman AL, Pearl PL, Shevell (Eds). The cerebellum and the hereditary ataxias. Swaiman's Pediatric Neurology: Principles and Practice, 6th edition. Amsterdam, Netherlands: Elsevier; 2014. p. e1564-94.

Altered Sensorium

94

Section Editor: **Kripasindhu Chatterjee**
Section Co-Editors: **Atanu Bhadra, Ashim Kumar Ghosh**
Authors: **Jasodhara Chaudhuri, Atanu Bhadra**

Introduction

- Altered sensorium is a common symptom in pediatric critical care units.
- There is a wide range of differential diagnoses, which may range from reversible (toxin-induced) to permanent (hypoxic injury-related).

Etiology

- Altered sensorium is caused by diffuse neuronal dysfunction due to decreased glycemic supply to brain/lack of oxygenation from vascular compromise as a result of structural or nonstructural causes.
- Etiology of the altered sensorium is given in **Box 1**.

BOX 1: Etiology of the altered sensorium.

NEUROLOGICAL CAUSES	TOXIC METABOLIC CAUSES
• Trauma	• Drugs
• Tumors	• Toxin
• *Vascular:* Stroke	• Anticonvulsant overdose
• Meningitis	• Hypoxia
• Encephalitis	• Hypercapnia
• *Seizures:* Postictal and nonconvulsive status epilepticus	• Hepatic encephalopathy
• Autoimmune encephalitis	• Uremic encephalopathy
• Posterior reversible encephalopathy syndrome	• Hashimoto's encephalopathy
• Osmotic demyelination syndrome	• Environmental toxin
• Primary demyelinating disease	• Heat stroke

Steps to Arrive at a Diagnosis

- *Step 1:* Rapid assessment and stabilization
  - *Establish and maintain airway:* Intubate if Glasgow Coma Scale (GCS) score <8, impaired airway reflexes, abnormal respiratory pattern, signs of raised intracranial pressure (ICP), oxygen saturation <92% despite high flow oxygen, and fluid refractory shock.
  - Provide ventilation and oxygenation.
  - *Circulation:* Establish intravenous (IV) access, take samples [complete blood count (CBC), blood sugar, kidney function test (KFT), liver function test (LFT), electrolytes, blood gas, lactate, peripheral smear (PS) and rapid diagnostic tests (RDT) for malarial parasite, and serology for viruses], administer fluid bolus if in circulatory failure (20 mL/kg NS), and inotropes if required.
- *Step 2:* Clinical evaluation
  - *History and examination:* A careful and rapid history regarding perinatal history, developmental milestones, pre-existing illness, and medication history is taken. Any preceding event like a history of fever, its onset, duration, course, whether associated with seizures, family history of seizures, any accidental intake of medicine, immunization status, and dietary history is noted.
  - The general physical examination may provide pointers.
  - Pallor may indicate cerebral malaria and intracranial bleed.
  - *Icterus:* Possibility of leptospirosis, hepatic encephalopathy, or cerebral malaria
  - *Skin rashes:* Meningococcemia, dengue, measles, varicella, rickettsial diseases, arboviral diseases, and enteroviral encephalitis
  - *Petechiae:* Meningococcemia, dengue, and viral hemorrhagic fevers
  - Record the neurological examination documents, the level and localization of brain dysfunction, and information about the potential causes. Record the level of consciousness on an objective scale, like the GCS. A modified GCS should be used for infants and young children.
  - Pupillary size, shape, symmetry, and response to light provide valuable clues to brainstem and third nerve dysfunction. Topical administration of mydriatics must be avoided, but if done, should be documented to avoid confusion in interpretation. Unilateral pupillary dilatation in the comatose patient indicates evidence of oculomotor nerve compression from ipsilateral uncal herniation, unless proved otherwise. Look for extrapyramidal and pyramidal signs.

Investigations

- The protocol for investigations is given in **Table 1**.
- Start treatment after evaluation and investigations according to the probable etiology, always maintaining the vital parameters and airway protection.

TABLE 1: Protocol for investigation.

BASIC INVESTIGATIONS	TARGETED INVESTIGATIONS	FURTHER INVESTIGATION
Blood counts	*Neuroimaging:* MRI brain preferred	EEG (especially if there are seizures)
Blood glucose, hepatic, and renal profile	CT scan brain in emergency situation	Lactate
Serum electrolytes and chest X-ray	CSF study, if no contraindication	Ammonia
Dengue and malaria tests	Neuroviral panel	Metabolic profile
Toxicology screen	Autoimmune profile	Brain biopsy

CSF: cerebrospinal fluid; CT: computed tomography; EEG: electroencephalography; MRI: magnetic resonance imaging

Red Flags

- Unexplained injuries/marks on the body
- History of weight loss in recent past and acidotic breathing
- Unequal pupil size and abnormal pattern of breathing, posturing
- *Clinical pearls:* In a child with altered sensorium, a protocol-based rapid evaluation and an appropriated treatment based on the probable etiology are required.

Approach

The approach to the management of altered sensorium in a child is given in **Flowchart 1**.

FLOWCHART 1: Approach to altered sensorium in a child.

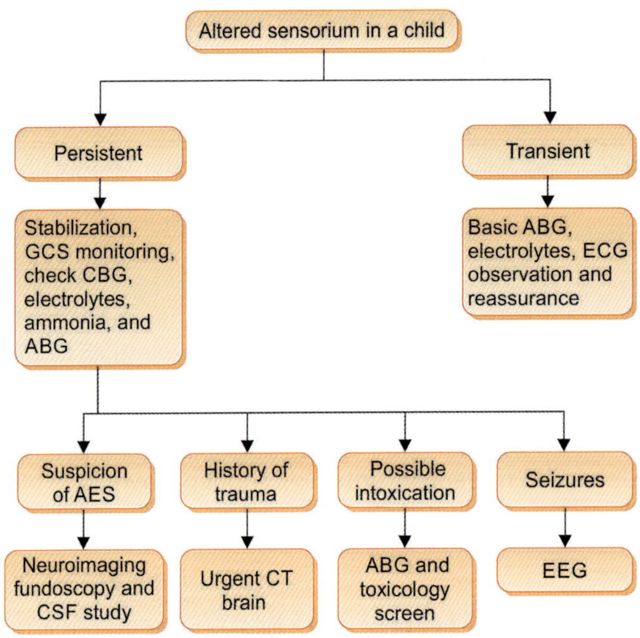

ABG: arterial blood gas; AES: acute encephalitis syndrome; CBG: capillary blood glucose; CSF: cerebrospinal fluid; CT: computed tomography; ECG: electrocardiography; EEG: electroencephalography; GCS: Glasgow coma scale

Suggested Reading

- Cashen K, Martin A, Aly A. Child with Altered Mental Status. In: Kamat DM, Sivaswamy L (Eds). Symptom-Based Approach to Pediatric Neurology. Cham, Germany: Springer; 2022.
- Davies E, Connolly DJ, Mordekar SR. Encephalopathy in children: An approach to assessment and management. Arch Dis Child. 2012;97(5):452-8.
- Kanich W, Brady WJ, Huff JS, Perron AD, Holstege C, Lindbeck G, et al. Altered mental status: Evaluation and etiology in the ED. Am J Emerg Med. 2002;20(7):613-7.
- Karmarkar SA, Aneja S, Khare S, Saini A, Seth A, Chauhan BK. A study of acute febrile encephalopathy with special reference to viral etiology. Indian J Pediatr. 2008;75(8):801-5.
- MacNeill EC, Vashist S. Approach to syncope and altered mental status. Pediatr Clin North Am. 2013;60(5):1083-106.
- Sharma S, Mishra D, Aneja S, Kumar R, Jain A, Vashishtha VM; Expert Group on Encephalitis, Indian Academy of Pediatrics. Consensus guidelines on evaluation and management of suspected acute viral encephalitis in children in India. Indian Pediatr. 2012;49(11):897-910.

Seizures and Epilepsy in Childhood

95

Section Editor: **Kripasindhu Chatterjee**
Section Co-Editors: **Atanu Bhadra, Ashim Kumar Ghosh**
Author: **Sheffali Gulati**

Definitions and Etiology

- *Seizure:* It is the transient occurrence of signs and symptoms due to abnormal, excessive, or synchronous neuronal activity in the brain characterized by abrupt and involuntary skeletal muscle activity. There is a clear onset and remission in a seizure.
- *Febrile seizure:* Seizures that occur in children aged between 1 month and 6 years with temperature rise over 38°C and without signs of infectious disease of the central nervous system.
- *Epilepsy:* The International League Against Epilepsy (ILAE) Task Force proposed the operational (practical) clinical definition of epilepsy as a disease of the brain defined by any of the following conditions:
    - At least 2 unprovoked (or reflex) seizures occurring >24 hours apart
    - 1 unprovoked (or reflex) seizure and a probability of further seizures similar to the general recurrence risk (at least 60%) after 2 unprovoked seizures, occurring over the next 10 years
- *Status epilepticus:* This occurs due to the failure of the mechanisms responsible for the termination of seizure the initiation of a mechanism, leading to abnormally prolonged seizures (for ≥5 minutes). It can have long-term consequences (>30 minutes) including neuronal death, neuronal injury, and alteration of neuronal network, depending on the type and duration of seizures.

Etiology Based on Onset of Seizures

- *Acute seizures:* Due to hypoglycemia, hypocalcemia, and hyponatremia; central nervous system infections like meningitis or any systemic or toxic insult; febrile seizures
- *Recurrent unprovoked seizures:* Complex interplay of multiple etiologies—structural brain lesions, neurometabolic/neurodegenerative disorders, and genetic predisposition

Red Flags

- Head injury with delayed seizure
- Associated developmental delay or regression
- Headache prior to the seizure
- Presence of bleeding disorder and anticoagulation therapy
- Presence of meningeal signs
- Presence of focal signs
- Drug use

International League Against Epilepsy 2017 Classification of Seizures

SEIZURE TYPE		
Focal onset	Generalized onset	Unknown onset

⬇

EPILEPSY TYPE			
Focal	Generalized	Combined focal and generalized	Unknown

EPILEPSY SYNDROMES			
Focal onset		***Generalized onset***	
Aware	***Impaired awareness***	***Motor***	***Nonmotor absence***
Motor onset • Automatism • Atonic • Clonic • Epileptic spasm • Hyperkinetic • Myoclonic • Tonic	*Nonmotor onset* • Autonomic • Behavior arrest • Cognitive • Emotional • Sensory	• Tonic–clonic • Tonic • Clonic • Myoclonic • Myoclonic–atonic • Atonic • Epileptic spasm	• Typical • Atypical • Myoclonic • Eyelid myoclonia

Algorithmic Approach

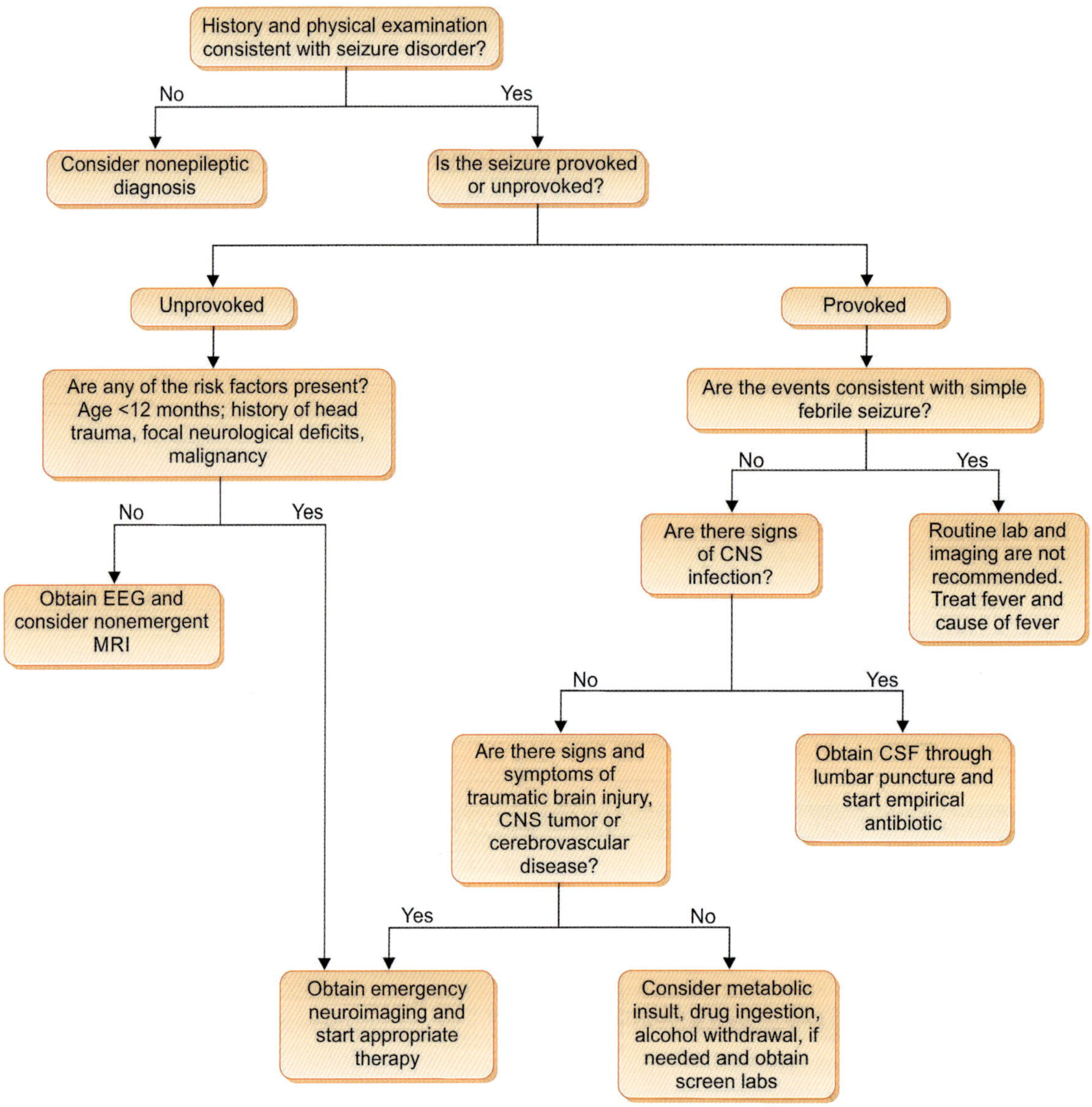

CNS: central nervous system; CSF: cerebrospinal fluid; EEG: electroencephalogram; MRI: magnetic resonance imaging

Suggested Reading

- American Academy of Pediatrics, Provisional Committee on Quality Improvement, Subcommittee on Febrile Seizures. Practice parameter: The neurodiagnostic evaluation of the child with a first simple febrile seizure. Pediatrics. 1996;97(5):769-72.
- Gulati S, Kalra V, Sridhar MR. Status epilepticus in Indian children in a tertiary care center. Indian J Pediatr. 2005; 72(2):105-8.
- Gulati S, Kaushik JS. How I treat a first single seizure in a child. Ann Indian Acad Neurol. 2016;19(1):29-36.
- Riviello JJ Jr, Ashwal S, Hirtz D, Glauser T, Ballaban-Gil K, Kelley K, et al.; American Academy of Neurology Subcommittee; Practice Committee of the Child Neurology Society. Practice parameter: diagnostic assessment of the child with status epilepticus (an evidence-based review): Report of the Quality Standards Subcommittee of the American Academy of Neurology and the Practice Committee of the Child Neurology Society. Neurology. 2006;67(9):1542-50.
- Scheffer IE, Berkovic S, Capovilla G, Connolly MB, French J, Guilhoto L, et al. ILAE classification of the epilepsies: Position paper of the ILAE Commission for Classification and Terminology. Epilepsia. 2017;58(4):512-21.
- Sourbron J, Auvin S, Arzimanoglou A, Cross JH, Hartmann H, Pressler R, et al. Medical treatment in infants and young children with epilepsy: Off-label use of antiseizure medications. Survey Report of ILAE Task Force Medical Therapies in Children. Epilepsia Open. 2023;8(1):77-89.

Microcephaly

96

Section Editor: **Kripasindhu Chatterjee**
Section Co-Editors: **Atanu Bhadra, Ashim Kumar Ghosh**
Author: **Anita Sharma**

Introduction

Microcephaly is defined as head circumference over three standard deviations (SD) below the mean for that age, gender, and race.

Etiology

Microcephaly is classified as:

- Primary (genetic)
- Secondary (nongenetic)

The etiology of primary and secondary microcephaly is given in **Table 1**.

TABLE 1: Etiology of primary and secondary microcephaly.

FEATURES	PRIMARY MICROCEPHALY	SECONDARY MICROCEPHALY
Microcephaly present	Since birth	Normal at birth and then drops
Etiology	• *Genetics:* AR, AD, and X-linked—Associated with brain malformations • *Syndromes:* Trisomy (21,18, and 13), Cri-du-chat syndrome, Williams syndrome, and Seckel syndrome	• *Perinatal insult:* Hypoxia, hypoglycemia, and meningitis • *Congenital infections:* Cytomegalovirus, rubella, toxoplasmosis, HIV, and Zika virus • Malnutrition and hypothyroidism • Birth injuries • Phenylketonuria • Maternal intake (alcohol and phenytoin) and illness (toxemia, hypothyroidism, and diabetes) • Rett syndrome

AD: autosomal dominant; AR: autosomal recessive, HIV: human immunodeficiency virus

Red Flags

Symptoms

- Consanguinity
- Positive family history

Predisposing factors:

- Development delay and intellectual disability
- Visual, hearing, and speech abnormality
- Seizures
- Neurological deficit/Neuroregression
- Episodic vomiting, ataxia, encephalopathy, and neuroregression
- Female child, autistic, hand-washing movement, indicating Rett syndrome

Signs

- Microcephaly
- Progressive head circumference decline
- Tone abnormality

New neurological signs and symptoms:

- Facial dysmorphism
- Organomegaly

Differential Diagnosis

The differential diagnosis of microcephaly is given in **Table 2**.

TABLE 2: Differential diagnosis of microcephaly.

	MICROCEPHALY	CRANIOSYNOSTOSIS
Skull shape	Normal	Abnormal
Bony ridges along sutures	None	Palpated
Intracranial pressure	Normal	Raised

Important Pointers

- Regular follow-up
- Head circumference:
  - Measure serially the head circumference
  - Head circumference of siblings, parents, and other family members
- Early identification of comorbidities for timely intervention:
  - Cerebral palsy
  - Global developmental delay/intellectual disability
  - Vision and hearing disorders
  - Speech and language delay
  - Epilepsy
  - Hyperactivity
  - Failure to thrive
- Genetic counseling

Investigations

The following investigations are done based on history and examination:

- Screening for infections and thyroid
- Karyotype, fluorescence in situ hybridization (FISH), and chromosome microarray for chromosomal disorder
- *X-ray skull/computed tomography (CT) head:* Calcification
- *Magnetic resonance imaging (MRI) brain:* More sensitive and safe, indicated if the diagnosis is unclear after a comprehensive evaluation
- Metabolic screen
- *Unexplained microcephaly with normal MRI:* Check maternal serum phenylalanine.

Approach

The approach to the management of children with microcephaly is given in **Flowchart 1**.

FLOWCHART 1: Approach to the management of children with microcephaly.

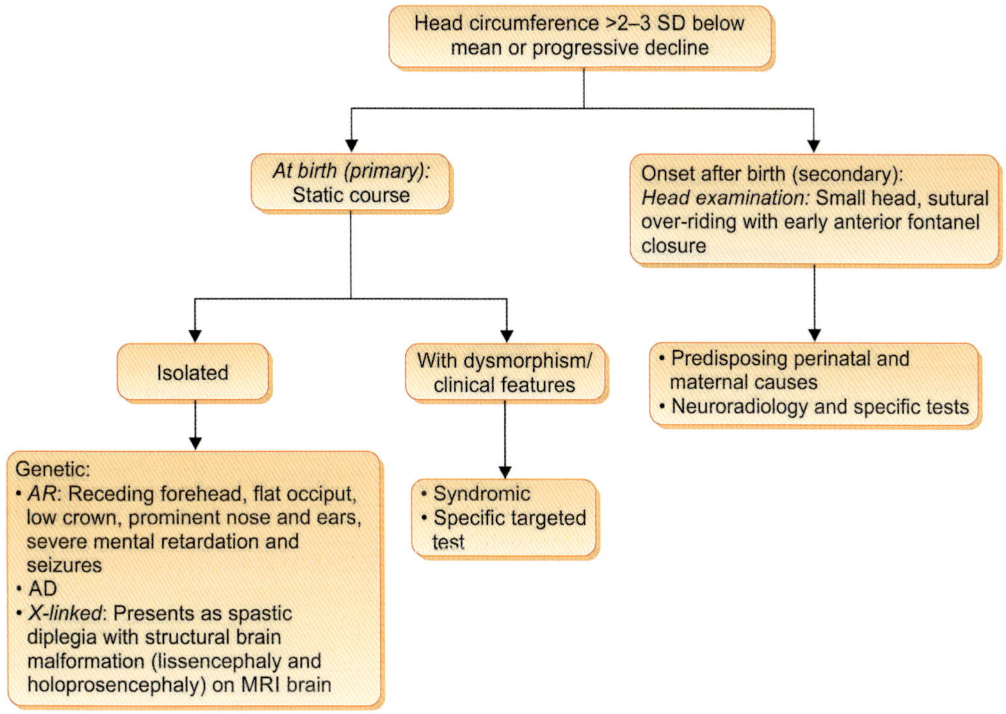

AD: autosomal dominant; AR: autosomal recessive; MRI: magnetic resonance imaging; SD: standard deviations

Suggested Reading

- Ashwal S, Michelson D, Plawner L, Dobyns WB; Quality Standards Subcommittee of the American Academy of Neurology and the Practice Committee of the Child Neurology Society. Practice parameter: Evaluation of the child with microcephaly (an evidence-based review): Report of the Quality Standards Subcommittee of the American Academy of Neurology and the Practice Committee of the Child Neurology Society. Neurology. 2009;73(11):887-97.
- Becerra-Solano LE, Mateos-Sánchez L, López-Muñoz E. Microcephaly, an etiopathogenic vision. Pediatr Neonatol. 2021;62(4):354-60.
- Hagen MVD, Pivarcsi M, Liebe J, von Bernuth H, Didonato N, Hennermann JB, et al. Diagnostic approach to microcephaly in childhood: A two-center study and review of the literature. Dev Med Child Neurol. 2014;56(8): 732-41.

Facial Dysmorphism

97

Section Editor: **Nehal Patel**
Section Co-Editor: **Jay T Dhirwani**
Authors: **Urvi Sanghvi, Ashka Prajapati**

Introduction

- Dysmorphology refers to the study of abnormal patterns of human growth and the recognition and study of congenital human structural anomalies and patterns of birth defects.
- Neonatologists/pediatricians are often the first physicians to evaluate and therefore must be familiar with various physical differences so that further screening for occult malformations, diagnostic testing, and counseling can be done appropriately.

Etiology

- Maybe associated with multiple malformations.
- *Syndromic/genetic:* Chromosomal/single gene disorder/teratogenic/vascular factors/congenital infection related
- As a part of association [like vertebral anomalies, anorectal malformations, cardiovascular anomalies, tracheoesophageal fistula, esophageal atresia, renal and/or radial anomalies, limb defects (VACTERL)], or sequence like Pierre Robin syndrome
- *Isolated abnormality:* Syndromic—single gene defect/sporadic/familial (nongenetic/sporadic)
- *Environmental:* Infections/teratogenic exposure
- *Polygenic:* Isolated cleft palate/lip

History

- Consanguinity
- Family history
- Antenatal scan abnormalities
- Maternal history for teratogenic exposure/medication (e.g., valproate and phenytoin)
- Fetal movements

Examination

- *Overall impression (gestalt):* Each part of the face is to be examined for size, shape, and position and then define abnormalities using human phenotyping ontology.
- Divide the face into sections such as forehead, midface, and oral region. View face from front and side.
- Lateral profile better for depth/height of structures like nasal bridge, position of mandible relative to maxilla, and midface development for the exact description of each feature
- Face round, elongated, doll-like, and asymmetric
- Check from above to below in a systematic manner.
- Abnormality in skin like—birthmarks (café-au-lait, strawberry angioma, and port wine stain
- Examine parents alongside to rule out familial traits.

Key points (checkpoints) to look for:

- *Skull:* Abnormal shape (brachycephaly/dolichocephaly), craniosynostosis, bulging of anterior fontanel (AF), sloping forehead, and hair growth/texture/color
- Frontal bossing, bitemporal narrowing, and eyebrows (arched, straight, and synophrys)
- *Eye:* Size (microphthalmia/anophthalmia), palpebral fissure (upslant/downslant, and elongate), blepharophimosis, ptosis—internal parts for coloboma/lens, corneal defect, heterochromia (color of iris), etc.
- *Other features:* Hypertelorism/hypotelorism
- *Ear:* Posterior rotated, low set, microtia/anotia, dysplastic ear, and preauricular tag
- *Nasal bridge:* Depressed, prominent, and broad base
- *Nose:* Size (short, tubular, columella (hanging/short), and anteverted nares
- *Mouth:* Small, large, tented upper lip/cleft lip, and asymmetric
- *Lips:* Thin/thick, everted, and tented/cleft lip
- *Oral cavity:* Cleft palate, high arched, gum hypertrophy/large protruded tongue, and teeth for abnormal shape/discoloration
- *Maxillary region:* Hypoplastic maxilla
- *Mandibular region:* Micrognathia/retrognathia, and small chin

Investigations

- *Look for underlying systemic involvement:* Two-dimensional (2D) echocardiogram, ultrasound abdomen, neuroimaging, endocrine, and X-rays/infantogram
- *For the genetic etiology:* Karyotype/microarray
- *Single gene sequencing/next-generation sequencing (NGS) based assay:* Whole exome sequencing
- Toxoplasmosis, Other agents, Rubella, Cytomegalovirus, and Herpes Simplex (TORCH) assay

Red Flag Signs

- Bulging AF
- Craniosynostosis
- Anophthalmia/microphthalmia
- Severe dysplastic ear
- Vascular birthmark
- Cleft palate
- Pierre Robin sequence

Approach

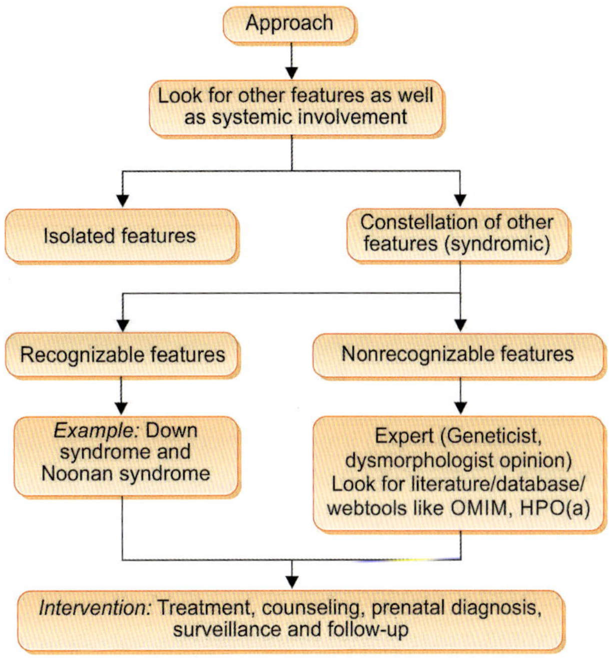

Suggested Reading

- Allanson JE, Cunniff C, Hoyme HE, McGaughran J, Muenke M, Neri G. Elements of morphology: Standard terminology for the head and face. Am J Med Genet A. 2009;149A(1):6-28.
- Biesecker LG, Aase JM, Clericuzio C, Gurrieri F, Temple IK, Toriello H. Elements of morphology: Standard terminology for the hands and feet. Am J Med Genet A. 2009;149A(1):93-127.
- Jones KL, Jones MC, del Campo M. Smith's Recognizable Patterns of Human Malformations, 7th edition. Philadelphia: Elsevier Saunders; 2013. pp. 133-4.

Vision Impairment

98

Section Editor: **Sumitha Nayak**
Section Co-Editor: **Priya Shivalli**
Author: **Prashanth SN**

Introduction

- Vision impairment can have profound and irreversible consequences if not diagnosed and treated on time. Lately, the incidence is increasing mainly due to the overuse of digital screens and visual accommodation for near work.
- Low vision in children can cause challenges in attaining milestones of development, educational goals, social interactions, and self-independence. Symptoms can vary with age.
- It can also be mistaken for intellectual disability and behavioral disorders, and may be masked by concomitant systemic health issues.

Definition

As per the American Academy of Ophthalmology's Preferred Practice Patterns for Vision Rehabilitation, vision impairment is described as an "irreversible visual loss or impairment in a person younger than 21 years that does not improve with refractive correction, medical treatment, or surgical intervention".

Etiology

- The causes of pediatric low vision includes:
  - *Ocular structural abnormality:* Malformed/maldeveloped eyes
  - *Secondary to other ocular pathology:* Myopia, hypermetropia, pediatric cataract, retinoblastoma, squint, and retinopathy of prematurity
  - As manifestations of a genetic/systemic syndrome
  - Cerebral visual impairment (CVI)
  - Nystagmus
  - Optic atrophy
- Any structural abnormality of the eye, from anterior to posterior can be responsible. This includes corneal opacification, congenital cataract, primary aphakia, chorioretinal coloboma, optic nerve hypoplasia, and foveal hypoplasia.
- Pathology in the eyes includes deficiency of limbal stem cells, congenital nystagmus, aniridia, retinal dystrophy, trauma, and may be iatrogenic.

Signs and Symptoms

Milestones of visual development:

- *Birth–4 months:* Light adjustment and focusing on objects in front.
- *5–8 months:* Perceiving depth and recognizing faces
- *9–12 months:* Hand–eye coordination and gross spatial recognition
- *In older children:* Blurry vision, eye strain, and headaches
- *By school age:* Difficulty in reading, commonly mistaken for a learning disability

Red Flag Signs

- Low sensitivity to bright lights
- Absent/delayed eye contact
- Delayed development of social smile
- Unaware of own hands
- No goal-directed hand movements
- No fixation on familiar objects, toys, and faces
- Clumsy crawling
- Difficulty reaching out for toys
- Holding objects extremely close
- Any delays in motor development

Evaluation

- *Premature neonates:* Assess and treat as per protocols for retinopathy of prematurity (ROP) screening.
- *Older children:* Refer for assessment at the earliest.
- Most children are sent to ophthalmology around school age/whenever they can vocalize symptoms of blurry vision. Sometimes, caregivers seek earlier evaluation for abnormal visual behavior of their child.

Ophthalmic investigations required are as follows:

- Vision and refraction
- Color vision and contrast sensitivity
- Visual field assessment
- Ophthalmologist's examination including dilated retinal evaluation
- Ocular coherence tomography (OCT)
- Visual evoked potential (VEP)
- Electroretinogram (ERG)
- Electrooculogram (EOG)

Referral to a neurologist in case of unexplained visual loss and to diagnose cortical blindness/intracranial pathologies.

Approach to a Child with Low Vision

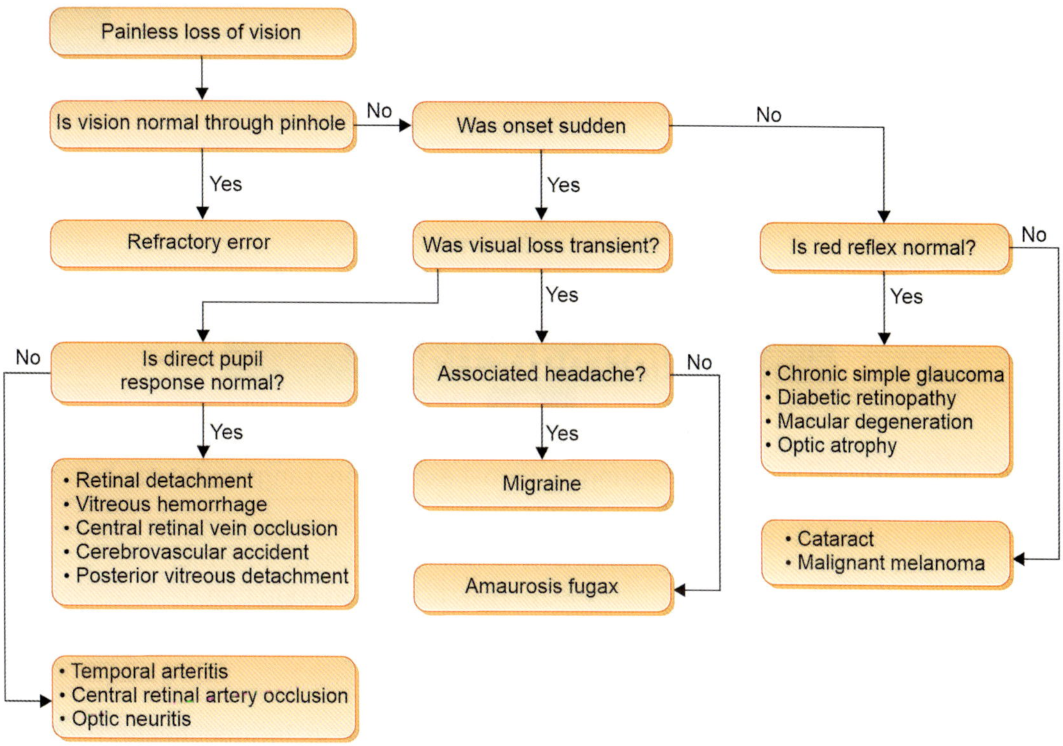

Suggested Reading

- Khurana AK, Khurana A, Khurana B. Comprehensive Ophthalmology, 9th edition. New Delhi: Jaypee Brothers Medical Publishers (P) Ltd; 2023.
- Salmon JF. Kanski's Clinical Ophthalmology: A Systematic Approach, 9th edition. Amsterdam, Netherlands: Elsevier; 2019.
- Sihota R, Tandon R. Parsons diseases of the eye, 24th edition. India: Elsevier Health Sciences; 2024.
- Yanoff M, Duker JS. Ophthalmology, 6th edition. Amsterdam, Netherlands: Elsevier; 2022.

Speech Delay

99

Section Editor: **Sumitha Nayak**
Section Co-Editor: **Priya Shivalli**
Authors: **Somashekar AR, Saloni A Thakur**

Introduction

- Speech is the motor act of communicating by verbal expression. Language is the knowledge of a symbol system used for interpersonal communication.
- Language and speech are two main domains of neurodevelopment, together with gross and fine motor skills, social and personal skills, activities of daily living, and cognition.
- Speech and language delay may be:
  - *Primary:* No associated comorbidity for the delay
  - *Secondary:* Attributed to another condition/syndrome; these include hearing loss, Down's syndrome, etc.

Etiology

Common causes of speech delay include:

- Hearing loss
- Slow development
- Intellectual disability
- *Genetic disorders:* Psychosocial deprivation twins, autism, elective mutism, and cerebral palsy

Red Flags

- No babbling by 12 months
- Using <3 words by 15 months
- Not saying "mamma" and "dadda" by 18 months
- Not using at least 25 words by 2 years of age/at least 200 words by 3 years of age

Developmental Milestones for Language and Speech in Children

AGE	RECEPTIVE	EXPRESSIVE
6 months	Turns to rattling sound and turns to voices	• Laughs • Vocalizes (cooing)
9 months	–	• Babbles single syllables, Says "mamma" or "dadda" • Waves bye-bye
12 months	Follows one-step command	• Babbles • Imitates vocalizations and sounds • Says one word • Waves bye-bye
15 months	–	• Says one word • Says three words
18 months	Points to at least one body part	• Says three words • Says six words
2 years	Points to two pictures and follows two-step command	• Combines words • Names one picture
2.5 years	Points to six body parts	• Knows two actions • Names one picture • Speech half understandable
3 years	–	• Knows two adjectives • Names four pictures • Names one color
4 years	–	• Speech all understandable • Defines five words • Names four colors • Speech all understandable

Physical Examination and Screening Tests

- Measurement of height, weight, and head circumference
- Note any dysmorphic features/abnormal physical findings
- A complete neurologic examination including vision and hearing evaluations

Screening Tests

- The early language milestone scale
- Peabody picture vocabulary test revised
- Denver developmental screening test

Early Language Milestone Scale

- Simple tool for those <3 years of age
- Focuses on expressive, receptive, and visual language
- Helps clinicians identify developmental needs of children from birth till the age of 3

Peabody Picture Vocabulary Test—Revised

- For children 2.5–18 years of age
- Is an untimed, individual intelligence test that measures receptive (hearing) vocabulary and provides a quick estimate of their verbal ability or aptitude.

Denver Developmental Screening Test

- Is the most popular screening test in use for infants and young children.
- It screens for the cognitive and behavioral problems in preschool children.

Speech Assessment Tools

- *Dynamic evaluation of motor speech skill (DEMSS) (>3 years):* To assess reduced phonemic and/or phonetic inventories, vowel or prosodic errors, poor speech intelligibility, and/or little-to-no verbal communication
- *Motor speech examination (3–11 years):* Identifies deviant speech characteristics
- *CHOCSLAT (1–4 years):* Emphasis on the grammatical classification and meanings of children's statements.
- *Bayley-III (1–42 months):* Diagnosing early developmental delays
- *CELF-4 (5–21 years):* Overall core language, receptive and expressive language, language content, language structure, working memory indices, various levels of the linguistic rule system, metalinguistic skills, and phonological awareness
- *PLS-5 English (0–7 years):* Total language, auditory comprehension, expressive communication standard scores, growth scores, percentile ranks, and language age equivalents
- *Tabby Talks (4–16 years):* Prosodic, voice quality, and pronunciation
- *LEST (0–6 years):* Screening tool for language delay

Diagnostic Evaluation

- *Audiometry:* All children
- Tympanometry
- *An auditory brainstem response:* A definitive and quantitative physiologic means of ruling out peripheral hearing loss
- *Functional magnetic resonance imaging:* To study the brain lobe activity in speech delayed children
- Additional tests should be ordered only when they are indicated.
- Karyotyping for chromosomal abnormalities rule out fragile X syndrome.
- Electroencephalogram is done in case of associated seizures.

Algorithmic Approach

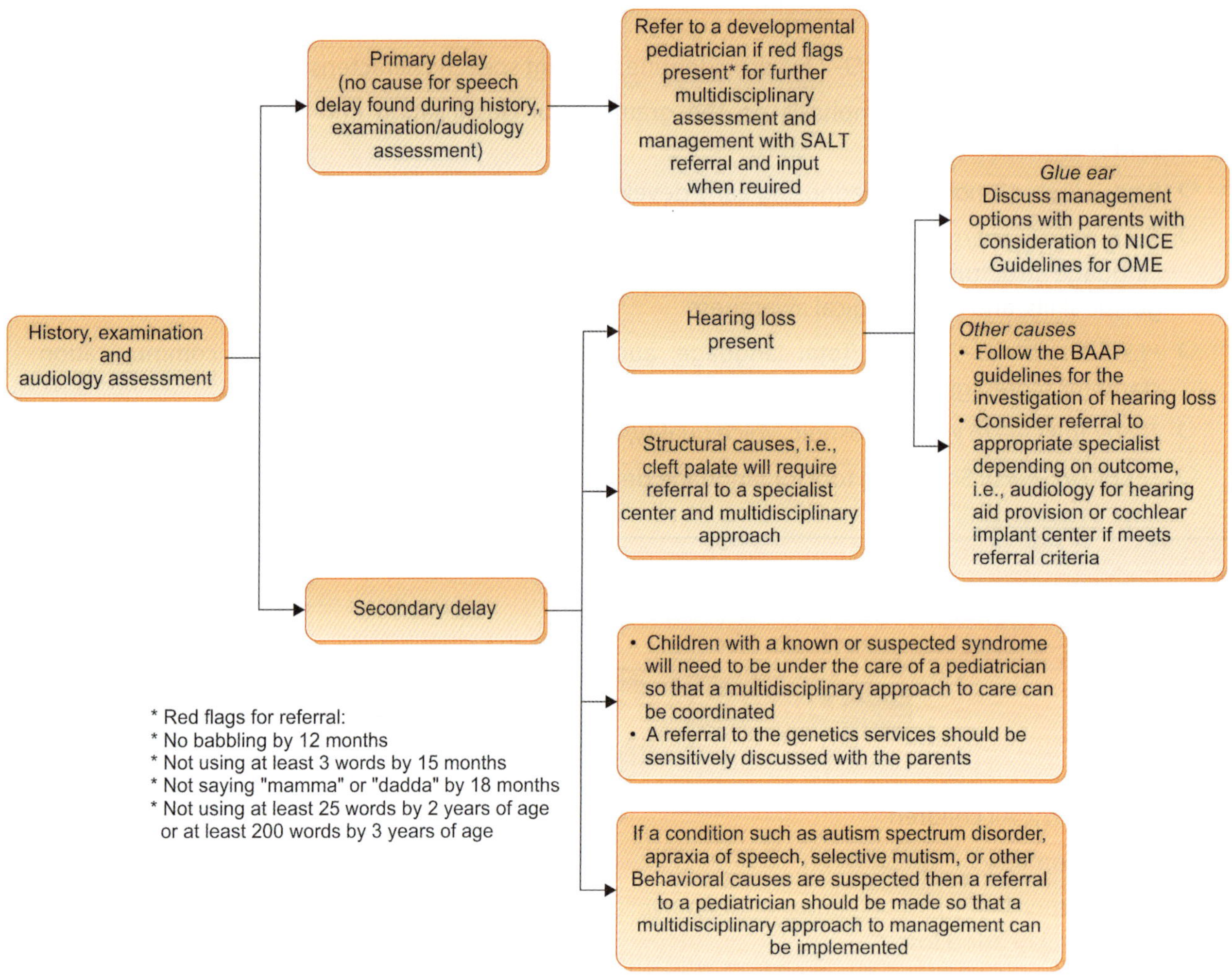

BAAP: British Association of Audiovestibular Physicians; NICE: National Institute for Health and Care Excellence; OME: otitis media with effusion; SALT: speech and language therapists

Suggested Reading

- Illingworth RS. In: Jain N, Nair MKC Russell P, Swamidhas P (Eds). Illingworth's The development of the infant and young child: Normal and abnormal. New Delhi: Elsevier; 2021.
- Jullien S. Screening for language and speech delay in children under five years. BMC Pediatr. 2021;21:362.
- Lawrence R, Bateman N. 12-minute consultation: An evidence-based approach to the management of a child with speech and language delay. Clin Otolaryngol. 2013;38(2):148-53.
- Usha GP, Alex JSR. Speech assessment tool methods for speech impaired children: A systematic literature review on the state-of-the-art in Speech impairment analysis. Multimed Tools Appl. 2023;1-38.

Breath-holding Spells

100

***Section Editor:* Sumitha Nayak**
***Section Co-Editor:* Priya Shivalli**
***Author:* Shrikiran Aroor Hebbar**

Introduction

- Breath-holding spells are paroxysmal self-limiting events.
- They are a result of provocation (pain, anger, or frustration).
- They result in crying followed by apnea during the expiration phase of crying.
- It could be followed by occurrence of either cyanosis (cyanotic type) or pallor (pallid type).
- There may be a loss of consciousness and altered body tone for a brief period usually lasting for 1 minute during or after the spell.
- They are seen in up to 10% of healthy babies between the age group of 6 months and 6 years, though the typical age of onset is between 6 months and 18 months.
- It is also termed infantile syncope.
- The cyanotic type is more common and follows anger or frustration.
- The pallid type is rarer and usually results from sudden fright or pain.
- A mixed type may also occur.

Etiology

- The etiology of breath-holding spells is not definite. Recent research suggests genetically mediated dysregulation of autonomic nervous system reflex is responsible for the spells.
- Pallid type is supposedly secondary to cardiac asystole similar to vasovagal attack.
- Cyanotic type results from a rise in intrathoracic pressure leading to impaired cerebral circulation.
- Anemia due to the compensatory mechanism of the autonomic system results in cerebral hypoxia.

Red Flag Signs

- Absence of provocating factors like anger
- Presence of prolonged altered sensorium
- Late onset of cyanosis
- Presence of baseline cyanosis
- Prolonged duration of cyanosis
- Presence of clubbing
- Prolonged tonic–clonic movements

Approach

- History related to age group
- History of provoking factors
- Previous history of seizures
- Details of cyanosis
- Occurrence of tonic–clonic movements
- Examination for clubbing in the hands
- Baseline pallor/cyanosis
- Neurodeficits
- Cardiac examination

Algorithm

- *Diagnosis:* Detailed clinical description is sufficient to make a diagnosis most of the time. Workup for iron deficiency must be done.
- An electroencephalogram (EEG) is indicated only if the manifestations are not classical.

- The algorithmic approach to the management of breath-holding spells is given in **Flowchart 1**.

FLOWCHART 1: Approach to breath-holding spells.

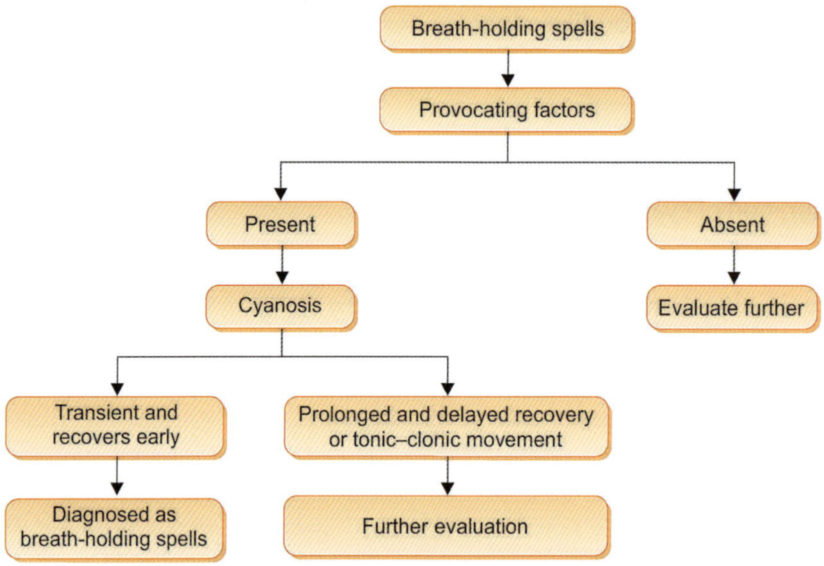

Suggested Reading

- Gupta P (Ed). UG Textbook of Pediatrics. New Delhi: Jaypee Brothers Medical Publishers (P) Ltd; 2023. pp. 84-5.
- Gupte S (Ed). The Short Textbook of Pediatrics, 13th edition. New Delhi: Jaypee Brothers Medical Publishers (P) Ltd; 2020. p. 107.
- Gupta P, Menon PSN, Ramji S, Lodha R (Eds). PG Textbook of Pediatrics, 3rd edition. New Delhi: Jaypee Brothers Medical Publishers (P) Ltd; 2022. pp. 766-7.

Palpitation

101

Section Editor: **Nehal Patel**
Section Co-Editor: **Jay T Dhirwani**
Authors: **Bhadra Trivedi, Ritesh Sukharamwala**

Definition

- Palpitation is defined as awareness about one's heartbeats.
- Its common causes are fever, anxiety, physical exertion, and arrhythmia.

Etiology

- *Hyperdynamic circulation:* Fever, infection, anemia, hyperthyroidism, hypoglycemia, and pheochromocytoma.
- *Sympathetic system stimulation:*
  - Physical exercise, stress, anxiety, psychological disturbances, and panic attacks cause overstimulation of sympathetic system.
  - *Central nervous system stimulants:* Caffeine-containing products, anticholinergic medications, and cough/cold remedies
- *Arrhythmias:*
  - Sinus tachycardia, premature atrial contractions, premature ventricular contractions, supraventricular tachycardia are the common causes of arrhythmia-induced palpitation.
  - *Electrolyte imbalances*: Hypokalemia causes arrhythmia and palpitation.
- *Structural heart disease:* This includes volume overload conditions like ventricular septal defect, patent ductus arteriosus, and mitral valve regurgitation trigger palpitation. Atrial septal defect, tricuspid valve atresia cause right atrium dilatation and palpitation due to sinoatrial (SA) node excitation.

Red Flag Signs

- Loss of consciousness/near syncope/convulsion
- Shortness of breath
- Loss of appetite
- Hypertension
- Perspiration

Evaluation of Palpitation

- *Detailed history:* Vague abdominal pain, chest pain, general uneasiness are common presenting complaints.
- Palpitation beginning abruptly is often due to arrhythmia. It may occur without exertion (if related to arrhythmia), while exertion may trigger arrhythmia. Premature atrial/ventricular contractions followed by compensatory pauses are described as "heart stops momentarily".
- *Arrhythmia in long QT syndrome:* Palpitation with syncope.
- Postural orthostatic tachycardia syndrome (POTS) while changing posture, getting off the bed, standing up after a long period of sitting, causes palpitations. This is rare in children.
- History suggesting viral or bacterial infection is essential to manage palpitations. Family history is significant in cases of long QT syndrome and hypertrophic cardiomyopathy.

Examinations

- A child experiencing palpitation for the first time will be anxious looking. Psychological evaluation for anxiety disorder should be done only after the control of palpitations.
- Heart rate indicates tachyarrhythmia or bradyarrhythmia, if it is >200 beats/minute. This requires immediate evaluation for supraventricular tachycardia. Very low heart rate with syncope can cause heart blocks. An increment in heart rate of 30 beats/minute from the baseline with a change in posture indicates postural orthostatic tachycardia.
- Bounding pulses with warm skip and tachycardia indicate psychotropic drug ingestion, hyperthyroidism, and pheochromocytoma.
- Murmur and abnormal heart sounds may be due to an underlying congenital heart disease.

Investigations

- Detailed blood counts, C-reactive protein (CRP), random blood sugar (RBS), thyroid-stimulating hormone (TSH), serum creatinine, serum electrolytes, serum calcium, serum glutamic oxaloacetic transaminase (SGOT), serum glutamate pyruvate transaminase (SGPT), and 12-lead electrocardiogram
- A detailed pediatric 2D echocardiogram to rule out congenital heart disease.

Approach to Palpitation

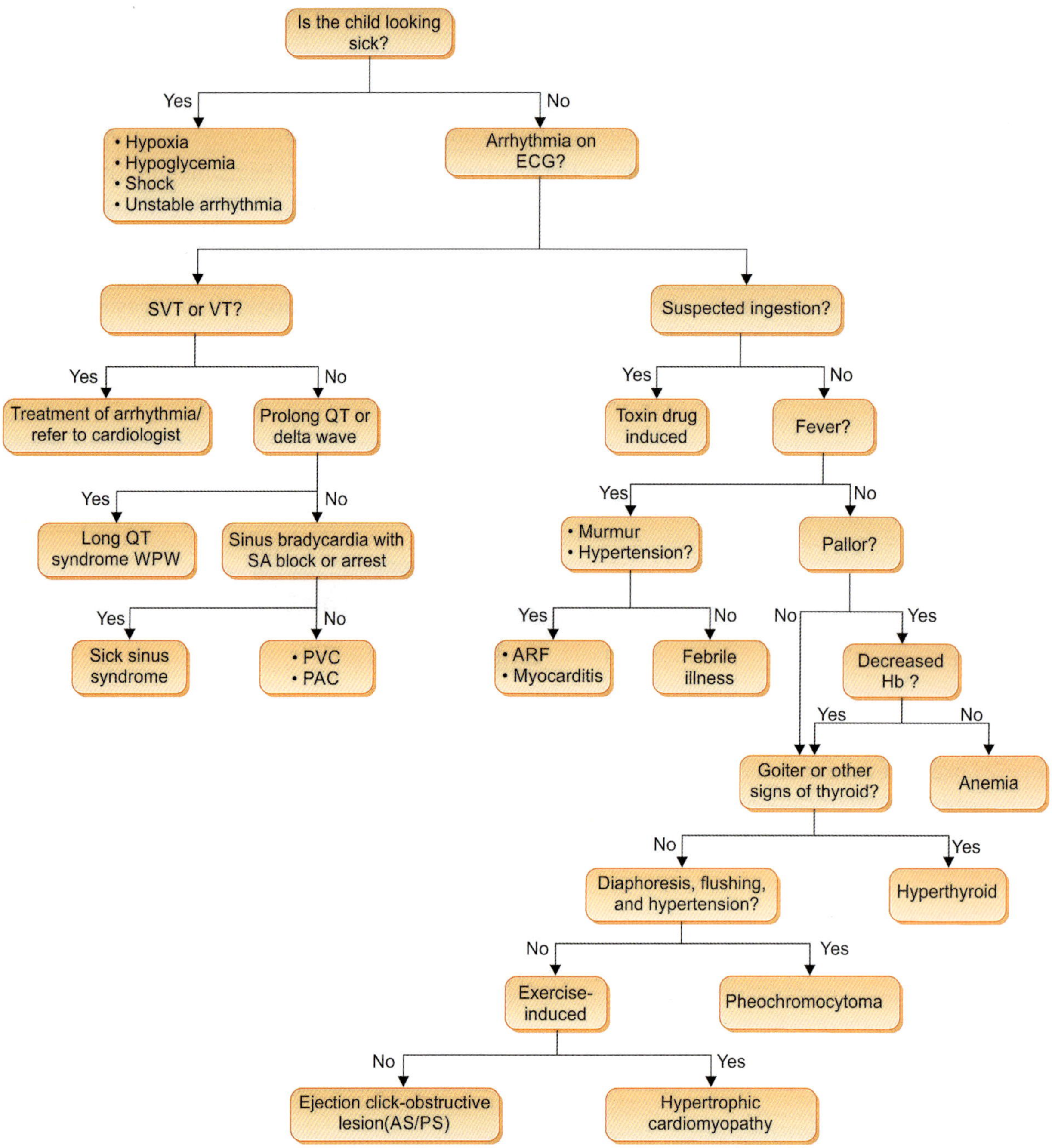

AS: aortic stenosis; ARF: acute rheumatic fever; PS: pulmonary stenosis; PAC: premature atrial contractions; PVC: premature ventricular contractions; SA: sinoatrial; SVT: supraventricular; VT: ventricular; WPW: Wolff Parkinson White Syndrome

Evaluation of Child with Irregular Heart Rhythm

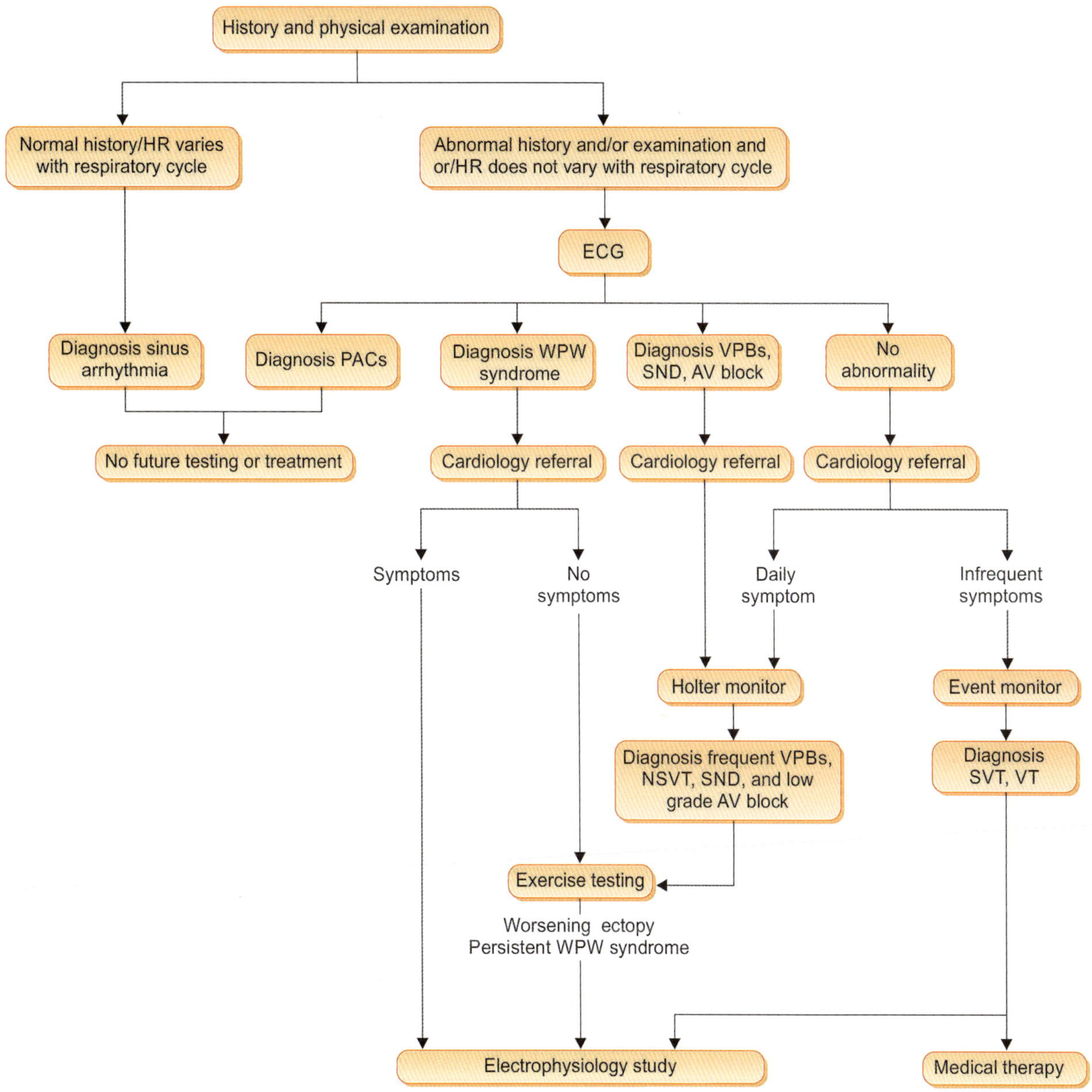

AV: atrioventricular; ECG: electrocardiography; HR: heart rate; NSVT: nonsustained ventricular tachycardia; PAC: premature atrial contractions; SND: sinus node dysfunction; SVT: supraventricular; VPBs: ventricular premature beats; WPW: Wolff Parkinson White syndrome

Suggested Reading

- Doniger SJ, Sharieff GQ. Pediatric dysrhythmias. Pediatr Clin North Am. 2006;53(1):85-105.
- Drago F, Battipaglia I, Di Mambro C. Neonatal and pediatric arrhythmias: Clinical and electrocardiographic aspects. Card Electrophysiol Clin. 2018;10(2):397-412.
- Wren C. Concise Guide to Pediatric Arrhythmias. New Jersey, US: John Wiley & Sons Ltd; 2011

Birth Injuries

102

Section Editor: **Nehal Patel**
Section Co-Editor: **Jay T Dhirwani**
Author: **Srinivasa Murthy D**

Introduction

- Injuries to the baby during the process of delivery are referred to as birth injuries.
- Mechanical forces operating during the labor are the cause of birth injury.
- The severity ranges from insignificant to catastrophic depending on the extent and organ injured.
- The incidence of birth injuries is approximately 2%. Mortality is about 2% of major injuries when associated with perinatal asphyxia.
- Most have few long-term consequences but cause significant parental anxiety.

Etiology

Mechanical forces acting on the baby during the labor **(Fig. 1)**.

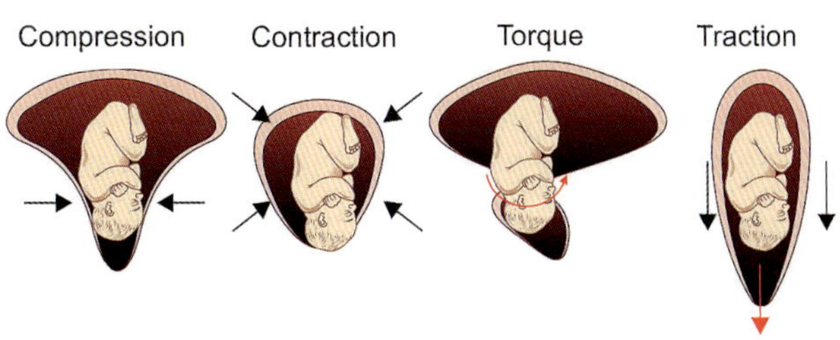

FIG. 1: Mechanical forces acting on the baby during labor.
Courtesy: Dr Srinivasa Murthy D, Karnataka, India

Predisposing Factors

Predisposing factors are given in **Table 1**.

TABLE 1: Predisposing factors.

MATERNAL	FETAL	OTHERS
• Primigravida • Cephalopelvic disproportion (CPD) • Pelvic anomalies	• Large baby • Small baby • Abnormal presentation/deep transverse arrest • Oligohydramnios	• Prolonged delivery • Rapid/precipitous delivery • Instrumental delivery • Versions

Types of Injuries

Various types of injuries are listed in **Table 2.**

TABLE 2: Types of injuries.

SKIN AND SOFT-TISSUE INJURIES	FRACTURES	BLEEDS (HEMORRHAGES)	NERVE PALSIES
• Abrasions • Bruising • Lacerations • Subcutaneous fat necrosis	• Clavicle (common) • Long bones • Skull • Vertebral (rare)	• Eyes • Soft-tissue • Extracranial • Intracranial • Visceral	• Facial palsy • Vocal cord palsy • Radial nerve palsy • Phrenic nerve palsy • Horner syndrome

- *Skin and soft-tissue injuries:* These are caused, generally, due to grazing of fetal parts to maternal pelvis and have good prognosis. Lacerations if severe, need suturing. Bruising and edema takes several days to heal. These injuries may need pain relief with oral analgesics.
- *Fractures:* These are caused by significant mechanical force. Excessive crying due to pain and loss of movement are classical symptoms. Fractures in neonates heal within 2–3 weeks.

- *Bleeding:* Subconjunctival hemorrhage occurs in babies born by normal vaginal delivery. They are benign and resolve over few weeks. No active intervention is needed. Black eye indicates associated skull fracture which needs urgent intervention by surgeons.

  Head bleed both intracranial and extracranial are common **(Fig. 2)**. Cephalohematoma needs close observation for jaundice. Hemorrhagic caput should be managed conservatively. Other head bleeds need imaging and supportive management. Anemia and cardiac failure are not uncommon with severe bleeding.

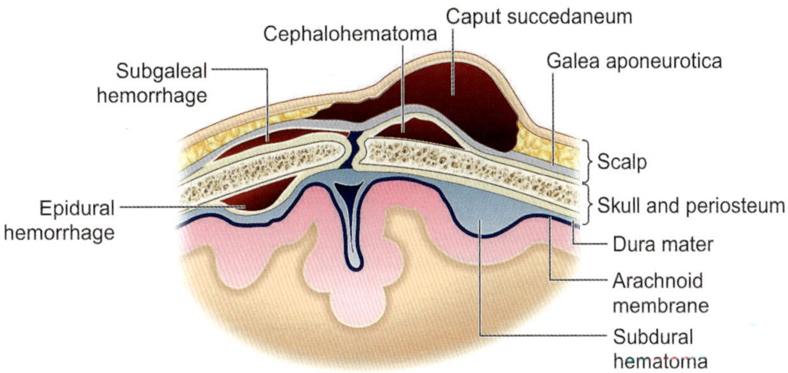

FIG. 2: Types of head bleed.
Courtesy: Dr Srinivasa Murthy D, Karnataka, India

- *Nerve injuries:* Traction during labor can cause partial or complete avulsion (10% of nerve injuries) of nerves. Commonest is brachial plexus injury. Erb's palsy followed by Klumpke's paralysis are results of brachial plexus injury.

  Facial nerve injury causes facial asymmetry which should be differentiated from hypoplasia of depressor anguli oris and abnormal position due to asynclitism.

  Bilateral recurrent laryngeal nerve injury can cause respiratory distress needing mechanical ventilation.

  Nerve injuries take 4–6 weeks, sometimes up to 1 year for recovery. Prevention of contractures, protection of eyes, and other supportive measures along with physiotherapy results in good outcomes.

Approach

The approach to management of birth injuries is illustrated in **Flowchart 1**.

FLOWCHART 1: Approach to management of birth injuries.

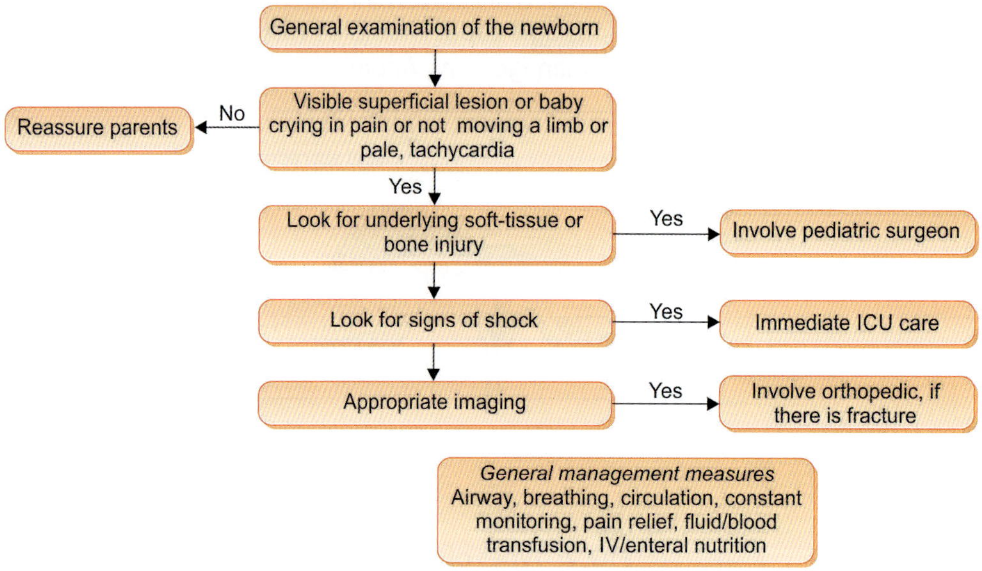

ICU: intensive care unit

Red Flag Signs

The following signs at presentation are red flag signs:

- Appearing pale
- Excessive crying
- Not moving limbs (pseudoparalysis)
- Tachycardia/bradycardia
- Convulsions

Suggested Reading

- Papanagiotou P, Rohrer T, Roth C, Politi M, Zimmer A, Reith W. Cranial birth trauma. Radiologe. 2009;49(10):913-7.
- Prabhu RS, Sajjid M, Anandan H. Incidence and predisposing factors of birth trauma in a tertiary care hospital in Chennai, India: A Prospective Study. Int J Sci Study. 2017;4(10):29-33.
- Ray S, Mondal R, Samanta M, Hazra A, Sabui TK, Debnath A, et al. Prospective study of neonatal birth trauma: Indian perspective. J Clin Neonatol. 2016;5:91-5.

Acne Vulgaris

103

Section Editor: **Gnanamurthy Narasimha**
Section Co-Editor: **Nagalatha Chidananda**
Author: **Preeti M Galagali**

Introduction

- Acne vulgaris is a chronic inflammatory skin disorder affecting face, arms, shoulders, chest, back, and neck.
- It may begin in preadolescence and usually subsides in adulthood.
- It commonly presents in the T-zone of face (forehead, nose, and chin) where the sebaceous glands are maximally located.

Etiopathogenesis

- *Multifactorial and complex etiopathogenesis:* Microcomedones are keratin plugs with corneocytes. These may progress into closed comedones (white head) or open comedones with an enlarged follicular orifice and melanin deposition/oxidation of the keratin plug (blackhead).
- Rupture of follicles with release of proinflammatory cytokines and bacteria into the dermis can cause inflammatory lesions.

Types

- *Noninflammatory:* Open and closed comedones
- *Inflammatory:* Papules, pustules, nodules, and cysts

Factors Affecting Acne

Factors affecting acne are illustrated in **Flowchart 1.**

FLOWCHART 1: Factors affecting acne.

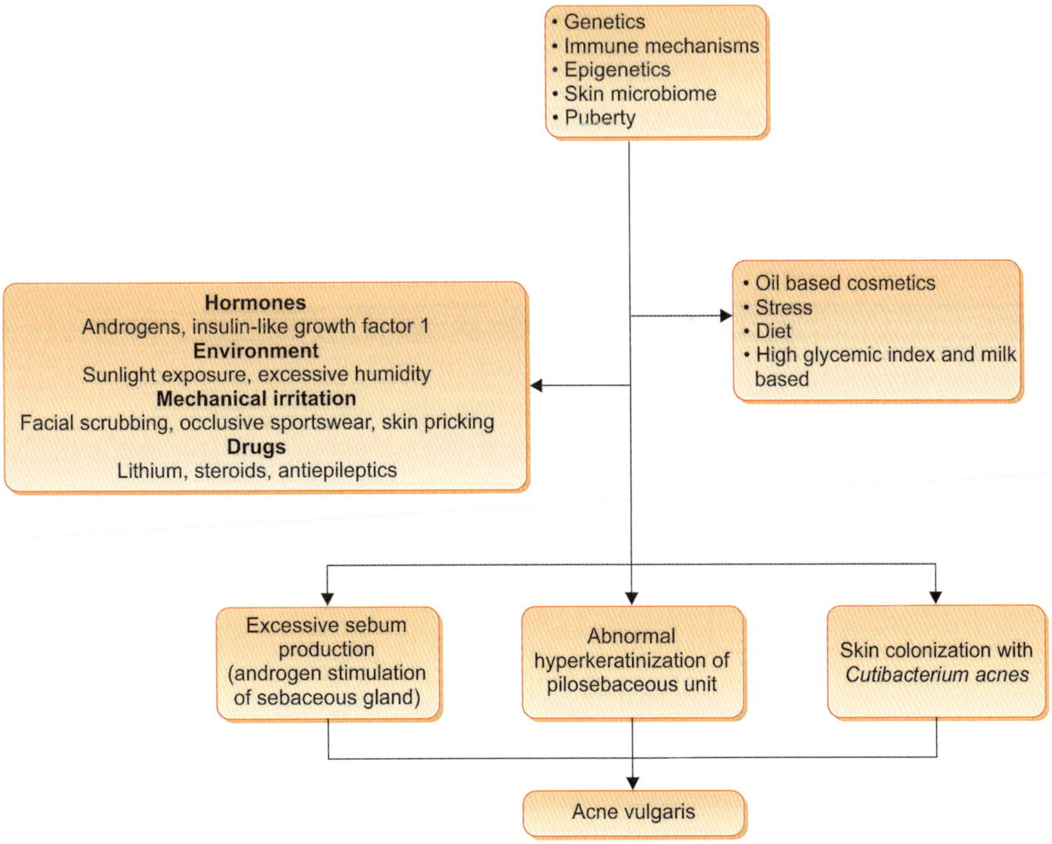

Grading

Lesions can be graded from 1–4 **(Table 1)**.

TABLE 1: Grades of acne and their severity.

GRADES OF ACNE	LESIONS	SEVERITY
Grade 1	Comedones	Mild
Grade 2	Papules	Moderate
Grade 3	Pustules	Severe
Grade 4	Nodules and cysts	Severe

Variants and Syndromes

Rare skin diseases are given in **Table 2**.

TABLE 2: Variants and syndromes.

VARIANTS/SYNDROME	CLINICAL FEATURES
• Infantile acne	• Appears at 3–6 months of age
• Acne conglobata	• Severe nodulocystic acne
• Acne fulminans	• Painful ulcerating hemorrhagic acne with fever and polyarthritis
• Acne excoriée	• Scarring associated with mild acne
• SAPHO syndrome	• Synovitis, Acne, pustulosis, hyperostosis, and osteitis
• PAPA syndrome	• Sterile pyogenic arthritis, pyoderma gangrenosum, and acne

Red Flag Signs

Red flag signs are given in **Table 3**.

TABLE 3: Red flag signs.

SIGNS	PROBABLE DIAGNOSIS
Preadolescent acne, severe resistant acne with oligomenorrhea, hirsutism, acanthosis nigricans, female pattern balding, with/without obesity	Polycystic ovarian syndrome
Preadolescent acne, signs of virilization, deepening of voice, male pattern balding, and clitoral enlargement	• Congenital adrenal hyperplasia • Adrenal or ovarian tumors • Ergogenic steroid use
Severe psychological distress	*Mental disorders:* Anxiety, depression, and body dysmorphic disorder

Comorbidities and Sequelae of Acne Vulgaris

Comorbidities and sequelae of acne vulgaris are given in **Table 4**.

TABLE 4: Comorbidities and sequelae.

COMORBIDITIES	SEQUELAE
• Mental health issues • Psychological distress • Body image concerns • Mental disorders (depression anxiety, and substance use disorder) • Suicidal Behavior • Hyperandrogenic states • Polycystic ovarian syndrome • Congenital adrenal hyperplasia • Adrenal or ovarian tumors • Ergogenic steroid use	• Acne fulminans • Hyperpigmentation • Gram-negative folliculitis • Abscess • Morbihan's disease (facial edema) • Permanent scarring • Keloid • School absenteeism • Unemployment • Poor quality of life

Approach

- A thorough and detailed history
- Physical, systemic, and mental health examination to assess acne severity and postacne sequelae
- Biochemical investigations and hormonal profile

Approach to management of acne vulgaris is given in **Flowchart 2**.

FLOWCHART 2: Approach to management of acne vulgaris.

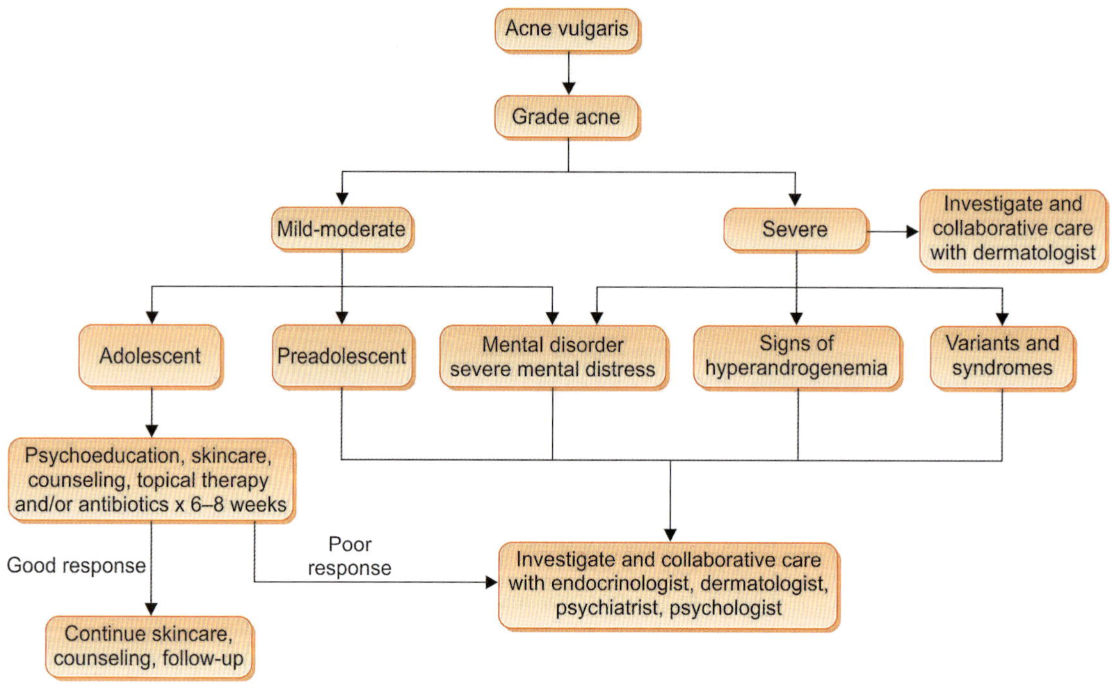

Suggested Reading

- Greydanus DE, Azmeh R, Cabral MD, Dickson CA, Patel DR. Acne in the first three decades of life: An update of a disorder with profound implications for all decades of life. Dis Mon. 2021;67(4):101103.
- Habeshian KA, Cohen BA. Current issues in the treatment of acne vulgaris. Pediatrics. 2020;145(Suppl 2):S225-30.
- Moosa AS, Lim SF, Koh YLE, Aau WK, Tan NC. The management of acne vulgaris in young people in primary care: A retrospective cohort study. Front Med (Lausanne). 2023;10:1152391.
- Sutaria AH, Masood S, Saleh HM, Schlessinger J. Acne Vulgaris. In: StatPearls [Internet]. Treasure Island (FL): StatPearls Publishing; 2023. [online] Available from https://www.ncbi.nlm.nih.gov/books/NBK459173/ [Last accessed July, 2024].
- Vasam M, Korutla S, Bohara RA. Acne vulgaris: A review of the pathophysiology, treatment, and recent nanotechnology-based advances. Biochem Biophys Rep. 2023;36:101578.

Angioedema

104

Section Editor: **Gnanamurthy Narasimha**
Section Co-Editor: **Nagalatha Chidananda**
Authors: **Balachandra BV, Sumalatha Soppa**

Definition

Angioedema means collection of fluid in the localized region in the deep dermal/subcutaneous tissue or submucosal tissue due to increased vascular permeability **(Fig. 1)**.

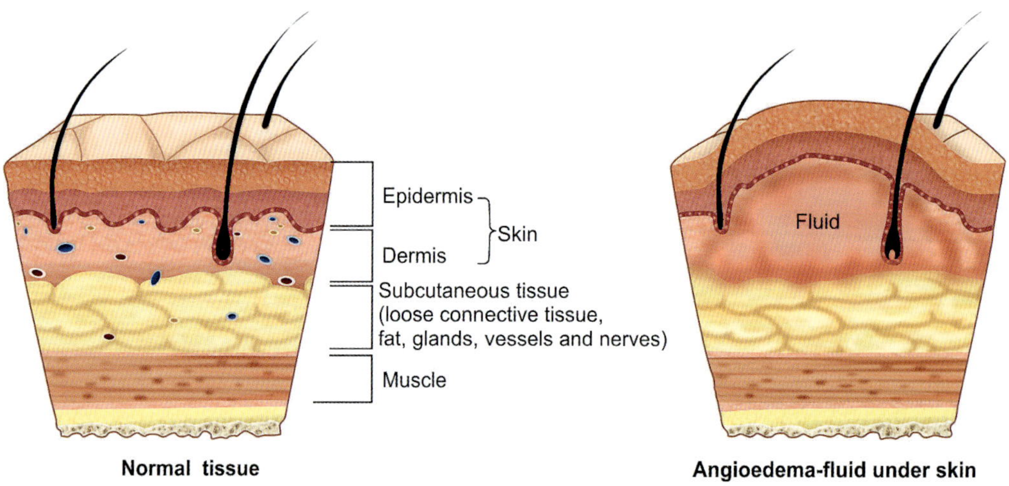

FIG. 1: Normal tissue versus angioedema.

Characteristics

- Nonpitting
- Nondependent
- Onset in minutes to hours and spontaneous resolution in hours to a few days.
- Asymmetric distribution
- Face, lips, extremities, genitals, larynx, and bowels are usually involved
- Present in ~40% of patients with urticaria
- Rarely angioedema can be a part of anaphylaxis process

Classification

Classification based on the mechanism of angioedema **(Table 1)**:

TABLE 1: Classification based on mechanism.

Bradykinin-induced AE				*Mast-cell-mediator-induced AE*		*Unknown mediator*
C1-INH deficiency/defect		*C1-INH normal*		*IgE-mediated*	*Non-IgE-mediated*	
Inherited	Acquired	Inherited	Acquired			
• HAE-1 • HAE-2	AAE-C1-INH	HAE nC1-INH (HAE-FXII, HAE-ANGPTI, HAE-PLG, HAE-UNK)	ACEI-AE	• Angioedema with anaphylaxis • Urticaria	Angioedema with urticaria	Idiopathic AE

[AAE-C1-INH: acquired angioedema due to C1-inhibitor deficiency; ACEI-AE: angiotensin-converting enzyme inhibitor-induced angioedema; ANGPTI: angiopoietin; FXII: factor XII; HAE-1: hereditary angioedema due to C1-inhibitor deficiency; HAE-2 hereditary angioedema due to C1-inhibitor dysfunction; HAE nC1-INH: hereditary angioedema with normal C1-inhibitor levels, either due to a mutation in *FXII*, *ANGPTI*, *PLG* or unknown (*HAE-FXII*, *HAE-ANGPTI*, *HAE-PLG*, and *HAE-UNK*); PLG: plasminogen]

Classification of angioedema based on etiology **(Table 2):**

TABLE 2: Classification based on etiology.

IgE-mediated angioedema	*Associated with chronic urticaria*	*C1 esterase inhibitor deficiency*	*Acquired angioedema*	*Idiopathic angioedema*
Food allergy: Milk, shellfish, eggs, tree nuts, peanuts, etc.	*Chronic inducible urticaria:* Cold urticaria, cholinergic urticaria, and vibratory angioedema	• Hereditary angioedema type 1 • Hereditary angioedema type 2 • Hereditary angioedema type 3 • Acquired angioedema	Hypertension medications, intake of ACE inhibitors	Unknown etiology –
Insect bite allergy: Honey bees, yellow jacket, hornets, wasp, and fire ants	*Chronic spontaneous urticaria:* Either autoimmune or idiopathic	–	–	–
Drug allergy: Penicillin and sulfa drugs, nonsteroidal anti-inflammatory drug (NSAID), angiotensin-converting-enzyme (ACE) inhibitors, and radiocontrast agents	–	–	–	–

Differentiation between Mast-cell-mediated and Bradykinin-mediated Angioedema

The difference between mast-cell-mediated and bradykinin-mediated angioedema is given in **Table 3.**

TABLE 3: Bradykinin-mediated angioedema versus mast-cell-mediated angioedema.

Bradykinin-mediated angioedema	*Mast-cell-mediated angioedema*
Slower evolution angioedema	Faster evolution of angioedema
Longer duration	Shorter duration
No urticaria	Urticaria
Itching absent	Itching present
No response to antihistamines	Response to antihistamines
May present with abdominal symptoms due to bowel wall edema	May present as a part of an allergic reaction—anaphylaxis

Features of bradykinin-mediated hereditary angioedema—an autosomal dominant condition:

- A positive family history
- Onset of symptoms in childhood/adolescence
- Recurrent and painful abdominal symptoms
- Occurrence of upper airway edema
- Failure to respond to antihistamines, glucocorticoids, and epinephrine
- Prodromal signs/symptoms before swellings
- The absence of urticaria

Features of bradykinin-mediated acquired angioedema:

- Negative family history.
- Onset of symptoms above 40 years
- Patient may be on angiotensin-converting-enzyme (ACE) inhibitors
- Symptoms related to lymphoma or benign monoclonal gammopathy

Red Flag Signs

- Family history
- Childhood onset
- With/without urticaria as a part of acute allergic reactions
- Slow progression over 2–3 days and resolves slowly over 3–5 days
- Without itching
- Unresponsive to antihistamines

Diagnostic Approach

FLOWCHART 1: Diagnostic approach to angioedema.

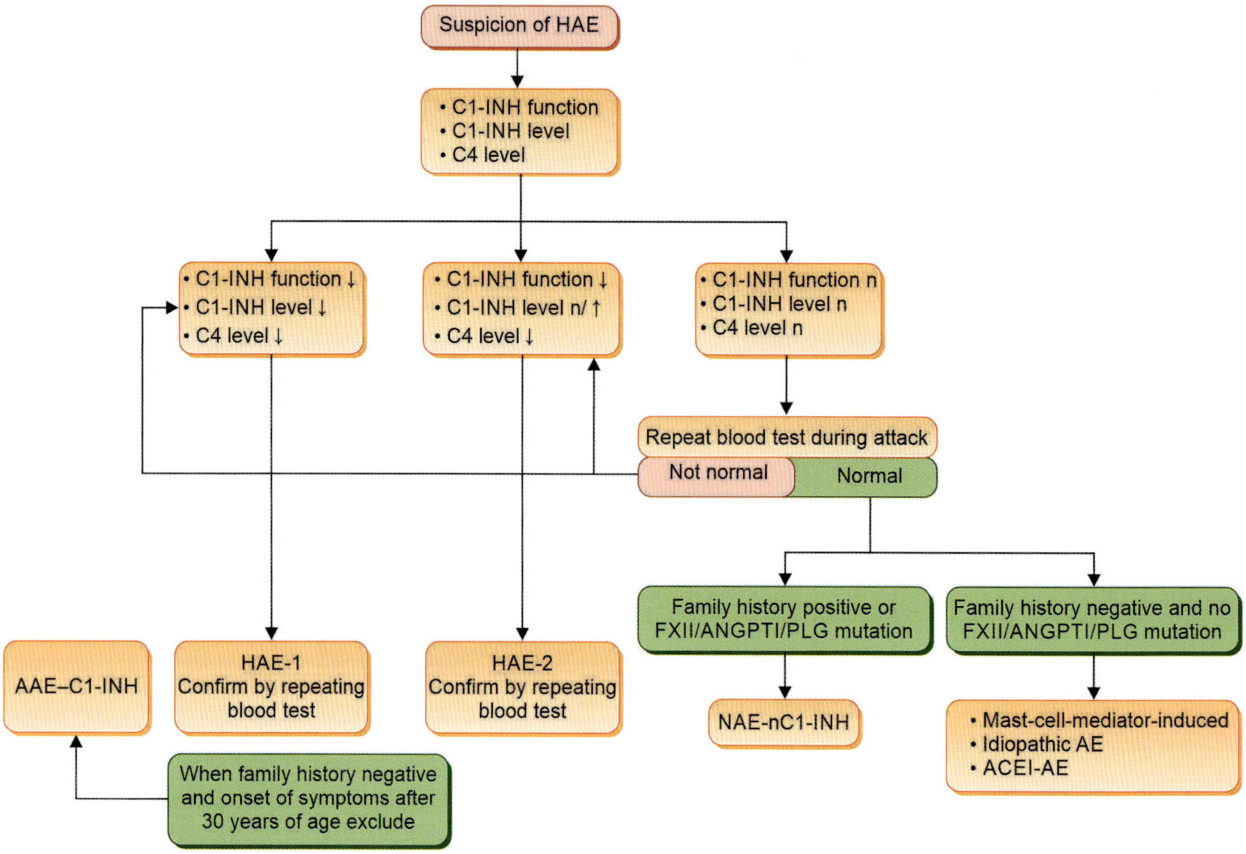

(ACEI-AE: angiotensin-converting enzyme inhibitor-induced angioedema; ANGPTI: angiopoietin; C1-INH: C1 esterase inhibitor; C4: complement 4; FXII: factor XII; HAE: hereditary angioedema; PLG: plasminogen)

Step 1: Good history to differentiate between mast-cell-mediated or nonmast-cell-mediated angioedema.

Step 2: Good history to differentiate between bradykinin-mediated hereditary or bradykinin-mediated acquired angioedema.

Step 3: For confirming hereditary angioedema or acquired angioedema, investigate with:

- Complement 4 levels
- C1 esterase quantitative
- C1 esterase functional assay

Step 4: If abnormal values, follow **Flowchart 1**.

Step 5: If all the values are normal, do genetic studies to identify mutations in factor XII, angiopoietin (ANGPTI) or plasminogen (PLG).

Step 6: If all the above results are inconclusive then probably the patient fits in to idiopathic angioedema of unknown mechanism.

Suggested Reading

- Burks AW, O'Hehir RE, Broide DH, Holgate ST, Bacharier LB, Khurana GK, Peebles RS (Eds). Urticaria and angioedema. Middleton's Allergy: Principles and Practice, 9th edition. Amsterdam, Netherlands: Elsevier; 2020.
- Maurer M, Magerl M, Ansotegui I, Aygören-Pürsün E, Betschel S, Bork K, et al. The international WAO/EAACI guideline for the management of hereditary angioedema–The 2017 revision and update. Allergy. 2018;73(8): 1575-96.

Clubbing

105

***Section Editor:* Nehal Patel**
***Section Co-Editor:* Jay T Dhirwani**
***Authors:* Nitin Rao, Yogesh Chintaman Sathe, Srujan Reddy Salukati**

Introduction

Clubbing is a bulbous enlargement of fingers/toes, resulting from chronic hypoxia. It is characterized by soft-tissue swelling of the terminal phalanx, flattening of the angle between the nail bed and the nail, with an increase in the anteroposterior and lateral diameters of the nails of fingers/toes. It is often predictive of serious underlying pathologic conditions.

Etiology

Clubbing is associated with:

- *Cardiac causes of chronic hypoxia:* Congenital cyanotic heart diseases (CCHD), infective endocarditis, atrial myxoma, carcinoid tumors, and venovenous collaterals
- *Pulmonary:* Carcinoma lung, bronchiectasis, lung abscess, interstitial lung diseases, cystic fibrosis, empyema, idiopathic pulmonary fibrosis, sarcoidosis, and pleural tumors like mesothelioma, complicated tuberculosis, and pulmonary arteriovenous malformation
- *Gastrointestinal:* Malabsorption, inflammatory bowel disease, celiac disease, cirrhosis—especially primary biliary cholangitis and ascariasis
- *Endocrine:* Graves disease (autoimmune hyperparathyroidism)/thyroid acropathy, severe secondary hyperparathyroidism, and growth hormone secreting tumors
- *Drug induced:* Laxative overdose, prolonged prostaglandin infusion, and interferon alpha 2a
- Idiopathic/congenital

Variants

- *Pseudoclubbing:* An over curvature of the nails in the longitudinal and transverse axes, with preservation of a normal Lovibond angle. It is associated with chronic kidney disease, hyperparathyroidism, sarcoidosis, scleroderma, subungual hematoma, and chromosome deletion.
- *Unilateral clubbing:* It may be due to aortic arch anomalies, aortic or subclavian artery aneurysm, pulmonary hypertension with patent ductus arteriosus (PDA), and brachial arteriovenous aneurysm or fistula.
- *Differential cyanosis and clubbing:* It is seen more in lower limbs than in the upper—seen in PDA with severe pulmonary hypertension and indicates shunt reversal.
- *Special form of clubbing:* Hypertrophic pulmonary osteoarthropathy (HPOA), also known as Pierre Marie–Bamberger syndrome is the combination of clubbing and thickening of the periosteum and synovium, and maybe diagnosed as arthritis. It is commonly associated with lung cancer.

Clinical Features

- *Lovibond angle:* The angle between the proximal nail fold and the nail at a location of the exit of the nail from the nail fold. Normal <180° **(Fig. 1)**.

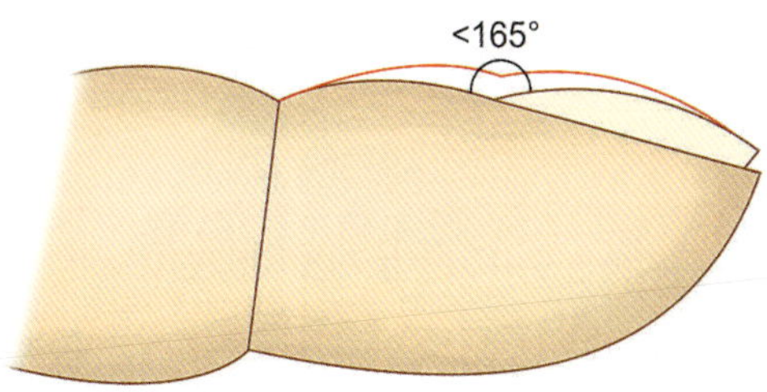

FIG. 1: Clubbing of the fingernail—the red line shows the outline of a clubbed nail.

- The phalangeal depth ratio (the ratio of digit's depth), measured at the nail and the distal interphalangeal (DIP) joint, is another objective sign to assess clubbing. The depth at the DIP joint is normally greater than that of the nail. A ratio of >1, favors clubbing **(Figs. 2 and 3)**.

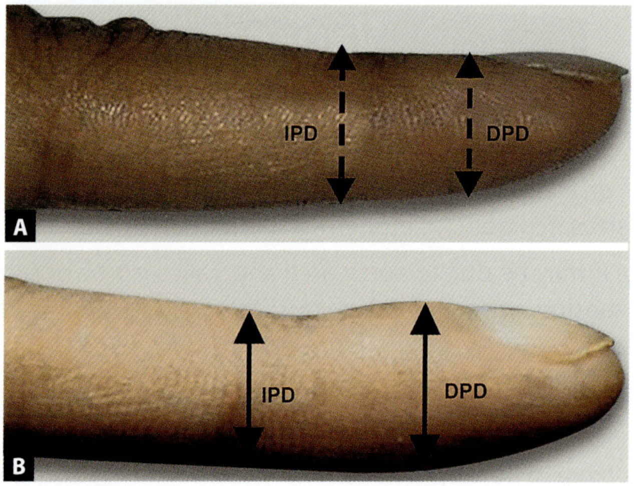

FIGS. 2A AND B: The depth at the nail bed is greater than the depth at distal interphalangeal joint—typical feature in clubbing.

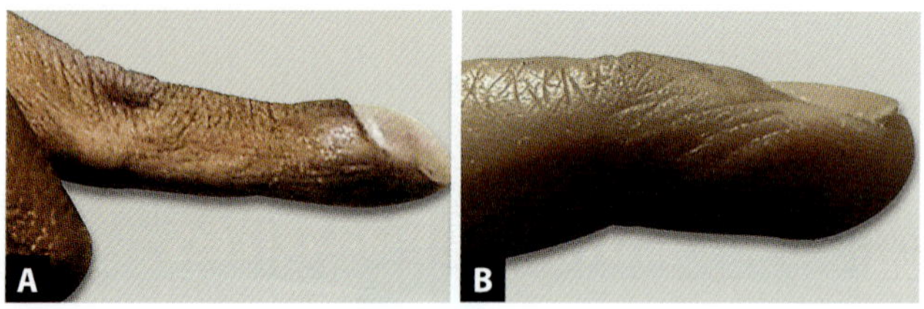

FIGS. 3A AND B: (A) Clubbed finger; (B) Normal finger.

- *Schamroth sign:* Obliteration of the diamond-shaped window normally produced when the dorsal surfaces of the corresponding finger of each hand are opposed is diagnostic **(Figs. 4A and B)**.

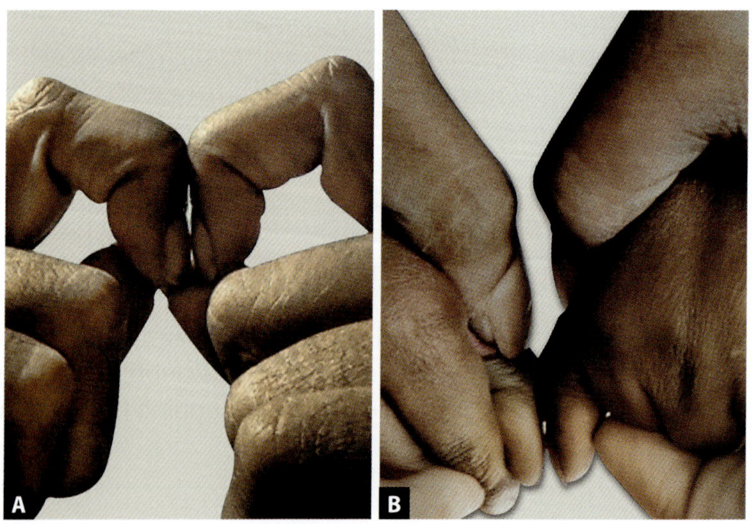

FIGS. 4A AND B: Schamroth window test for nail clubbing. (A) Normal—diamond-shaped window; (B) Clubbing—obliterated window.

Staging and Clinical Examination

Clubbing is classified into grades 1–5 **(Figs. 5A to E)**.

- *Grade 1:* Fluctuation and softening of nail bed
- *Grade 2:* Increase in the angle between nail bed and proximal nail fold
- *Grade 3:* Accentuated convexity of nail
- *Grade 4:* Clubbed appearance of finger
- *Grade 5:* Shiny change in nail with longitudinal striations/hypertrophic osteoarthropathy

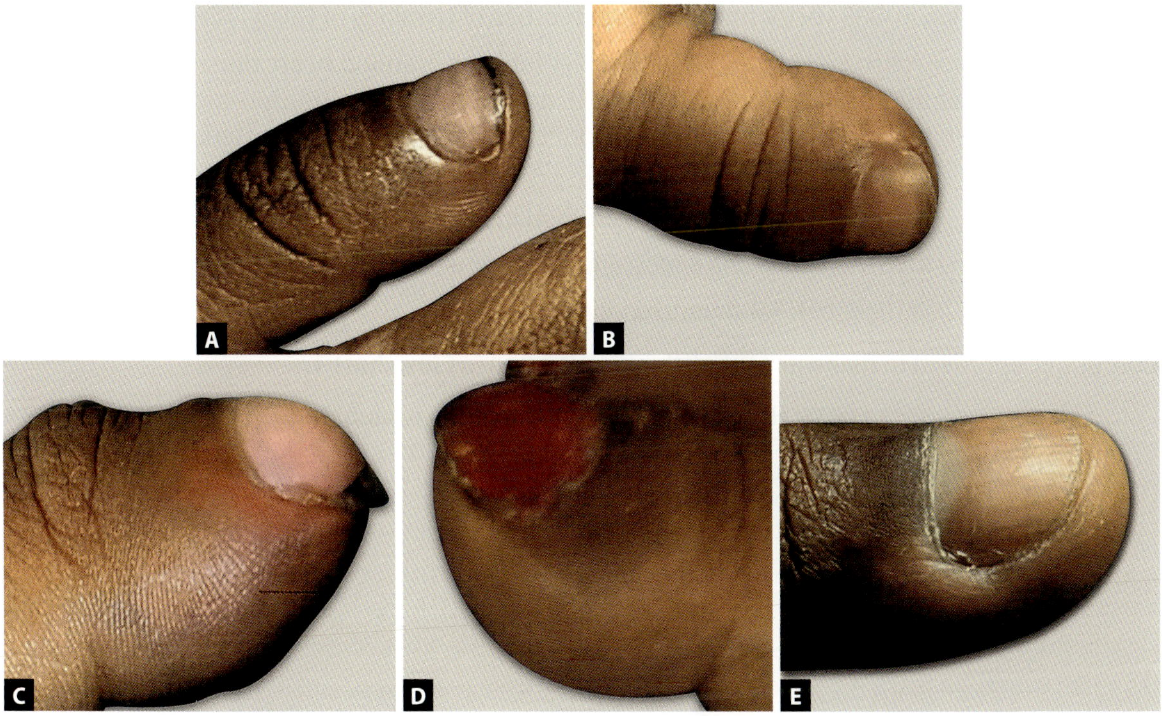

FIGS. 5A TO E: Grades of clubbing: (A) Grade 1; (B) Grade 2; (C) Grade 3; (D) Grade 4; (E) Grade 5.

Approach and Diagnosis

- Exclude pseudoclubbing before making the diagnosis.
- Detailed history with particular references to lung, heart, and gastrointestinal conditions should be taken.
- Thorough clinical examination is required.

Relevant investigations/studies should include:

- *Chest X-ray:* For cardiomegaly/pulmonary artery anatomy/pulmonary oligemia or plethora/lung fields
- *Electrocardiography (ECG):* For clues
- *Some typical ECG features for certain lesions:* Absent left ventricular (LV) forces in tricuspid atresia, sudden transition in QRS vector from V1–V2 suggestive of tetralogy of Fallot (TOF).
- *Two-dimensional echocardiography (2D echo):* Features of cyanotic heart diseases—R→L shunts, right ventricular (RV) outflow obstruction (TOF), admixture lesions [transposition of great vessels (TGA), totally anomalous pulmonary venous connection (TAPVC), truncus arteriosus, and tricuspid atresia], and infective endocarditis (rarely)
- *Computed tomography (CT)-scan chest:* Any cardiopulmonary disease
- *Ultrasonography (USG) Abdomen and Endoscopy:* Cirrhosis and features of Crohn's disease
- *Pertinent blood investigations:* For thyrotoxicosis

Algorithmic approach to management of clubbing is given in **Flowchart 1**.

FLOWCHART 1: Algorithmic approach to clubbing.

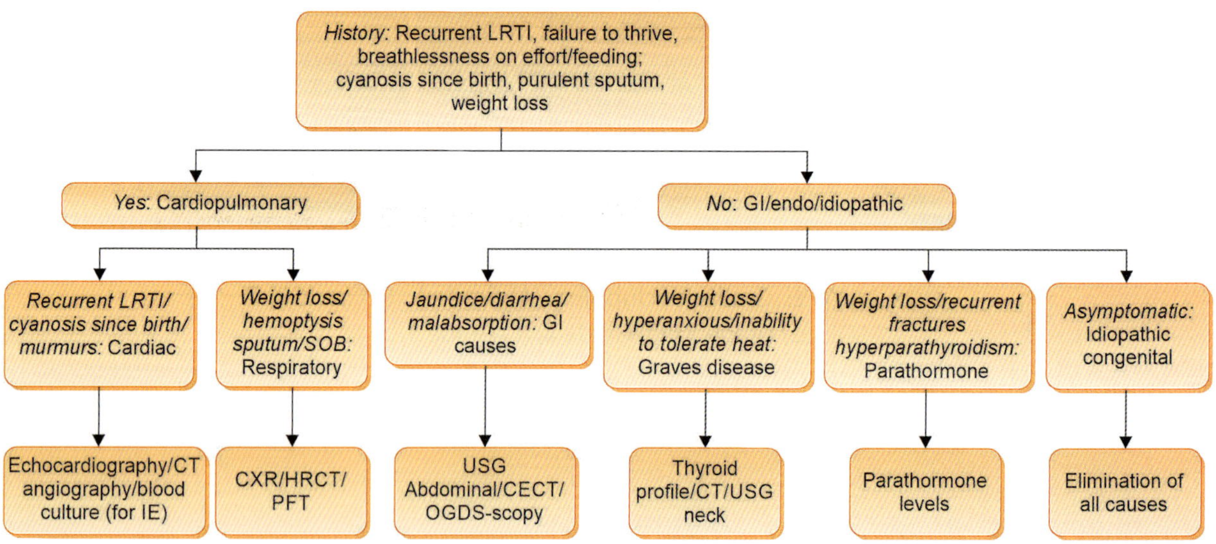

CECT: contrast-enhanced computed tomography; CT: computed tomography; CXR: chest X-ray; GI: gastro-intestinal; HRCT: high-resolution computed tomography; LRTI: lower respiratory tract infection; OGDS-SCOPY: oesophago-gastro-duodenoscopy-scopy; PFT: pulmonary function test; USG: ultrasound; SOB: shortness of breath

Red Flag Signs

- *Intense cyanosis (SpO_2 <60):* Complex CCHD
- Persistent fever and constitutional symptoms
- Persistent fever/purulent sputum
- Hemoptysis/constitutional symptoms/weight loss
- Gastrointestinal (GI) symptoms

Suggested Reading

- Clarke S, Barnsley L, Peters M, Morgan L, Van Der Wall H. Hypertrophic pulmonary osteoarthropathy without clubbing of the digits. Skeletal Radiol. 2001;30(11):652-5.
- Jyotsna M, Tharakan J. Clinical Sign: Clubbing. Indian J Cardiovasc Dis Women. 2017;2(3):e1–9.
- Marrie TJ, Brown N. Clubbing of the Digits. Am J Med. 2007;120(11):940-1.
- Rutherford JD. Digital clubbing. Circulation. 2013;127(19):1997-9.
- Spicknall KE, Zirwas MJ, English JC 3rd. Clubbing: An update on diagnosis, differential diagnosis, pathophysiology, and clinical relevance. J Am Acad Dermatol. 2005;52(6):1020-8.

Eczema

106

Section Editor: **Gnanamurthy Narasimha**
Section Co-Editor: **Nagalatha Chidananda**
Authors: **Chidananda NK, Gnanamurthy Narasimha**

Introduction

Eczema indicates an inflammation of the skin. It is often used interchangeably with the word dermatitis.

Definition

Eczema refers to skin eruptions characterized by acute symptoms of erythema, edema, and pruritus. When chronic, it presents as dryness, scaling, lichenification, and nodules.

Types

- Eczema can be of two types: *Acute and chronic.*
- There can be a waxing–waning course with acute changes on chronic lesions and vice versa.

Etiology

- *With genetic disorders:* For example, Wiskott–Aldrich syndrome and hyperimmunoglobulin E syndrome
- *Associated systemic illness:* For example, psoriasis, Langerhans cell histiocytosis (LCH), and seborrhea
- *Allergy:* For example, atopic dermatitis (AD)/allergic contact dermatitis
- *Infections*: For example, human immunodeficiency virus (HIV)/candida/tinea/impetigo

Approach to Clinical Diagnosis

History

Detailed history includes:

- *Age:* Different distribution patterns in different age groups
- *Type of skin lesion:* White patch/roughness/darkening of skin
- *Affected areas:* Cheeks/face/scalp/flexural areas/diaper area, etc.
- Precipitating factors
- Presence/absence of pruritus
- *Symptoms of chronicity:* Darkening of skin—lichenification
- *Associated systemic features if any*: Consider systemic diseases manifesting with eczema
- Family history of eczematous diseases

Red Flag Signs

- Persistent/recurrent lesions recalcitrant to general therapeutic measures
- Recalcitrant diaper rash with seborrhea, nail pitting, and intergluteal erythema
- Intractable seborrhea like dermatitis with chronic diarrhea and failure to thrive (FTT)
- Dermatitis with recurrent infections and petechiae
- Recalcitrant diaper dermatitis with petechiae
- Perioral, anogenital, and extremities involvement with irritability, diarrhea, and FTT

Specific Diagnostic Pointers (Pattern Recognition)

CLUE	DIAGNOSIS
Greasy scaly lesions on the scalp in infants	Cradle cap (seborrhea)
Perioral lesions	Lip licker's dermatitis
Facial dermatitis with involvement of eye lids	Nail polish sensitivity
Erythematous scaly patches subsiding to leave white patches without well demarcated margins usually on the face	Pityriasis alba
Rashes that itch: Family history of atopy with chronic or chronically relapsing, typical age-matching distribution of pruritic lesions	Atopic dermatitis (AD)
Small gray–white papules in extensor areas of arms, thighs, and buttocks with a family history (atopic)	Keratosis pilaris
Linear vesiculobullous	Rhus dermatitis (poison ivy/oak/sumac)
Recurrent/seasonal vesicular lesions of palms and soles (tapioca like vesicles)	Pompholyx (dyshidrotic eczema)
Clustered lesions occurring at varied intervals in various stages of healing over exposed areas like extremities, head, and neck	Papular urticaria
Peeling of the skin in palms and soles	Keratolysis exfoliativa
Pruritic coin-shaped lesions usually on buttocks, shoulders, or extensor areas—no raised edges/well demarcated margins	Nummular eczema
Hypo/hyperpigmented sharply demarcated macules over the trunk, with fine scales and do not tan on sun exposure	Tinea versicolor
Eczema—site of involvement—ear lobule/belt buckle area/tattoo/back of buttocks and thighs (toilet seat)	Contact dermatitis
Beefy red with satellite lesions and involvement of the groin (concavity)	Candida dermatitis
Symmetric involvement of dorsum/soles of feet/digits with sparing of interdigital spaces	Shoe dermatitis
Sweaty feet with painful/itchy fissures/glazed appearance	Juvenile plantar dermatosis (JPD)
Triad of eczema, recurrent skin/pulmonary infections, and increased immunoglobulin E (IgE), they can develop skeletal and dental abnormalities later	Hyper IgE syndrome
Chronic eczema, recurrent infections, and thrombocytopenia with small platelets	Wiskott–Aldrich syndrome
Eczema, diffuse hypopigmentation, photosensitivity, and seizures	Phenylketonuria (PKU)

Investigations

Investigations have limited role:

- *Histology:* Often nonspecific, majority have intraepidermal edema (spongiosis)
- *Potassium hydroxide (KOH) preparation:* To distinguish tinea from nummular eczema
- *Skin patch test in older children:* Allergic contact dermatitis
- Alkaline phosphatase (Zinc-dependent enzyme): Low in acrodermatitis enteropathica
- *Systemic/genetic disorders:* Human immunodeficiency virus (HIV)/Langerhans cell histiocytosis (LCH)/ Wiskott–Aldrich/phenylketonuria (PKU), etc., investigate as required

Algorithmic Approach

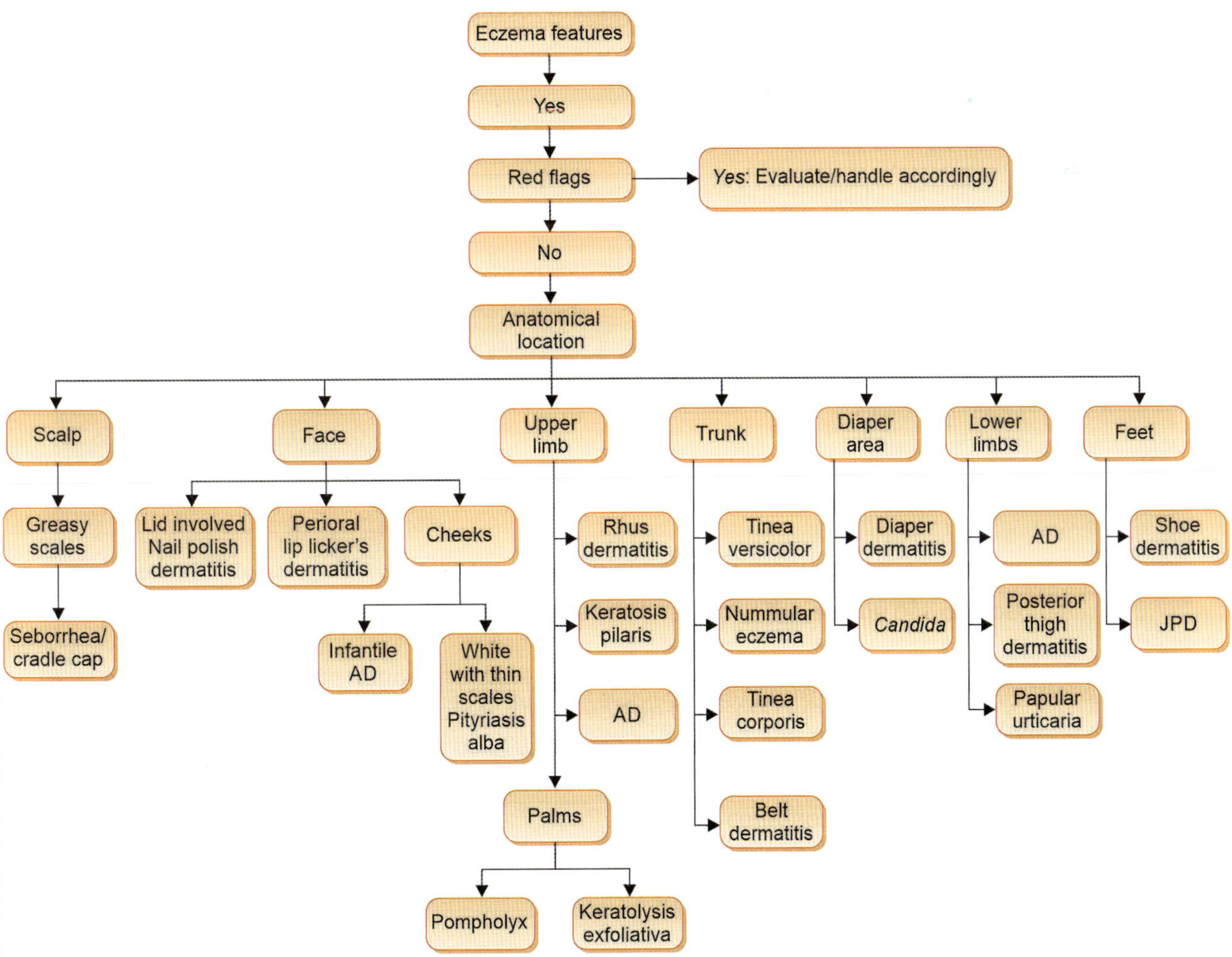

AD: atopic dermatitis; JPD: Juvenile plantar dermatosis

Suggested Reading

- Dhar S, Srinivas SM. Color Atlas & Synopsis of Pediatric Dermatology. New Delhi: Jaypee Brothers Medical Publishers (P) Ltd; 2021.
- Kay Shou-Mei Kane, Nambudiri VE, Stratigos AJ. Color Atlas and Synopsis of Pediatric Dermatology, 3rd edition. New York, United States: McGraw Hill Professional; 2016.
- Kliegman RM, Stanton B, St Geme JW, Schor NF, Behrman RE, Nelson WE (Eds). Nelson Textbook of Pediatrics, 21st edition. Philadelphia: Elsevier; 2020.

Inattention and Impulsivity

107

Section Editor: **Sumitha Nayak**
Section Co-Editor: **Priya Shivalli**
Author: **Shamik Ghosh**

Introduction

- Children often have inattention, impulsivity, and hyperactivity presenting as attention deficit hyperactivity disorder (ADHD).
- Prevalence of ADHD in India is 5.7%; it is higher in males, 9–10 years of age group, and lower socioeconomic class.

Etiology

Two types of attention occur in humans:

1. *Automatic attention:* While doing something that's interesting or engaging
2. *Directed attention:* For something that is tiring/of low interest

Directed attention skills that are mediated by the frontal lobe of the brain tend to be weaker in ADHD.

Red Flag Signs

- Interrupting frequently
- Unable to finish tasks
- Impulsivity
- Inability to sit still
- Problems in staying organized

Approach and Diagnosis

- Assessment of:
  - Parents
  - Child
  - Child's teachers and other caregivers
- Look for *comorbidities*
  - Depression
  - Anxiety
  - Obsessive–compulsive disorder (OCD)
  - Oppositional defiant disorder (ODD)
  - Learning disabilities

Diagnostic and Statistical Manual of Mental Disorders, Fifth Edition, Text Revision Pointers to Diagnosis

- Symptoms must occur in two or more settings (home, school, and/or social situations) and impair their ability to function in daily activities.
- Child's provider must identify the presence or absence of six or more symptoms (mentioned later in this chapter).
- Symptoms must have started before the child turned 12 years old.
- Symptoms persist for at least 6 months.

Types of Attention Deficit Hyperactivity Disorder

Predominantly Inattentive Presentation

Diagnostic and Statistical Manual of Mental Disorders, Fifth Edition, Text Revision (DSM-5-TR) guidelines:

Child must display at least *six of the following nine behaviors.*

1. Trouble paying attention to details/making careless mistakes
2. Issues remaining focused on tasks and activities
3. Difficulty listening well, daydreaming, or seeming distracted
4. Trouble with following instructions and/or finishing tasks
5. Difficulty with organizing tasks and activities
6. Avoiding/disliking tasks requiring continuous mental effort
7. Losing things frequently
8. Easily distracted by outside stimuli
9. Forgetfulness in daily activities

Predominantly Hyperactive/Impulsive Presentation

The DSM-5-TR Guidelines

Child must display at least *six of the following nine behaviors.*

1. Fidgeting with/tapping hands or feet/squirming frequently
2. Leaving their seat when remaining seated is expected
3. Running/climbing when it is not appropriate
4. Trouble playing or engaging in leisure activities quietly
5. Always seeming "on the go" or "driven by a motor"
6. Talking too much
7. Blurting out answers before questions are completed
8. Frequent trouble waiting for their turn
9. Often interrupting or intruding on others' conversations or games

Combined Presentation

Combined presentation includes behaviors from both the inattentive and hyperactive/impulsive categories.

The DSM-5-TR Guidelines

Children must display at least 12 of the total behaviors (at least six inattentive behaviors and six hyperactive/impulsive behaviors).

Algorithmic Approach

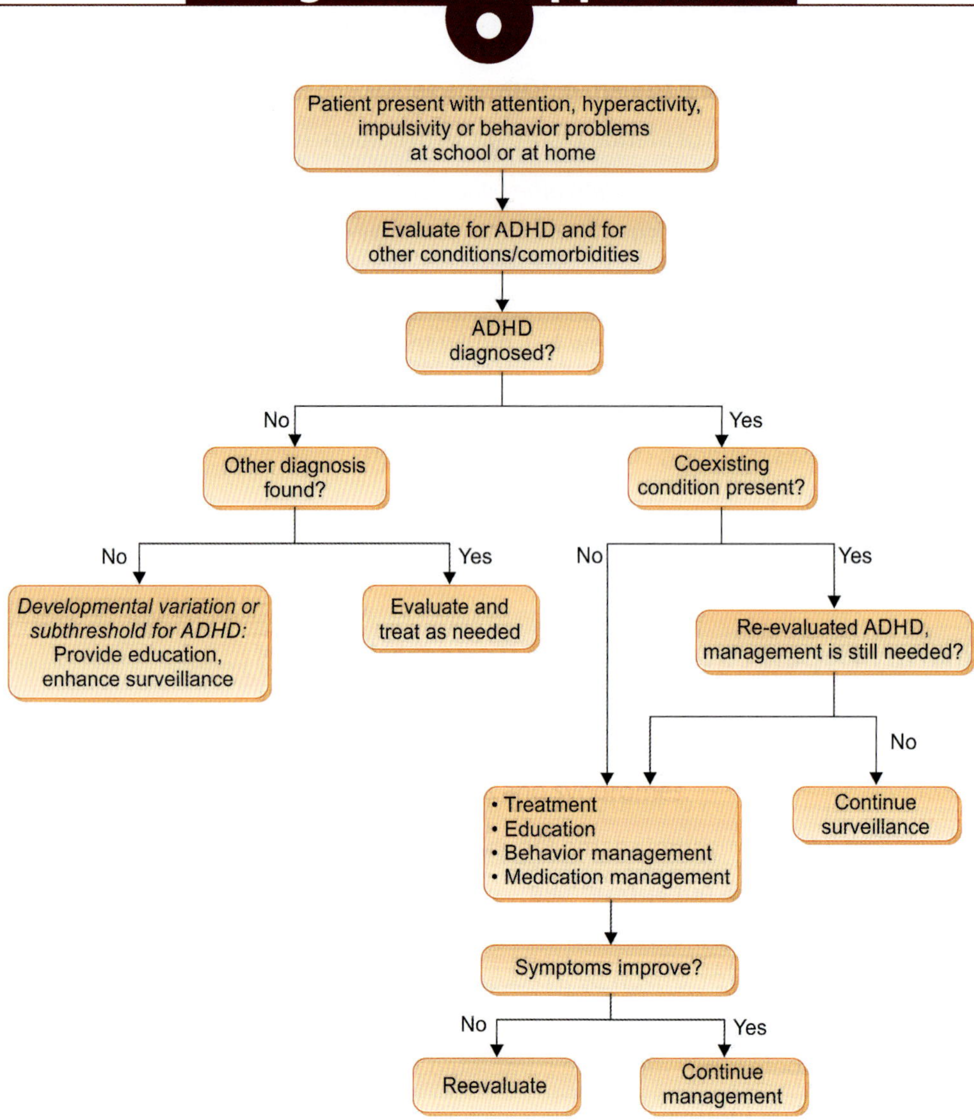

ADHD: attention deficit hyperactivity disorder

Suggested Reading

- National Consultation Meeting for Developing IAP Guidelines on Neuro Developmental Disorders under the aegis of IAP Childhood Disability Group and the Committee on Child Development and Neurodevelopmental Disorders; Dalwai S, Unni J, Kalra V, Singhi P, Shrivastava L, Nair MKC, et al. Consensus statement of the Indian Academy of Pediatrics on evaluation and management of attention deficit hyperactivity disorder. Indian Pediatr. 2017;54(6):481-8.
- Schellack N, Meyer H. The management of attention-deficit/hyperactivity disorder in children. S Afr Pharm J. 2021;79(9):12-20.
- Shah R, Grover S, Avasthi A. Clinical Practice Guidelines for the assessment and management of attention-deficit/hyperactivity disorder. Indian J Psychiatry. 2019;61(Suppl2):176-93.
- Substance Abuse and Mental Health Services Administration. DSM-5 Changes: Implications for Child Serious Emotional Disturbance [Internet]. Rockville (MD): Substance Abuse and Mental Health Services Administration (US); 2016.
- Venkata JA, Panicker AS. Prevalence of attention deficit hyperactivity disorder in primary school children. Indian J Psychiatry. 2013;55(4):338-42.

Hyperhidrosis

108

Section Editor: **Gnanamurthy Narasimha**
Section Co-Editor: **Nagalatha Chidananda**
Authors: **Sahana M Srinivas, Puneetha B**

Introduction

- Hyperhidrosis is a chronic autonomic disorder characterized by excessive sweating beyond the physiological need to maintain normal thermoregulation.
- Those affected have difficulties in holding a pen, handing utensil, keeping papers dry, gripping the handlebar of a bicycle, using computer mouse, or using a video game controller which affects their psychosocial development and well-being. Early diagnosis and therapy improve the quality of life.

Types

Hyperhidrosis is classified into the following types:

- *Primary:* It starts early at an average age of 14–25 years and is usually idiopathic. Causes are genetic usually. It occurs without a sweating trigger, results from excessive neurogenic activity of normal eccrine sweat glands.
- *Secondary:* It occurs in response to a stimulus, usually due to adverse effects of medications or systemic disorders, particularly neurologic.

Diagnostic Criteria for Primary Hyperhidrosis

- Excessive sweating >6 months
- Sweating involves axilla, palms, soles, and/or face
- Bilateral and symmetric sweating
- Decreased/no sweating at night
- Sweating episodes last at least 7 days
- The individual is <25 years of age
- Positive family history
- Sweating impairs daily living activities

Causes for Secondary Hyperhidrosis

- *Physiological:* Hot weather, exercise, anxiety, obesity, ingestion of spicy, citrus food or alcohol
- *Endocrine:* Hyperthyroidism, hypopituitarism, diabetes, menopause, hypoglycemia, pregnancy, pheochromocytoma, carcinoid syndrome, and acromegaly
- *Neurologic:* Parkinson's disease, spinal cord injury and stroke, vasovagal syncope, hypothalamic hyperhidrosis, and reflex sympathetic dystrophy
- *Neoplastic:* Tumors of central nervous system (CNS), Hodgkin's disease, myeloproliferative diseases, and cancer of thoracic cavity
- *Infectious:* Tuberculosis, malaria, and septicemia
- *Drugs:* Fluoxetine, venlafaxine, doxepin, opioids, amitriptyline, insulin, nonsteroidal anti-inflammatory drugs (NSAIDS)
- *Toxicity:* Alcoholism and substance abuse
- *Iatrogenic:* Postoperative compensatory sweating (sympathectomy and cardiac surgery).

Constitutional symptoms of fever, weight loss, anorexia, palpitations suggest systemic disease and clinical evidence of thyroid or neurological disease.

Spinal cord damage and reflex sympathetic dystrophy causes regional hyperhidrosis.

Focal secondary hyperhidrosis occurs in Frey syndrome, gustatory sweating, eccrine nevus, social anxiety disorder, and unilateral focal hyperhidrosis (e.g., neurological disorder or tumor).

Red Flag Signs

- Diffuse or generalized excessive sweating
- Sweating at night/during sleep
- Constitutional symptoms of fever, weight loss, anorexia, and palpitations

Approach to Evaluation

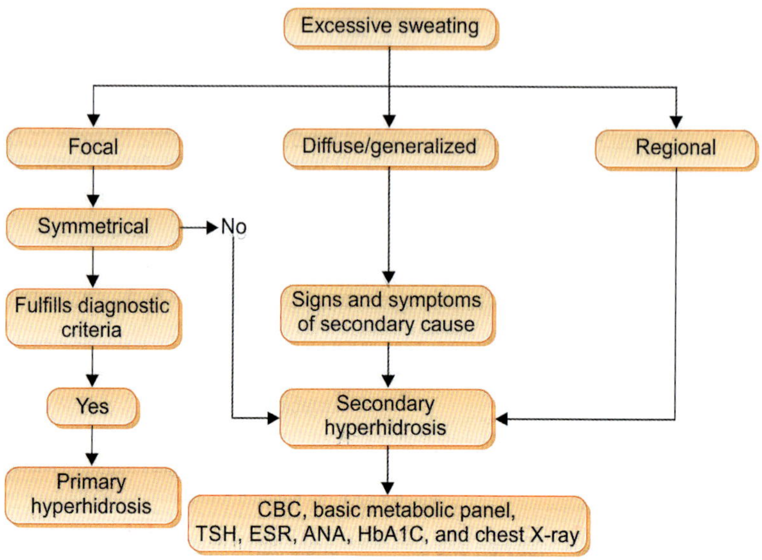

ANA: antinuclear antibody; CBC: complete blood count; ESR: erythrocyte sedimentation rate; HbA1C: glycated hemoglobin; TSH: thyroid-stimulating hormone

Suggested Reading

- Bohaty BR, Hebert AA. Special considerations for children with hyperhidrosis. Dermatol Clin. 2014;32(4):477-84.
- Brackenrich J, Fagg C. Hyperhidrosis. In: StatPearls [Internet]. Treasure Island (FL): StatPearls Publishing; 2024. [online] Available from https://www.ncbi.nlm.nih.gov/books/NBK459227/ [Last accessed July, 2024].
- Hornberger J, Grimes K, Naumann M, Glaser DA, Lowe NJ, Naver H, et al.; Multi-Specialty Working Group on the Recognition, Diagnosis, and Treatment of Primary Focal Hyperhidrosis. Recognition, diagnosis, and treatment of primary focal hyperhidrosis. J Am Acad Dermatol. 2004;51(2):274-86.
- Pradhan S, Madke B, Sirka CS. Review of oral anticholinergics in the treatment of palmoplantar hyperhidrosis. Indian J Drugs Dermatol. 2019;5(2):75-82.
- Remington C, Ruth J, Hebert AA. Primary hyperhidrosis in children: A review of therapeutics. Pediatr Dermatol. 2021;38(3):561-7.
- Wong NS, Adlam TM, Potts GA, Farshchian M. Hyperhidrosis: A review of recent advances in treatment with topical anticholinergics. Dermatol Ther (Heidelb). 2022;12(12):2705-14.

Hemangiomas

109

Section Editor: **Gnanamurthy Narasimha**
Section Co-Editor: **Nagalatha Chidananda**
Authors: **Nagesh A, Rashmi Agarwal**

Introduction

Hemangiomas (strawberry marks) are benign tumors of infancy resulting from endothelial cell proliferation. They can be congenital or infantile.

International Society for the Study of Vascular Anomalies Classification of Vascular Tumors

International Society for the Study of Vascular Anomalies (ISSVA) classification of vascular tumors is given in **Flowchart 1**.

FLOWCHART 1: Classification of vascular tumors.

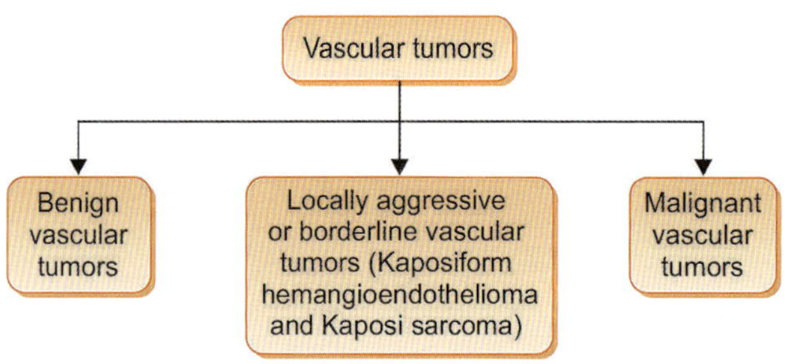

International Society for the Study of Vascular Anomalies (ISSVA) classification of benign vascular tumors is given in **Flowchart 2**.

FLOWCHART 2: Classification of benign vascular tumors.

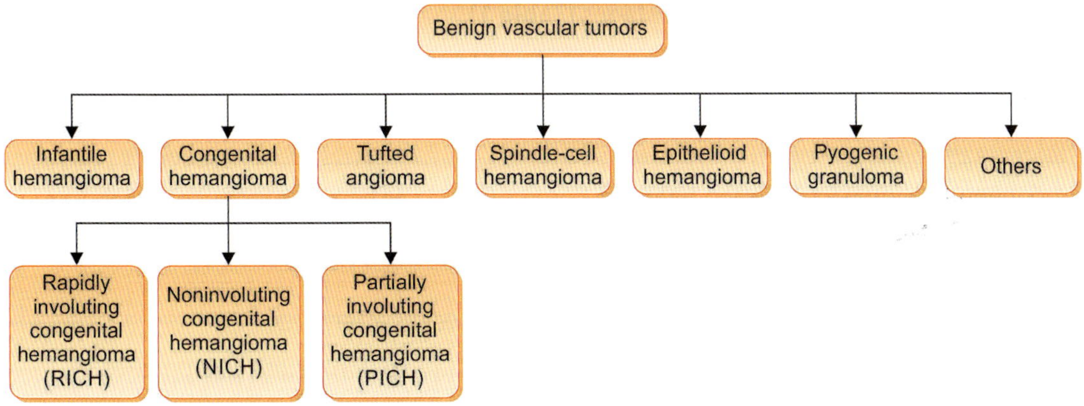

Etiology of Infantile Hemangioma

The risk factors of infantile hemangioma are given in **Box 1**.

BOX 1: Risk factors for infantile hemangioma.

- Low birth-weight babies
- Premature babies
- Female infants
- Multiparous pregnancies
- Estrogen use during pregnancy
- Positive family history
- Caucasian race
- In vitro fertilization
- Maternal smoking
- Older maternal age
- Placental anomalies
- Gestational diabetes/hypertension
- Vaginal bleeding in the first trimester
- Amniocentesis/chorionic villus sampling

The exact etiology of infantile hemangiomas has several hypotheses:

- Hypoxic stress upregulates expression of GLUT1 and VEGF leading to the mobilization of endothelial progenitor cells.
- Placental trophoblasts may serve as the origin of stem cells for hemangiomas.
- Vasculogenesis and angiogenesis

Clinical Features

Hemangiomas are characterized by three stages **(Table 1)**.

TABLE 1: Three stages of hemangioma.

PROLIFERATIVE PHASE	PLATEAU PHASE	INVOLUTION PHASE
Most rapid growth in the first 3–4 months followed by gradual growth that may continue up to 12 months of age	Between 6 and 12 months	Regression starts around 1 year of age; 90% of hemangioma involution is complete by the age of 4 years

- A hemangioma, usually, becomes apparent within 1–4 weeks after birth.
- *Precursor lesions:* Pale area of vasoconstriction/telangiectatic patch/bruise-like patches
- *Site:* Predilection for the head and neck; can occur anywhere in the skin, mucous membranes, and internal organs

Types of Hemangiomas

Types of hemangiomas are given in **Flowchart 3.**

FLOWCHART 3: Types of hemangiomas.

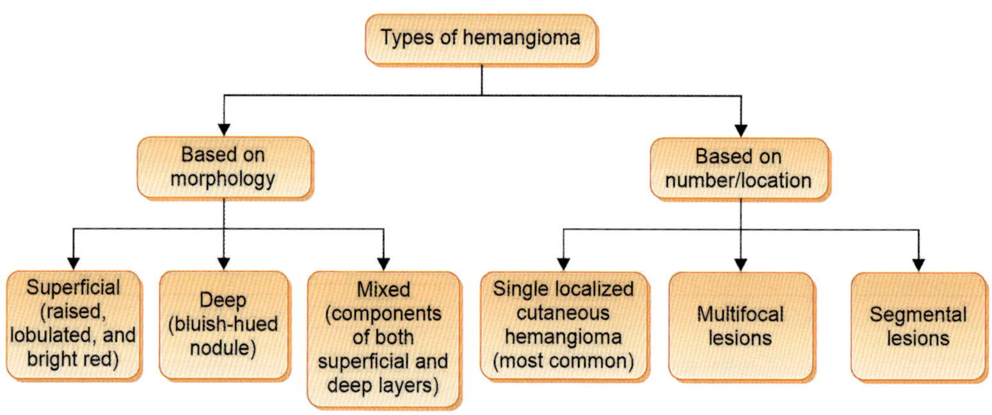

Evaluation of Hemangiomas

The approach to evaluation of hemangiomas is given in **Flowchart 4.**

FLOWCHART 4: Evaluation of hemangiomas.

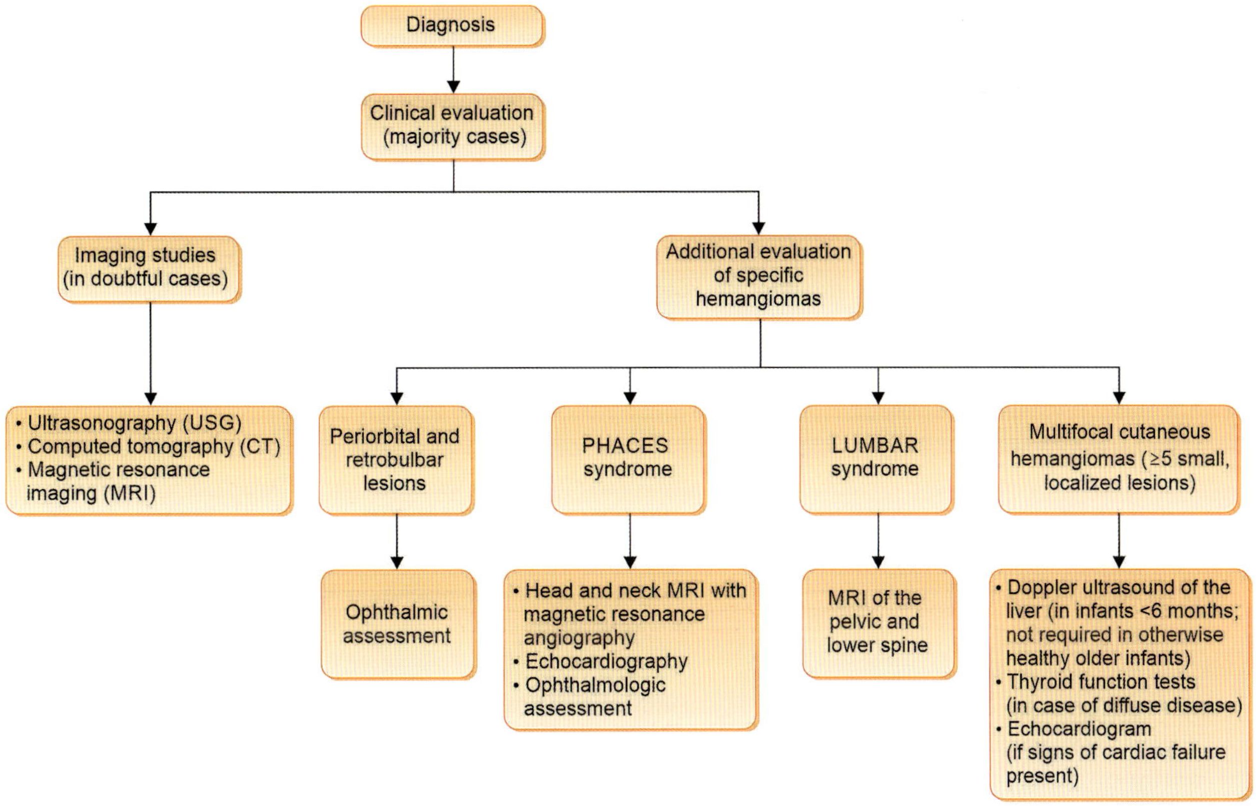

PHACE: Posterior fossa malformations, Hemangioma, Arterial anomalies, Coarctation of the aorta/cardiac defects, and Eye abnormalities; LUMBAR: Lower-body hemangioma, Urogenital abnormalities/ulceration, Myelopathy (severe compression) of the spinal cord, Bony deformities, Anorectal malformations and arterial anomalies, Renal anomalies

Red Flag Signs

The anatomic location of the hemangioma and their associated risks are given in **Table 2.**

TABLE 2: Red flag signs of infantile hemangiomas.

ASSOCIATED RISK	ANATOMIC LOCATION
Cosmetic disfigurement/scarring	Nasal tip, ear, perioral, and large facial lesions
Functional impairment	
Ophthalmic complication (astigmatism, amblyopia, myopia, tear-duct occlusion)	Periorbital and retrobulbar
Airway obstruction (nasal, subglottic and laryngeal passages)	Segmental "beard area" and central neck
Feeding difficulties	Perioral and oral lesions
Associated structural anomalies	
PHACES syndrome	*P*osterior fossa anomalies, *h*emangioma (large, segmental hemangioma on the face/head), *a*rterial anomalies, *c*ardiac anomalies, and *e*ye anomalies
LUMBAR syndrome	*L*ower-body hemangioma and other cutaneous defects; *u*rogenital anomalies/*u*lceration; *m*yelopathy, *b*ony deformities; *a*norectal malformations, *a*rterial anomalies; and *r*enal anomalies
Ulceration	Perineal, axilla, neck, and perioral
Visceral involvement (liver and gastrointestinal tract)	Multifocal cutaneous hemangiomas (≥5 small, localized lesions)
Very large (≥5 cm), rapidly growing cutaneous hemangiomas	–

Referral is recommended during the early hemangioma proliferation phase, ideally by 1 month of age, to a pediatric dermatologist/vascular anomalies team for infantile hemangiomas with potential risk for complications.

Suggested Reading

- George A, Mani V, Noufal A. Update on the classification of hemangioma. J Oral Maxillofacial Pathology. 2014; 18(Suppl 1):S117-20.
- Jung HL. Update on infantile hemangioma. Clin Exp Pediatr. 2021;64(11):559.
- Rodríguez Bandera AI, Sebaratnam DF, Wargon O, Wong LC. Infantile hemangioma. Part 1: Epidemiology, pathogenesis, clinical presentation and assessment. J Am Acad Dermatol. 2021;85(6):1379-92.
- Sebaratnam DF, Rodríguez Bandera AL, Wong LC, Wargon O. Infantile hemangioma. Part 2: Management. J Am Acad Dermatol. 2021;85(6):1395-404.
- Tiemann L, Hein S. Infantile hemangioma: A review of current pharmacotherapy treatment and practice pearls. J Pediatr Pharmacol Ther. 2020;25(7):586-99.

Rashes

110

Section Editor: **Gnanamurthy Narasimha**
Section Co-Editor: **Nagalatha Chidananda**
Authors: **Sahana M Srinivas, Hania Qamar Khan**

Introduction

Rashes in children can be due to infections and inflammation of skin, or underlying multisystem disorder, or may be a cutaneous sign of sinister problems like internal malignancies.

Types

They may be of different types **(Box. 1)**:

BOX 1: Types of rashes.

- *Macules:*
  - Changes in skin color
  - Hyperpigmented
  - Hypopigmented
- *Papules and plaques:*
  - *Papules:* Raised lesions <1 cm
  - *Plaques:* Raised lesions >1 cm
- *Vesicles and bullae:*
  - Fluid filled lesions
  - Vesicles <1 cm
  - Bullae >1 cm
- *Nodules:*
  - Deep-seated lesions
  - Better felt than seen
- *Petechiae and purpura:*
  - Extravasated blood in skin
  - *Petechiae:* Pinpoint
  - *Purpura:* <1 cm

Etiology and Presentation

Macular Rash

- *Hypopigmented macules* ***(Box 2)***:

BOX 2: Presentation and etiology of hypopigmented macules.

- *Nevus depigmentosus:* Birthmark characterized by well-defined hypopigmented macule; onset is at birth or early infancy; the lesions are usually single but may be multiple.
- *Vitiligo:* Depigmented macules present over skin; may be associated with depigmented hair (leukotrichia) and other autoimmune disorders
- *Pityriasis alba*: A form of low-grade eczema characterized by ill-defined hypopigmented macules most commonly on the face in young children.
- *Hansen's disease:* Dry-looking, hypoaesthetic macules; often feeding nerves may be present,
- *Pityriasis versicolor*: Caused by yeast *Malassezia furfur*, present with fine, scaly hypo- or hyperpigmented macules usually over the chest and back (seborrheic distribution).

- *Hyperpigmented macules* ***(Box 3)***:

BOX 3: Etiology and presentation of hyperpigmented macules.

- *Freckles:* Irregular, small, dark colored spots, seen over the sun-exposed parts in light-colored individuals.
- *Lentigines:* These are characterized by well-defined pigmented macules, larger than freckles. They may be isolated or part of genetic syndromes such as:
  - LEOPARD syndrome
  - Carney complex—associated with myxoma
  - Peutz–Jeghers syndrome
  - Gardner syndrome
- *Café-au-lait macules (CALMs):* These are well-defined coffee-brown spots with onset at birth or early childhood. They can be seen in normal individuals (<6 CALMs). Associated disorders are:
  - Neurofibromatosis
  - Tuberous sclerosis
  - McCune–Albright syndrome
  - Legius syndrome
  - Multiple endocrine neoplasia (MEN) syndrome
  - Noonan syndrome
  - Bloom syndrome

- *Erythematous macules:*
  - Hemangioma
  - Capillary malformation (port-wine stain/nevus simplex)

Papules and Plaques

The commonly seen causes of papules are depicted in **Flowchart 1**.

FLOWCHART 1: Commonly seen causes of papules.

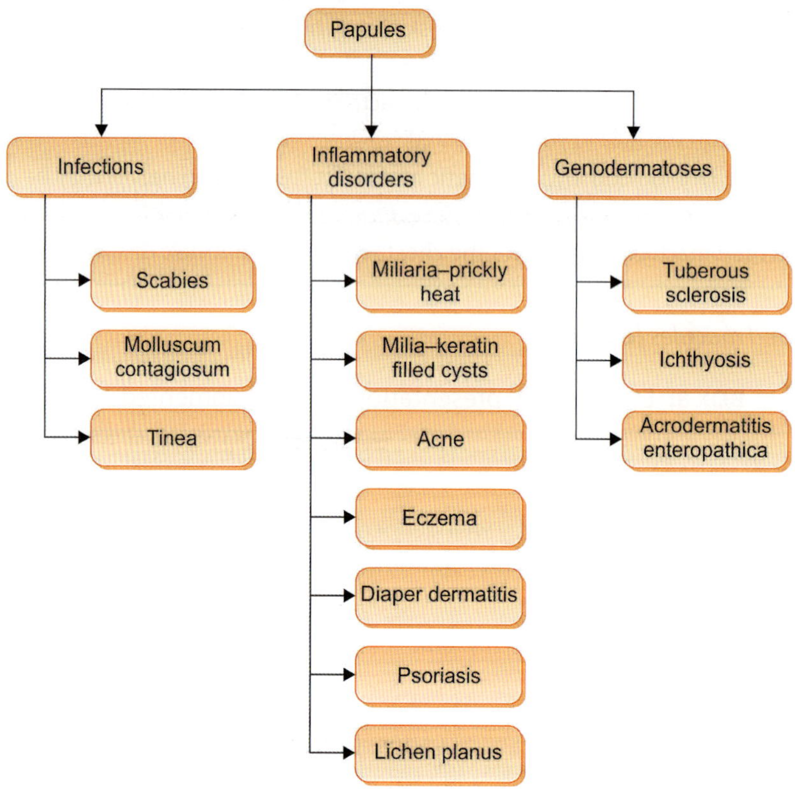

Vesicles and Bullae

Commonly seen conditions presenting as vesicles and bullae are given in **Flowchart 2**.

FLOWCHART 2: Commonly seen conditions presenting as vesicles and bullae.

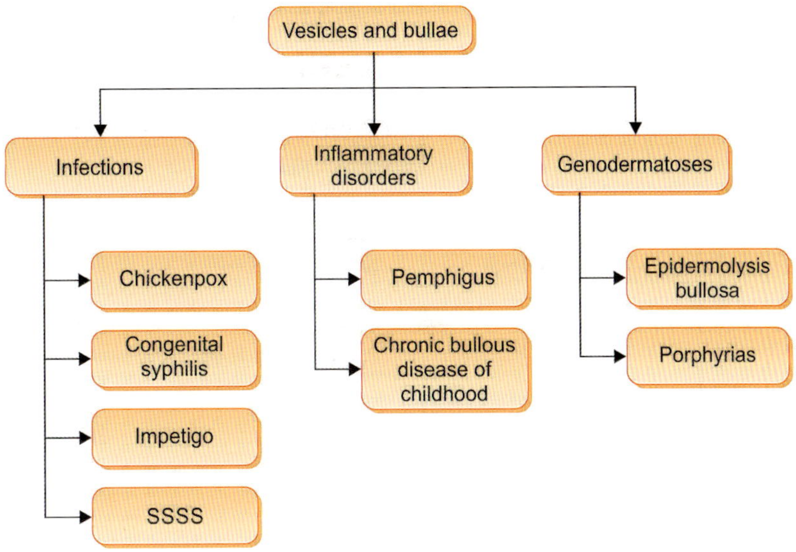

SSSS: Staphylococcal scalded skin syndrome

Petechiae and Purpura

- *Diascopy:* Lesion does not blanch on pressing with glass slide.
- *Purpura fulminans:*
  - Life-threatening emergency
  - Symmetrical diffuse purpura due to disseminated intravascular coagulation
  - *Causes **(Flowchart 3)**:*
    - *Neonatal:* Clotting defects
    - *Acute infections:* Meningococcus, rickettsia, leptospirosis, etc.
    - *Idiopathic:* 7–10 days after streptococcal infection

FLOWCHART 3: Causes of purpura.

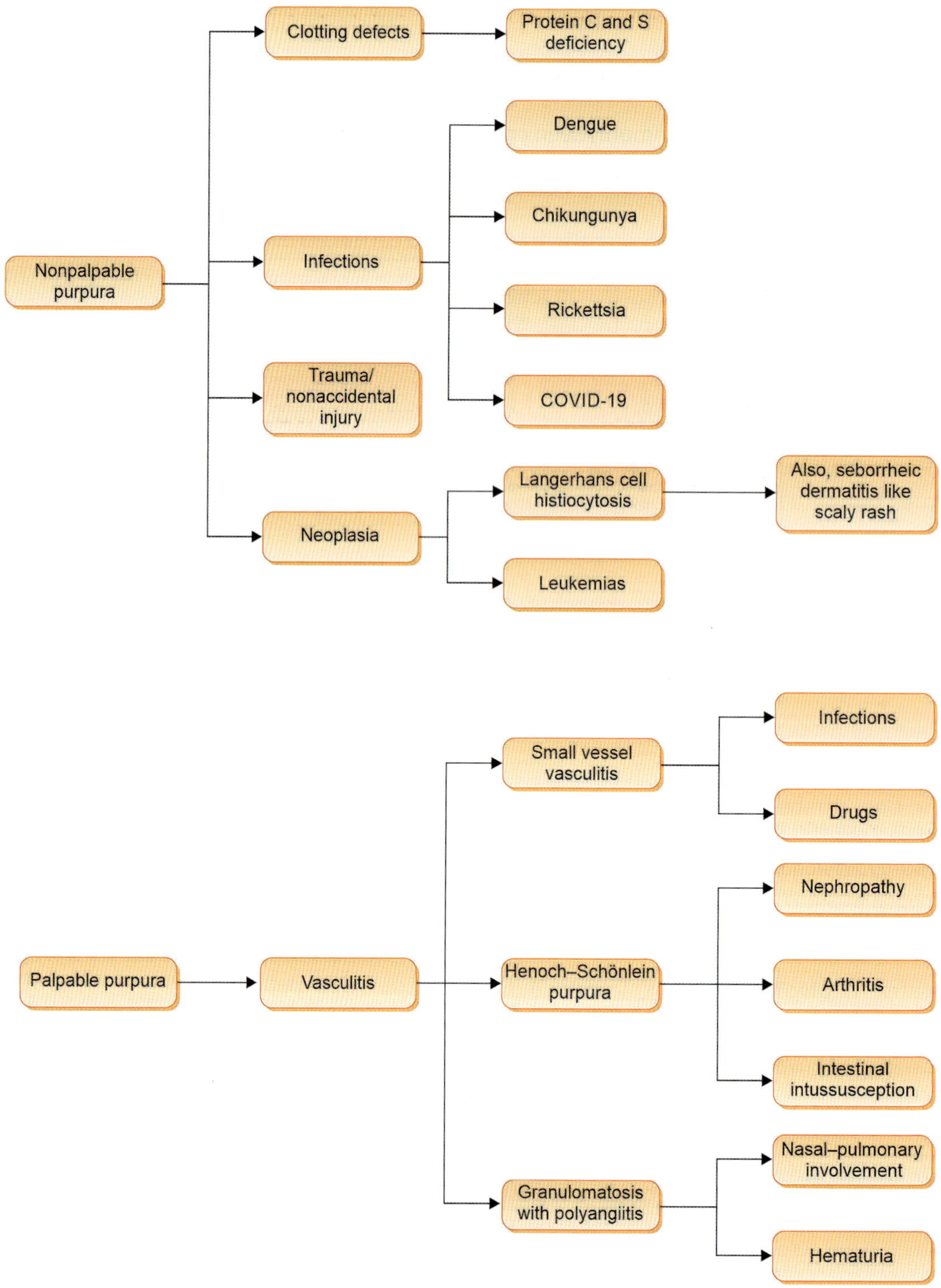

COVID: coronavirus disease

Nodules

The common causes of nodules to be known by pediatricians are given in **Flowchart 4**.

FLOWCHART 4: Common causes of nodules.

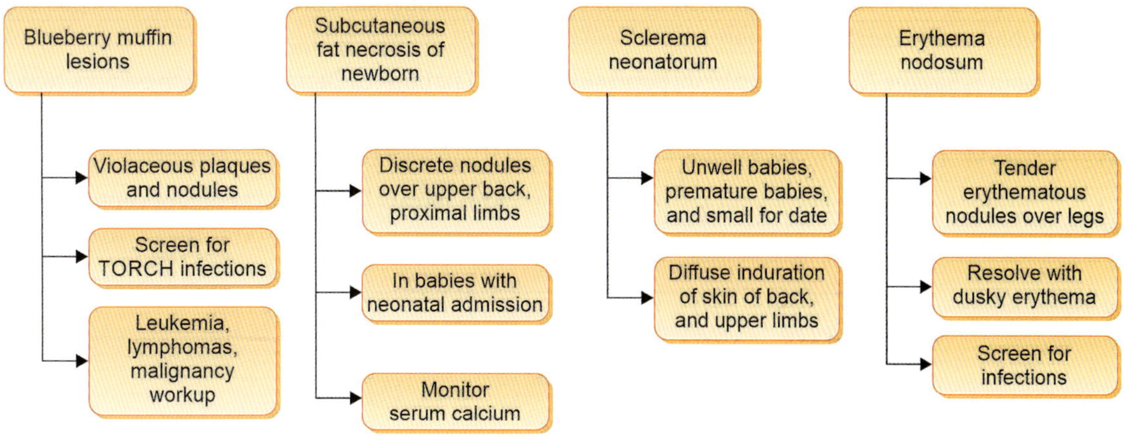

TORCH: toxoplasmosis, others (syphilis, hepatitis B), rubella, cytomegalovirus, herpes simplex

Red Flag Signs in Pediatric Rashes

Erythroderma: Erythema and scaling involving over 90% body surface area.

The red flag signs are given in **Table 1**.

TABLE 1: Red flag signs in pediatric rashes.

CONDITIONS	NEONATAL	INFANTILE
Ichthyosis	• Netherton syndrome • Congenital ichthyosiform erythroderma • Nonbullous ichthyosiform erythema	
Eczema	Seborrheic sermatitis	Atopic eczema
Metabolic disorders	• Holocarboxylase deficiency • Biotinidase deficiency • Essential fatty acid deficiency	
Immunodeficiency syndromes	Hyper IgE syndrome	
Inflammatory disorders		Psoriasis
Infections	• Congenital candidiasis • Staphylococcal scalded skin syndrome	• Neonatal candidiasis • Dermatophytosis
Drugs	–	Toxic epidermal necrolysis
Malignancies		• Langerhans cell histiocytosis • Leukemia • Cutaneous lymphomas

Suggested Reading

- Dhar S, Srinivas S. Color Atlas and Synopsis of Pediatric Dermatology, 4th edition. New Delhi: Jaypee Brothers Medical Publishers (P) Ltd; 2021.
- Sacchidanand S, Savitha AS, Shilpa K, Shashi Kumar BM. IADVL Textbook of Dermatology, 5th edition. New Delhi: Bhalani Publishing House; 2022.
- Sarkar R, Garg VK. Erythroderma in children. Indian J Dermatol Venereol Leprol. 2010;76(4):341-7.
- Sarkar R, Mishra K, Garg VK. Fever with rash in a child in India. Indian J Dermatol Venereol Leprol. 2012;78(3): 251-62.

Bleeding Neonate

111

Section Editor: **Nehal Patel**
Section Co-Editor: **Jay T Dhirwani**
Authors: **Vishnu Mohan PT, Manikumar S**

Introduction

- *Neonatal* bleeding can be life threatening.
- Thrombocytopenia is the most frequent abnormality.
- 6% of neonatal intensive care unit (NICU) admissions have severe thrombocytopenia of <50/nL

Approach

In neonates, plasma concentrations of many factors are low by nearly 50% and increase to adult levels by 6 months of age.

- *Sick neonates:* Think of acquired coagulation defects
- *Healthy neonates:* Think of inherited coagulation defects

Clinical presentations of neonatal bleeding are given in **Box 1**.

BOX 1: Clinical presentations.

- Extracranial (subgaleal bleed and cephalohematoma)
- Puncture sites (heel prick, newborn screen, or immunizations)
- Intracranial
- Skin bleeds (petechiae, purpura, and ecchymosis)
- Persistent oozing from umbilical stump
- Bleeding from gastrointestinal tract (GIT), urinary tract, and respiratory tract are rare

Various mimics of serious bleeding disorders are given in **Box 2**.

BOX 2: Mimics of serious bleeding disorders.

- Gastrointestinal tract (GIT) bleeding from swallowed maternal blood—'Apt test' to differentiate
- Ecchymoses on presenting part especially in breech presentation
- Mosquito-bite spots versus petechiae (true skin bleeds would not blanch completely)
- Vulval bleeding at 3–7 days of life in a female
- Pink urine from urate crystals in the first 3 days of life/beyond
- Extracranial bleeds (high risk when both forceps/vacuum attempted); needs evaluation if increasing in size
- Umbilical bleeding from slipped ligature
- Isolated intraventricular hemorrhage in the 1st week of life in a very preterm neonate

Apt test: Fetal hemoglobin is resistant to alkali. Mix 1 part of vomitus with 5 parts of saline. Centrifuge at 2,000 rpm for 10 minutes. Add 4 mL of 10% sodium hydroxide (NaOH) to 1 mL supernatant. Brown color indicates maternal blood and pink indicates fetal blood.

Sampling errors/spurious values need to be ruled out **(Box 3)**.

BOX 3: Causes of Sampling errors/spurious values.

- Common in neonates, especially if polycythemic (high hematocrit reduces plasma to citrate ratio in the sample)
- Tissue factor activation in a sample may mask severe factor VIII deficiency.
- Difficult venipuncture results in contamination and activation by tissue factor.

Three-generation pedigree for known Mendelian inheritance is required **(Box 4)**.

BOX 4: Family history.

- *X-linked recessive inheritance:* Hemophilia A (factor VIII deficiency) and B (factor IX deficiency)
- *Autosomal dominant:* von Willebrand disease, dysfibrinogenemia, and hemorrhagic telangiectasia
- *Autosomal recessive:* Other factor deficiencies

One third of hemophilia A cases result from spontaneous mutations.

Approach to a neonate with thrombocytopenia is illustrated in **Flowchart 1.**

FLOWCHART 1: Approach to a neonate with thrombocytopenia.

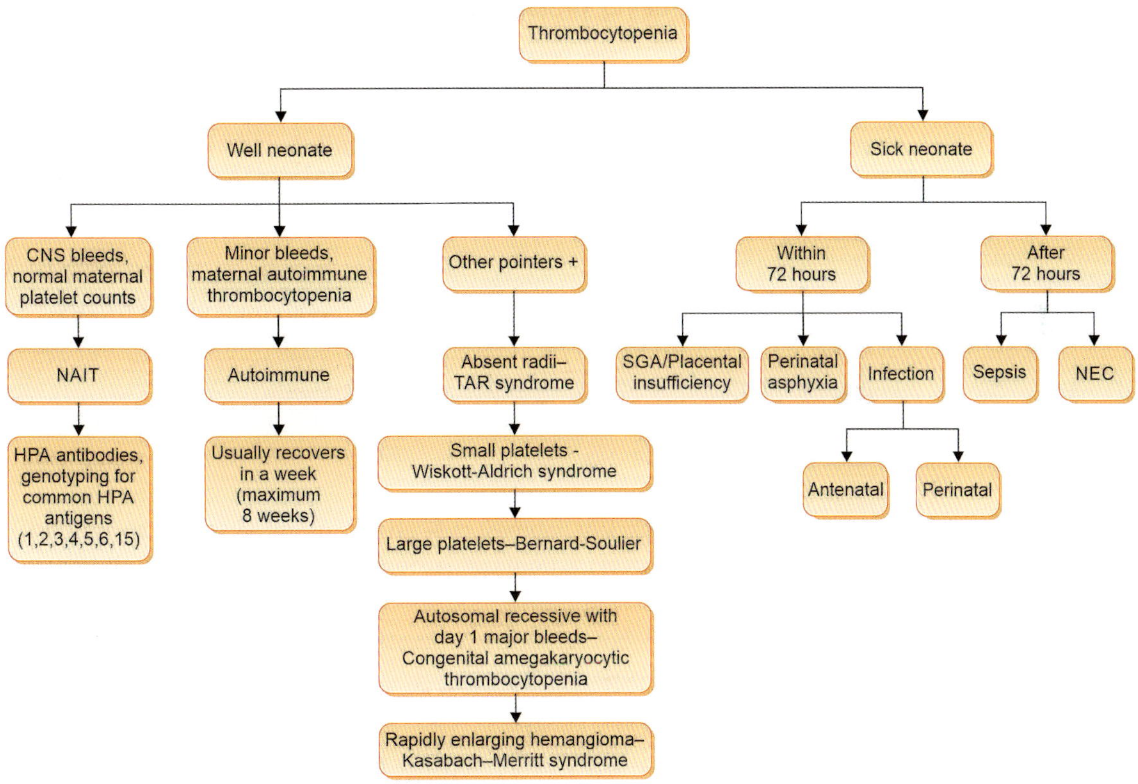

CNS: central nervous system; HPA: human platelet antigens; NEC: necrotizing enterocolitis; NAIT: neonatal alloimmune thrombocytopenia; SGA: small for gestational age; TAR: thrombocytopenia absent radius

Approach to a neonate with coagulation abnormality is illustrated in **Figure 1**.

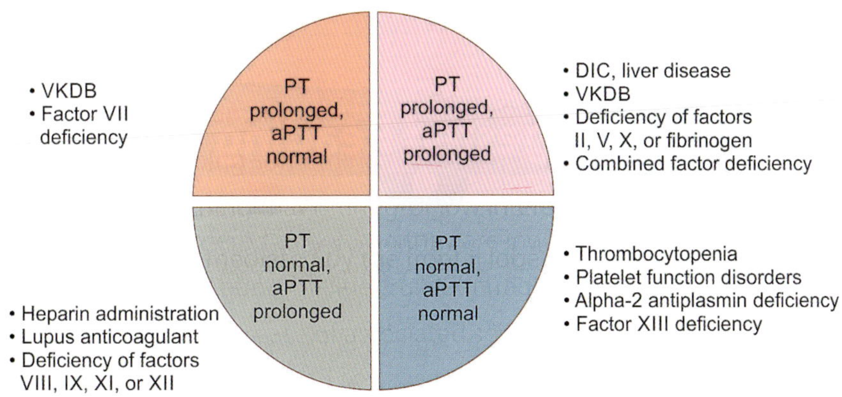

FIG 1: Approach to a neonate with coagulation abnormality.

Note: VKDB, DIC, liver disease, heparin administration, lupus anticoagulant, and thrombocytopenia are acquired coagulation defects typically seen in sick neonates.

The rest are inherited coagulation defects typically seen in healthy neonates.

aPTT: activated partial thromboplastin time; DIC: disseminated intravascular coagulation; PT: prothrombin time; VKDB: vitamin K deficiency bleeding

Vitamin K Deficiency Bleeding

A major cause of preventable serious bleeding in a neonate is vitamin K deficiency bleeding (VKDB). It manifests with prothrombin time (PT) being prolonged and disproportionate to the activated partial thromboplastin time (aPTT).

Features of VKDB are given in **Table 1**.

TABLE 1: Features of vitamin K deficiency bleeding.

FEATURE	EARLY VKDB	CLASSIC VKDB	LATE VKDB
Onset	Within 24 hours	1–7 days	>7 days–6 months
Incidence	6–12% without maternal prophylaxis	0.25–1.7% if no prophylaxis at birth, <0.2/100,000 with prophylaxis	80 infants per 100,000 births in LMIC without prophylaxis, 6/100,000 with prophylaxis
Presentation	Cranial, intrathoracic, and GIT	Often mild bleeds gastrointestinal, nasal, and skin	Often major bleeds 50% intracranial bleed, and 69% multifocal hemorrhages
Etiology	Maternal drugs affecting vitamin K metabolism	Low placental transfer, deficient in breast milk, and lack of gastrointestinal flora	Those who have not received prophylaxis, may suggest an underlying malabsorption or hepatic dysfunction
Protection offered by vitamin K birth dose	Some reduction	81% reduction in moderate-to-severe bleeding	97% reduction
Outcome	CNS bleeds have poor prognosis (50%)	Usually favorable	20–50% mortality and 42.8% neurologic deficits

CNS: central nervous system; GIT: gastrointestinal tract; LMIC: low-and middle-income countries; VKDB: vitamin K deficiency bleeding

Suggested Reading

- Campbell SE, Bolton-Maggs PH. Congenital and acquired bleeding disorders in infancy. Earl Hum Dev. 2015;91(11):637-42.
- Sankar MJ, Chandrasekaran A, Kumar P, Thukral A, Agarwal R, Paul VK. Vitamin K prophylaxis for prevention of vitamin K deficiency bleeding: A systematic review. J Perinatol. 2016;36(Suppl 1):S29-35.

Fever of Short Duration

112

Section Editor: **B Rajsekhar**
Section Co-Editor: **Suchitra Pusapati**
Authors: **G Sudhakar, Sinchana Bhat**

Introduction

Fever of short duration is defined as rectal temperature >100.4°F lasting <7 days. A comprehensive approach will rule out occult bacteremia and serious bacterial infections (SBI).

Etiology (Table 1)

Based on the cause:

- *Infections:*
  - *Viral:* Respiratory syncytial virus (RSV) and influenza
  - *Gastrointestinal:* Acute watery diarrhea and bacillary dysentery
  - *Bacterial:* Urinary tract infection (UTI), pneumonia, acute otitis media (AOM), and meningitis
  - *Tropical:* Dengue, malaria, scrub typhus, leptospirosis, and enteric fever

TABLE 1: Diagnostic pointers to an etiology of fever.

ETIOLOGY	DIAGNOSTIC POINTERS
Family history of fever, daycare attendance, well between fever spikes	Viral fever
Excessive crying during micturition, costovertebral tenderness with high-grade fever	• UTI • Pyelonephritis
Altered sensorium, inconsolable cry, bulging fontanelle, and meningismus (older children)	Meningitis
Inconsolable cry, congestion/bulging of the tympanic membrane, and crying in sleep	Acute otitis media
Congested throat, exudates pharyngitis, petechiae on soft palate and uvula, strawberry tongue, and cervical adenopathy	• Acute pharyngitis • Scarlet fever
Painful cervical lymph nodes	Acute cervical lymphadenitis
• Tachypnea and grunting toxic appearance • Well-appearing with respiratory distress	• Bacterial pneumonia • Bronchiolitis
Right-sided abdominal pain, and toxic appearance	Right lower lobe pneumonia
• Loose stools, vomiting, and abdominal pain • Tender hepatomegaly and icterus • Palpable soft spleen	• Acute gastroenteritis • Viral hepatitis • Enteric fever
Tachycardia, hypotension, and petechiae on skin	Dengue fever
Strawberry tongue, unilateral lymphadenopathy, and fissuring of lips	Kawasaki disease
Swollen painful joint/limb, decreased range of movement, and Paradoxical crying on holding	Septic arthritis/osteomyelitis
Rash: Maculopapular and vesicular	HMFD, measles, dengue, rickettsia and varicella

(HFMD: hand-foot-and-mouth disease; UTI: urinary tract infection)

- *Noninfective:*
  - *Inflammatory:* Kawasaki disease
  - *Postvaccination:* Within 24–48 hours and in case of measles vaccine—after a week
  - Heatstroke
  - *Toxins:* Cocaine, methamphetamine, and tricyclic antidepressants
- *Based on the age:*
  - *1–3 months:* Occurs commonly, self-limiting viral infection, 5% may be in an early phase of an SBI.
  - *3–36 months:* Occurs commonly in viral infections; risk of SBI in well-appearing, partially immunized/unimmunized children is around 1%; *Streptococcus pneumoniae*, *Staphylococcus aureus*, *Neisseria meningitidis*, *Haemophilus influenzae* type B are common organisms; completely immunized children have a risk of bacteremia <0.5%.
  - *>36 months:*
    - *Viruses:* RSV, influenza, parainfluenza, enterovirus, and varicella
    - *Bacteria: Streptococcus*, pneumococcus, *Staphylococcus*, *Haemophilus*, and *Mycoplasma*

Red Flag Signs

- Altered sensorium/excessive irritability/lethargy/seizures
- Impaired circulation/mottled skin/cyanosis
- Warm body with cool extremities
- Disproportionate tachycardia/respiratory rate
- Not feeding well
- Severe dehydration
- Respiratory distress/failure/SpO_2 <94% in room air

Approach

The approach to managing fever of short duration is given in **Flowchart 1**.

FLOWCHART 1: Approach to the management of fever of short duration.

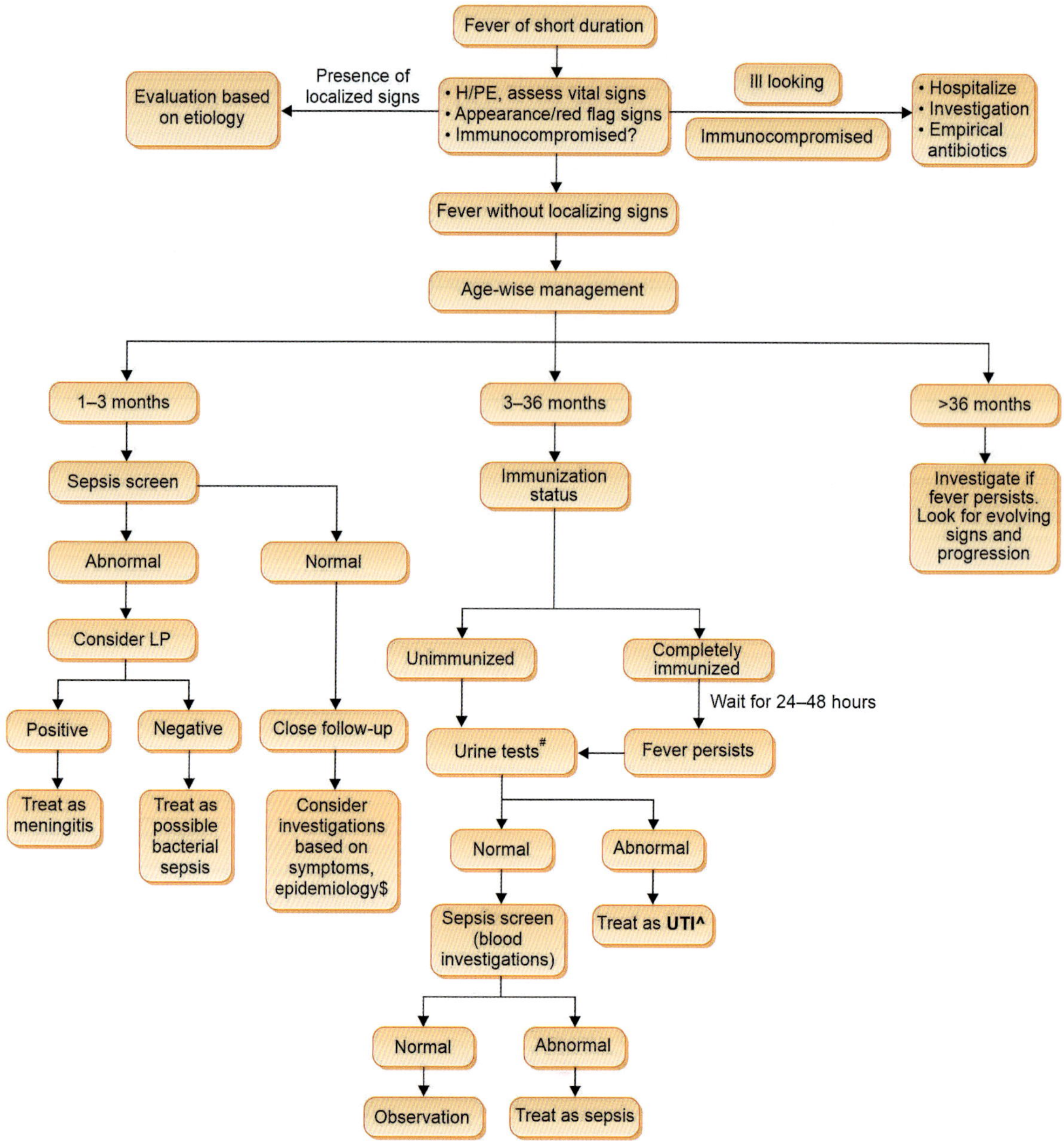

(H/PE: history and physical examination; LP: Lumbar puncture, Abx: antibiotics, UTI: urinary tract infection)

Note: $: possible tropical etiology workup

Contd...

Contd...

#Risk factors for UTI—circumcised boys <6 months, uncircumcised <12 months, girls <2 years, previous UTI, and anomalies of urinary tract

Cultures, LP should be done before beginning antibiotics. LP indicated in sick infants/in well-looking positive septic screen (<3 months)/if strong suspicion of meningitis/neurological signs in older children.

Septic Screen: Complete blood count (CBC), absolute neutrophil count (ANC), C-reactive protein (CRP), procalcitonin*, urine analysis and culture, and blood culture

**Highly sensitive and specific, however subject to availability and cost affordability*

Chest X-ray [If respiratory signs are present/white blood cell (WBC) count >15,000/cu mm]

Suggested Reading

- Barbi E, Marzuillo P, Neri E, Naviglio S, Krauss BS. Fever in Children: Pearls and Pitfalls. Children (Basel). 2017;4(9):81.
- For Academic College of Emergency Experts in India (ACEE-INDIA)–INDO US Emergency and Trauma Collaborative; Mahajan P, Batra P, Thakur N, Patel R, Rai N, Trivedi N, et al. Consensus Guidelines on Evaluation and Management of the Febrile Child Presenting to the Emergency Department in India. Indian Pediatr. 2017;54(8):652-60.
- NICE Guideline Updates Team (UK). Fever in under 5s: Assessment and initial management (NICE guideline, No. 143). London: National Institute for Health and Care Excellence; 2019.
- Pantell RH, Roberts KB, Adams WG, Dreyer BP, Kuppermann N, O'Leary ST, et al. Clinical Practice Guideline: Evaluation and management of well-appearing febrile infants 8 to 60 days old. Pediatrics. 2021;148(2):e2021052228.

Fever with Joint Pains

113

***Section Editor:* B Rajsekhar**
***Section Co-Editor:* Suchitra Pusapati**
***Author:* Abhay Shivpuri**

Introduction

Fever with joint pains can present in children of any age. Before diagnosing a child with inflammatory arthritis and commencing steroids, it is vital to rule out other causes such as infections, neoplasias, and immunodeficiencies.

History

- *Characteristics of joint pains and fever:*
  - *Acute:* Trauma, infections, and reactive arthritis
  - *Inflammatory pains:* Early morning stiffness >30 minutes in joints and aggravation of pain after rest
- *Precipitating factors:* Trauma and preceding illness
- *Associated symptoms:*
  - *Acute rheumatic fever:* Migratory arthralgia/arthritis
  - *Inborn errors of immunity (IEI):* Recurrent skin, lung, ear infections; frequent hospitalizations; or history of sibling deaths
  - *Systemic autoinflammatory diseases (SAID):* Early age at onset, recurrent fevers, unexplained rashes, and family history of recurrent fevers
- *Associated co-morbidities:* Inflammatory bowel disease (IBD), psoriasis, uveitis, connective tissue diseases (CTD) like systemic lupus erythematosus (SLE), juvenile dermatomyositis (JDM), sarcoidosis, scleroderma, etc.
- *Ask about family history suggesting:* Psoriasis, IBD, spondyloarthropathies, periodic fevers, history of tuberculosis (TB) contact

Physical Examination

- *General appearance:* Failure to thrive, height and weight for age
- *Skin examination:*
  - *SLE:* Malar rash and hair loss
  - *JDM:* Heliotrope rash and Gottron's papules
  - *Systemic juvenile idiopathic arthritis (SJIA):* Evanescent pink maculopapular rashes
  - *IgA vasculitis [Henoch–Schönlein purpura (HSP)]:* Lower extremity palpable purpura
  - *Acute rheumatic fever:* Erythema marginatum and subcutaneous nodules
  - *Kawasaki disease:* Polymorphous rashes, subcutaneous edema, and skin peeling
- *Eye examination:*
  - *Oligoarticular JIA:* Silent chronic uveitis
  - *Enthesitis-related arthritis:* Acute symptomatic uveitis
  - *Kawasaki disease:* Nonsuppurative conjunctival injection, and perilimbal sparing
- *Oral examination:*
  - *SLE:* Oral ulcers and palate mucositis
  - *Kawasaki disease:* Mucositis and strawberry tongue
- *Respiratory examination:*
  - *IEI:* Recurrent pneumonias
  - *SLE/scleroderma/SJIA:* Pleuritis and interstitial lung disease
- *Cardiovascular examination:*
  - *SLE/SJIA/acute rheumatic fever (ARF):* Pericarditis
  - *SLE/Scleroderma*: Raynaud phenomenon
  - *Kawasaki disease:* Myocarditis and coronary aneurysms
- *Gastrointestinal examination:*
  - *IBD:* Poor growth, weight loss, diarrhea, and abdominal pains
  - *Reactive arthritis:* Preceding infectious gastroenteritis
  - *IgA vasculitis:* Intermittent colicky abdominal pains
  - *Periodic fevers:* Episodes of pain in abdomen during fevers
- *Genitourinary examination:*
  - *Gonococcal arthritis*: Pustular urethritis or cervicitis
  - *Reactive arthritis:* Nongonococcal urethritis

- *Neurologic examination:*
  - *SLE:* Seizures, psychosis, emotional lability, and stroke
  - *Kawasaki disease:* Severe irritability or asymmetric polyneuropathy
  - *Childhood vasculitis:* Stroke
  - *JDM:* Proximal muscle weakness
- *Joint examination:*
  - Referred pain (e.g., knee pain due to hip synovitis)
  - Pediatric gait, arms, legs, and spine (p-GALS) screening for joint examination

Approach to Diagnosis and Management

A simplified approach is shown in the **Flowchart 1**.

FLOWCHART 1: A simplified approach to diagnosis and management of fever with joint pains.

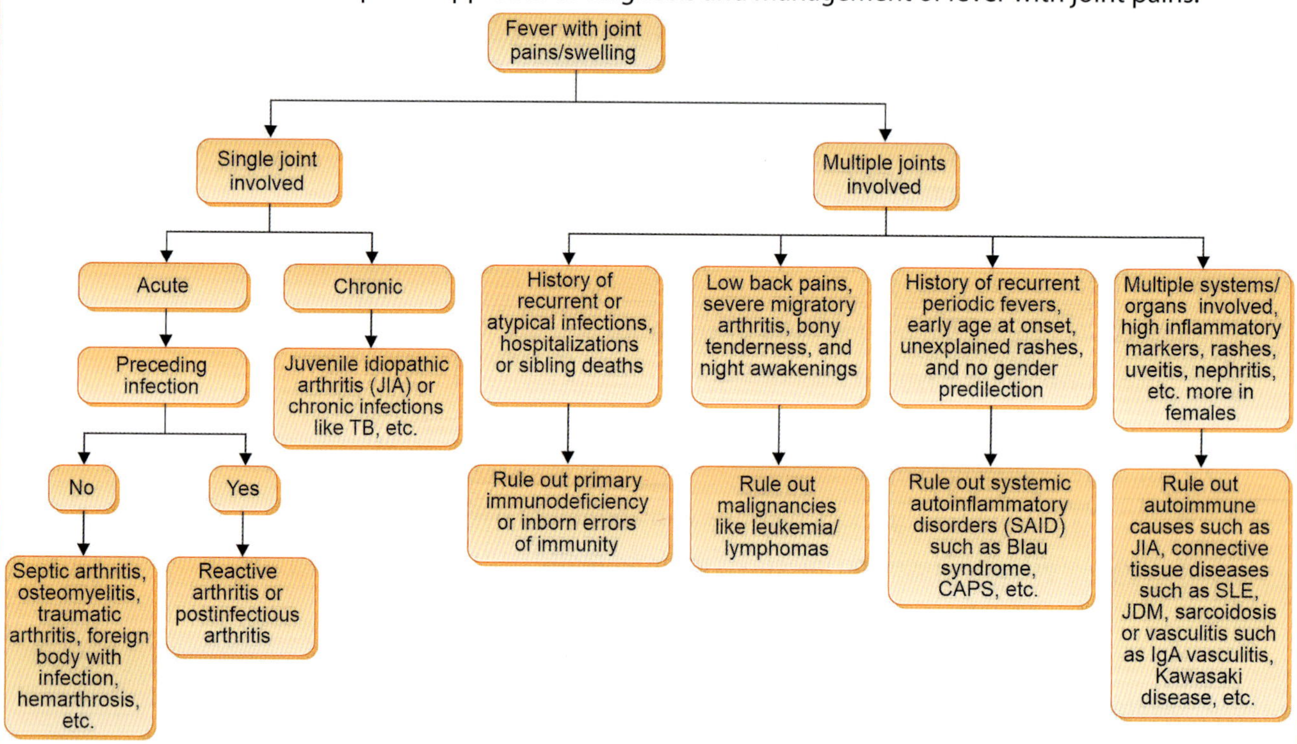

(CAPS: cryopyrin-associated autoinflammatory syndromes; JDM: juvenile dermatomyositis; SLE: systemic lupus erythematosus; TB: tuberculosis)

Red Flag Signs

- Severe night pains and awakenings
- Migratory arthritis/arthralgias
- Bony tenderness, low back pain, and periarthritic pain
- Reduced appetite and weight loss
- *Blood reports:* Cytopenias, lymphocytic predominant white blood cells (WBC), raised uric acid, lactate dehydrogenase (LDH) or an abnormal blood film showing blast cells
- Reduced appetite, fatigue, weight loss, organomegaly, and lymphadenopathy
- Investigations showing cytopenias, leukocytosis, lymphocytic predominant differential counts, raised uric acid and LDH, and blast cells in blood film

Suggested Reading

- Balan S. Approach to joint pain in children. Indian J Pediatr. 2016;83(2):135-39.
- Haines KA. The Approach to the child with joint complaints. Pediatr Clin North Am. 2018;65(4):623-38.
- Sen ES, Clarke SL, Ramanan AV. The child with joint pain in primary care. Best Pract Res Clin Rheumatol. 2014;28(6):888-906.

Fever of Unknown Origin 114

Section Editor: **B Rajsekhar**
Section Co-Editor: **Suchitra Pusapati**
Authors: **Bhaskar Shenoy, Harshini T Reddy**

Introduction

- Fever of unknown origin (FUO) is characterized by a prolonged fever without a discernible source following a thorough evaluation.
- There should be a documented temperature >38°C (100.4°F) by a healthcare provider, with no identifiable cause despite 8 days of thorough evaluation.

Classification

CLASSIC	HEALTHCARE-ASSOCIATED	IMMUNODEFICIENT	HIV-ASSOCIATED
• *Temperature:* ≥38°C • *Duration:* 3 weeks • *No cause identified with:* – 1 week IP investigations – ≥2 OPD visits	• *Temperature:* ≥38°C • *Duration:* After 1 week of hospitalization • Not present/ in incubation at admission	• *Temperature:* ≥38°C • *Duration:* ≥1 week • Negative culture after 48 hours	• In HIV patients • *Temperature:* ≥38°C • *No cause identified with:* – ≥1 week IP investigations – ≥3 weeks of OPD evaluation

(HIV: human immunodeficiency virus; IP: inpatient; OPD: outpatient department)

Etiology

- Etiology includes the following:
  - Infections
  - Rheumatologic (connective tissue or autoimmune)
  - Autoinflammatory
  - Oncologic
  - Neurologic
  - Genetic
  - Factitious
  - Iatrogenic
- Most FUOs are atypical presentations of common diseases.
- Sometimes, the presentation is characteristic yet a definitive diagnosis is established only after prolonged observation; initial clinical manifestations and lab results are normal/negative.
- At every clinical encounter, review for any "red flag" signs.

Red Flag Signs

- Weight loss
- Increased lethargy
- Drenching night sweats
- Inability to perform activities of daily living
- Changes in other symptomatology and physical examination

Diagnostic Clues

CONDITIONS	CLUES FROM HISTORY AND PHYSICAL EXAMINATION
Brucellosis	Contact/consumption of products from infected goats, pigs, buffalo, cows, and unpasteurized milk; hepatosplenomegaly, suppurative musculoskeletal lesions, uveitis, hepatitis, and pancytopenia
Enteric fever	Consumption of contaminated food/water; headache, arthritis, hepatosplenomegaly, leukopenia, and relative bradycardia
Leptospirosis	Occupational exposure in rice/sugarcane fields, recreational water sports; bitemporal and frontal headache, calf and lumbar muscle tenderness, conjunctival suffusion, and hepatic and renal failure
Juvenile idiopathic arthritis	Hepatosplenomegaly, lymphadenopathy, evanescent rash, anemia, and elevated inflammatory markers
Sarcoidosis	Fatigue, weight loss, leg pain, anemia, elevated inflammatory markers, uveitis, and mediastinal lymphadenopathy
Dress syndrome	Prescription/nonprescription exposure of drugs; exanthem, eosinophilia, and organ dysfunction

Approach to Fever of Unknown Origin in Children more than 3 Months of Age

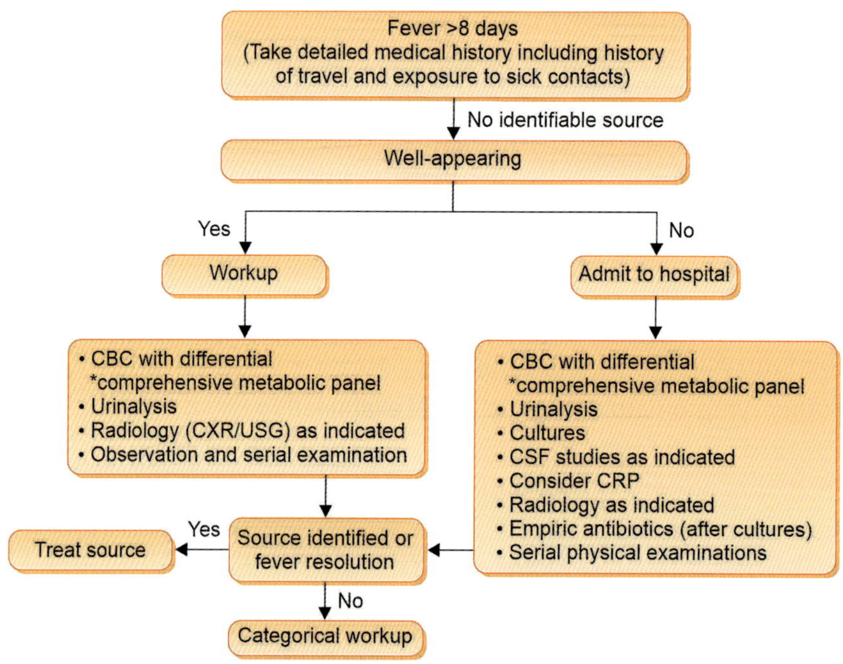

Comprehensive metabolic panel: Calcium, glucose, liver and renal function tests, and electrolytes
(CBC: complete blood count; CRP: C-reactive protein; CSF: cerebrospinal fluid; CXR: chest X-ray; USG: ultrasonography)

Second-line Investigations

- Bone marrow examination
- *Infectious disease workup:* Serology [Epstein–Barr virus (EBV) and human immunodeficiency virus (HIV)], molecular diagnostics [multiplex polymerase chain reaction (PCR)], specific cultures [tuberculosis (TB) and prolonged incubation for *Brucella*], and rule out HIV
- Autoantibody profiles for rheumatologic and autoimmune conditions
- Advanced imaging modalities [computed tomography (CT), magnetic resonance imaging (MRI), and positron emission tomography (PET)] are to be considered if initial imaging is equivocal or negative based on clinical suspicion.
- Specialist opinion

Suggested Reading

- Kliegman R, Stanton B, St Geme JW, Schor NF, Behrman RE, Nelson WE (Eds). Nelson Textbook of Pediatrics, 21st edition. Philadelphia PA: Elsevier; 2020.

Headache

115

Section Editor: **Janani Shankar**
Section Co-Editor: **Arathi Srinivasan**
Authors: **Mounika B, Arijit Chattopadhyay**

Introduction

Headache is a common complaint that is encountered in the outpatient department. It is a leading cause of disability in adolescents and young adults (10–24 years).

Etiology

Most often the headache is primary—migraine, tension headache, and trigeminal autonomic cephalalgias.

The causes of secondary headaches are as follows:

- *Infection:*
  - *Localized:* Upper respiratory/face/eyes/ear infections
  - *Central nervous system (CNS):* Meningitis/brain abscess
- *Ingestion:*
  - Medications like oral contraceptive pills (OCPs), steroids, selective serotonin reuptake inhibitors (SSRI), and serotonin and norepinephrine reuptake inhibitors (SNRI)
  - Growth hormone, tetracyclines, vitamin A, and steroids withdrawal are associated with idiopathic intracranial hypertension.

- Head injuries
- Cranial/cervical vascular disorders
- Nonvascular intracranial disorders
- Intracranial tumor
- *Cranial neuropathies:*
  - Trigeminal neuralgia
  - Glossopharyngeal neuralgia
  - Facial nerve entrapment
- *Systemic conditions:*
  - Hypoxia/hypercapnia
  - High altitude
  - Hypertension
  - Pheochromocytoma
- *Psychiatric disorders:*
  - Somatization disorder
  - Psychotic disorder

Red Flag Signs

SYMPTOMS	SIGNS
Vomiting	Abnormal neurological examination
Blurring of vision	Lethargic, ataxia, and altered level of consciousness
Unsteadiness of gait	Increased autonomic symptoms
Irritability	Hypertension/Hypotension
Refusal of feeds	Bradycardia
Seizures	Diplopia
	Papilledema/retinal hemorrhage
	Neurocutaneous markers
	Bruit of head, neck, and eyes [arteriovenous (AV) malformation]

Approach

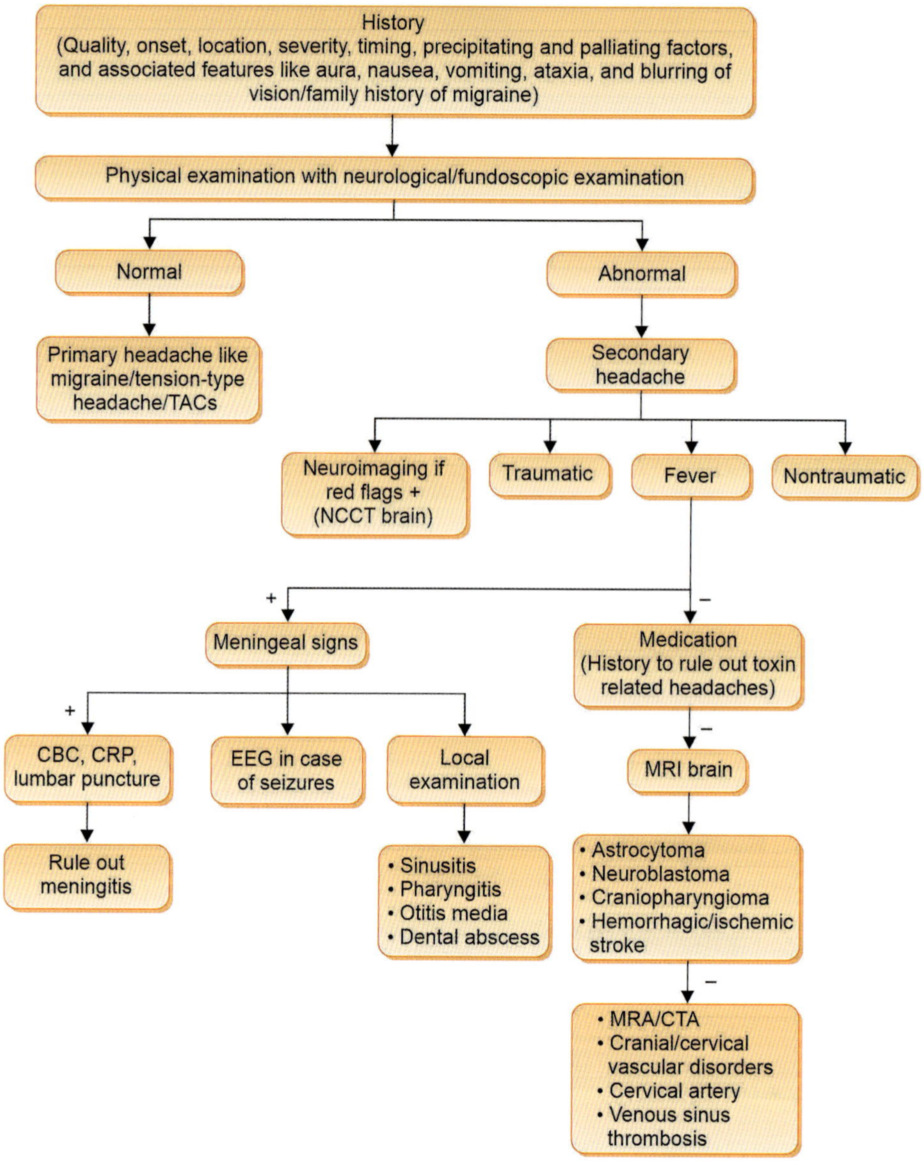

Note: The presence of an abnormal neurologic examination or unusual neurologic symptoms is a key clue that additional investigation is warranted.

Laboratory investigations does not contribute much to the diagnosis

(CBC: complete blood count; CRP: C-reactive protein; CTA: computed tomography angiography; NCCT: noncontrast computed tomography; MRA: magnetic resonance angiography TACs: trigeminal autonomic cephalalgias)

Neuroimaging in Headache

- Abnormal neurological features (History/examination)
- *Systemic symptoms:* Syndromic/growth delay
- Acute onset severe headache
- Acute change in chronic headache

Suggested Reading

- Headache Classification Committee of the International Headache Society (IHS). The International Classification of Headache Disorders, 3rd edition. Cephalalgia. 2018;38(1):1-211.

Hematemesis

116

Section Editor: **B Rajsekhar**
Section Co-Editor: **Suchitra Pusapati**
Authors: **Prasad BS, Suraj S Shetty**

Introduction

Hematemesis refers to the vomiting of blood/coffee ground-like material. It is the usual presentation of upper gastrointestinal (UGI) bleeding, from structures proximal to the ligament of Treitz.

Etiology

Etiology includes the following **(Table 1)**:

TABLE 1: Etiology of hematemesis from different sites.

CAUSES	NEONATES AND INFANTS	CHILDREN
Esophagus	• Esophagitis • Trauma during nasogastric tube insertion	• Esophageal varices • Mallory–Weiss tear
Stomach	• Swallowed maternal blood • Stress gastritis	• Gastric varices • Gastric ulcer • Henoch–Schönlein purpura • Vascular malformation
Duodenum	Duodenitis	• Duodenal ulcer • Hemosuccus pancreaticus
Systemic causes	Vitamin K deficiency	Bleeding and clotting disorders

- *Neonate and infant:*
  - *Swallowed maternal blood:* Apt–Downey test—used to distinguish maternal blood from gastro-intestinal (GI) bleed
  - Esophagitis/stress gastritis
  - Vitamin K-dependent bleeding or hemorrhagic disease of newborns is prevented by vitamin K prophylaxis
  - Trauma during nasogastric tube insertion
  - Congenital anomalies
  - Coagulopathy
- *Child and adolescent:*
  - Gastric/esophageal varices
  - Vascular malformations
  - Mallory–Weiss tear—longitudinal mucosal lacerations in the distal esophagus, usually after forceful retching
  - Peptic ulcer disease
  - Drug-induced ulcers [Nonsteroidal anti-inflammatory drugs (NSAIDs)]
  - Vasculitis (e.g., Henoch–Schönlein purpura)
  - Bleeding/clotting disorders
  - Foreign bodies

Note:

- Red dye/food colorings may be confused with blood, after vomiting.
- Munchausen syndrome by proxy caregivers, when administered blood or blood-like substance.

Red Flag Signs

- Associated melena
- Severe pallor/hemoglobin <8 g/dL
- Hypotension and tachycardia
- Orthostatic hypotension
- Decompensation with the appearance of encephalopathy in liver diseases

History

- The time course of the bleeding episode, estimated blood loss, and presence of pain in abdomen
- The presence of melena/hematochezia may suggest significant GI bleed.
- *Drug history:* NSAIDs, ibuprofen, corticosteroids, and tetracyclines
- History of liver disease or jaundice
- *Nasopharyngeal bleeding:* Recent/recurrent epistaxis
- *History of easy bruising/bleeding from other sites:* bleeding/ clotting disorder.

Physical Examination

- Examination of the skin and mucus membranes for bruising, petechiae, and mucosal bleeding
- *Cutaneous signs of generalized vascular malformations:* Five or more may suggest possibility of GI hemangiomatosis
- *Abdominal examination:* Signs of portal hypertension, splenomegaly, and prominent veins over abdomen

Approach

- *Emergency care:*
  - *Airway and breathing:* Supplemental oxygen/intubation
  - *Circulation:* IV access (two large cannulas)
  - *Fluid resuscitation:* Crystalloids/ionotropes
  - *Blood resuscitation:* Packed red blood cells (PRBC) if hemoglobin <8g/dL; transfuse blood at 1:1:1 ratio of PRBC: FFP: Platelets if massive transfusion required
  - Correction of coagulopathy/metabolic/electrolyte abnormality
  - No oral consumptions
  - Ryle's tube insertion and aspiration if active bleeding is suspected.

- *Investigations:*
  - Complete blood count (decrease in hemoglobin >2 g/dL is significant), coagulation parameters, urea/creatinine, electrolytes, liver function test, blood grouping/cross-matching, immediate venous blood gas to assess pH, lactate, base excess, and hematocrit
  - Upper GI endoscopy
  - *Ultrasonography:* Liver disease, portal hypertension, or large vascular anomalies

The approach to the management of a child with hematemesis is illustrated in **Flowchart 1**.

FLOWCHART 1: The approach to a child with hematemesis.

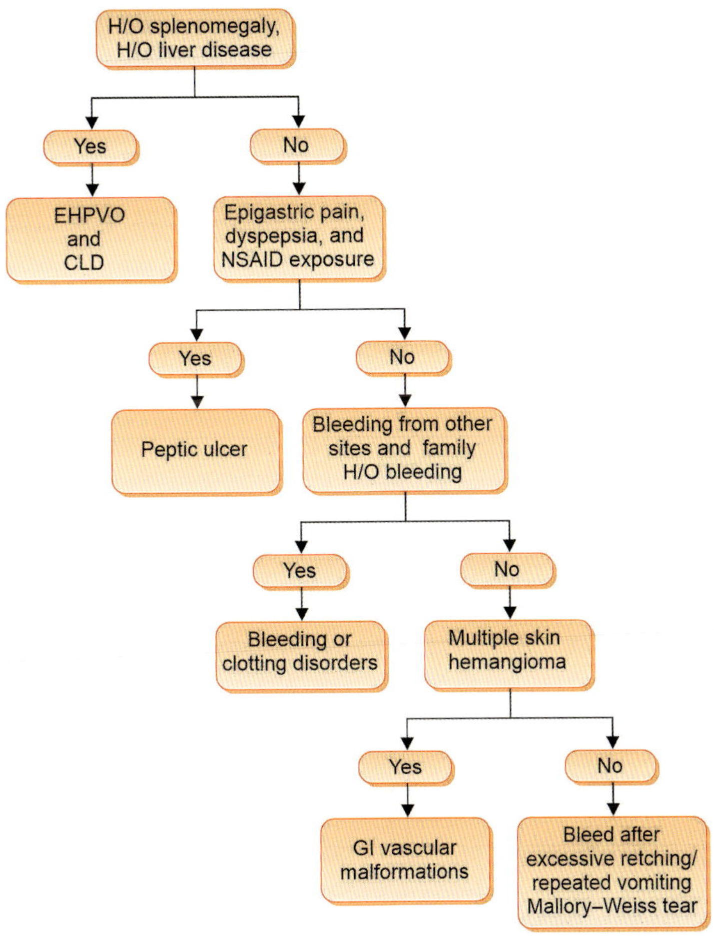

(CLD: chronic liver disease; EHPVO: extrahepatic portal vein obstruction; GI: gastrointestinal; H/O: history of; NSAID: nonsteroidal anti-inflammatory drugs)

Suggested Reading

- Feldman M, Friedman LS, Brandt LJ. Sleisenger and Fortran's Gastrointestinal and liver disease,11th edition. Philadelphia: Elsevier; 2021. pp. 283-98.
- National Institute for Health and Care Excellence. (2012). Acute upper gastrointestinal bleeding in over 16s: Management. [online] Available from: http://guidance.nice.org.uk/CG141/NICE Guidance/ pdf/English. [Last accessed August, 2024].

Lymphadenopathy

117

***Section Editor:* Janani Shankar**
***Section Co-Editor:* Arathi Srinivasan**
***Authors:* Raja Rajeswari, Pooja Gujjal Chebbi, Nuthan Kumar MK**

Introduction

- Lymphadenopathy (or "swollen glands") is a common entity found in children; the cause is reactive in most cases.
- The presence of this can be due to various causes such as infection, inflammation, or an underlying hematological malignancy, and thus detailed history and examination are crucial for the approach.

Definitions

- *Lymphadenitis:* A lymph node that is enlarged due to an infective or inflammatory etiology that may be warm and tender to touch and erythematous. Systemic signs may or may not be present.
- *Lymphadenopathy:* Enlarged lymph node(s), which is >2 cm and has an increased chance of being caused by serious underlying conditions.

  Lymphadenopathy is a condition when lymph nodes are abnormal in size, shape, and consistency.

  If the size of the palpable lymph nodes is >1.5 cm in the inguinal region and >1 cm anywhere else, it is considered to be significant.

  However, when cervical lymph nodes that are palpable are >2 cm in size, it is unlikely to be a serious condition.

Based on the involvement of lymph nodes, lymphadenopathy can be classified into the following two types:

1. *Localized lymphadenopathy:* Nodes that are enlarged and confined to one particular region
2. *Generalized lymphadenopathy:* Nodes that are enlarged and found in two or more noncontiguous areas

Lymphadenopathy can be classified into the following types on the basis of the duration it lasts for:

- Acute lymphadenopathy: <1 week
- Subacute lymphadenopathy: 1–3 weeks
- Chronic lymphadenopathy: >4 weeks

Approach

The etiology and approach to diagnosing lymphadenopathy are given in **Flowchart 1**.

FLOWCHART 1: Etiology and approach to lymphadenopathy.

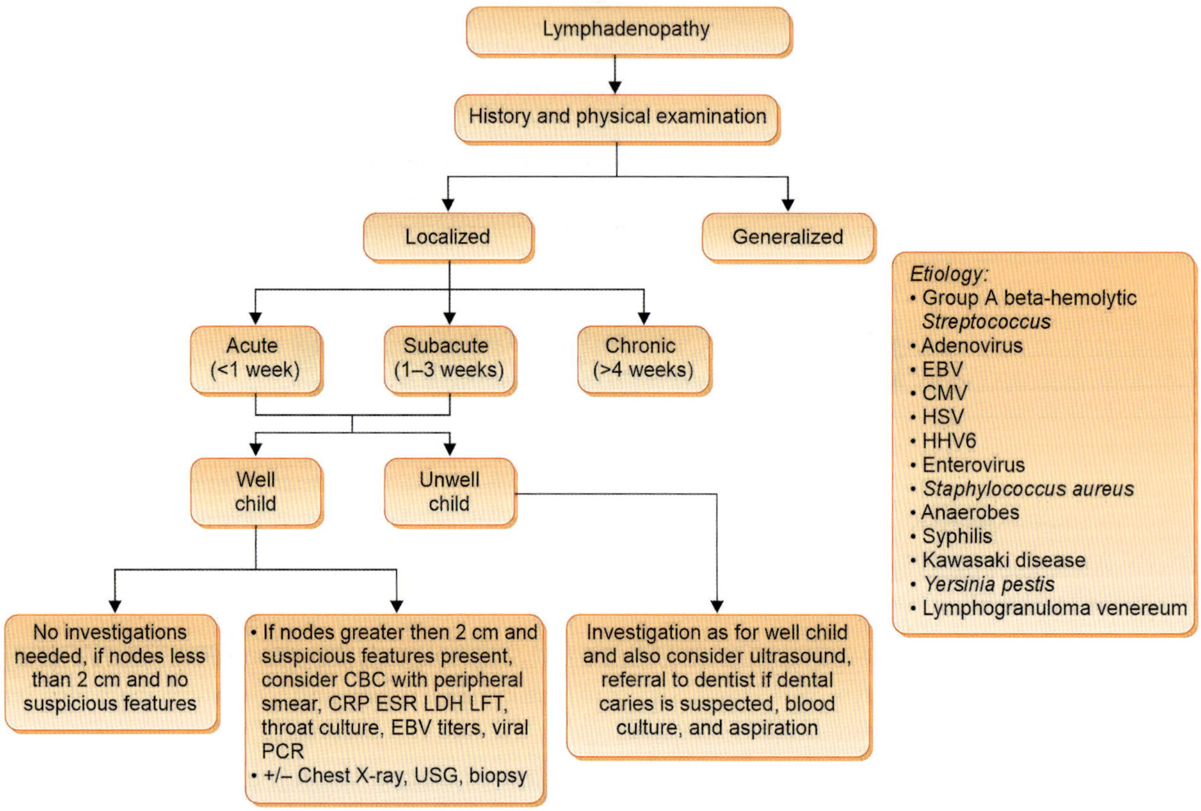

(CBC: complete blood count; CMV: cytomegalovirus; CRP: c-reactive protein; EBV: Epstein–Barr virus; ESR: erythrocyte sedimentation rate; HSV: herpes simplex virus; HHV6: human herpesvirus 6; LDH: lactate dehydrogenase; LFT: liver function tests; PCR: polymerase chain reaction; USG: ultrasonography)

The etiology and approach to diagnosing chronic lymphadenopathy are given in **Flowchart 2**.

FLOWCHART 2: Approach to chronic lymphadenopathy.

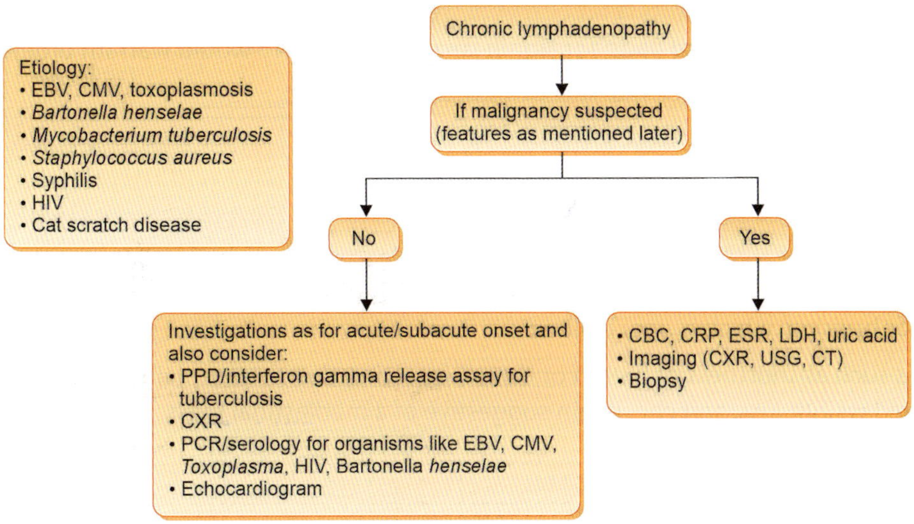

(CT: computed tomography; CBC: complete blood count; CMV: cytomegalovirus; CRP: c-reactive protein; CXR: chest X-ray; EBV: Epstein–Barr virus; ESR: erythrocyte sedimentation rate; HIV: human immunodeficiency virus; LDH: lactate dehydrogenase; PCR: polymerase chain reaction; PPD: purified protein derivative; USG: ultrasonography)

The etiology and approach to diagnosing generalized lymphadenopathy are given in **Flowchart 3**.

FLOWCHART 3: Approach to generalized lymphadenopathy.

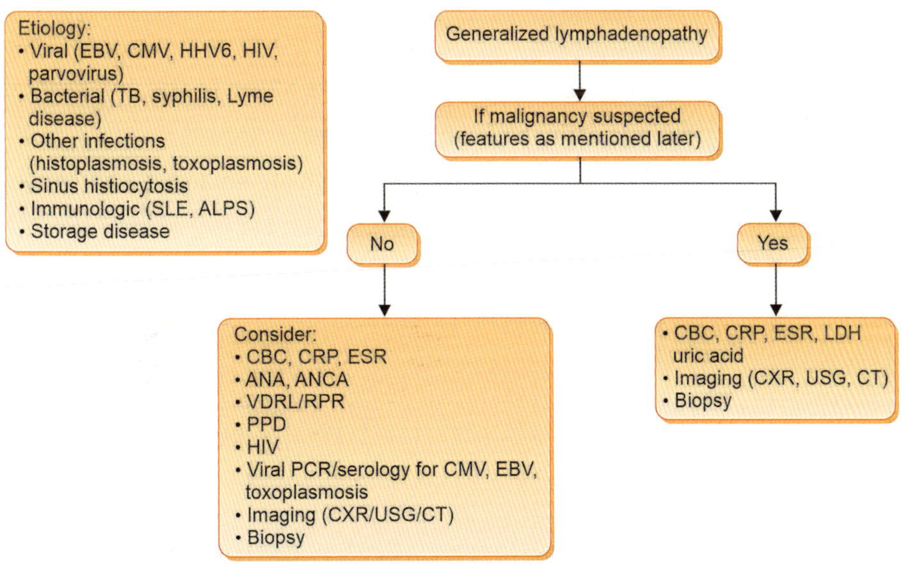

(ALPS: autoimmune lymphoproliferative syndrome; ANA: antinuclear antibody; ANCA: antineutrophil cytoplasmic antibodies; CT: computed tomography; CBC: complete blood count; CMV: cytomegalovirus; CRP: c-reactive protein; CXR: chest X-ray; EBV: Epstein–Barr virus; ESR: erythrocyte sedimentation rate; HIV: human immunodeficiency virus; LDH: lactate dehydrogenase; PCR: polymerase chain reaction; PPD: purified protein derivative; RPR: rapid plasma reagin; SLE: systemic lupus erythematosus; USG: ultrasonography; VDRL: venereal disease research laboratory)

Red Flag Signs

The following are considered "red flags" for significant pathology and would warrant urgent referral:

- Severe pallor
- Loss of weight
- Loss of appetite
- Fatigue
- Fever or any signs of sepsis
- Bleeding or bruising, which is unexplained
- Symptoms such as shortness of breath or discomfort lying down, unexplained fever or night sweats, unexplained weight loss, and chest pain suggestive of a mediastinal mass

Investigations

Most children with just a single node palpable need not be evaluated for the same.

The indications for detailed evaluation include:

- Cervical lymph nodes that are palpable over 2 weeks and are >2 cm in size and progressing
- Unexplained inguinal lymphadenopathy >1.5 cm in diameter
- Axillary, epitrochlear, and supraclavicular lymph nodes which are enlarged >1.5 cm and are not due to any obvious underlying cause
- Symptoms of the red flags mentioned earlier

When to Suspect Malignancy?

A single lymph node >2 cm in diameter with any of the following additional features may prompt a detailed evaluation:

- Absence of definite infectious cause
- Node significantly enlarged >2 cm, present for over 6 weeks or more, not reducing in size
- Extensive distribution
- Firm/hard consistency and immobile on palpation
- Not tender

Clinical criteria for referral regardless of the size of the palpable lymph nodes:

- Supraclavicular nodes
- Splenomegaly, loss of weight, and night sweats
- Associated bone pain and limping
- Chest X-ray showing mediastinal widening

Suggested Reading

- Maini R, Nagalli S. Lymphadenopathy. In: StatPearls [Internet]. Treasure Island (FL): StatPearls Publishing; 2024. Available from https://www.ncbi.nlm.nih.gov/books/NBK558918/ [Last accessed August, 2024].
- Pomeranz AJ, Sabnis S, Busey SL, Kliegman RM. Lymphadenopathy. Pediatric Decision-Making Strategies, 2nd edition. Philadelphia: Elsevier Saunders; 2016. pp. 28-230.
- Rajasekaran K, Krakovitz P. Enlarged neck lymph nodes in children. Pediatr Clin North Am. 2013;60(4):923-36.
- Rosenberg TL, Nolder AR. Pediatric cervical lymphadenopathy. Otolaryngol Clin North Am. 2014;47(5):721-31.
- Sahai S. Lymphadenopathy. Pediatr Rev. 2013;34(5):216-27.

Oliguria

118

Section Editor: **Gnanamurthy Narasimha**
Section Co-Editor: **Nagalatha Chidananda**
Author: **Shashikiran KB**

Definition

- Oliguria is defined as urine output <1 mL/kg per hour in infants. In children urine output <0.5 mL/kg per hour for over 6 hours.
- Anuria is defined as the absence of any urine output.
- Acute kidney injury (AKI) can be defined by kidney disease improving global outcome (KDIGO) as:
  - Increase in serum creatinine by ≥0.3 mg/dL from baseline within 48 hours, or
  - Increase in serum creatinine to ≥1.5 times baseline within the prior 7 days, or
  - Urine volume ≤0.5 mL/kg/h for 6 hours
- Serum creatinine does not accurately reflect the glomerular filtration rate (GFR) in a patient whose kidney function is changing. Hence, decreased urine output is the most visible sign of AKI. The degree of oliguria strongly correlates with poor outcomes in children with AKI.

Risk Factors

- Common in hospitalized patients (50% patients in ICU)
- Intravascular volume depletion
- Prior history of renal disease
- Receiving mechanical ventilation
- Nephrotoxic agents and vasoconstrictive drugs
- Comorbidities, for example, congestive heart failure and liver disease

Etiology

The causes of oliguria/anuria are given in **Table 1**.

TABLE 1: Causes of oliguria/anuria.

MECHANISM	ETIOLOGY
Prerenal	
↓Intravascular volume	Dehydration, blood loss, diuretics, burns, and nephrotic syndrome
↓Cardiac function	Heart failure and arrhythmias
Peripheral vasodilatation	Sepsis, anaphylaxis, and antihypertensive medications
Renal vasoconstriction	Sepsis, NSAIDs, and ACE-I
Intrinsic renal	
Acute tubular injury	Prolonged ischemia, nephrotoxins, and sepsis
Renal vascular diseases	HUS, vasculitis, and thrombosis
Interstitial diseases	Interstitial nephritis and infections
Glomerular diseases	PSGN, RPGN, HSP
Postrenal	
Obstruction to urine flow	Posterior urethral valve, PUJ obstruction, and calculi neurogenic bladder

(ACE-I: angiotensin-converting enzyme inhibitors; HSP: Henoch–Schölein purpura; HUS: hemolytic uremic syndrome NSAIDs: nonsteroidal anti-inflammatory drugs; PSGN: poststreptococcal glomerulonephritis; PUJ: pelviureteric junction; RPGN: rapidly progressive glomerulonephritis)

Evaluation

The evaluation of oliguria is given in **Table 2.**

TABLE 2: Evaluation of oliguria.

History	
History of fluid loss	Vomiting, diarrhea, burns, and surgery
Exposure to nephrotoxic agents	NSAIDs and aminoglycosides
Features of glomerular diseases	Skin lesions/rash, joint pains, purpura, bloody diarrhea, and hematuria
Features suggesting obstruction	Anuria, poor stream, and lower abdominal pain
Physical examination	
Volume loss signs	Dry mucosa, reduced skin turgor, tachycardia, hypotension, prolonged CRT, and weak peripheral pulses
Fluid overload signs	Edema, hypertension, and heart failure features
Systemic causes	Skin rash, purpura, features of arthritis, and healed skin lesions.
Signs of obstruction	Poor urinary stream, and enlarged palpable bladder

(CRT: capillary refill time; NSAIDS: nonsteroidal anti-inflammatory drugs)

Laboratory Tests and Imaging

- Estimation of serum creatinine and serum electrolytes
- Urinalysis
- Fractional sodium excretion to differentiate between pre and intrinsic AKI
- Kidney ultrasound

Serum creatinine may not rise until a 50% or more reduction in GFR occurs.

Diagnostic Fluid Challenge

Diagnostic fluid challenge differentiates prerenal fluid responsive from intrinsic causes **(Table 3)**.

Indication:

- When cause not ascertained from history and examination
- History suggestive of prerenal cause but duration of insult is unknown

Procedure:

10–20 mL/kg of normal saline is administered over 20–30 minutes:

- Improvement in clinical status and a reduction in blood urea/serum creatinine—prerenal etiology
- Absent improvement (and/or the development of fluid overload)—intrinsic AKI

Fluid challenge is *contraindicated* in patients with obvious volume overload/heart failure.

TABLE 3: Urinary indices to differentiate prerenal from intrinsic causes.

MEASUREMENT	PRERENAL	INTRINSIC RENAL
Urine specific gravity	>1.020	<1.010
Urine to serum creatinine ratio	>40	<20
Urine sodium	<20 mEq/L	>40 mEq/L
FENa	<1%	>2%
FEUrea	<35%	>50%

(FENa: fractional excretion of sodium; FEUrea: fractional excretion of urea)

Red Flag Signs

- Anuria
- Advanced azotemia
- Features of fluid overload, hyperkalemia, and metabolic acidosis
- Features of systemic illness affecting the kidneys

Approach

The approach to a child presenting with oliguria/anuria is given in **Flowchart 1**.

FLOWCHART 1: Approach to a child presenting with oliguria/anuria.

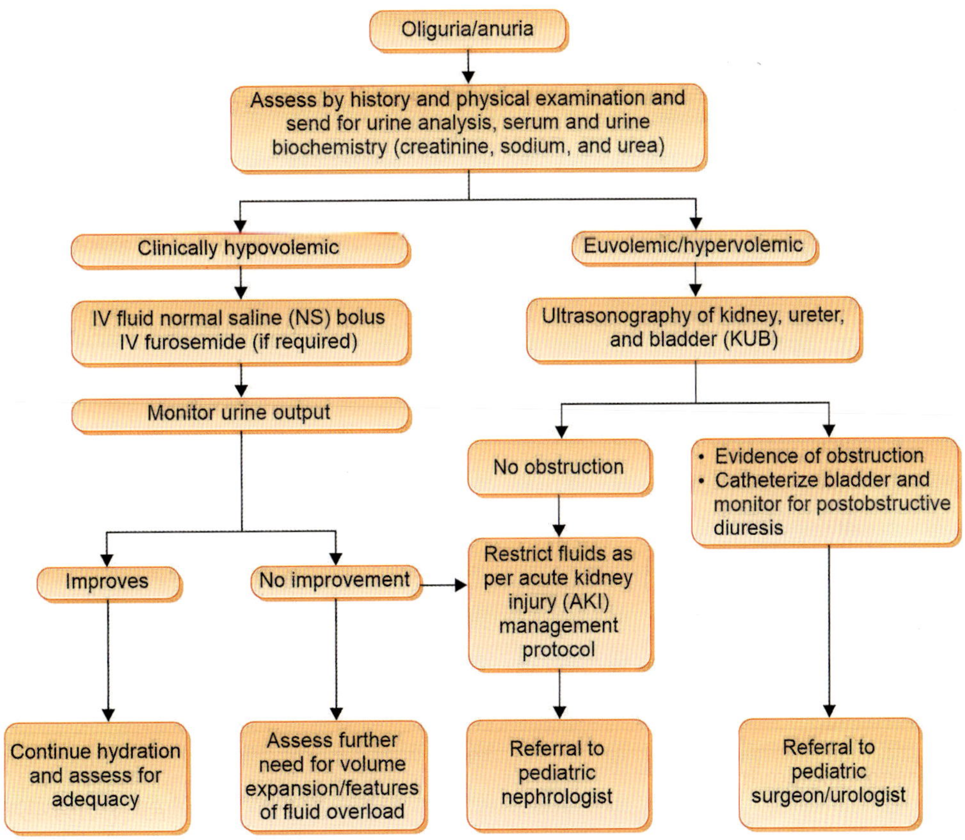

Suggested Reading

- Jain A, Mattoo TK. Oliguria and Anuria. In: McInerny TK, Adam HM, Campbell DE, DeWitt TG, Foy JM, Kamat DM, Baum R, Kelleher KJ (Eds). Textbook of Pediatric Care. US: American Academy of Pediatrics; 2016.
- Sethi SK, Bunchman T, Chakraborty R, Raina R. Pediatric acute kidney injury: New advances in the last decade. Kidney Res Clin Pract. 2021;40(1):40–51.

Polyuria

119

Section Editor: **Gnanamurthy Narasimha**
Section Co-Editor: **Nagalatha Chidananda**
Author: **Saumil Gaur**

Introduction

- Polyuria in children is defined as urine output >2 L/m²/day and >3 L/day in adults.
- Mechanisms of polyuria are classified as:
  - *Water diuresis:* Defective urine concentration by kidneys
  - *Solute diuresis:* Increased loss of solutes enhancing water loss
  - *Increased fluid intake:* Polydipsia

Causes

- *Solute diuresis:* Glucosuria, urea diuresis, sodium diuresis
  - *Glucosuria:* In diabetes mellitus
  - *Urea diuresis:* Resolution of azotemia, glucosteroid therapy leading to increased metabolism, and administration of large amounts of protein causing ureagenesis
  - *Sodium diuresis:* Volume expansion with large amounts of IV saline infusion/release of bilateral urinary tract obstruction
  - *Mannitol:* In case of raised intracranial pressure (ICP), it can create osmotic diuresis

- *Water diuresis:* Maybe primary polydipsia, arginine vasopressin (AVP) deficiency, and AVP resistance
  - *AVP deficiency (AVP-D) due to:*
    - *Genetics:* Autosomal recessive/autosomal dominant forms; DIDMOAD (diabetes insipidus, diabetes mellitus, optic atrophy, and deafness syndrome)/Wolfram syndrome
    - *Malformations:* Septo-optic dysplasia, holoprosencephaly, and anencephaly
    - *Central nervous system (CNS) causes:* Head trauma, brain death; tumors like craniopharyngioma, pinealoma, germinoma; sarcoidosis; histiocytosis; pituitary surgery; and hypoxic–ischemic injury
  - *AVP-resistance:* Hereditary, V2 receptor gene mutations, aquaporin 2 mutations, hypercalcemia, hypokalemia, bilateral urinary tract obstruction, sickle cell disease/trait, craniopharyngioma surgery, Bardet–Biedl syndrome, and Bartter syndrome

Evaluation

- *Confirmation:* Strict input/output volume chart for 2–3 days.
- Disproportionate urine output >2 L/m^2/day is confirmative.
- *Laboratory samples:* Urine osmolality, serum osmolality, sodium, potassium, chloride, creatinine, urea nitrogen, arterial blood gas (ABG), and random blood sugar (RBS).

History

- *Age of onset:* In the first month of life—hereditary and in first year—familial AVP-D type
- *Rapidity of onset with weight loss*: Diabetes mellitus
- *Failure to thrive with weight loss*: AVP-R
- *Head trauma, cranial malignancy, and meningitis:* AVR-D
- *Constipation and paraesthesia:* Hypercalcemia
- *Failure to thrive, bony changes, anemia:* Chronic kidney disease
- *Failure to thrive, acidotic breathing, constipation, bony changes:* Renal tubular acidosis

Interpretation

- *Psychogenic polydipsia:* Low serum osmolality, normal/low serum osmolality, low serum sodium, positive response to water deprivation test.
- *Water diuresis due to AVP-D/AVP-R:* Elevated serum osmolality (>300 mOsm/L), low urine osmolality (<300 mOsm/L), urine specific gravity (<1.005), and serum sodium (>145 mosm/L)
- *Solute diuresis:* Confirmed by measuring the urine osmolality >400–600 mOsmol/kg and calculating *the total daily osmolar output* (>1,000 mOsmol).

$$\text{Total daily osmolar output} = \text{Urine osmolality} \times \text{24-hour urine volume}$$

An algorithmic approach to normonatremia is illustrated in **Flowchart 1**.

FLOWCHART 1: Algorithmic approach to normonatremia.

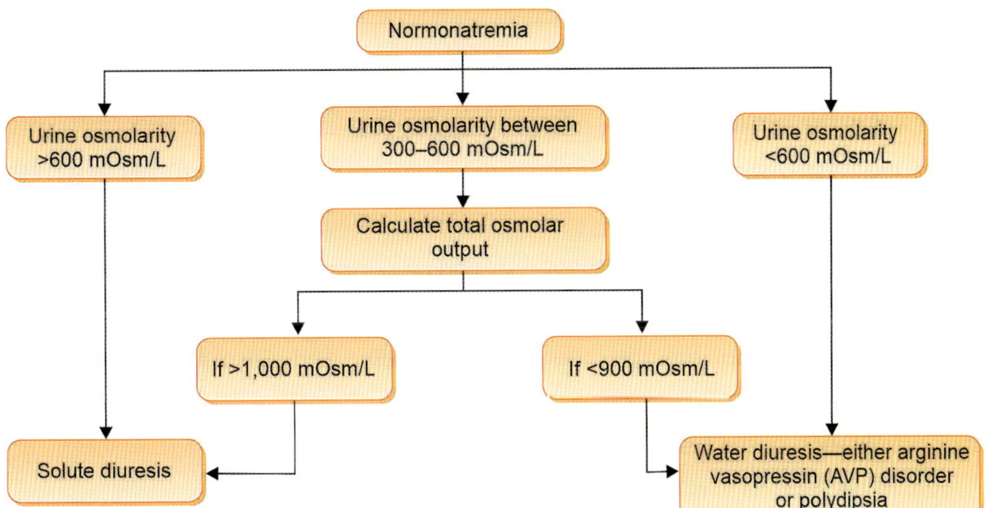

An algorithmic approach to hypernatremia is illustrated in **Flowchart 2**.

FLOWCHART 2: Algorithmic approach to hypernatremia.

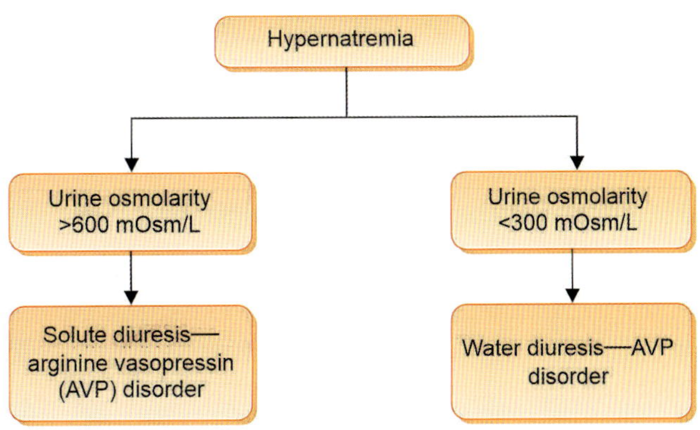

An algorithmic approach to hypernatremia is illustrated in **Flowchart 3**.

FLOWCHART 3: Algorithmic approach to hyponatremia.

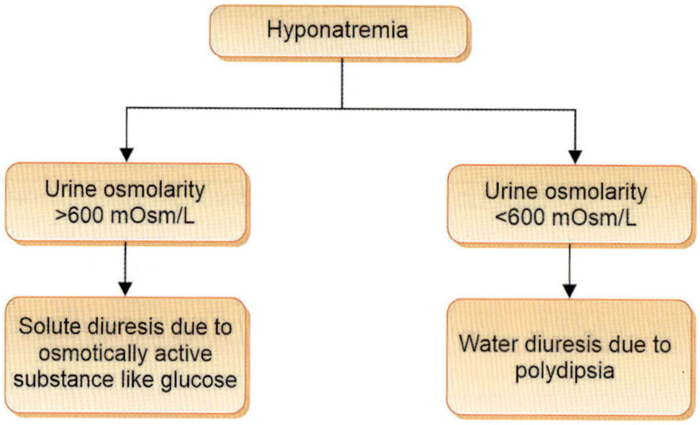

Special tests useful in the evaluation of polyuria:

- *Water deprivation test:* Distinguishes between psychogenic polydipsia and AVP-R or AVP-D defects
- *Desmopressin response test:* Distinguishes between AVP-R versus AVP-D.

Water deprivation test for older infants and children should be performed under close medical supervision.

The patient should not be allowed to lose >5% of their body weight. Monitor vital signs (temperature, pulse, and blood pressure), body weight, laboratory tests, urine and plasma osmolarities, and plasma sodium concentration.

Endpoints for termination of the test:

- Urine osmolality is ≥600 mOsmol/kg.
- Urine specific gravity ≥1.020.
- Plasma osmolality exceeds 295 or 300 mOsmol/kg.
- Plasma sodium is 145 mEQ/L or higher.

Desmopressin response test: Desmopressin is administered (5–10 µg by nasal insufflation or 2–4 µg intravenously/subcutaneously) and serial measurements of serum and urine osmolarity along with serum sodium are taken.

- *AVP-D:* >50% increase in baseline urine osmolality
- *Complete AVP-R:* <10–15% increase in baseline urine osmolality
- *Partial AVP-R:* Around 35–45% increase in baseline urine osmolality

Red Flag Signs

- Severe hypernatremia with features of dehydration
- Maintained urine output despite being in shock/severe dehydration

Suggested Reading

- Bhasin B, Velez JC. Evaluation of polyuria: The roles of solute loading and water diuresis. Am J Kidney Dis. 2016;67(3):507-11
- Christ-Crain M, Winzeler B, Refardt J. Diagnosis and management of diabetes insipidus for the internist: An update. J Intern Med. 2021;290(1):73-87.
- Huynh T, Signal D, Christ-Crain M. Paediatric perspectives in the diagnosis of polyuria-polydipsia syndrome. Clin Endocrinol (Oxf). 2024.

Unusual Urine Color and Odor

120

Section Editor: **Gnanamurthy Narasimha**
Section Co-Editor: **Nagalatha Chidananda**
Author: **Vikram Sakaleshpur Kumar**

Introduction

- The urinalysis is frequently ordered in pediatric clinical tests, primarily owing to the simplicity of urine collection and examination.
- A simple gross examination of urine, including an assessment of odor and color, plays a crucial role in understanding various disease conditions.

Pediatric Conditions Associated with Unusual Urine Odors

The normal urine odor is described as "Urinoid".

The varied urine odors and associated compounds and disorders are given in **Table 1.**

TABLE 1: Disorders and compounds associated with various unusual urine orders.

ODOR	COMPOUND	DISORDER
Strong smell		Dehydration/prolonged room temperature
Pungent or fetid		Urinary tract infection
Fruity/sweet		Diabetic ketoacidosis
Ammoniacal		Prolonged bladder retention

Contd...

Contd...

ODOR	COMPOUND	DISORDER
Maple syrup/burnt sugar	2-Oxoisocaproic acid	Maple syrup urine disease
Sweaty feet	Isovaleric acid	• Isovaleric acidemia • Multiple acyl-coenzyme A (CoA) dehydrogenase deficiency (glutaric aciduria type II) • 3-Hydroxy-3-methyl glutaric aciduria
Cat urine	3-Hydroxyisovaleric acid	• 3-Methylcrotonyl-CoA carboxylase deficiency • Multiple carboxylase deficiency
Cabbage-like	2-Hydroxybutyric acid	• Tyrosinemia type 1 • Methionine malabsorption
Rancid butter	2-Oxo-4-methiolbutyric acid	Tyrosinemia type 1
Acid smell	Methylmalonic acid	Methylmalonic acidemia
Sulfurous	Hydrogen sulfide	Cystinuria
Fish market	Trimethylamine	Trimethylaminuria
Fecal smell		Gastrointestinal-bladder fistula
Sulfuric smell		Cystine decomposition
Swimming pool		Hawkinsinuria

Varied Urine Colors

- A freshly voided urine sample typically has a normal appearance, being clear and ranging from pale to dark yellow.
- Various medications and foods can potentially alter the color of urine. Substances responsible for abnormal urine color can impact the accuracy of reagent strip tests, leading to false-positive or false-negative results.
- Cloudiness in urine may be due to prolonged exposure to room temperature (beyond an hour), presence of triphosphate crystals in alkaline urine, elevated urates, urinary tract infection (UTI), pyuria, or highly concentrated urine.
- If cloudy urine is obtained with no suspicion of a UTI based on clinical presentation or initial urinalysis, conduct a repeat urinalysis with microscopy using a freshly voided specimen.

The varied urine colors and associated compounds and disorders are given in **Table 2.**

TABLE 2: Disorders and compounds associated with various unusual urine colors.

COLOR	COMPOUND	DISORDER/CAUSES
Blue	Indican	Hartnup disorder
Blue/brown	Homogentisic acid	Alkaptonuria
Brown	Methemoglobin	Myoglobinuria
Red/brown	Hemoglobin/methemoglobin	Hemoglobinuria and myoglobinuria
Light red	Urates	Hyperuricosuria
Red	Erythrocytes	Hematuria
Cloudy	Phosphaturia, pyuria, chyluria, lipiduria, and hyperoxaluria	Diet high in purine-rich foods (hyperuricosuria)
Brown	Bile pigments and myoglobin	Fava beans
Brownish-black	Bile pigments, melanin, and methemoglobin	Cascara, levodopa, methyldopa, and senna
Green or blue	Pseudomonal UTI and biliverdin	Amitriptyline, indigo carmine, IV cimetidine, IV promethazine, methylene blue, triamterene, and indomethacin
Orange	Bile pigments	Phenothiazines, phenazopyridine, rifampin, and vitamin C
Red	Hematuria, hemoglobinuria, myoglobinuria, and porphyria	Beets, blackberries, and rhubarb
Red		Phenolphthalein and rifampin
Dark Yellow	Concentrated urine	Carrots
Red on standing	Porphobilinogen	Suggests the presence of porphobilinogen, which is increased in acute porphyrias

Red Flag Signs

- Parental concern about peculiar color and odor of the child's urine
- Evidence of edema
- *Hematuria:*
  - Recurrent hematuria
  - Hematuria associated with multisystemic symptoms
  - Hematuria with a history of recent streptococcal infection
  - Hematuria with bloody diarrhea
  - Hematuria in a child with sickle cell disease

Algorithmic Approach to Urine Color

An algorithmic approach to urine color is given in **Flowchart 1**.

FLOWCHART 1: Approach to urine color.

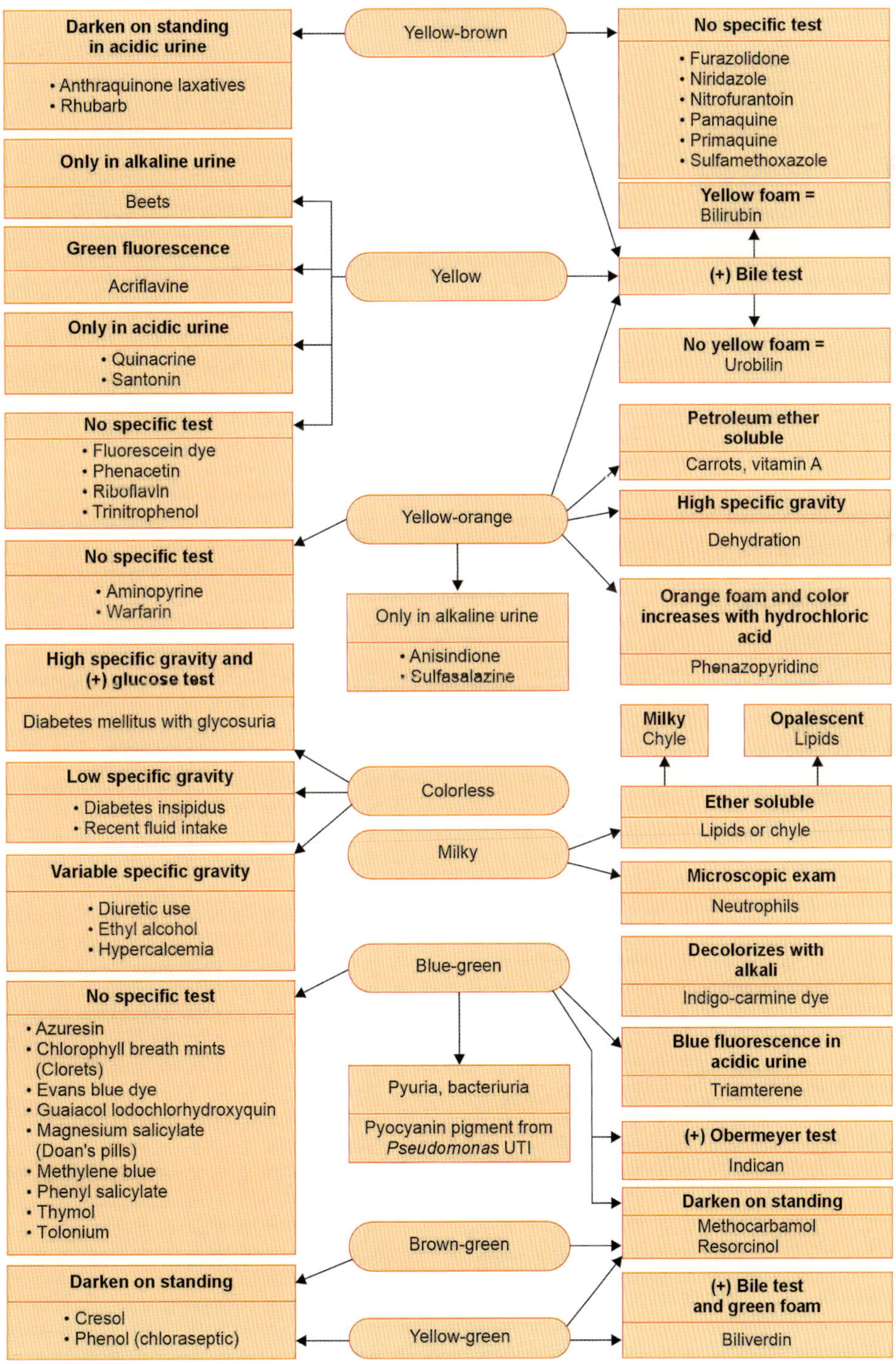

Contd...

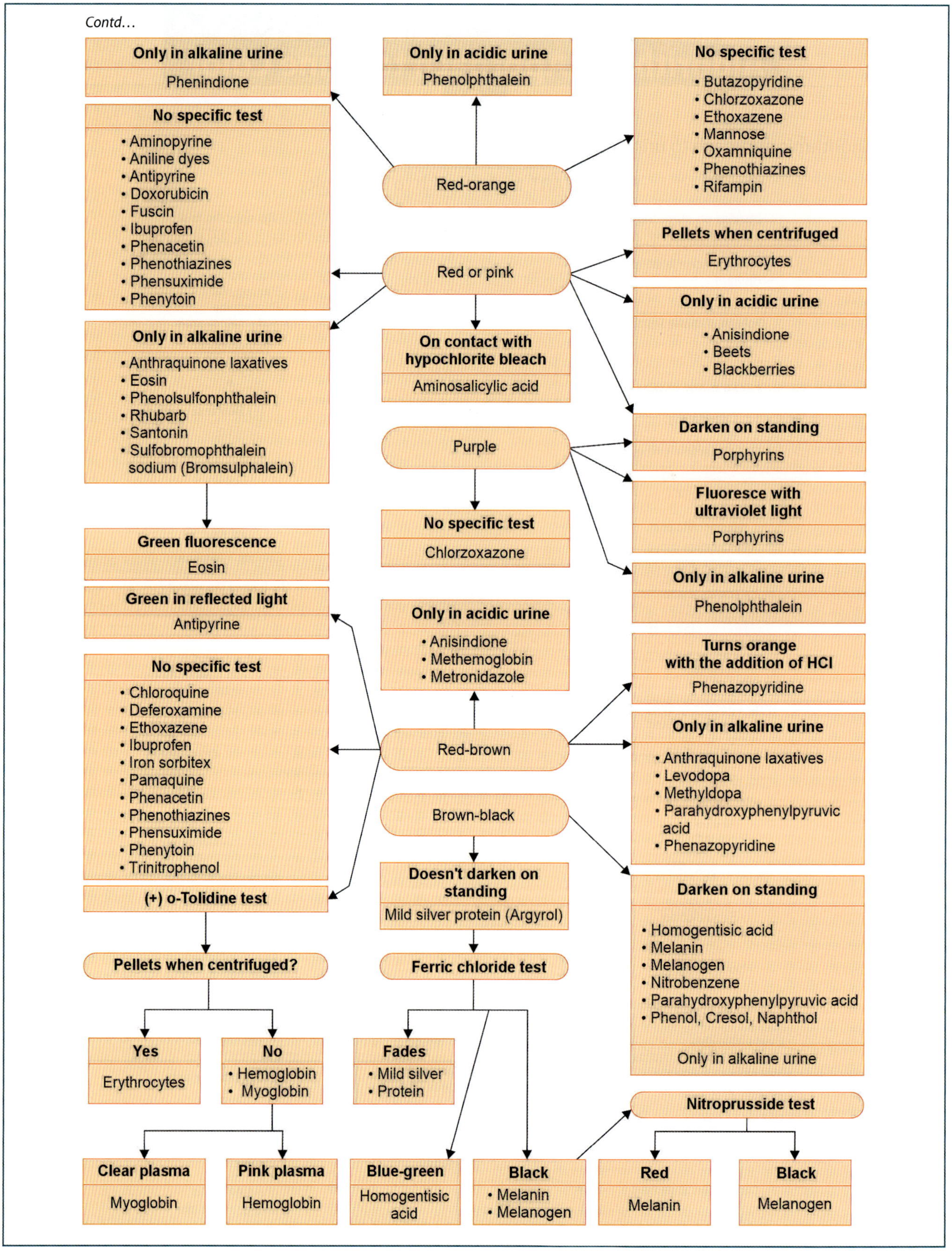
Contd...
Only in alkaline urine
Phenindione
Only in acidic urine
Phenolphthalein
No specific test
• Butazopyridine
• Chlorzoxazone
• Ethoxazene
• Mannose
• Oxamniquine
• Phenothiazines
• Rifampin
No specific test
• Aminopyrine
• Aniline dyes
• Antipyrine
• Doxorubicin
• Fuscin
• Ibuprofen
• Phenacetin
• Phenothiazines
• Phensuximide
• Phenytoin
Red-orange
Pellets when centrifuged
Erythrocytes
Red or pink
Only in acidic urine
• Anisindione
• Beets
• Blackberries
Only in alkaline urine
• Anthraquinone laxatives
• Eosin
• Phenolsulfonphthalein
• Rhubarb
• Santonin
• Sulfobromophthalein sodium (Bromsulphalein)
On contact with hypochlorite bleach
Aminosalicylic acid
Darken on standing
Porphyrins
Purple
Fluoresce with ultraviolet light
Porphyrins
Green fluorescence
Eosin
No specific test
Chlorzoxazone
Only in alkaline urine
Phenolphthalein
Green in reflected light
Antipyrine
Only in acidic urine
• Anisindione
• Methemoglobin
• Metronidazole
Turns orange with the addition of HCl
Phenazopyridine
No specific test
• Chloroquine
• Deferoxamine
• Ethoxazene
• Ibuprofen
• Iron sorbitex
• Pamaquine
• Phenacetin
• Phenothiazines
• Phensuximide
• Phenytoin
• Trinitrophenol
Red-brown
Only in alkaline urine
• Anthraquinone laxatives
• Levodopa
• Methyldopa
• Parahydroxyphenylpyruvic acid
• Phenazopyridine
Brown-black
Doesn't darken on standing
Mild silver protein (Argyrol)
Darken on standing
• Homogentisic acid
• Melanin
• Melanogen
• Nitrobenzene
• Parahydroxyphenylpyruvic acid
• Phenol, Cresol, Naphthol
Only in alkaline urine
(+) o-Tolidine test
Pellets when centrifuged?
Ferric chloride test
Yes
Erythrocytes
No
• Hemoglobin
• Myoglobin
Fades
• Mild silver
• Protein
Nitroprusside test
Clear plasma
Myoglobin
Pink plasma
Hemoglobin
Blue-green
Homogentisic acid
Black
• Melanin
• Melanogen
Red
Melanin
Black
Melanogen

Suggested Reading

- Enns GM, Packman S. Diagnosing inborn errors of metabolism in the newborn: Clinical features. Neoreviews. 2001;2(8):e183-91.
- Patel HP. The abnormal urinalysis. Pediatr Clin North Am. 2006;53(3):325-37.
- Raymond JR, Yarger WE. Abnormal urine color: Differential diagnosis. South Med J. 1988;81(7):837-41.

Temper Tantrums

121

Section Editor: **Sumitha Nayak**
Section Co-Editor: **Priya Shivalli**
Author: **Mahima Mittal**

Introduction

- Any behavior that comes across as unpleasant, disruptive, or associated with emotional outbursts are referred to as temper tantrums.
- They usually occur in response to the child's unmet needs or desires.
- Younger children who cannot express their needs/control their emotions are commonly affected.
- These occur at least once a day, lasting approximately 3 minutes in children below 5 years of age.

Etiology

- In toddlers, temper tantrums occur due to a need for parental attention.
- These are a result of desire for independence with limited capacity to self-regulate.

Children who have difficulty in expression due to language deficits may have more frequent and aggressive tantrum behaviors.

Presentation

- Temper tantrums may occur in varied forms such as episodes of excessive crying, loud screaming, flailing, hitting self/objects, throwing large items, breath-holding and going limp, head banging, pushing objects/others, biting people/objects.
- The tantrum usually lasts anywhere between 0.5 and 1 minute. The behavior and mood are normal between episodes.

Red Flag Signs

- Children >5 years with a repeated pattern
- Episodes lasting >15 minutes
- Occurring over five times per day
- Extreme aggression with physical injury/destruction of property
- Associated sleep disorders, enuresis, or negative moods between episodes

Associated Features

Temper tantrums may be associated with the following:

- Deficits of behavior development
- *Psychiatric problems:* Disruptive impulse control
- *Conduct disorders:* Oppositional defiant disorder
- *Trauma-related disorders:* Post-traumatic stress disorder
- *Neurodevelopmental problems:* Attention deficit hyperactivity disorder, autistic features, learning disorders, and vision/hearing deficits

Approach to Diagnosis

- Detailed history
- Thorough physical examination
- An assessment of family dynamics and their reaction to the tantrum

The approach to diagnosis and managing temper tantrums is given in **Flowchart 1**.

FLOWCHART 1: Approach to temper tantrums in children.

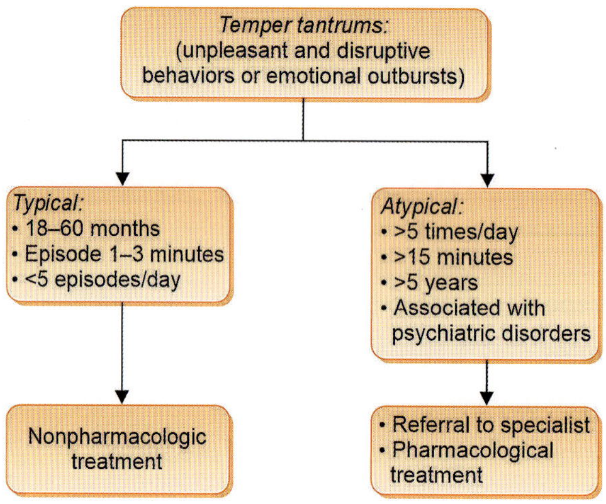

Nonpharmacological Approach

- *RIDD strategy:*
  - *R*emain calm: Keep a neutral voice with a quiet approach and emphasize redirection and distraction.
  - *I*gnore: Do not pay too much attention.
  - *D*istract the child/leave the area with the child.
  - *Do* say "yes" to ensure child's physical and safety needs, but do not give in to demands as it may reinforce undesired behaviors.
- Parent–child interaction therapy (PCIT) can be used to decrease behavioral problems in children aged 2–7 years.

Suggested Reading

- Bruno A, Celebre L, Torre G, Pandolfo G, Mento C, Cedro C, et al. Focus on disruptive mood dysregulation disorder: A review of the literature. Psychiatry Res. 2019;279:323-30.
- Daniels E, Mandleco B, Luthy KE. Assessment, management, and prevention of childhood temper tantrums. J Am Acad Nurse Pract. 2012;24(10):569-73.
- Sisterhen LL, Wy PAW. Temper Tantrums. In: StatPearls [Internet]. Treasure Island (FL): StatPearls Publishing; 2023. Available from https://www.ncbi.nlm.nih.gov/books/NBK544286/ [Last accessed August, 2024].

Anorexia

122

Section Editor: **Kripasindhu Chatterjee**
Section Co-Editors: **Atanu Bhadra, Ashim Kumar Ghosh**
Authors: **Sukanta Chatterjee, Shilpi Siddhanta Talukdar**

Introduction

- Anorexia refers to a prolonged lack of appetite.
- The hypothalamus houses the hunger and satiety centers. The afferent nerves from the gastrointestinal (GI) tract to these centers determine the anorexia that characterizes stomach and intestinal disorders. Other factors affecting satiety are ghrelin, leptin, and plasma glucose, which also reflect intestinal function.

Etiology

The etiology may be acute or chronic:

- Acute (<3 months), e.g., infection, trauma, and burns
- Chronic (≥3 months), e.g., chronic lung disease, cancer, and chemotherapy

It can be also classified as caused by:

- *Infections:* Urinary tract infections, GI tract and liver infections, viral fever, and parasitic infestations
- *Micronutrient deficiencies:* Zinc deficiency and wet beriberi (vitamin B_1 deficiency)
- *Electrolyte abnormalities:* Hyponatremia, and hypocalcemia
- Cancers and side effects of chemotherapy

- Burns
- *Systemic diseases:* Thyroid disorders, Addison's disease, increased intracranial pressure, hypothalamic dysfunction, rheumatologic diseases, abdominal migraine, and nephrotic syndrome
- Heavy metal intoxication
- *Behavioral, socioeconomic, or environmental:*
  - Parental dietary beliefs lead to inappropriately restricted diets; drinking excessive amounts of fruit juice
  - Child abuse/nonaccidental injuries
- *Anorexia nervosa:* 0.5–1% prevalence
- *Others:* Constipation
- Side effects of medications, for example, antibiotics
- Psychiatric causes

Red Flag Signs

- Severe weight loss
- Hypothermia
- Bradycardia
- Hypotension
- Weakened immune system/anemia
- Orthostatic changes in pulse and blood pressure
- Recurrent infections
- Arrhythmias
- Seizures

Approach

Ask for the following: Onset, duration, progress, timing, vomiting, nausea, dysuria, precipitating and palliating factors, history of any major illness, fever, medications, pain in abdomen, and HEADSSS (Home, Education/Employment, Activities, Drugs, Sex and relationships, Self-harm and depression, Safety and abuse) assessment in adolescents **(Flowchart 1)**

FLOWCHART 1: Approach to anorexia.

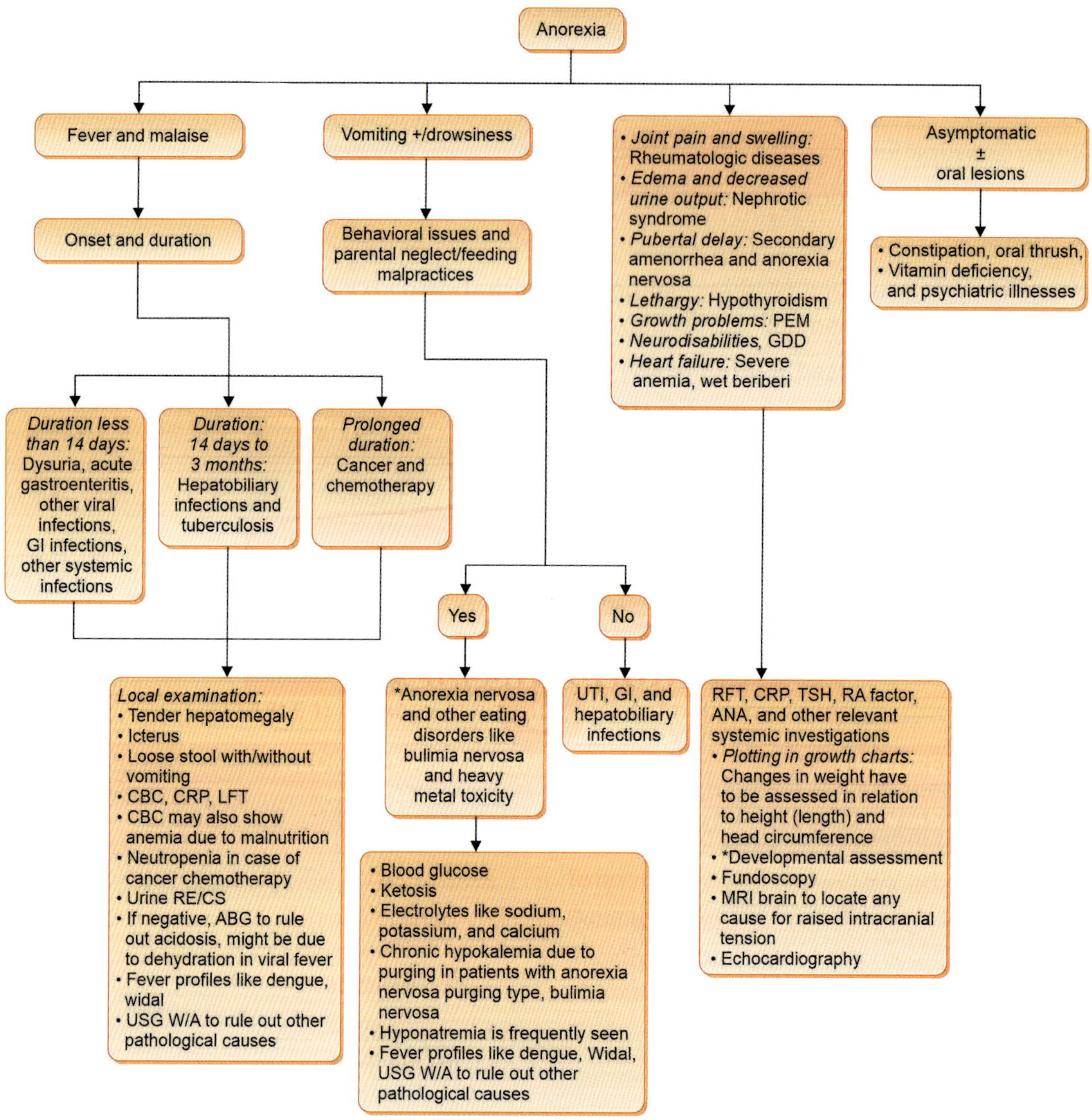

(ABG: arterial blood gas; ANA: antinuclear antibodies; CBC: complete blood count; CRP: C-reactive protein; GI: gastrointestinal; GDD: global developmental delay; LFT: liver function test; MRI: magnetic resonance imaging; PEM: protein-energy malnutrition; RA: rheumatoid arthritis; RE/CS: routine examination and culture sensitivity; RFT: renal function tests; TSH: thyroid-stimulating hormone; USG: ultrasonography; UTI: urinary tract infection; W/A: whole abdomen)

Suggested Reading

- Mammen P, Russell S, Russell PS. Prevalence of eating disorders and psychiatric comorbidity among children and adolescents. Indian Pediatr. 2007;44(5):357-9.
- Nivedita N, Sreenivasa G, Sathyanarayana Rao TS, Malini SS. Eating disorders: Prevalence in the student population of Mysore, South India. Indian J Psychiatry. 2018;60(4):433-7.
- Sravanti L, Velusamy AJP, Karki U, Kommu JVS, Girimaji SC. Clinical profile of children and adolescents diagnosed with anorexia nervosa in Indian context. Asian J Psychiatr. 2022;71:103077.
- Vaidyanathan S, Kuppili PP, Menon V. Eating Disorders: An Overview of Indian Research. Indian J Psychol Med. 2019;41(4):311-7.

Antenatally Detected Renal Anomalies

123

Section Editor: **Gnanamurthy Narasimha**
Section Co-Editor: **Nagalatha Chidananda**
Authors: **P Anil Kumar, Soundharya S, Ramesh Santhana Krishnan**

Introduction

- Renal anomalies are among the most common congenital anomalies as the development of urogenital system is complex.
- The structural abnormalities may or may not be associated with functional abnormality.

Etiology

The new evidence demonstrates that genetic and molecular changes impact embryonic kidney and urinary tract development. Congenital anomalies of the kidney and urinary tract (CAKUT) can present as an isolated renal condition or as part of a clinical syndrome.

Classification

The classification of antenatal renal anomalies is given in **Flowchart 1**.

FLOWCHART 1: Classification of antenatal renal anomaly.

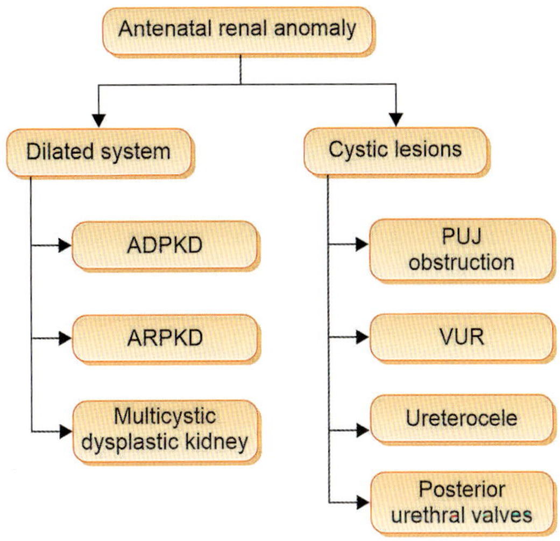

(ADPKD: autosomal dominant polycystic kidney disease; ARPKD: autosomal recessive polycystic kidney disease; PUJ: pelviureteric junction; VUR: vesicoureteral reflux)

Investigations

- *Fetal ultrasonography (USG):* A common modality for screening
- *Fetal magnetic resonance imaging (MRI):* It plays an important role where ultrasound is inconclusive. It overcomes the obstacles posed by a lack of amniotic fluid and has added value in terms of refining, modifying, or adding to the diagnostic information provided by ultrasound.

Referral Criteria for Antenatal and Postnatal Renal Anomalies

Fetal intervention: Currently, fetal surgery is considered only in the case of posterior urethral valves (PUV).

Termination of pregnancy is indicated in:

- Bilateral renal agenesis
- Associated with aneuploidy
- Cystic lesions in kidney with loss of corticomedullary differentiation

An important common entity requiring regular monitoring is antenatally detected hydronephrosis. The simple practical approach is mentioned in **Table 1**.

Antenatal assessment: This is to assess the degree of hydronephrosis and prognostication.

TABLE 1: A practical approach to the antenatal assessment of hydronephrosis.

BASED ON PELVIC APD			SFU CLASSIFICATION		UTD CLASSIFICATION	
	Second trimester	Third trimester	SFU1	Urine barely split pelvis	UTDA1	Central or no calyceal dilatation
Mild	4–6 mm	7–9 mm	SFU2	Moderate renal pelvis splitting confined to renal border with dilated major calyces		
Moderate	7–10 mm	10–15 mm	SFU3	Pelvis distended beyond renal border, major and minor calyces dilated, and parenchyma spared	UTDA2–3	*Any one of the following:* Peripheral calyceal dilatation, abnormal parenchymal thickness/ appearance, ureters abnormal, bladder abnormal, and unexplained hydramnios
Severe	>10 mm	>15 mm	SFU4	Parenchyma thinned		

(APD: anteroposterior diameter; SFU: Society of Fetal Urology; UTD: urinary tract dilatation)

Postnatal Evaluation

Clinical examination and investigations:

Physical Examination

- *A palpable abdominal mass:*
    - Multicystic dysplastic kidney (MCDK)
    - Ureteropelvic junction (UPJ) obstruction
    - Autosomal recessive polycystic kidney disease (ARPKD)

- *Absent abdominal wall musculature with bilateral undescended testes:* Suggests diagnosis of prune belly syndrome
- *Palpable bladder:*
  - PUV
  - Urethral atresia
  - Urethral stricture
- *A palpable abdominal mass:* Severe bilateral hydronephrosis or severe unilateral hydronephrosis in a single functioning kidney warrants immediate postnatal evaluation with a renal sonogram and voiding cystourethrogram (VCUG)

Postnatal investigations indicated in:

- *MCDK:* Usually resolves
- Polycystic kidney disease (PCKD) is of two types:
  1. *Autosomal dominant:* Manifests later in life and can lead to renal failure later
  2. *Autosomal recessive:* Manifests early in childhood and is incompatible with life, requiring kidney transplant in early childhood
- *Ureterocele, cysts, duplication anomalies, etc.:* Do not require any intervention; only postnatal evaluation and management are needed.
- *Antenatally diagnosed hydronephrosis*—Requires close monitoring

Managing Antenatally Diagnosed Hydronephrosis

The degree of hydronephrosis indicates the necessity of postnatal assessment and intervention.

- *Mild hydronephrosis:* No intervention
- *Moderate hydronephrosis:* Postnatal assessment and some intervention
- *Severe hydronephrosis:* Definite postnatal assessment and intervention as required.

Postnatal assessment of children with antenatal hydronephrosis:

- Unilateral hydronephrosis
  - Postnatal USG is done after 3 days of life as there is physiologic oliguria for the first 48 hours.
  - In case of persistent hydronephrosis on the postnatal USG after 72 hours, do isotope scintigraphy after 1 month.
  - In case of massive hydronephrosis with a palpable kidney, renal scintigraphy [ethylene dicysteine (EC) scan] needs to be done immediately.

- *Bilateral hydronephrosis* needs prompt assessment:
  - Assess for a palpable bladder/any other clinical clue for PUV
  - USG to rule out PUV in male babies
  - Bladder catheterization and a micturating cystourethrogram
  - If PUV is diagnosed, refer to a pediatric surgeon.
  - If PUV is ruled out, assess for other causes such as bilateral pelviureteric junction (PUJ) obstruction, ureteroceles, neurogenic bladder, urethral atresia, etc., and refer to surgeon.
- *Renal function tests:* Progressive daily increase in the creatinine values are indicative of a severe degree of renal failure.
- *The role of isotope scintigraphy:*
  - *Diethylenetriamine pentaacetate (DTPA):* After 4–6 weeks, if no red flag signs
  - *EC/mercaptoacetyltriglycine-3 (MAG 3):* The scan of choice in cases of severe hydronephrosis either in a single system/palpable kidney
  - *Dimercaptosuccinic acid (DMSA) scan* is a measure of cortical function and scarring if any. No use in cases of hydronephrosis

Red Flag Signs

- Oligohydramnios (timing and severity)
- Renal cortical cysts
- Renal size and poor corticomedullary differentiation
- Fetal renal pelvis anteroposterior diameter 6 mm or over at 24 weeks; and 10 mm or more at 30 weeks
- Bilateral hydronephrosis with distended bladder and dilated ureters
- Single kidney with moderate-to-severe hydronephrosis

An algorithmic approach to postnatal management of antenatally detected renal anomaly is given in **Flowchart 2**.

FLOWCHART 2: Postnatal management of antenatally detected renal anomaly.

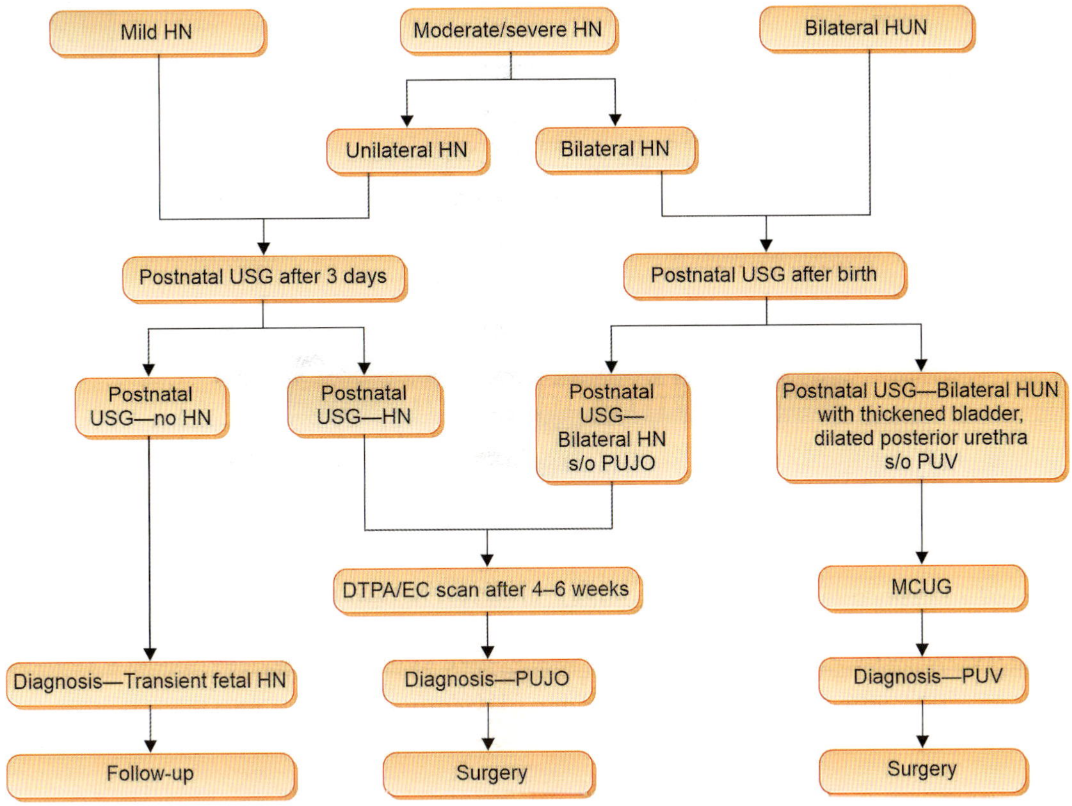

(DTPA: diethylenetriamine pentaacetate; EC: ethylene dicysteine; HN: hydronephrosis; HUN: hydroureteronephrosis; MCUG: micturating cystourethrogram; PUV: posterior urethral valves; PUJO: pelviureteric junction obstruction; USG: ultrasonography)

Suggested Reading

- Dias T, Sairam S, Kumarasiri S. Ultrasound diagnosis of fetal renal abnormalities. Best Pract Res Clin Obstet Gynaecol. 2014;28(3):403-15.
- Prasad P, Agar C, Harrison C. Congenital renal tract abnormalities: A neonatal perspective. Infant. 2017;13(3):100-4.

Fatigue and Weakness

124

Section Editor: **Kripasindhu Chatterjee**
Section Co-Editors: **Atanu Bhadra, Ashim Kumar Ghosh**
Authors: **Kaustav Nayek, Taraknath Ghosh**

Introduction

- Fatigue is defined as unusual tiredness due to an inability to increase the supply of energy or blood flow with exertion.
- Weakness is mainly due to muscular/neurological causes but could be due to psychological causes. Prevalence in the pediatric age group is around 4.4% with the highest frequency among adolescent females. The prevalence is 21% in children suffering from chronic diseases.

Etiology of Fatigue

INFANCY	CHILDHOOD	ADOLESCENTS
Congenital heart diseases	Upper respiratory tract infection	Anxiety or depression
Severe anemia	Otitis media and sinusitis	JIA and IBD
Congenital hypothyroidism	Hepatitis	Malignancy
	AIDS and malignancies	Diabetes, hypothyroidism, hypopituitarism, Addison's disease, and severe obesity
	Renal disease	Pulmonary diseases
	Obstructive sleep apnea	Drug abuse
	Chronic asthma and allergies	Fibromyalgia

(AIDS: acquired immunodeficiency syndrome; IBD: inflammatory bowel disease; JIA: juvenile idiopathic arthritis)

Weakness in Infancy

- Spinomuscular atrophy
- Down syndrome
- Congenital hypothyroidism
- Infant botulism
- Congenital myasthenia

Weakness in Childhood and Adolescence

CENTRAL CAUSE	NERVE CAUSE	NMJ CAUSE	MUSCLE CAUSE
Childhood multiple sclerosis	Motor neuron disease	Myasthenia gravis	Myopathy
CVA	Peripheral neuropathy	Botulism	Muscular dystrophy
CNS infections			Dermatomyositis
Tumor			
Traumatic brain injury			
Spinocerebellar ataxia			
Migraine			
Mitochondrial diseases			

(CNS: central nervous system; CVA: cerebrovascular accidents; NMJ: neuromuscular junction)

Drug-related fatigue: Consumption of benzodiazepines, antiepileptics, neuroleptic, and selected antihypertensives, can produce drug-related fatigue.

Red Flag Signs

- Bone pain, weight loss, and night sweats—consider leukemia and lymphoma
- Abdominal pain, vomiting, diarrhea, weight loss; failure to thrive—rule out inflammatory bowel disease (IBD) and celiac disease.
- Shortness of breath—due to cardiac or pulmonary causes

Algorithm for Approach

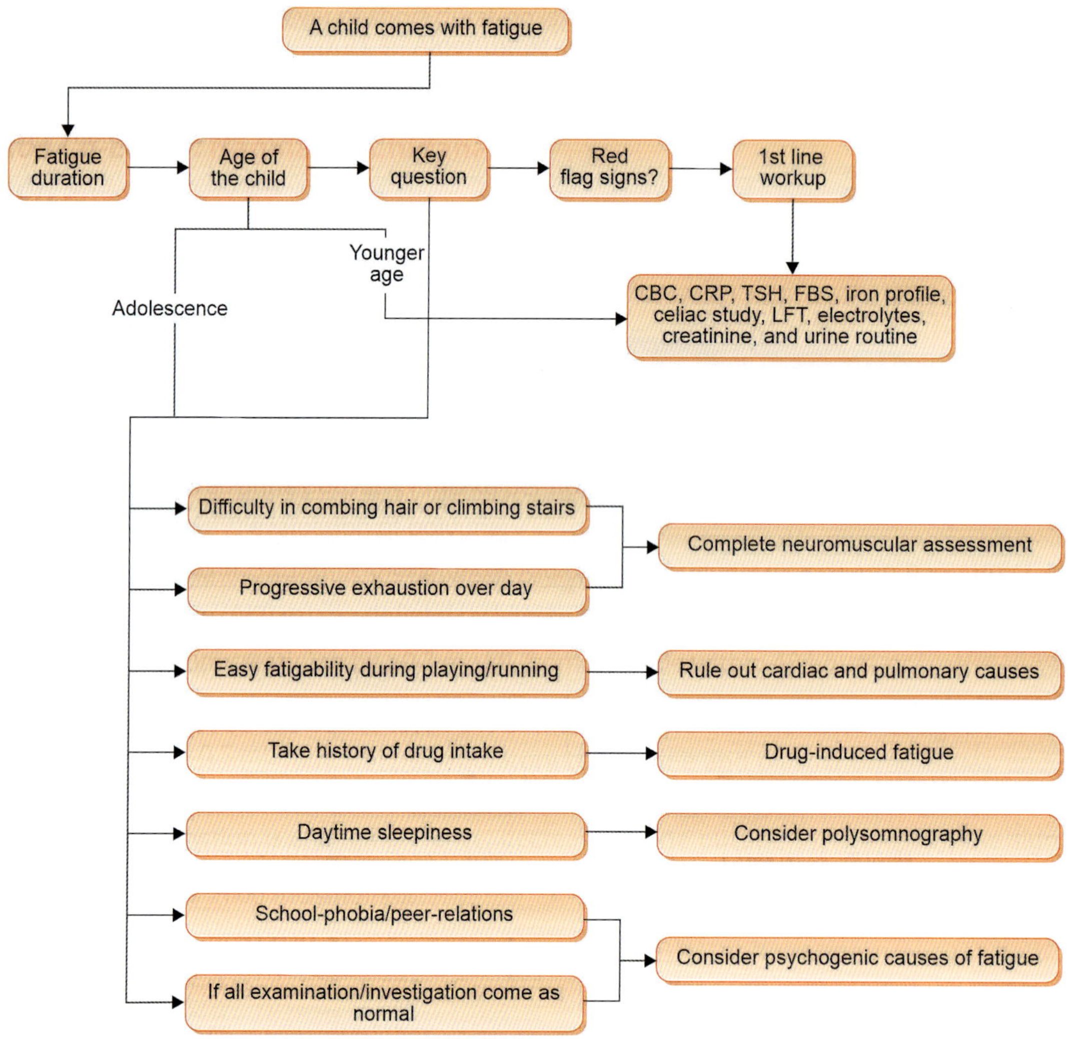

(CBC: complete blood count; CRP: C reactive protein; FBS: fasting blood sugar; LFT: liver function tests; TSH: thyroid-stimulating hormone)

Suggested Reading

- De Nardi L, Lanzetta MA, Ghirigato E, Barbi E, Gortani G. Approach to the child with fatigue: A focus for the general pediatrician. Front Pediatr. 2022;10.
- Farmer A, Fowler T, Scourfield J, Thapar A. Prevalence of chronic disabling fatigue in children and adolescents. Br J Psychiatry. 2004;184(6):477-81.
- Magnusson MR. Chronic fatigue syndrome. In: Kliegman RM, Geme JW, Blum NJ, Tasker RC, Shah SS, Wilson KM, Behrman RE, Nelson WE (Eds). Nelson Textbook of Pediatrics, 21st edition. Philadelphia: Elsevier Inc; 2020. pp. 1093-6.
- Nap-van der Vlist MM, Dalmeijer GW, Grootenhuis MA, van der Ent K, van den Heuvel-Eibrink MM, Swart JF, et al. Fatigue among children with a chronic disease: A cross-sectional study. BMJ Paediatrics Open. 2021;5(1):e000958.
- Van de Vijver E, Van Gils A, Beckers L, Van Driessche Y, Moes ND, van Rheenen PF. Fatigue in children and adolescents with inflammatory bowel disease. World J Gastroenterol. 2019;25(5):632-43.

Medically Unexplained Symptoms

125

Section Editor: **Kripasindhu Chatterjee**
Section Co-Editors: **Atanu Bhadra, Ashim Kumar Ghosh**
Authors: **Mandira Roy, Kripasindhu Chatterjee**

Introduction

- Medically unexplained symptoms (MUS) or medically unexplained physical symptoms (MUPS) are a group of symptoms with no organic medical explanation despite methodical physical examination and rational investigation.
- The terminology can be misleading because the degree of impairment of function outweighs the concerned symptom, shadowing the presence of a medical cause.
- Also known as somatoform symptoms, somatization symptoms, functional symptoms, etc., these symptoms are grouped together into a single entity called "somatic symptoms and related disorders (SSRDs)" in the latest Diagnostic and Statistical Manual of Mental Disorders, Fifth Edition (DSM5).
- Approximately 10–25% of children and adolescents report chronic somatic complaints and around 68% of children who present for medical treatment have psychological factors associated with somatic complaints.

Etiology

The etiology is not fully understood. Evidence supports a complex interplay of physiological, psychological, and interpersonal factors. Some important etiological factors are:

- *Physiological:* Relatively, normal physiological bodily sensations may feel excessive. For example, normal peristaltic movement may seem abnormal as a manifestation of a life-threatening disease.
- *Biological:* Genetically, predetermined pain thresholds and tolerance. Females are more prone to MUS than males. A family history of MUS in parents or grandparents may occur.

- *Psychological:* A deficit in cognitive development of a child leads to a lack of coping skills, emotional dysregulation, distorted perceptions of reality, and difficulties with emotional expression. These are the most common causes. The presence of pre-existing psychiatric comorbidities like anxiety disorder, obsessive–compulsive disorder, and depressive disorders may coexist.
- *Family environment:* Financial hardship, abusive parents, alcohol/drug addiction in the family, Emotionally unavailable parents or caregivers
- *School environment*: Bullying, physical or emotional abuse in school, and fear of academic failure

Red Flag Signs

- Prolonged history with several doctor visits and unnecessary surgeries
- Unusual anxiety in patients as well as caregivers
- Severe impairment of diet, sleep, and other daily activities
- Unresponsiveness to standard treatment
- Signs of physical, mental, and sexual abuse, especially in adolescents

Diagnosis

- The diagnosis is made after excluding all other causes
- The spectrum of MUS can be broad and needs proper clinical classification and a stepped-care approach **(Table 1)**.

TABLE 1: Spectrum of medically unexplained symptoms (MUS).

TYPE	SYMPTOMS	APPROACH
Mild	Self-limiting	No investigations needed; observation
Moderate	Recurrent and involves multiple systems	Needs standard investigations
Severe	Severe, distressing, and impairing activities of daily living	May need hospitalization and a thorough workup

Approach to Diagnose Medically Unexplained Symptoms

The approach to diagnosing MUS is given in **Flowchart 1**.

FLOWCHART 1: Approach to diagnose medically unexplained symptoms (MUS).

Step 1: Detailed medical history—onset, frequency, progression, and specific system involvement

↓

Step 2: Detailed psychosocial history (may need separate session with the child and caregivers), family environment, school environment, and family history of psychiatric illness

↓

Step 3: Thorough physical examination according to the systems involved

↓

Step 4: Judicious workup to rule out potential organic pathology

↓

Step 5: Referral to a psychiatrist, if some psychiatric comorbidities like depression or anxiety are suspected

Suggested Reading

- American Psychiatric Association. Diagnostic and Statistical Manual of Mental Disorders, Fifth Edition. United States: American Psychiatric Association; 2013. pp. 311-27.
- Hadji-Michael M, McAllister E, Reilly C, Heyman I, Bennett S. Alexithymia in children with medically unexplained symptoms: A systematic review. J Psychosom Res. 2019;123:109736.
- Hughes T, Meredith F, Monteregge S, Bennett S, Shafran, R. Medically unexplained symptoms in children: An experimental investigation of the impact of internet searching on parental responses. Behav Cogn Psychother. 2021;49(1):91-103.
- Leaviss J, Davis S, Ren S, Hamilton J, Scope A, Booth A, et al. Behavioural modification interventions for medically unexplained symptoms in primary care: Systematic reviews and economic evaluation. Health Technol Assess. 2020;24(46):1-490.

Picky Eating

126

Section Editor: **Kripasindhu Chatterjee**
Section Co-Editors: **Atanu Bhadra, Ashim Kumar Ghosh**
Author: **Subhasish Bhattacharyya**

Introduction

- Picky eating is a common behavior in early childhood. The accepted definition of picky eating, proposed by Dovey et al., refers to children "who consume an inadequate variety of foods though rejection of a substantial amount of food that are familiar (as well as unfamiliar) to them".
- At around 2–3 years of age, up to 20% of children are picky eaters irrespective of ethnicity and socioeconomic status. There may be an associated family-dysfunctional environment. Boys and girls are equally affected.

Etiology

Causes of picky eating include:

- Early feeding difficulties/late introduction of lumpy foods at weaning/pressure to eat
- Parents/caregiver's pressure to eat more
- Erratic appetite
- Attention-seeking behavior
- Dysfunctional family
- Excessive intake of carbonated drinks juice and sweets
- Copying parents and older children
- Meals between the meals
- Early choosiness, especially if the mother is worried by this

Some are very sensitive to taste, smell, and texture. Others develop picky-eating habits by modeling their parent's fussy eating habits.

Red Flag Signs

- Being underweight/overweight, poor growth patterns, and zinc, iron, vitamins, and other micronutrients deficiency disorders
- Associated developmental difficulties
- Chronic and recurrent constipation
- Susceptibility to chronic illness and infection

Differentiate from food allergies/intolerance, lactose intolerance, gastroesophageal reflux disease (GERD), celiac sprue, emotional disorders, functional dysphagia, and post-traumatic feeding disorder.

Approach

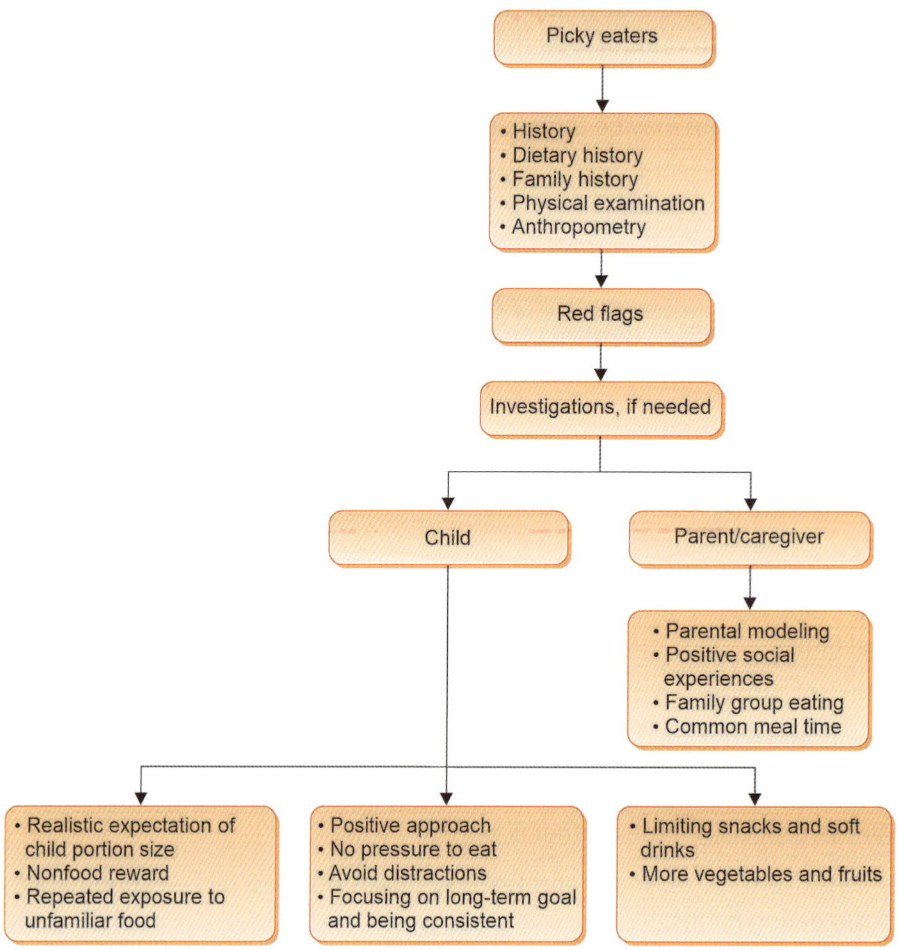

Suggested Reading

- Cunliffe L, Coulthard H, Williamson IR. The lived experience of parenting a child with sensory sensitivity and picky eating. Matern Child Nutr. 2022;18(3):e13330.
- Diamantis DV, Emmett PM, Taylor CM. Effect of being a persistent picky eater on feeding difficulties in school-aged children. Appetite. 2023;183:106483.
- Elizabeth KE. Picky eating. In: Nutrition and Child Development, 6th edition. New Delhi: Paras Medical Publisher; 2022. pp. 103-8.
- Kamarudin MS, Shahril MR, Haron H, Kadar M, Safii NS, Hamzaid NH. Interventions for picky eaters among typically developed children-A scoping review. Nutrients. 2023;15(1):242.
- Taylor CM, Emmett PM. Picky eating in children: Causes and consequences. Proc Nutr Soc. 2019;78(2):161-9.
- Walton K, Kuczynski L, Haycraft E, Breen A, Haines J. Time to re-think picky eating? A relational approach to understanding picky eating. Int J Behav Nutr Phys Act. 2017;14(1):62.

Substance Use

127

Section Editor: **Kripasindhu Chatterjee**
Section Co-Editors: **Atanu Bhadra, Ashim Kumar Ghosh**
Authors: **Joydeep Das, Mandira Roy**

Introduction

- Substance use is commonly seen in adolescence and is showing an increasing trend in both urban and rural India. Overdose can cause substantial disability, mortality, and also other medical complications, such as hepatitis C virus, HIV, and bacterial infections which continue to surge among young adults who use opioids and other criminalized drugs as well.
- This is also a known risk factor for the development of neuropsychiatric symptoms in adolescence and substance-use disorders (SUDs) in adulthood.

Etiology

Etiology is multifactorial, ranging from individual personal characteristics (e.g., cognitive development, psychological factors, physical craving) and genetics predisposition to socioenvironmental factors (e.g., peer pressure, parenting, family and school environment, community traditions, and other structural factors).

Commonly Used Substances

Some commonly used substances are given in the following text.

Alcohol

Alcohol is one of the most commonly used recreational drugs all over the world, with adolescents being a large group of consumers.

Alcohol has neurotoxic effects and possibly modifies a number of structures and circuits in the brain, most commonly the meso-corticolimbic and striatal systems. Stress-related psychopathologies are more common in adolescent alcohol exposure (AAE) than other substance abuse and are associated with increased rate and severity of the attacks. Adolescents are also notably less sensitive than adults toward many of the intoxication cues that suppress drinking, such as hangover, sedation, and motor impairment, and are more prone to the reinforcing effects of alcohol, such as social facilitation.

Cannabis

Cannabis is being more accessible and available in recent times, because of its both recreational and medical legality. Its perception as a potentially addictive and harmful substance is decreasing over the last few decades.

Adolescent cannabis exposure (ACE) has been linked to multiple neuropsychiatric disorders and is being identified as a risk factor in schizophrenia and psychosis. It has also been linked to depression, anxiety, and addiction toward other agents.

Nicotine

Electronic e-cigarette products have led to an increase in the use of nicotine among adolescents. Nicotine has multiple harmful effects on cognitive development and behavior.

Adolescent nicotine exposure (ANE) is associated with increased risk mood and anxiety disorder. ANE increases the likelihood of continued use of nicotine, cannabis, and alcohol. Nicotine also modulates multiple neurotransmitter system pathways, including gamma-aminobutyric acid (GABA), glutamate, dopamine, acetylcholine, and serotonin which play a key role in the adolescence neurodevelopment.

Polyuse

Cannabis, alcohol, and nicotine use are often directly related to each other. All three are often used in combination, because of reinforcing properties of each other and persistent use of one drug might cause relapse of another.

Red Flags

- Persistence changes in mood (anger outburst, irritability, defensiveness)
- Poor scholastic performance (absenteeism, low grades, loss of attention skills)
- Changing companions, friends, and reluctance to disclose their identity to family members
- Constant demand for money; sometimes stealing
- Lack of engagement in former interests like sports or family events; general low energy
- Substances with abuse potential (drug or alcohol) can be found in youth's room or personal effects
- Physical or mental changes (clumsy gait, memory lapses, lack of eye–hand coordination, slurring of speech)
- Physical changes like sudden weight loss, frequent nose bleeding, involuntary movements, tremors. Multiple injection wounds.
- Lack of personal hygiene and difficulties doing daily living activities

Screening

CRAFFT (Car, Relax, Alone, Forget, Family/Friends, Trouble) questionnaire screening tool has been developed for early screening of substance abuse in adolescents and young people (aged 12–21 years), which can alert healthcare providers and parents to take life-saving interventions at early stages **(Box 1)**.

BOX 1: CRAFFT Questionnaire.

Part A

- During the past 12 months, did you drink alcohol (more than a few sips)?
- During the past 12 months, did you smoke any marijuana or hashish?
- During the past 12 months, did you use anything else to get high?
- If the answer is "no" to all three opening questions, the doctor will only ask the first question of Part B, while those who respond with a "yes" to any of the opening questions will be asked all six CRAFFT queries.

Part B: The six CRAFFT questions:

- *C:* Have you ever ridden in a CAR driven by someone (including yourself) who was "high" or had been using alcohol or drugs?
- *R:* Do you ever use alcohol or drugs to RELAX, feel better about yourself, or fit in?
- *A:* Do you ever use alcohol/drugs while you are by yourself, or ALONE?
- *F:* Do you ever FORGET things you did while using alcohol or drugs?
- *F:* Do your FAMILY or FRIENDS ever tell you that you should cut down on your drinking or drug use?
- *T:* Have you gotten into TROUBLE while you were using alcohol or drugs?

- **Intervention:** Excessive consumption of nicotine, alcohol and cannabis or other substances can have long-lasting effects on the brain and body. Continued screening at outpatient behavioral health setting is essential to isolate the predictors, mechanisms, and consequences of adolescent drug use. Efficacious treatment options and preventive interventions should be adopted parallely.
- **Bridge clinics** whether hospital-based or outpatient clinics, offer immediate access to medications for opioid use disorder (MOUD) and other SUDs treatment and are increasingly being available in recent times.
- **Preventive and therapeutic interventions** to reduce adolescent substance abuse should be incorporated at global, national and local levels. Integration of adolescent mental health into national and regional policies, strategies and programs should be implemented in day to day practice. Family, schools, peers, community, health services, and other institutions play important roles in the multidisciplinary management.
- Influential people and community leaders, health care providers and other components of the the health system, and policymakers should actively participate to reduce the burden of the disease at each level of

FLOWCHART 1: Algorithm to approach a case of substance use.

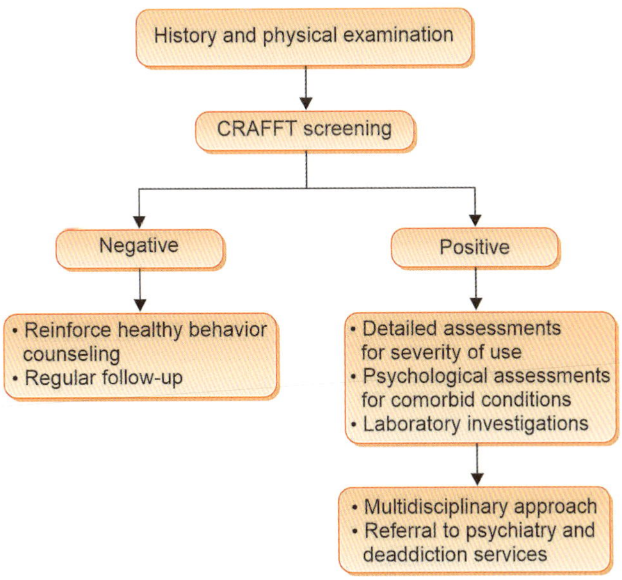

Suggested Reading

- Belay LM, Sendekie TY, Eyowas FA. Quality of multiple-choice questions in medical internship qualification examination determined by item response theory at Debre Tabor University, Ethiopia. BMC Med Educ. 2022;22(1):635.
- Knight JR, Shrier LA, Bravender TD, Farrell M, Vander Bilt J, Shaffer HJ. A new brief screen for adolescent substance abuse. Arch Pediatr Adolesc Med. 1999;153(6):591-6. doi: 10.1001/archpedi.153.6.591. PMID: 10357299.
- National Health Mission. Orientation programme for Medical Officers to provide Adolescent-Friendly Health Services: Handouts. [online] Available from https://nhm.gov.in/images/pdf/programmes/RKSK/Medical_Officer_Training_Manual/Resource_Book_Medical_Officer.pdf.
- Park E-A, Jung A-R, Choi S. Analysis of related factors for adolescents' intention to use alcohol in Korea. PLoS One. 2022;17(10):e0275957.
- Song Y, Kim H, Park SY. An item response theory analysis of the Korean version of the CRAFFT scale for alcohol use among adolescents in Korea. Asian Nurs Res. 2019;13(4):249-56.
- World Health Organization. Adolescent mental health. [online] Available from https://www.who.int/news-room/fact-sheets/detail/adolescent-mental-health.

Failure to Thrive

128

Section Editor: **Kripasindhu Chatterjee**
Section Co-Editors: **Atanu Bhadra, Ashim Kumar Ghosh**
Author: **Susrut Das**

Introduction

- Failure to thrive (FTT)/failure to gain weight is a descriptive diagnostic term that describes a child below 5 years not gaining weight as per the peer group.
- While describing FTT, stature or height is usually not considered. When both weight and height are affected, it is considered growth failure.

Definition

Failure to thrive (FTT) is described as less than 3rd centile in growth chart. But, as small-for-gestational-age (SGA) babies below 2 years, preterm babies, and children with short stature could not be categorized under this definition, a newer definition is available.

New Definition

Failure to thrive is defined as "Deceleration of growth curve crossing 2 major centile lines in a serial growth plotting. When serial growth plotting is NOT available, FTT is defined as <80% of ideal body weight OR <3rd centile as per weight per height chart".

Etiology

- A significant percentage of cases that are described as FTT are a category of pseudo or perceived FTT because of a lack of serial growth recordings.
- The etiology of true FTT is classified into two categories **(Table 1)**.

TABLE 1: Etiology of true failure to thrive.

NONORGANIC	ORGANIC
• Poverty • Lack of parenting knowledge • Poor nutritional practices • Abuse and neglect	• *GIT:* GERD, malabsorption (celiac disease, etc.), and IBD. • *CNS:* Cerebral palsy, mental retardation, and developmental disorders • *CVS:* Congenital heart disease • *Renal:* Renal tubular acidosis and chronic kidney disease • *Endocrine:* Diabetes mellitus and hypothyroidism • *Pulmonary:* Cystic fibrosis and bronchial asthma • *Infections:* Tuberculosis, HIV, chronic parasitic infections, and recurrent antibiotic abuse • *Genetic:* Inborn error of metabolism and chromosomal anomalies • *Others:* Micronutrient deficiency, drug-induced, pollutants, and poisoning

(CNS: central nervous system; CVS: cerebrovascular system; GIT: gastrointestinal tract; GERD: gastroesophageal reflux disease; HIV: human immunodeficiency virus; IBD: inflammatory bowel disease)

Red Flag Signs

- Symptomatic organic causes
- Persistent FTT despite nutritional intervention
- Overt electrolyte imbalance
- Severe anemia
- Severe malabsorption syndromes
- Immunocompromised child
- Signs of abuse and neglect

Approach

A practical approach to a case of FTT in clinical practice is shown in **Flowchart 1**.

FLOWCHART 1: Diagnostic algorithm for management of a child with failure to thrive (FTT).

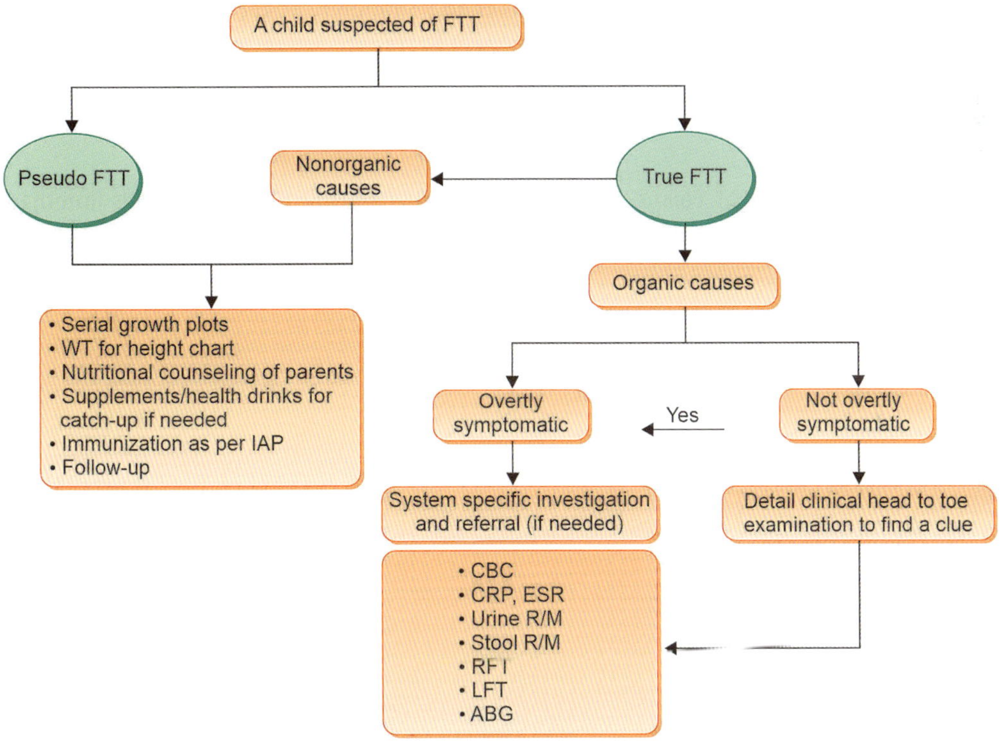

(ABG: arterial blood gas; CBC: complete blood count; CRP: c-reactive protein; ESR: erythrocyte sedimentation rate; IAP: Indian Academy of Pediatrics; LFT: liver function test; RFT: renal function test; R/M: routine and microscopy)

Suggested Reading

- Franceschi R, Rizzardi C, Maines E. Liguori A, Soffiati M, Tornese G. Failure to thrive in infant and toddlers: A practical flowchart-based approach in a hospital setting. Ital J Pediatr. 2021;47(1):62.
- Homan GJ. Failure to Thrive: A Practical Guide. Am Fam Physician. 2016;94(4):295-9.
- Maiti P, Mondal B. IMNCI Guidelines. An Ultimate Guide to Community Medicine. New Delhi: Jaypee Brothers Medical Publishers (P) Ltd; 2016
- Parthasarathy A, Menon PSN, Agarwal RK, Thacker N, Choudhury P, Ugra D, Nair MKC, Gupta P, Agrawal RC, Amladi T (Eds). IAP Textbook of Pediatrics, 4th edition. New Delhi: Jaypee Brothers Medical Publishers (P) Ltd; 2009. pp. 111-5.
- Smith AE, Shah M, Badireddy M. Failure to Thrive. [Updated 2023 Nov 12]. In: StatPearls [Internet]. Treasure Island (FL): StatPearls Publishing; 2023. Available from https://www.ncbi.nlm.nih.gov/books/NBK459287/ [Last accessed August, 2024].

Feeding Difficulties in Neonates

129

Section Editor: **Nehal Patel**
Section Co-Editor: **Jay T Dhirwani**
Authors: **Nagalatha Chidananda, Nehal Patel**

Introduction

Identifying feeding difficulties is important to prevent potential serious short- and long-term consequences in infants.

Causes

The main causes of feeding problems in the neonates are listed in **Flowchart 1**.

FLOWCHART 1: Causes of feeding problems in the neonates.

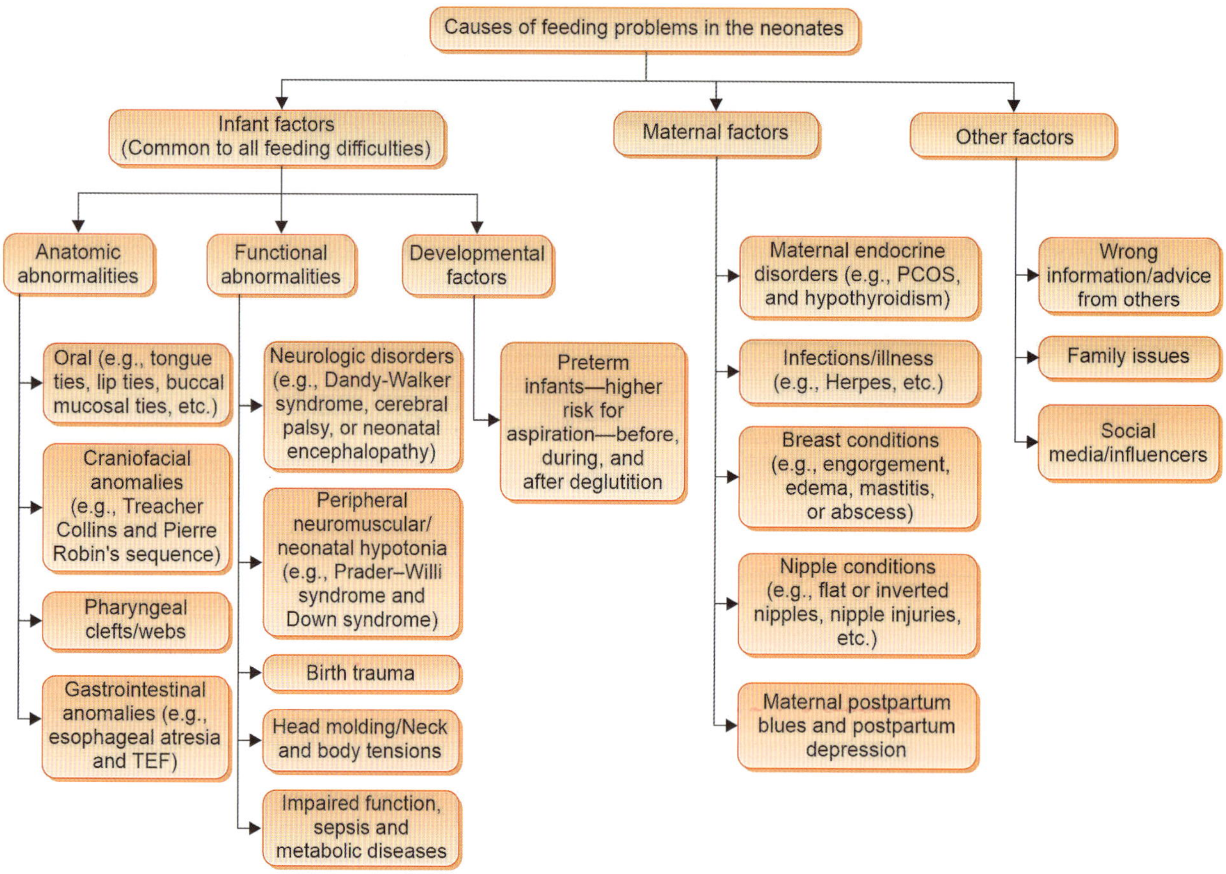

(PCOS: polycystic ovary syndrome; TEF: tracheoesophageal fistula)

Clinical Manifestations

The signs and symptoms of feeding disorders are given in **Table 1**.

TABLE 1: Clinical manifestations of feeding disorders.

FEEDING PATTERN/BEHAVIOR	RESPIRATORY SYMPTOMS/FINDINGS	FAILURE TO THRIVE
• Poor suck and inability to latch • Pooling of milk • Drooling • Prolonged feeding/passive at the breast • Fussiness, crying, and back arching • Apnea, choking, cyanosis or other acute events during feeding	• Significant cough • Noisy breathing • Aspiration pneumonia • Respiratory distress like cyanosis/increased respiratory rate	• Not gaining weight–regained birth weight by 10 days in term; not gaining weight in 15 days in preterm • *Dehydration:* Few/no stools, scanty urine, urate crystals, weak cry, dry mucous membrane, and sunken fontanelle • Lethargy, irritability, and less hunger cues

History

History related to feeding disorder in infant is given in **Flowchart 2**.

FLOWCHART 2: History related to feeding disorders in infants.

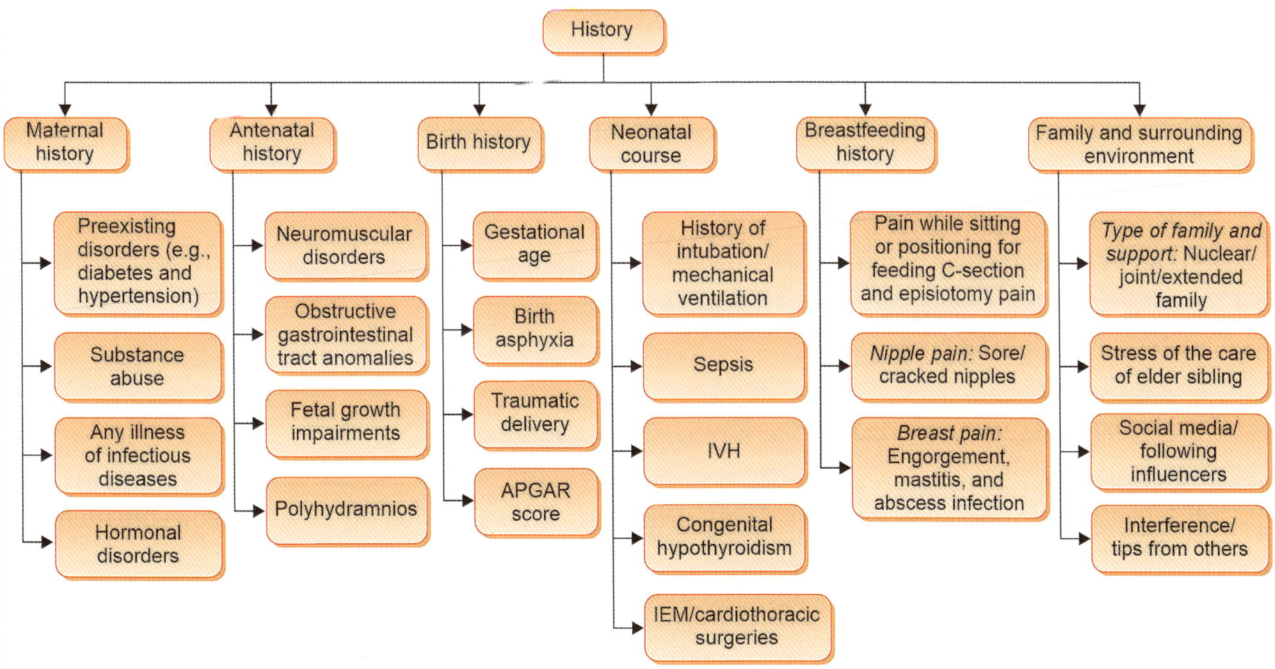

(APGAR: appearance, pulse, grimace, activity and respiration; IEM: inborn errors of metabolism; IVH: intraventricular hemorrhage)

Diagnostic Approach

The Physical Examination

Infant Examination

It includes:

- Weight/height—for severity
- Any systemic illness
- *Physical barriers:* Congenital diaphragmatic hernia (CDH), limb anomalies, etc.
- *Assessment of face:* Jaw, lips—cleft lip, hard and soft palate—cleft/high arched, tethered oral structure, lip tie/tongue tie; use Bristol tongue assessment score.
- Cranial nerve function involved in feeding.

Maternal Examination

- Any major illness/infection/endocrine disorder
- *Breast size/shape:*
  - Small/large breasts
  - *Examination of glandular tissue:* Hypoplastic breasts
  - Check breast compressibility.
- *Nipple examination:*
  - Small/large/flat
  - *Inverted nipple:* Check for protractility
- *Supply related:* Oversupply/under supply/overactive oxytocin reflex

Assessing Breastfeeding Technique

- *Prefeeding readiness:* Gestational age, medical stability, and prefeeding skills
- *Observation of a feed:*
  - Place/environment of the feed
  - Family support while mother readies herself
  - Interaction between baby and mother while feeding
  - Positioning and latching
  - Alignment of baby
  - *Breast holds:* C/U/(Scissoring—hold can cause improper latching)
- *Nutritive sucking:*
  - Infant's state of alertness, rooting reflexes; sucking/suck–swallow rhythm/Suck–swallow–breathing coordination in preterm
  - Observe the latch and various associated sounds
- *Post-feeding behaviors:*
  - Post-feeding breast/nipple changes
  - Crying/calm baby

Investigations

Investigations are required for infants with anatomical/neurological defects, red flag signs, mothers with certain conditions **(Flowchart 3)**.

FLOWCHART 3: Investigations.

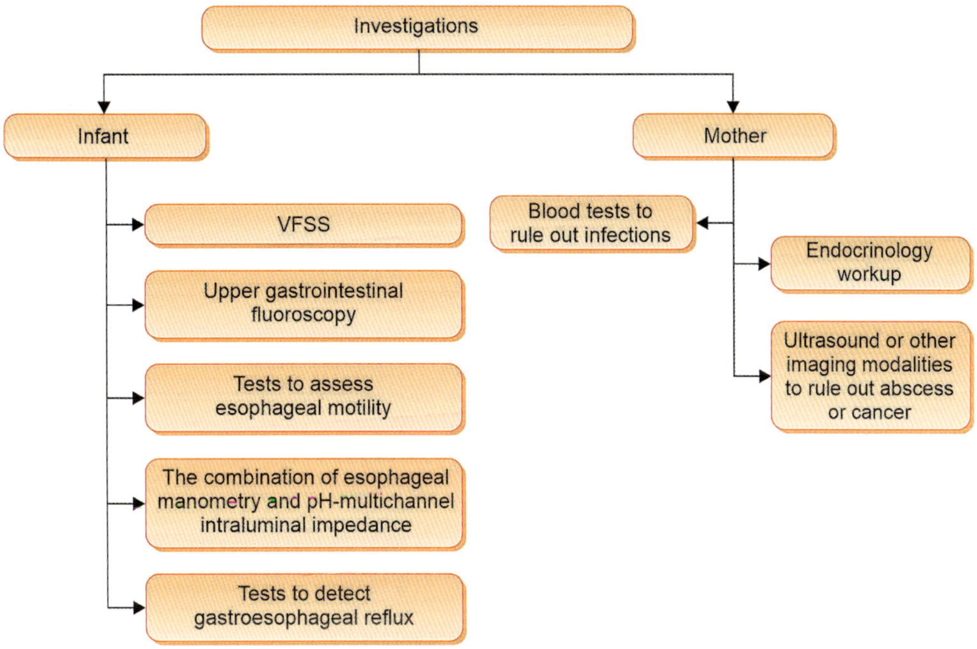

(VFSS: video fluoroscopic swallow study)

Red Flag Signs

Red flag signs include the following:

- Failure to thrive
- Episodes of apnea/choking
- Respiratory distress
- Cyanosis during/post-feeds

Approach to Evaluate the Child with Feeding Difficulty

The approach to evaluating a child with feeding difficulty is given in **Flowchart 4**.

FLOWCHART 4: Approach to evaluate the child with feeding difficulty.

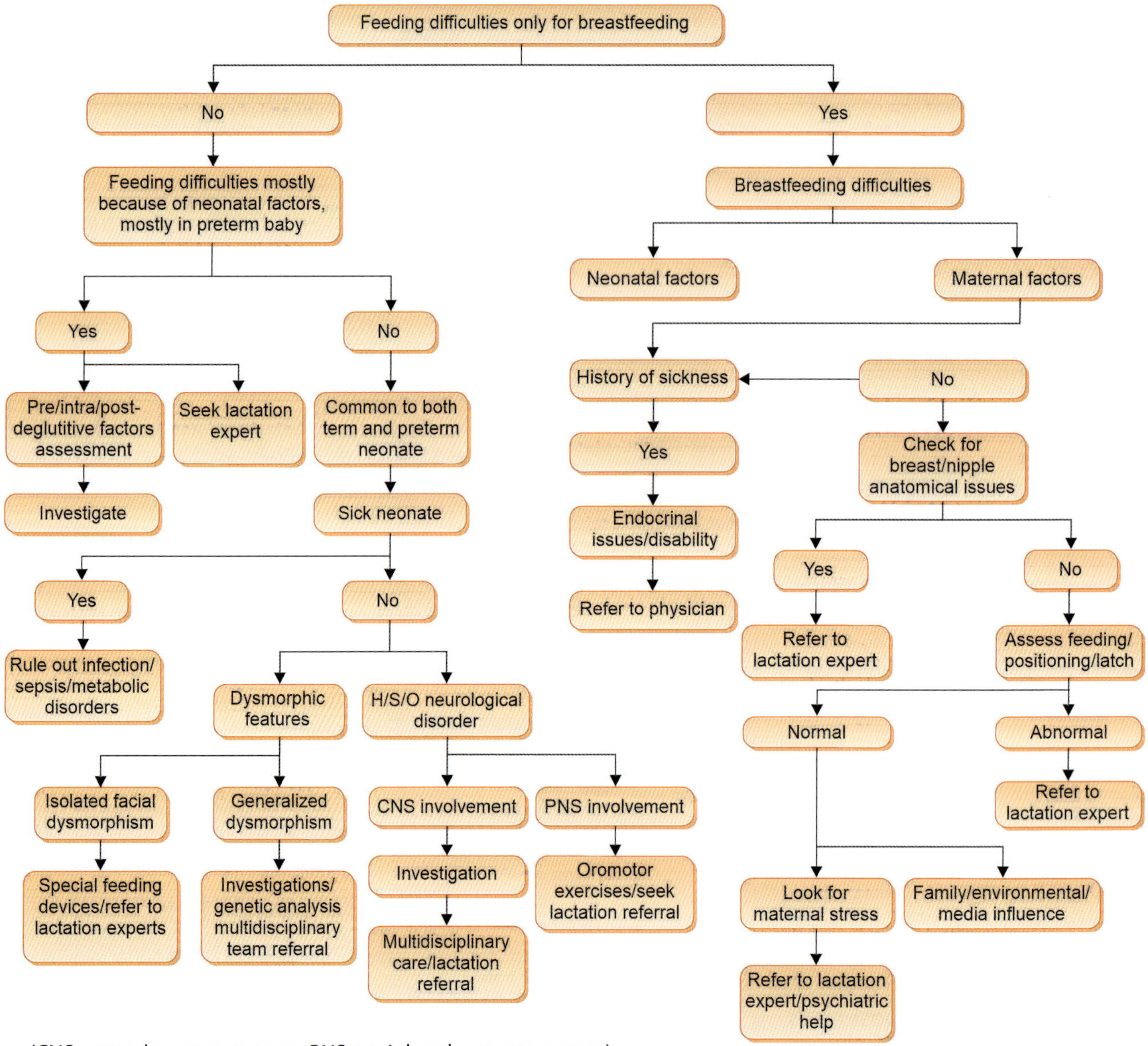

(CNS: central nervous system; PNS: peripheral nervous system)

Suggested Reading

- Jadcherla SR. Abrams SA, Hoppin AG (Eds). (2023). Neonatal oral feeding difficulties due to sucking and swallowing disorders. [online]. Available from https://medilib.ir/uptodate/show/4976 [Last accessed August, 2024].
- Lawrence N, Rosen-Carole C (Eds). Breastfeeding infants with problems. Breastfeeding, 9th edition. Philadelphia: Elsevier; 2022. pp. 457-501.

Congenital Orthopedic Disorders

130

Section Editor: **Nehal Patel**
Section Co-Editor: **Jay T Dhirwani**
Authors: **Maulin Shah, Joyance James Mammen**

Introduction

- A newborn with a misshapen limb requires early diagnosis of the congenital malformations and timely referral to the respective specialty.
- While some conditions like congenital muscular torticollis and radioulnar synostosis may become evident later, other conditions can readily be diagnosed.

Types of Orthopedic Deformities

- *Arthrogryposis multiplex congenita/amyoplasia:* It is characterized by the presence of multiple joint contractures. All children with any congenital limb malformation should have a visual inspection of the sacral region for stigmata of spinal dysraphism.
- *Left Sprengel's shoulder with elevated scapula:* Scapula at a higher level than the other side resulting in limited shoulder abduction.

  Management: Surgical lowering of the scapula after 2–3 years of age
- *Radial club hand with wrist deformity:* It is characterized by radially deviated wrist, short forearm with/without absent thumb, and lateral rays. It is associated with Fanconi anemia, thrombocytopenia-absent radius (TAR), VACTERL (vertebral defects, anal atresia, cardiac defects, tracheoesophageal fistula, renal anomalies, and limb abnormalities)/VATER syndrome.

  Management: Early splinting and distractor application followed by centralization of carpus over ulna—1st year of life.

- *Ulnar club hand with absent medial fingers:* Short forearm, with ulnar deviated wrist and absent medial rays

  Management: Early splinting and surgical intervention at 2 years.

- *Absent thumb:* Hypoplastic/absent thumb with/without radial club hand

  Management: Pollicization of the index finger by 3 years

- *Syndactyly: Fused 3rd and 4th fingers* or webbed or fused digits

  Management: Plastic surgical intervention to separate fingers and increase hand span

- *Bilateral congenital talipes equinovarus (CTEV)/Clubfeet*: Affected foot in plantar flexion with heel varus and foot in inversion, and forefoot adducted (foot resembles golf club)

  Management:

  - Early serial corrective casts by Ponseti method followed by abduction orthosis.
  - Referral in early neonatal period when recognized.
  - Needs to be differentiated from postural variants and metatarsus adductus.

- *Bilateral congenital dislocation of knee*: It is characterized by hyperextended knee joint. In severe cases, toes can project into the chest wall.

  Management: Serial corrective casts, some cases may require further surgery.

- *Right developmental dysplasia of hip (DDH)*: With short thigh segment and decreased hip abduction; Commonly associated with torticollis and metatarsus adductus

  Management: Pavlik harness to maintain the head in a reduced position; may require surgery in late diagnosed cases >6 months.

- *Right fibular hemimelia with ankle deformity:* Hypoplastic or absent fibula with/without absence of lateral rays; associated with congenital short femur and focal femoral deficiency

  Management: Early splinting; mostly, will require surgical intervention later

- *Posteromedial bowing of leg:* Short leg segment with a posterior bow, commonly associated with calcaneovalgus deformity

  Management: Bracing in infancy and limb lengthening late

- *Anterolateral bowing of leg:* Short leg segment with anterior bow

  - *Etiology:* Pseudoarthrosis of tibia, neurofibromatosis, and fibrous dysplasia.
  - *Management:* This needs bracing in walking age group and surgical intervention later. Bracing may prevent potential fractures.

- *Rocker-bottom foot of congenital vertical talus (CVT)*: Heel in equinus and valgus, forefoot dorsiflexed, rocker-bottom appearance; commonly seen in arthrogryposis and spina bifida

  Management: Serial corrective casts with reverse Ponseti method + surgery

Approach to a Child with Orthopedic Disorders

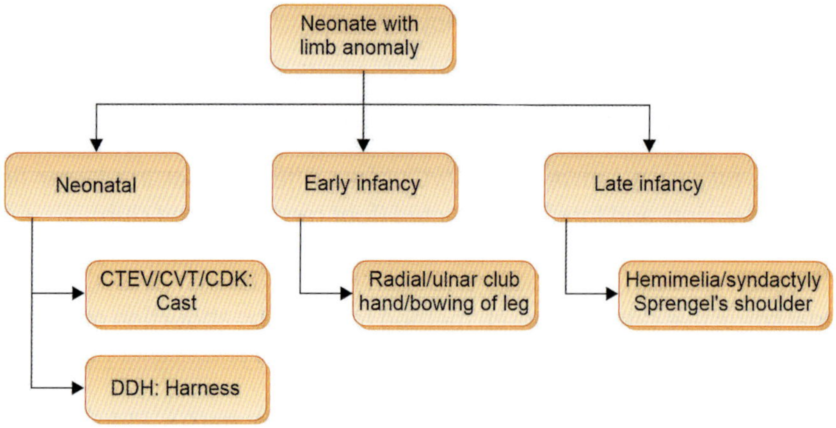

(CDK: congenital dislocation of knee; CVT: congenital vertical talus; CTEV: congenital talipes equinovarus; DDH: developmental dysplasia of hip)

Red Flag Signs

- Stigmata of spinal dysraphism should be evaluated further and treated accordingly along with the limb anomalies.
- Infants with multiple limb anomalies should be evaluated for syndromic associations and systemic involvement.

Suggested Reading

- Herring JA. Tachdjian's Pediatric Orthopaedics From the Texas Scottish Rite Hospital for Children, 6th edition. Amsterdam, Netherlands: Elsevier; 2022.
- Hefti F. Pediatric Orthopedics in Practice, 1st edition. Berlin: Springer; 2007.
- Joseph B, Nayagam S, Loder R, Torode I. Paediatric Orthopaedics A System of Decision-Making, 2nd edition. England, UK: Routledge; 2016
- Rockwood CA. Rockwood and Wilkins' Fractures in Children. Philadelphia: Lippincott Williams & Wilkins; 2010.
- Weinstein SL, Flynn JM. Lovell and Winter's Pediatric Orthopaedics, 7th edition. Philadelphia: Lippincott Williams & Wilkins; 2014.

Drooling

131

Section Editor: **B Rajsekhar**
Section Co-Editor: **Suchitra Pusapati**
Authors: **Sanjay KS, Arun YB**

Introduction

- Drooling, also known as sialorrhea, is defined as salivary incontinence/involuntary spillage of saliva over the lower lip.
- It maybe seen in healthy children till 2 years of age. It is common in neurologically impaired children. It maybe embarrassing, with considerable social stigma.

Approach

- *Detailed history:*
  - Age of onset, chronicity, and severity of drooling, with its consequent problems like feeding issues and speech problems
  - Any precipitating factors such as ingestion of drug/toxic material or teething
  - Detailed perinatal history, and developmental history in children with neurological deficits
- *Examination:*
  - Thorough examination of oral cavity, throat, and neurological assessment
  - Assess the severity of drooling and its impact on quality of life of the patient and caregivers.

The approach to the management of drooling is given in **Flowchart 1**.

FLOWCHART 1: Approach to the management of drooling.

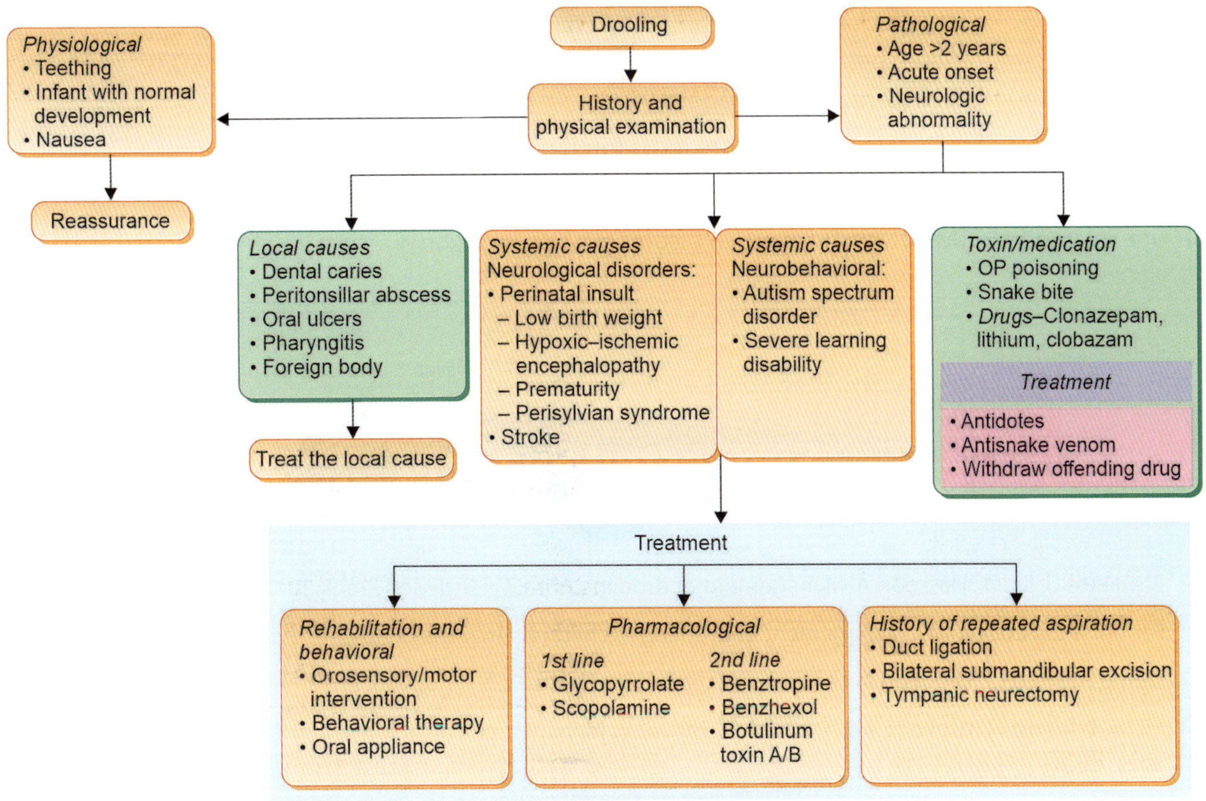

(OP: organophosphate)

Classification

- Drooling is classified as physiological or pathological based on the focused history with neurological and oropharyngeal examination.
- *Physiological:* It is often self-limited, below 2 years of age. Parental reassurance will suffice.
- *Pathological:* It could be due to several reasons. It maybe due to neurodevelopmental abnormality like pseudobulbar palsy, cerebral palsy, stroke; bulbar weakness like Bell's palsy, riboflavinopathy; and primary muscular disorders like congenital myopathies, spinal muscular atrophy, and myasthenic syndromes.
- Look for local causes like peritonsillar abscess, pharyngitis, and dental infections. Intoxication with organophosphate chemicals and snake bites can also be associated with drooling.
- Hyposensitivity of lips and oropharynx in autistic children often results in drooling.
- The sudden onset of drooling should raise suspicion of local causes like foreign body ingestion or toxin exposure.
- Certain antiseizure medications like clonazepam and clobazam cause hypersalivation and drooling.

Red Flag Signs

- Persistent drooling beyond 2 years of age
- Sudden onset of excessive drooling/choking—foreign body ingestion
- Drooling associated with fever, dysphonia, dyspnea, epiglottitis/peritonsillar abscesses
- Unexplained, sudden onset drooling—Poisoning

Suggested Reading

- Bavikatte G, Sit PL, Hassoon A. Management of drooling of saliva. Br J Med Pract. 2012;5(1):50712.
- Fairhurst CB, Cockerill H. Management of drooling in children. Arch Dis Child Educ Pract Ed. 2011;96(1):25-30.
- Leung AK, Kao CP. Drooling in children. Paediatr Child Health. 1999;4(6):406-11.
- Melo B, Araújo R, Azevedo MJ, Amorim R, Palhau L. Management of sialorrhea in children. Pediatric Oncall. 2021;18(3).

Hirsutism

132

Section Editor: **Gnanamurthy Narasimha**
Section Co-Editor: **Nagalatha Chidananda**
Authors: **Ravi Hiremagalur, Vani HN**

Definition

- Hirsutism is defined as excessive growth of terminal/coarse hair in androgen-dependent areas of the body.
- Hypertrichosis refers to generalized *excessive hair growth*, not confined to the androgen-dependent areas.

Etiology

- *Hyperandrogenic causes:*
  - Polycystic ovarian syndrome
  - Androgen-secreting tumors—ovarian and adrenal glands
  - Nonclassical congenital adrenal hyperplasia
- *Nonhyperandrogenic hirsutism causes:*
  - *Medications:* Include glucocorticoids, cyclosporine, and danazol
  - *Endocrinopathies:* Cushing's syndrome, hypothyroidism, hyperprolactinemia, and acromegaly
  - *Other causes:* Postmenopausal women and pregnant women
  - *Idiopathic:* Diagnosis of exclusion

Evaluation

- *History and physical examination:*
  - *Onset and progression:* Peripubertal in primary and secondary nontumoral hirsutism. Late-onset with rapid virilization and tumors
  - Menstrual cycle irregularities
  - *Signs of hyperandrogenism:* Acne, alopecia, female pattern hair loss, scoring of hirsutism using modified Ferriman–Gallwey method (≥8)
- *Biochemical tests*: In the early follicular phase (3rd–6th day)—total testosterone, dehydro-epiandrosterone sulfate (DHEAS), luteinizing hormone (LH), follicle-stimulating hormone (FSH), Free T4, thyroid-stimulating hormone (TSH), prolactin and 17-hydroxy progesterone (17-OHP), steroid hormone binding globulin (SHBG), adrenocorticotropic hormone (ACTH) stimulation test, and dexamethasone suppression test are done, if required.
- *Imaging:* Ultrasound and magnetic resonance imaging (MRI)/computed tomography (CT)—ovarian, adrenal, and pituitary tumors.

Red Flag Signs

- Sudden onset of hirsutism
- Rapid progression
- Clitoromegaly
- Galactorrhea
- Menstrual irregularities
- Signs and symptoms of hypo/hyperthyroidism, Cushing's syndrome, and acromegaly

Approach

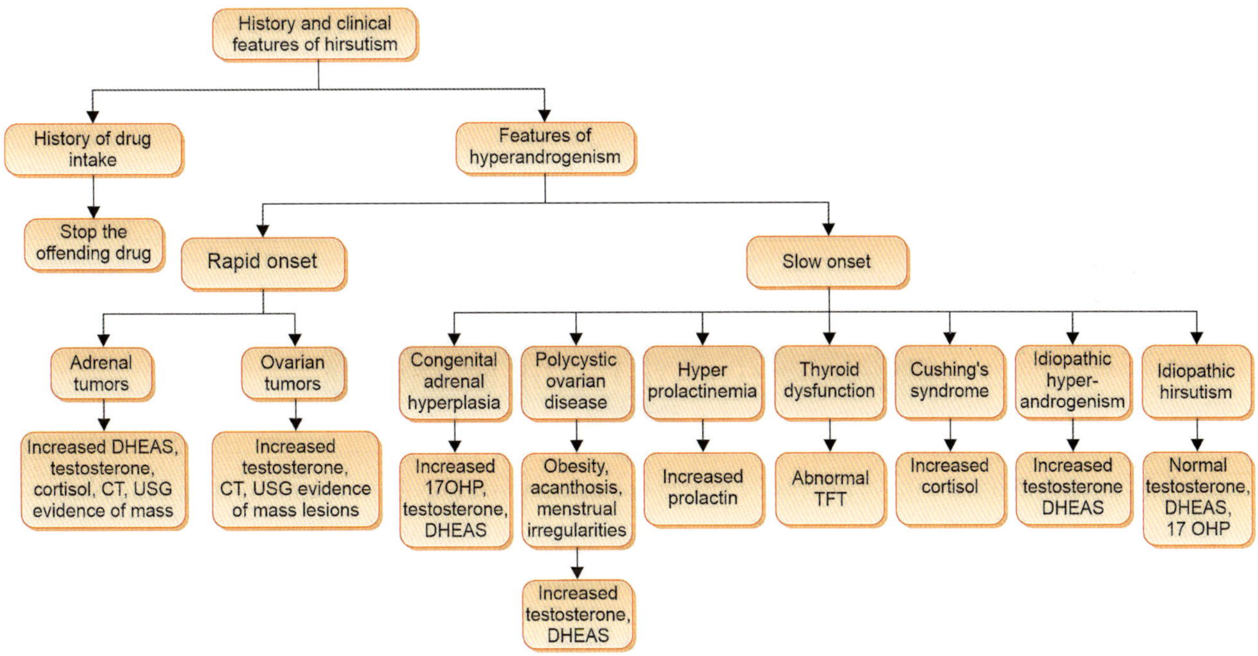

(CT: computed tomography, DHEAS: dehydroepiandrosterone sulfate; OHP: hydroxyprogesterone; TFT: thyroid function test; USG: ultrasonography)

Suggested Reading

- Cross AS, Moustafa M, Elder CJ. Fifteen-minute consultation: Approach to the adolescent presenting with hirsutism. Arch Dis Child Educ Pract Ed. 2024;109(2):66-72.
- De Kroon RWPM, den Heijer M, Heijboer AC. Is idiopathic hirsutism idiopathic? Clin Chim Acta. 2022;531:17-24.
- Heidelbaugh JJ. Endocrinology Update: Hirsutism. FP Essent. 2016;451:17-24.
- Lizneva D, Gavrilova-Jordan L, Walker W, Azziz R. Androgen excess: Investigations and management. Best Pract Res Clin Obstet Gynaecol. 2016;37:98-118.
- Oliveira TF, Comim FV. Understanding hirsutism in PCOS. Expert Rev Endocrinol Metab. 2024;19(2):103-10.
- Peña AS, Witchel SF, Hoeger KM, Oberfield SE, Vogiatzi MG, Misso M, et al. Adolescent polycystic ovary syndrome according to the international evidence-based guideline. BMC Med. 2020;18(1):72.

Cardiac Murmurs

133

Section Editor: **Nehal Patel**
Section Co-Editor: **Jay T Dhirwani**
Authors: **Munesh Tomar, Bhavi S Barchha**

Introduction

- Cardiac auscultation is tremendously helpful in evaluating patients with suspected heart disease.
- Cardiac murmurs result from turbulent blood flow across normal/abnormal orifices.

Types

Systolic Murmur

- *Pansystolic:* Murmur starts with the first heart sound (S1) (partially masking it), and ends with the second heart sound (S2) without change in character. It is soft and blowing. It is caused by ventricular septal defect (VSD), mitral regurgitation (MR), and tricuspid regurgitation (TR).
- *Ejection systolic (ESM):* Murmur audible during ejection, i.e., after S1, ending with/before the corresponding S2; crescendo-decrescendo, peak in mid/late systole. ESM is produced at the outflow tract (pulmonary/aortic) due to obstruction/increased flow across the normal valve.
- *Early systolic:* Murmur starts with S1, ending before mid-systole. Its causes include small muscular VSD closing in mid systole and mild TR.
- *Late systolic:* Starts late in systole ending with S2. Its causes include mitral valve prolapse with MR.

Diastolic Murmur

- *Mid diastolic (MDM):* It is low pitched, rumbling, and audible in tricuspid/mitral area. It occurs due to obstruction/increased flow across the respective valves.
- *Late diastolic/presystolic:* In the late diastolic phase, ending with S1, corresponding to atrial systole.
- *Early diastolic (EDM):* It starts with aortic/pulmonic component of S2. Indicates regurgitation of the respective semilunar valve.

Continuous Murmur

Continuous murmur begins in systole, and continues uninterrupted/without change in character through the S2, into diastole. It may occupy whole/part of the diastole.

Analyzing a Murmur

- *Timing:* Systole/diastole/continuous
- *Location:*
  - *Aortic valve:* 2nd intercostal space at right sternal border
  - *Pulmonary valve:* 2nd intercostal space at left sternal border
  - *Tricuspid valve:* 4th intercostal space at left sternal border
  - *Mitral valve:* 5th intercostal space at left midclavicular line
  - *Radiation:* Murmurs may radiate, heard at remote locations
- *Intensity:*
  - *Grade I:* Faint, barely audible
  - *Grade II:* Soft
  - *Grade III:* Easily audible, without a palpable thrill
  - *Grade IV:* Easily audible, with a palpable thrill
  - *Grade V:* Loud murmur, audible with stethoscope lightly touching the chest
  - *Grade VI:* Loudest murmur, audible with stethoscope touching the chest
- *Pitch:*
  - High/low frequency
  - *Other terms:* Blowing, harsh, musical, rumbling, and squeaky

- *Profile:*
  - *Crescendo:* Murmur increasing in intensity
  - *Decrescendo:* Murmur decreasing in intensity [aortic regurgitation (AR), pulmonary regurgitation (PR), and mitral stenosis (MS)]
  - *Crescendo–decrescendo:* Murmur initially increases in intensity, peaks, and then decreases in intensity [aortic stenosis (AS), pulmonary stenosis (PS)]
  - *Plateau:* Static intensity (MR and TR)
- *Dynamic auscultation:* Various maneuvers that alter loading conditions of the heart result in variations in murmur.
  - *Handgrip:* Increases afterload and increases murmur of AR, MR and VSD. The opposite effect is seen with hypertrophic obstructive cardiomyopathy (HOCM) and mitral valve prolapse (MVP).
  - *Squatting:* Increases preload; increases murmur of AS, MS, AR, and MR; and decreases murmurs of HOCM and MVP
  - *Valsalva:* Decreases preload and increases murmurs due to HOCM and MVP; decreases murmurs of AS, MS, AR, MR, and VSD
  - *Standing abruptly:* Decreases preload; same effects as Valsalva
  - *Respiration:* Right-sided murmur increases with inspiration and left-sided murmurs are more prominent with expiration.

The characteristic pathological murmurs are given in **Table 1**.

TABLE 1: Characteristic pathological murmurs.

LESION	MURMUR	LOCATION	SPECIFIC POINTS
ASD	Ejection systolic (pulmonary), MDR (tricuspid)	Left upper sternal border	S2 wide and fixed with MDR at LLSB
VSD	Pansystolic, harsh/loud in small defects; softer, less intense in large ones	• Left lower sternal area • Radiates to the entire precordium	S2 wide and variable with MDR at apex
PDA	Continuous, "machinery"	• Left infraclavicular region • Radiates to back	Peaking at S2 with MDR at apex
TOF	ESM	Left upper sternal area	• S2 single • Increasing cyanosis • Lesser intensity of murmur
MR	High pitched pansystolic	• At apex • Radiates to axilla	Reduces with hand grip
MS	Low-pitched diastolic, presystolic accentuation	At apex	*Heard with the bell of stethoscope with severity:* Gap between OS and S2 decreases, murmur duration increases

Contd...

Contd...

LESION	MURMUR	LOCATION	SPECIFIC POINTS
AR	High-pitch, EDM, begins with A2, length increases with increasing severity of AR	• Right upper parasternal area • Radiates to left mid sternum and apex	Increases with hand grip
AS	• ESM, crescendo–decrescendo • With increasing severity of stenosis, the peak occurs later	• Right upper parasternal area • Radiates to carotid	Reduces with handgrip and inspiration
PR (high pressure)	High-pitched, decrescendo	• 2nd left intercostal space • Radiates toward the mid-right sternal edge	Increases with inspiration (Graham Steell murmur)
PR (normal pressure)	Low pitched EDM	2nd left intercostal space	Increases with inspiration
PS	Harsh crescendo–decrescendo ESM, ends with P2	At left upper sternal edge	Increases with inspiration
TR	Pansystolic	Left LSB	Increases with inspiration
Functional murmur	Early/ejection systolic	Left lower sternal border	• S1, S2 normal • No thrill—anemia/hyperdynamic stage

(AR: aortic regurgitation; AS: aortic stenosis; ASD: atrial septal defect; ESM: ejection systolic murmur; EDM: early diastolic murmur; LSB: lower sternal border; LLSB: left lower sternal border; MDR: mid diastolic rumble; MS: mitral stenosis; MR: mitral regurgitation; OS: opening snap; PDA: patent ductus arteriosus; PR: pulmonary regurgitation; PS: pulmonary stenosis; TOF: tetralogy of Fallot's; TR: tricuspid regurgitation; VSD: ventricular septal defect)

Red Flag Signs

- Presence of abnormal pulses
- Central cyanosis
- Associated abnormal heart sounds
- Systolic murmur grade 3 or more
- Diastolic murmur
- Abnormal electrocardiogram (ECG) and chest X-ray (CXR)
- Any symptomatic child

Investigations

A systematic clinical examination is crucial in suspected cardiac disease. For final anatomic and functional diagnosis, also do:

- Electrocardiogram
- Chest X-ray
- Echocardiography
- Cardiac catheterization, computed tomography (CT) pulmonary angiography, and cardiac magnetic resonance imaging (MRI)—in selective cases

Approach

The approach to the management of systolic murmur is given in **Flowchart 1.**

FLOWCHART 1: Approach to systolic murmur.

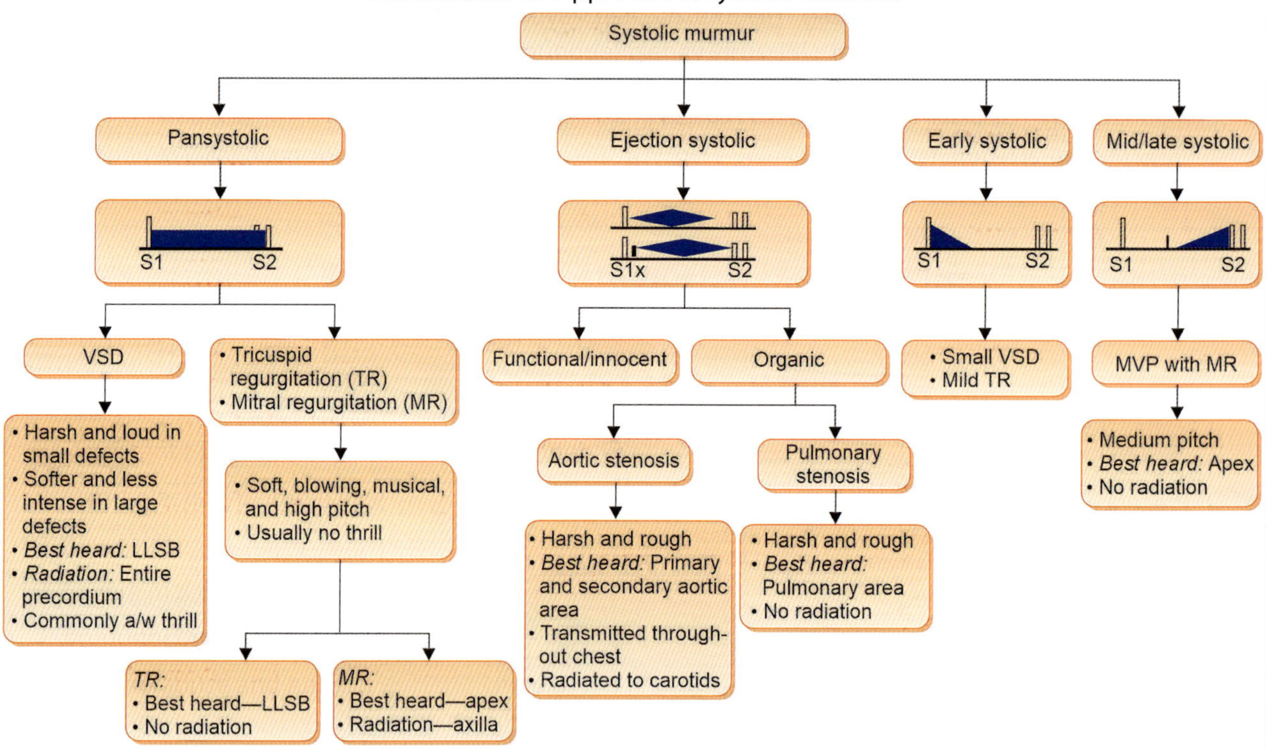

(LLSB: left lower sternal border; MVP: Mitral Valve Prolapse; VSD: ventricular septal defect)

The approach to the management of diastolic murmur is given in **Flowchart 2.**

FLOWCHART 2: Approach to diastolic murmur.

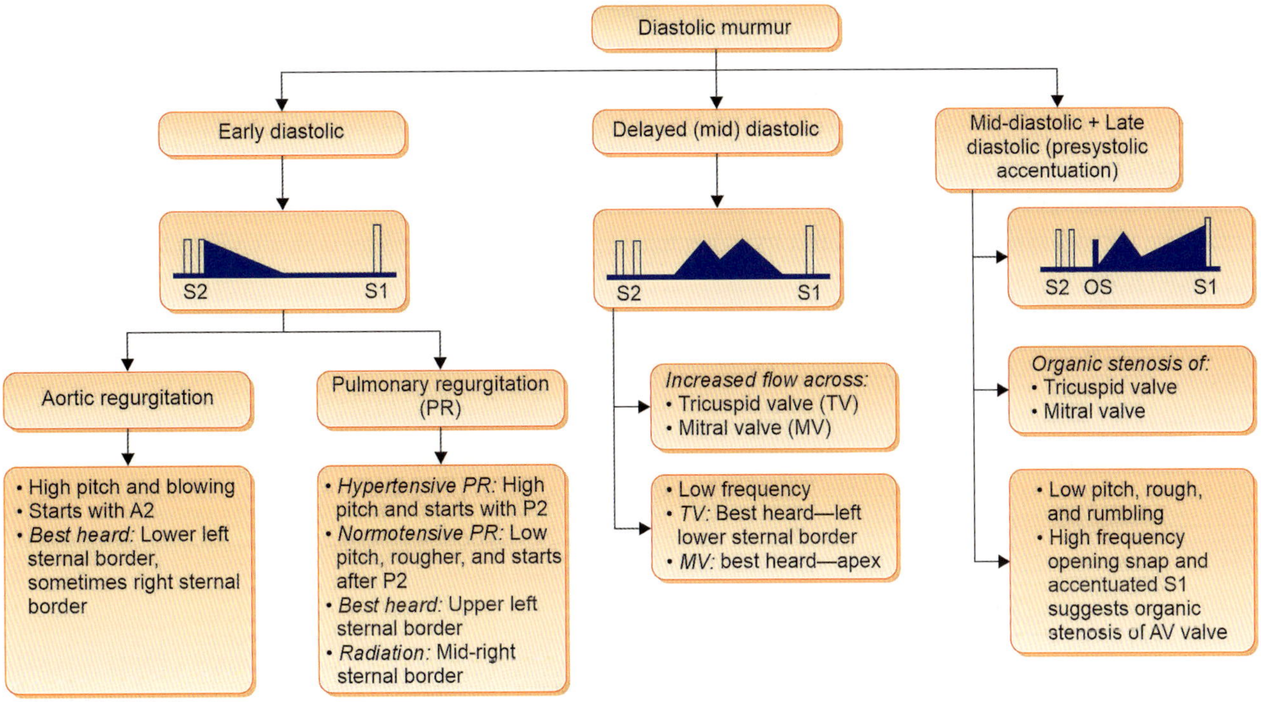

(AV: atrioventricular)

The approach to the management of continuous murmur is given in **Flowchart 3.**

FLOWCHART 3: Approach to continuous murmur.

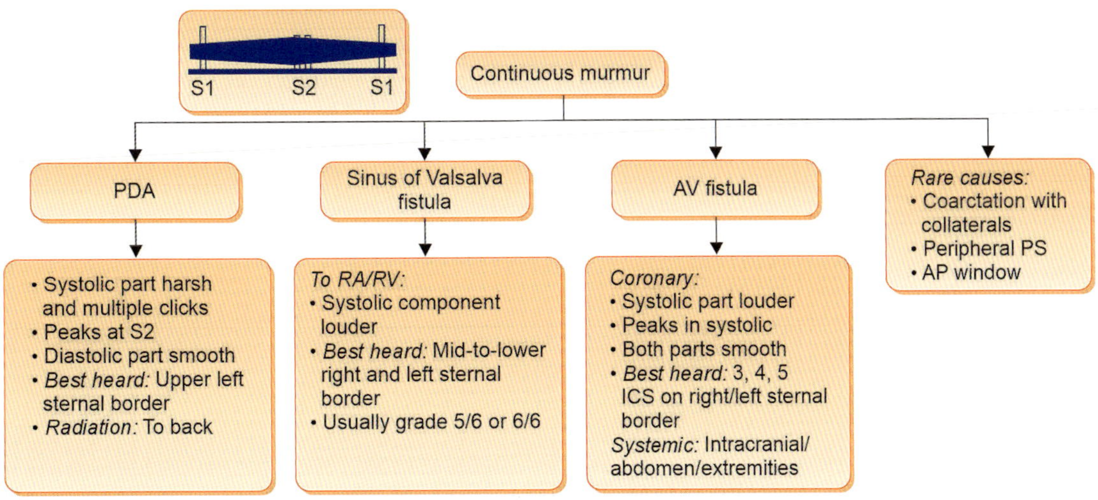

(AP: aortopulmonary; ICS: intercostal space; PDA: patent ductus arteriosus; PS: pulmonary stenosis; RA: right atrium; RV: right ventricle)

Suggested Reading

- Swartz MH (Ed). The heart. Textbook of Physical Diagnosis: History and Examination, 8th edition. Philadelphia, PA: Elsevier; 2021.
- Thomas SL, Heaton J, Makaryus AN. Physiology, Cardiovascular Murmurs. In: Stat Pearls [Internet]. Treasure Island (FL): StatPearls Publishing; 2024. Available from https://www.ncbi.nlm.nih.gov/books/NBK525958/ [Last accessed August, 2024].
- Voin V, Oskouian RJ, Loukas M, Tubbs RS. Auscultation of the heart: The basics with anatomical correlation. Clin Anat. 2017;30(1):58-60.

Steatorrhea

134

Section Editor: **B Rajsekhar**
Section Co-Editor: **Suchitra Pusapati**
Authors: **Aditi, GV Basavaraja**

Introduction

- Steatorrhea, or chronic fatty diarrhea, is excess oil in stools.
- It is either due to fat maldigestion or malabsorption.
- Maldigestion is defective intraluminal hydrolysis, while malabsorption is defective mucosal absorption of digested lipids.

Etiology and Pathogenesis

Steatorrhea is due to luminal, mucosal, or postmucosal causes **(Table 1)**. It maybe due to:

- *Reduced emulsification:* Due to less than the critical amount of intraluminal bile acids.
- *Decreased lipolysis:* Pancreatic enzyme deficiency causes decreased luminal hydrolysis of fat to monoglycerides.
- *Decreased mucosal absorption:* Mucosal diseases, with villous shortening and inflammation leads to reduced surface area, and hence defective uptake of free fatty acids.
- *Defective chylomicron formation:* Chylomicrons traffic the digested fats within enterocytes. Defective chylomicron formation accumulates lipids within enterocytes.
- *Defective lymphatic transport of chylomicrons:* Decreased transport of lipids via lacteals occurs due to postmucosal fat malabsorption.

TABLE 1: Etiology and pathogenesis of steatorrhea.

PATHOPHYSIOLOGICAL MECHANISM	MALABSORBED SUBSTRATE(S)	REPRESENTATIVE CAUSE(S)
	Maldigestion	
Bile-acid deficiency	Fat along with fat-soluble vitamins and calcium	• *Decreased synthesis and/or secretion of bile acids* – Inborn errors of bile acid synthesis – Cholestatic liver diseases – Biliary obstruction • *Intestinal loss of conjugated bile* – Ileal disease – Ileal sodium bile acid cotransporter defect • Luminal deconjugation of bile acids • Small intestinal bacterial overgrowth (SIBO)
Pancreatic insufficiency	Fat along with protein and carbohydrates	• Congenital deficiency of enzymes (lipase and colipase) • Congenital pancreatic insufficiency (cystic fibrosis, Shwachman syndrome, Johanson–Blizzard syndrome, and Pearson marrow pancreas syndrome • Chronic pancreatitis
	Malabsorption	
Reduced mucosal absorption	• Isolated fat malabsorption • Fat along with carbohydrates and proteins	• Congenital transporter defect (abetalipoproteinemia, chylomicron retention disease) • Generalized mucosal disease (celiac disease, Crohn's disease, and tropical sprue) • Infections like human immunodeficiency virus (HIV) and giardiasis
Decreased transport from the intestine	Fat and protein	• Primary intestinal lymphangiectasia (PIL) • Secondary (venous stasis, heart failure, Fontan surgery, tuberculosis, and lymphoma)

Red Flag Signs

The red flag signs are given in **Table 2.**

TABLE 2: Red flag signs.

SYMPTOM/SIGN	PATHOPHYSIOLOGY
Chronic diarrhea: Greasy pale bulky stools, floating of stools, and passing frank oil per rectum	Fat maldigestion/malabsorption
Absent subcutaneous fat, poor growth, preserved appetite, and rectal prolapse	Fat loss
Xerophthalmia and night blindness	Vitamin A deficiency
Bone pain, fractures, tetany, and muscle pain	*Malabsorption:* Vitamin D, calcium, magnesium, and phosphorus
Ataxia	Vitamin E deficiency
Easy bruisability and ecchymoses	Vitamin K deficiency
Dermatitis	Essential fatty acid and zinc deficiency
Pedal edema and ascites	Protein loss
Disease confirmation by genetics study	
Bloating and flatulence	Carbohydrate malabsorption
Anemia and koilonychia	Iron, folic acid, and vitamin B_{12} deficiency
Kidney stones	Increased colonic oxalate absorption

Approach

The approach to the management of a child with steatorrhea is given in **Flowchart 1**.

FLOWCHART 1: Approach to a child with steatorrhea.

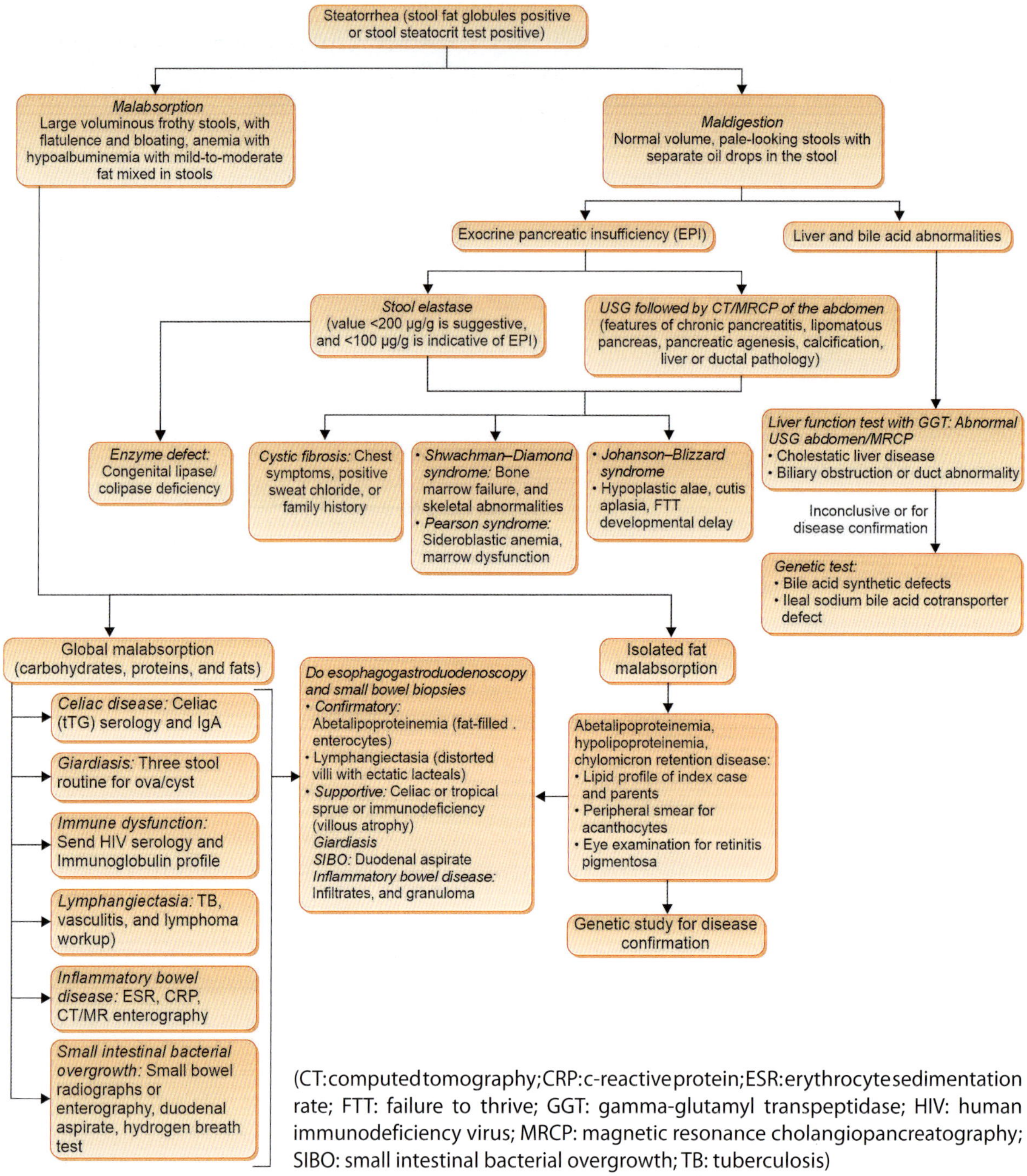

(CT: computed tomography; CRP: c-reactive protein; ESR: erythrocyte sedimentation rate; FTT: failure to thrive; GGT: gamma-glutamyl transpeptidase; HIV: human immunodeficiency virus; MRCP: magnetic resonance cholangiopancreatography; SIBO: small intestinal bacterial overgrowth; TB: tuberculosis)

Suggested Reading

- Feldman M, Friedman LS, Brandt LJ. Maldigestion and malabsorption. Sleisenger and Fordtran's gastrointestinal and liver disease: Pathophysiology, diagnosis, management, 11th edition. Amsterdam, Netherlands: Elsevier; 2021.
- Kleinman RE, Goulet OJ, Giorgi MV. Walker's Pediatric Gastrointestinal Disease: Physiology, Diagnosis, Management, 6th edition. Netherlands: Wolters Kluwer; 2018.
- Ulshen MH. Diarrhea and steatorrhea. In: Adam HM, Foy JM. Signs and Symptoms in Pediatrics. United States: American Academy of Pediatrics; 2015.

Torticollis

135

Section Editor: **Sumitha Nayak**
Section Co-Editor: **Priya Shivalli**
Author: **Priya Shivalli**

Introduction

Torticollis or *twisted neck* is due to contraction or contracture of the neck muscles resulting in the head tilting to one side. It is a nonspecific symptom.

Classification

Congenital

- *Commonest cause:* Congenital muscular torticollis (CMT)
- Due to the shortening and fibrosis of the sternocleidomastoid (SCM) muscle
- Rarer causes include malformations of cervical spine, Chiari malformations, and spina bifida
- May be associated with birth trauma/antenatal complications
- Often associated with craniofacial asymmetry

Causes

- *Osseous anomalies:* Hemivertebra, unilateral atlanto-occipital fusion, and Klippel–Feil Syndrome
- *Soft-tissue abnormalities:* Unilateral absence of SCM, and pterygium colli

Acquired

Generally, starts after 4–6 months. It maybe due to:

- Injury of SCM/trapezius muscle/inflammation
- Cervical muscle spasm/cervical nerve irritation
- Atlantoaxial rotatory subluxation (AARS) can present with SCM spasm on the ipsilateral side to which the chin is tilted.

Causes

- *Musculoskeletal:* Muscle spasm (wry neck)
- *Trauma:* Fracture/dislocation and spinal hematoma
- *Infection:*
  - *Head and neck:* Upper respiratory tract infections (URTI), mastoiditis, cervical adenitis, retro-pharyngeal abscess, and dental infection
  - *Spine:* Osteomyelitis
  - Central nervous system (CNS) infections
- *AARS:*
  - Injury/ligamentous laxity
  - Postsurgery
  - Grisel syndrome
- *Inflammation:* Juvenile idiopathic arthritis (JIA)
- *Oncologic:* CNS tumors and bone tumors
- *Dystonic syndrome:* Idiopathic spasmodic torticollis and drug reactions
- Ocular dysfunction
- Benign paroxysmal torticollis of infancy (BPTI)

Red Flag Symptoms

- Stiffness of neck/restricted neck extension
- Fever, drooling, and vomiting
- Increasing pain, unremitting or disturbing sleep
- Recent injury
- Poor progress in treatment
- Disturbed gait
- History of headaches, and behavioral change
- Photophobia, strabismus, and diplopia

Life-threatening Causes

- Retropharyngeal abscess
- Cervical spine injury
- *CNS tumors:* Posterior fossa and spinal
- Spinal epidural hematoma/suppurative jugular thrombophlebitis

Congenital Muscular Torticollis

Comorbidities:

- Congenital hip deformities
- Congenital deformities of head/spine/malformations of skull and face bones/feet

Approach

Typical presentations include lateral tilt of the head, contralateral chin rotation, and restricted movements of neck.

The approach to the evaluation and management of torticollis is given in **Flowchart 1**.

FLOWCHART 1: Evaluation and management of muscular torticollis.

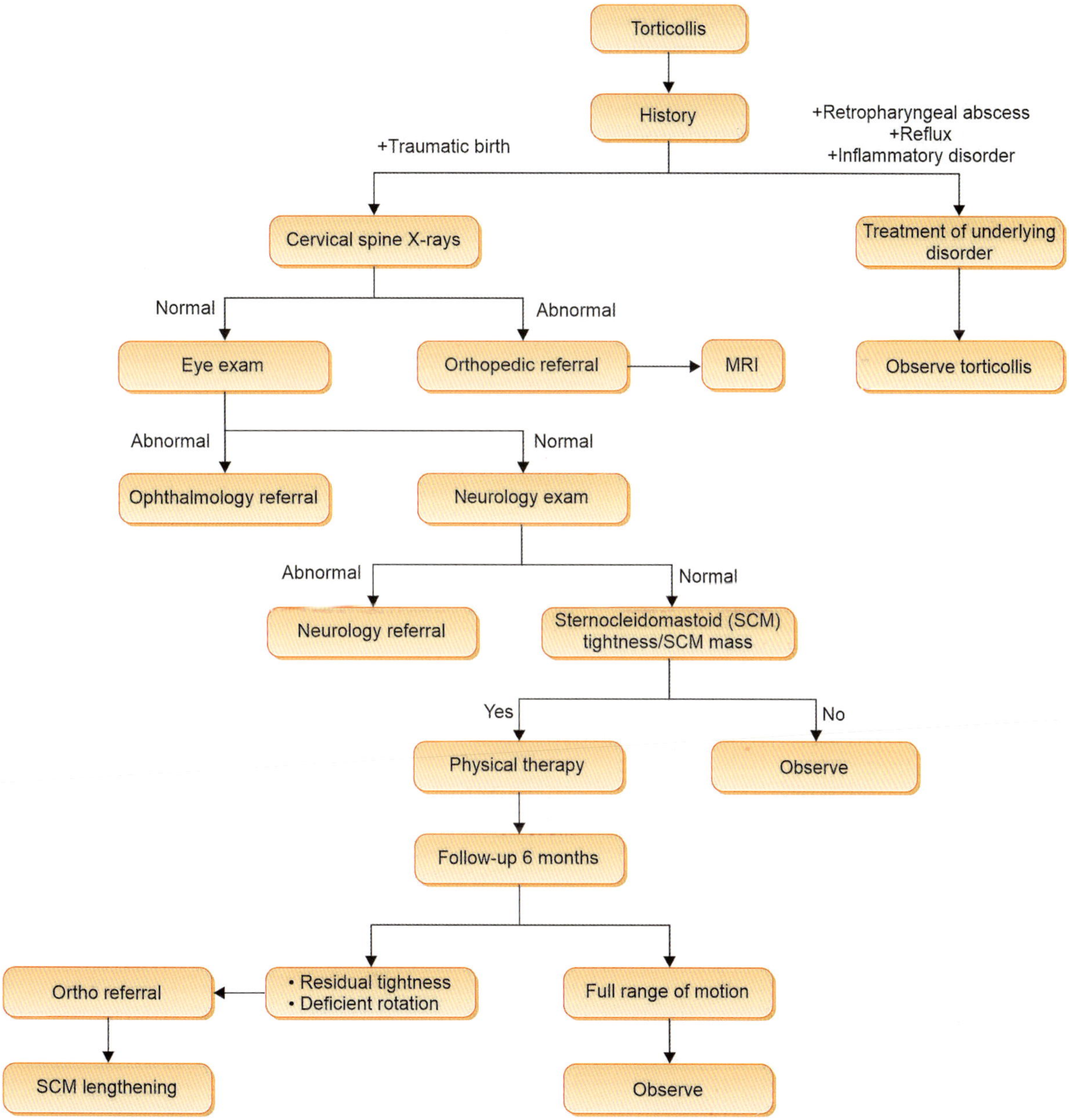

History

- Age of onset of symptoms and duration
- Abnormal head/neck position for prolonged time, for example, playing video games and sleeping posture
- Recent injury
- Fever, throat pain, and dysphagia
- Headache, vomiting, ataxia, seizures, disturbed gait, and pain in the back/neck
- Double vision and photophobia
- *Birth history:* Birth injury, oligohydramnios, and breech presentation
- Medications causing dystonia, for example, metoclopramide
- *Underlying conditions:* Down syndrome

Examination

- Position of head and chin
- SCM muscle mass maybe palpable in CMT along with plagiocephaly, motor delay/hip dysplasia
- Tenderness in muscle or in the midline C-spine
- ENT examination
- Range of *Active* movements of neck, without applying force
- Signs of space-occupying lesions and lymphadenopathy/tonsillitis/middle ear infection
- Eye movements

Imaging

Generally, imaging is not useful; however the following maybe considered:

- *Cervical spine plain X-ray:* For conditions with ligamentous laxity
- Ultrasonography (USG) neck in infants
- Computed tomography (CT) ± magnetic resonance imaging (MRI) neck ± brain

A new simple clinical assessment tool under the acronym PINCH is designed to aid pediatricians in diagnosing the etiology of torticollis **(Table 1)**.

TABLE 1: PINCH clinical assessment tool.

	PAINFUL	INTERMITTENT	NEUROLOGICAL SIGNS	CONGENITAL	HEAD SHAPE
Sternomastoid tumor	–	–	–	+	±
Positional plagiocephaly	–	–	–	–	+
Benign paroxysmal torticollis of infancy	–	+	+	–	–
Segmentation anomaly	–	–	–	+	–
Atlantoaxial rotatory subluxation	+	–	–	–	–
Dystonia	+	+	+	–	–
Neoplasm	–	–	+	–	–
Ocular	–	–	+	+	–

Suggested Reading

- Boston Children's Hospital. (2024). What is torticollis? [online]. Available from https://www.childrenshospital.org/conditions-and-treatments/conditions/t/torticollis [Last accessed August, 2024].
- Dayasiri K, Rao S. Fifteen-minute consultation: Evaluation of paediatric torticollis. Arch Dis Child Educ Pract Ed. 2023;108(1):17-21.
- Gundrathi J, Cunha B, Tiwari V, Mendez MD. Congenital Torticollis. In: StatPearls [Internet]. Treasure Island (FL): StatPearls Publishing; 2024. Available from https://www.ncbi.nlm.nih.gov/books/NBK549778/ [Last accessed August, 2024].
- Macias CG. Bachur RG, Phillips WA, Isaacson GC, Wiley JF (Eds). (2024). Acquired Torticollis in Children. [online]. Available from https://medilib.ir/uptodate/show/6462 [Last accessed August, 2024].
- NHSGGC Paediatrics for Health Professionals. Torticollis in children. [online]. Available from http://www.clinicalguidelines.scot.nhs.uk/ggc-paediatric-guidelines/ggc-guidelines/emergency-medicine/torticollis-congenital-and-acquired-in-children/ [Last accessed August, 2024].

Vaginal Discharge

136

Section Editor: **Gnanamurthy Narasimha**
Section Co-Editor: **Nagalatha Chidananda**
Author: **Nagalatha Chidananda**

Introduction

- The vaginal secretions are usually thin and clear to white in a variable amount.
- Malodorous, abnormal consistency of vaginal discharge accompanied by blood, pain, pruritus, or dysuria is usually pathologic.

Classification

AGE-WISE	ETIOLOGICAL CLASSIFICATION
Prepubertal	Physiological
Postpubertal	Pathological
	• *Infection:* Vulvovaginitis/cervicitis/UTI
	• *Infestation:* Pinworm
	• Inflammatory
	• Atrophic
	• *Malignant:* Rhabdomyosarcoma and endodermal tumors
	• Congenital anomaly
	• *Miscellaneous:* Foreign body/sexual abuse

(UTI: urinary tract infection)

Approach to Diagnosis

- *Onset/duration of symptoms:*
  - *Acute:* Infections
  - *Chronic:* Foreign body, and benign or malignant vaginal tumors
  - *Recurrent:* Recurrent candidiasis—juvenile-onset diabetes and immunosuppression
  - *Cyclical discharge:* Preceding menarche and physiologic discharge
- *Age:*
  - *Neonatal:* Physiological (up to 2 weeks postdelivery), if >2 weeks age—look for maternal infection (herpes simplex/*Trichomonas*)
  - *Prepubertal:* 2–3 months prior to menarche—normally small amount of whitish secretion
  - *Postpubertal:* Just prior to periods—small amount of whitish discharge
- *Risk factors:*
  - Tight clothing
  - Synthetic clothes
  - Wet swimming costumes
  - *Irritants:* Harsh chemical, perfumes, detergents, softeners, creams, and ointments
  - Poor personal hygiene
  - Obesity
- *Associated symptoms:*
  - Dysuria
  - *Pruritus:* Enterobius vermicularis, intense pruritus/lichen sclerosus
  - Infections of the respiratory tract and skin
  - History of foreign body
  - History of sexual abuse
  - History of systemic infections/chronic illness
  - *Type of secretion:* Color, quantity, and consistency
  - *Associated symptoms:* Itching and rashes

Examination

General Physical

- Tanner staging of sexual maturity
- Features of autoimmune diseases, atopic dermatitis, and eczema

Local Examination

- Inspect underwear for the presence of discharge and bleeding.
- Look for vulvar swelling, vesicular lesions, ulcerations, skin excoriation.
- Foreign body
- The presence of discharge, signs of inflammation, smegma, stool contamination, labial adhesions, and whitish discoloration
- Look for fistula, ectopic ureter, polyps, labial adhesions—requires vaginoscopy.
- Per rectal examination, as required
- Visualize the lower part of the vagina, vulva, and anus for signs of trauma such as scars, tears, loss of hymnal continuity that are indicative of sexual abuse.
- Colposcopy, if sexual abuse is suspected

Type of Secretion

DISCHARGE TYPE	DIAGNOSIS
Small, mucoid, whitish, and no odor	Normal physiological
Clear-to-purulent, large quantity, yellowish, greenish, and foul smell	Infection (vaginitis)
Mucopurulent and sometimes bloody discharge	*Shigella flexneri*
Thin, watery, and foul-smelling	*Escherichia coli*
Purulent, thick yellow discharge	*Neisseria gonorrhoeae*
Frothy, watery-yellow or green discharge, malodorous	*Trichomonas*
Painful vulvar eruptions and thin, watery vaginal discharge	Herpes simplex virus
Thick, white, cottage cheese-like, white plaques, and odorless	*Candida albicans*
Persistent, foul-smelling, bloody, or brown discharge	Foreign body
Discharge or bleeding on intravaginal examination	Malignancies

Investigations

TEST	RESULT	DIAGNOSIS
Vaginal cytology	Leukocytes	Infection (sensitive but not specific)
Vaginal smear/culture	Diphtheroids, *Bacteroides* and *Staphylococcus epidermidis*	Normal vaginal flora
	Haemophilus influenzae, group A and B Hemolytic streptococci and *Streptococcus pneumoniae*	Respiratory source
	Gram stain—intracellular pathogens	Gonococcus
	Multinucleated giant cells on vaginal cytology	Herpes
Other tests	Rising serum antibody titer	Herpes
	Sellotape test	Protozoal *Enterobius*
	Motile flagella seen on saline wet mount	*Trichomonas*
	KOH preparation—spores and hyphae	Fungal infection
	Biopsy of suspicious lesions	Malignancies

Red Flag Signs

- Persistent foul-smelling discharge ± blood
- Chronic discharge which bleeds on examination
- History of sexual abuse

Approach to Managing a Child with Vaginal Discharge

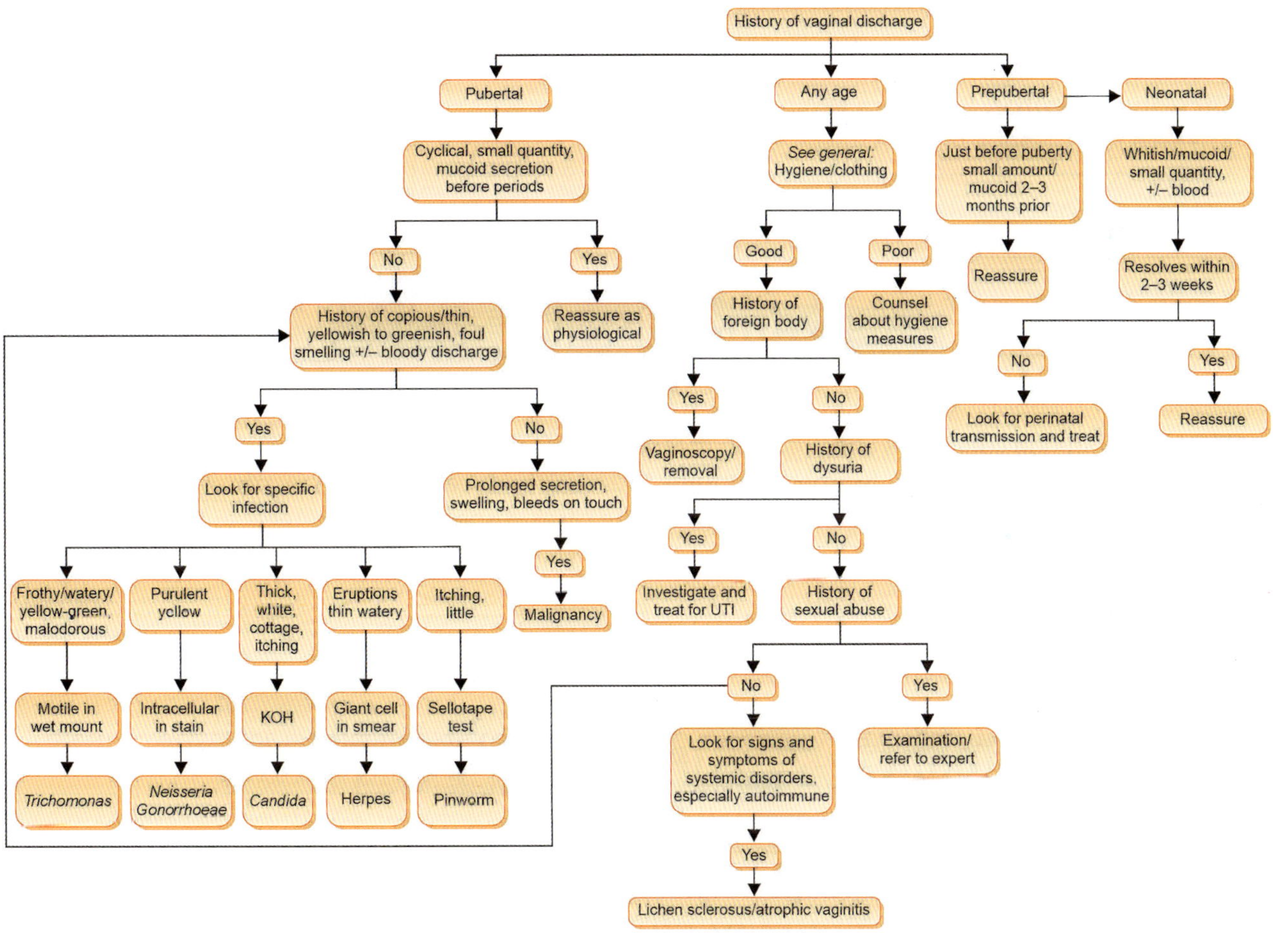

Suggested Reading

- Laufer MR, Emans SJ. In: Drutz JE, Woodward GA, Wiley JF (Eds). (2022). Overview of vulvovaginal conditions in the prepubertal child. [online] Available from https://medilib.ir/uptodate/show/6450 [Last accessed August, 2024].
- Makwela MR. Paediatric vaginal discharge. S Afr Fam Pract. 2007;49(7):30-1.

Skin Infection

137

Section Editor: **B Rajsekhar**
Section Co-Editor: **Suchitra Pusapati**
Author: **Srikrishna RSV**

Introduction

The most common conditions affecting skin in India are infections and infestations, seen in nearly half of the cases overall. Bacterial infections contribute to 27.29% and scabies to 10.16% of cases. Fungal and viral infections are observed in 4.65% and 3.68% of the cases, respectively.

Etiology, Presentation, and Treatment

Bacterial Infections

Pyodermas: Pyoderma is a superficial infection of the skin, caused by bacteria. This includes impetigo, folliculitis, furuncle, ecthyma, and several others.

Impetigo

- *Staphylococcus aureus* and *Streptococcus pyogenes* are the most common causes.
- Variants—bullous and nonbullous impetigo or impetigo contagiosa are the variants. It occurs on the face and the extremities. It evolves from small papulovesicles or pustules that rapidly rupture to form the typical lesions that seem like crusted plaques with honey-colored centers and surrounding erythema. It may have secondary impetiginization.
- Bullous impetigo presents as a thin-walled subcorneal blister that breaks down rapidly, leaving behind a red and moist erosion, surrounded by a typical peripheral remnant of blister roof.

Folliculitis and Furuncle

- It is a superficial infection of the follicular ostia caused by *Staphylococcus* which is seen on the perineum, buttocks, and scalp.
- The superficial red papules and pustules with perilesional erythema may occur without any other symptoms and are centered on the hair follicles.
- Furuncle is a deep-seated infection affecting hair follicles and their surrounding tissue. This leads to an abscess or a tender nodule.

For localized superficial infections, topical mupirocin or fusidic acid is administered until lesions heal. For multiple lesions and deeper infections, systemic antibiotics are prescribed for 7–10 days.

Abscess

- An abscess is a localized collection of pus due to an infection, mostly *S. aureus*.
- It is often painful and swollen, and the area around it can be red, warm, and tender. Pus is a mixture of dead tissue, bacteria, and white blood cells. Treatment is warm compresses to help drain the pus, incision and drainage, and antibiotics.

Cellulitis

- This is a potentially serious bacterial skin infection that affects the deeper layers of the skin, including the dermis and subcutaneous tissue. It is a red swollen area that feels warm and painful on the touch. There would be associated systemic symptoms like fever with chills and fatigue.
- Bacteria, including *Staphylococcus* and *Streptococcus*, cause it.
- Treatment involves local and systemic antibiotics with painkillers.

Rest and elevation of the area help in a quick resolution.

Fungal Infections

Tinea Capitis

- It is seen in prepubertal girls, caused by *Trichophyton tonsurans*.
- Single or multiple patches of hair loss with signs of inflammation seem like pustules or papules with crusting, scaling, and lymphadenopathy. Black dot tinea capitis and Kerion are variants.
- Oral Griseofulvin is the treatment of choice

Tinea Versicolor

- It is seen in young adolescents, caused by *Malassezia furfur*.
- Multiple macules are seen on the back, upper chest, and proximal upper extremities. These are hypopigmented and have scaling. Skin scraping using KOH reveals short, nonbranching hyphae and yeast cells.
- Topical selenium sulfide 2.5% lotion, imidazoles, ciclopirox olamine, and oral ketoconazole or fluconazole are used for treatment.

Viral Infections

Verruca Vulgaris (Common Warts)

- Human papillomavirus (HPV) 1, 2, 4, 7
- Skin- to flesh-colored hyperkeratotic rough surfaced papules on hands, fingers, periungual region, and feet
- Cryodestruction following paring of warts using liquid nitrogen via a spray gun or a cotton swab for 10–20 seconds. Cryotherapy is painful and not suitable for young children.
- Recalcitrant warts: Pulse dye laser, topical salicylic acid and 5-Fluorouracil 5% cream and Imiquimod

Verruca Plana (Plane Warts)

- HPV 3, 10, 28
- Small, flat-topped, skin-colored papules with granular surfaces anywhere on the body
- Koebnerization and autoinoculation are common.
- Topical retinoids for treatment

Plantar Warts

- These are seen on pressure points of metatarsal heads and ball of the foot.
- In contrast to other types of warts, plantar lesions are painful. They may resemble callosities and corn. The presence of typical findings of wart, the thrombosed capillaries, and punctate bleeding points help to differentiate them from other lesions.
- After a topical salicylic acid application for 4 months, aggressive therapy with repeated paring of the lesions was performed. Other options are cryosurgery, trichloroacetic acid, and laser.

Molluscum Contagiosum

- It is a poxvirus infection seen in school-aged children.
- Numerous flesh-colored or pearly white papules with central umbilication, without any other symptoms, are seen.

- Mainly, self-limiting treatment is required to prevent autoinoculation and further spread. Topical cantharidin, removal with a sharp curette, cryotherapy, topical tretinoin, and Imiquimod 5% cream are other options.

Viral Exanthems

- This includes a group of viral infections with maculopapular skin rashes and systemic symptoms like fever, cold, and cough.
- Measles, rubella, roseola, varicella, erythema infectiosum, and hand–foot–mouth disease are the common viral exanthems.
- Most viral exanthems are self-limiting and resolve on their own. Treatment is symptomatic with antipyretics like acetaminophen or ibuprofen, antihistamines or topical soothing lotions like calamine, and hydration and rest.

Parasitic Infections

Parasitic skin infections present as maculopapular rashes with itching caused by parasites.

Scabies

- This is caused by *Sarcoptes scabiei*, which appears as small, red papules with burrows in webs of fingers, wrists, and elbows. They have intense pruritus, and the rash spreads by sharing clothing.
- Treatment includes topical medications (e.g., permethrin cream or ivermectin) applied to the entire body. All household members and close contacts should also be treated.

Red Flags

- Fever with vesicles—needs isolation
- Fever with hemorrhagic rash—requires evaluation and hospitalization
- Fever with widespread rash and altered sensorium—needs admission
- Prolonged fever beyond two weeks with painful rash—further investigation

Algorithm for Evaluation

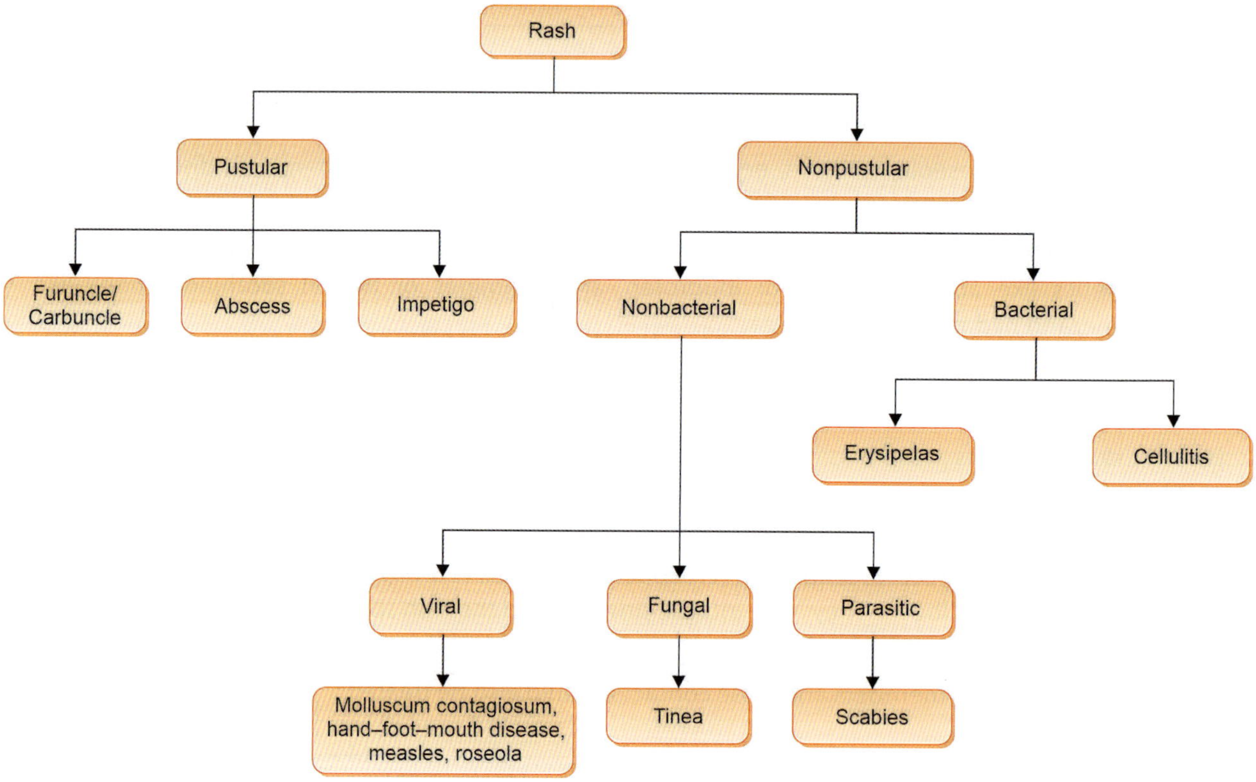

Signs	***Disease***
Koplik spots, morbilliform rash	Measles
Lymphadenopathy, rash after ampicillin	Infectious mononucleosis
Reticulate pattern, slapped cheek appearance	Erythema infectiosum
Lymphadenopathy, morbilliform rash	Roseola

Suggested Reading

- Nelson JSB, Stone MS. Update on selected viral exanthems. Curr Opin Pediatr. 2000;12:359-64.
- Sarkar R, Mishra K, Garg VK. Fever with rash in a child in India. Indian J Dermatol Venereol Leprol. 2012;78: 251-62.
- Sethuraman G, Bhari N. Common skin problems in children. Indian J Pediatr. 2014;81(4):381-90. doi: 10.1007/ s12098-013-1271-9.

Hypopigmented Skin Lesions

138

Section Editor: **Gnanamurthy Narasimha**
Section Co-Editor: **Nagalatha Chidananda**
Author: **C Vijayabhaskar**

Introduction

Hypopigmented skin lesions often trigger concerns among patients and caregivers. These pale patches vary in size and distribution.

Etiology

Hypopigmented skin lesions have several underlying causes:

- *Pityriasis alba:* Commonly seen in children; presents as round/oval hypopigmented patches, single/multiple, with scaling, on the face, sometimes involving the trunks. Is an endogenous eczema; tends to resolve by 15 years of age.
- *Tinea versicolor:* Caused by the yeast *Malassezia furfur*; this fungal infection manifests as hypopigmented or hyperpigmented macules on the trunk and extremities. Warm and humid climates contribute to its prevalence.
- *Polymorphous light eruption:* Occurs due to ultraviolet radiation from sunlight; manifests as scaly, itchy, burning sensation over the sun-exposed areas, especially the face.
- *Hansen's disease:* Due to *Mycobacterium leprae*; is more common in South India; manifests as a hypopigmented, anesthetic patch, involving the face and the body. Tuberculoid and borderline tuberculoid types are common among children.
- *Vitiligo:* A chronic autoimmune condition characterized by the destruction of melanocytes, leading to depigmented patches on the skin. Early vitiligo presents as hypopigmented patches. It affects individuals of all ages and ethnicities; prevalence is notably higher in South Asian populations.
- *Postinflammatory hypopigmentation:* Often follows conditions like eczema, impetigo, psoriasis, or atopic dermatitis.
- Topical steroids/demelanizing cream applications can lead to hypopigmentations.

Red Flag Signs

- Hypopigmented, hypoanesthetic patches—suspect Hansen's disease
- Hypopigmented patches turning to depigmented lesions
- Ashy leaf macule at the time of birth or later—tuberous sclerosis complex. Close follow-up required.
- Hypomelanosis of Ito—might be associated with central nervous system (CNS), skeletal and eye abnormalities—requires appropriate referral

Relevant Investigations

Mostly, hypopigmented patches are diagnosed clinically. In case of suspicion, the following investigations can be done:

- *KOH (potassium hydroxide) test:* To diagnose tinea versicolor by demonstrating the characteristic spaghetti and meatball appearance of hyphae and spores under microscopy
- *Skin biopsy:* Histopathological examination may be necessary for cases where diagnosis is uncertain, especially in distinguishing between Hansen's disease, vitiligo, and other hypopigmented conditions.
- *Wood's lamp examination:* Useful to differentiate between vitiligo and other hypopigmentary disorders. In vitiligo, affected areas fluoresce bright white under Wood's lamp due to absent melanin.

Approach to Hypopigmented Patches

Approach to hypopigmented patches is given in **Table 1**.

TABLE 1: Approach to hypopigmented patches.

APPROACH	CONDITIONS
Hypopigmented patches with scaling	• *Pityriasis alba*: Asymptomatic, hypopigmented scaly patches with an ill-defined border • *Pityriasis versicolor*: Well-defined hypopigmented patches with fine scales • *Polymorphous light eruption*: Varied morphology, hypersensitivity to UV radiation, with itching or burning sensation • *Seborrheic dermatitis*: Multiple scaly hypopigmented macules, associated with dandruff
Hypopigmented patches without scaling	• *Hansen's disease*: Impaired sensation • *Early vitiligo*: Difficult diagnosis. • *Postinflammatory hypopigmented patches*: Nonscaly patches over previous dermatoses • *Nevus anemicus or achromicus*: Present since birth • Steroid-induced hypopigmented patches
Hypopigmented patches with organ involvement	• *Hypomelanosis of Ito*: Hypopigmentation with skeletal, central nervous system (CNS), or eye abnormalities • *Tuberous sclerosis complex*: Ashy leaf macule at birth, other organ involvement

Approach to Managing Hypopigmented Skin Lesions

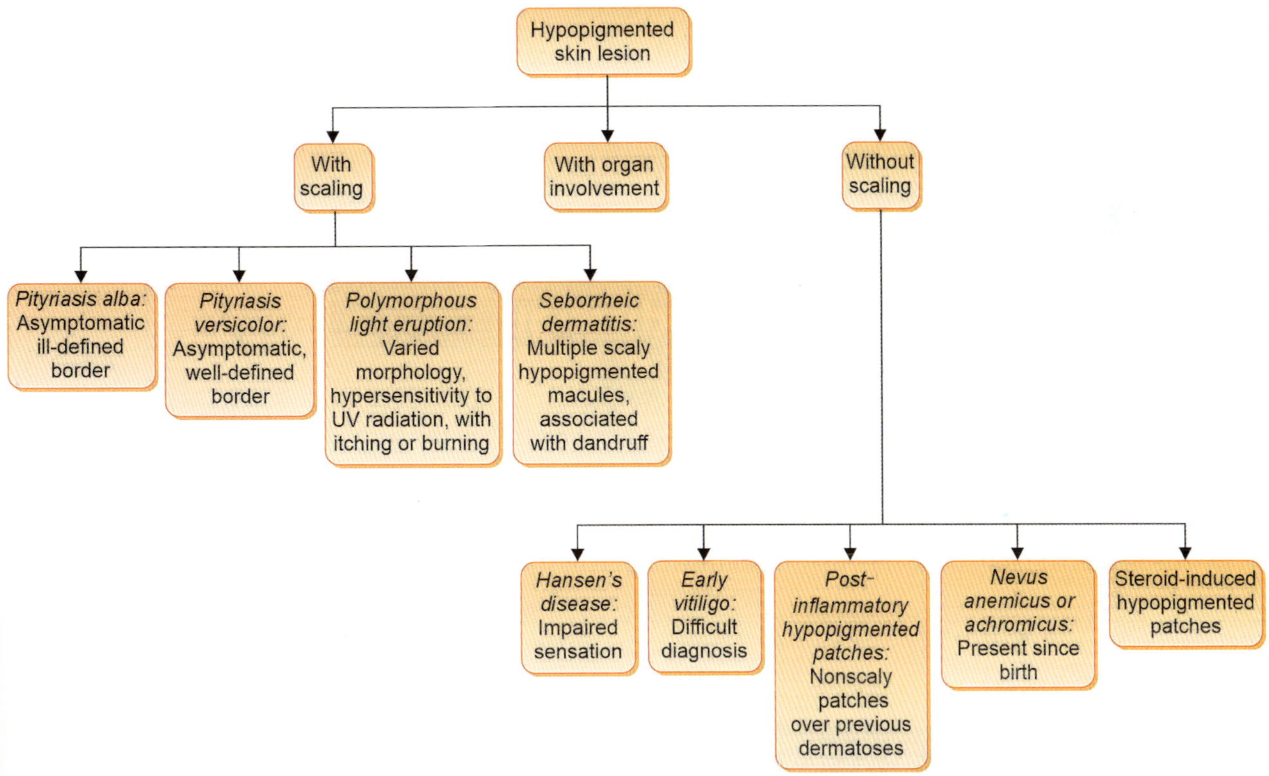

Suggested Reading

- Hill JP, Batchelor JM. An approach to hypopigmentation. BMJ. 2017;356:i6534.
- Madireddy S, Crane JS. Hypopigmented macules. [Updated 2023 Jun 28]. In: StatPearls [Internet]. Treasure Island (FL): StatPearls Publishing; 2024 Jan-. Available from https://www.ncbi.nlm.nih.gov/books/NBK556054/ [Last accessed September, 2024].
- Poon S, Beach RA. Localised hypopigmentation: clarification of a diagnostic conundrum. Br J Gen Pract. 2018;68(674):444-5.

Hyperpigmented Patches

139

Section Editor: **Gnanamurthy Narasimha**
Section Co-Editor: **Nagalatha Chidananda**
Author: **Gowri Somayaji**

Introduction

- Hyperpigmented rashes are patches of skin that are darker than the surrounding areas, often due to an excess of melanin.
- These may be *congenital* or acquired in childhood.
- The hyperpigmented patches may be diffuse or patchy in appearance.

Etiology

Etiology of hyperpigmented patches is given in **Table 1**.

TABLE 1: Etiology of hyperpigmented patches.

DIFFUSE	PATCHY	RETICULAR
Addison's	Café-au-lait macules	Tinea versicolor
Hemochromatosis	Freckle (ephelides)	Retained keratin
Ochronosis	Lentigo	Erythema ab igne
Chronic renal disease	Becker nevus	Reticulated/confluent papillomatosis
Drug or heavy metal—induced	*Mongolian spot*	Reticulated acropigmentation of Kitamura
Metastatic malignant melanoma	Nevus of Ota/Ito	Dowling–Degos disease
Bronze baby syndrome	Junctional melanocytic nevus	*Dyskeratosis congenita*
Vitamin B_{12} deficiency	Postinflammatory hyperpigmentation	Naegeli–Franceschetti–Jadassohn syndrome

Contd...

Contd...

DIFFUSE	PATCHY	RETICULAR
Familial progressive hyperpigmentation	Tinea versicolor	Hidrotic ectodermal dysplasia
Adrenoleukodystrophy	Melasma	
Lichen planus pigmentosus	Drug-induced	
Progressive systemic sclerosis	*Incontinentia pigmenti*	
	Morphea	
	Urticaria pigmentosa	
	Mosaic hypopigmentation	
	Phytophotodermatitis	
	Erythema dyschromicum perstans	
	Acanthosis nigricans	
	Chikungunya	
	Peutz–Jeghers syndrome	

Approach to Diagnosis

A detailed history is essential. It should include the following:

- Onset and duration
- *Associated symptoms:* Itching and pain
- *Systemic symptoms:* Neurologic, gastrointestinal (GI), renal, and endocrine symptoms
- Exposure to sun, vegetable matter, drugs, and toxins
- *Diet:* Nutrient deficiency, excessive calories, and fads
- *Preceding illness:* Fever and body ache
- Family history of similar lesions or other skin lesions
- *Lifestyle:* Sedentary and excessive sun exposure

Examination

- *Local examination:* Size, shape, number, texture, and surrounding erythema and areas involved
- *Systemic examination:* Body mass index (BMI)/weight/growth and development/nutritional status, and associated GI/renal/endocrine involvement

Investigations

- Most often, these rashes are benign, self-limiting, and do not require investigations.
- If an underlying systemic illness is suspected, investigate to establish the diagnosis and extent of illness
- Skin biopsies are rarely required
- Refer to endocrinologist/other specialists, as required

Red Flag Signs

- Dehydration/extreme fatigue/salt craving
- Neurological signs/symptoms like neuroregression, seizures, and progressive weakness
- Failure to thrive
- Multisystem involvement
- Positive family history

Algorithm to Management

The approach to management of hyperpigmented patches is given in **Flowchart 1.**

FLOWCHART 1: Approach to management of hyperpigmented patches.

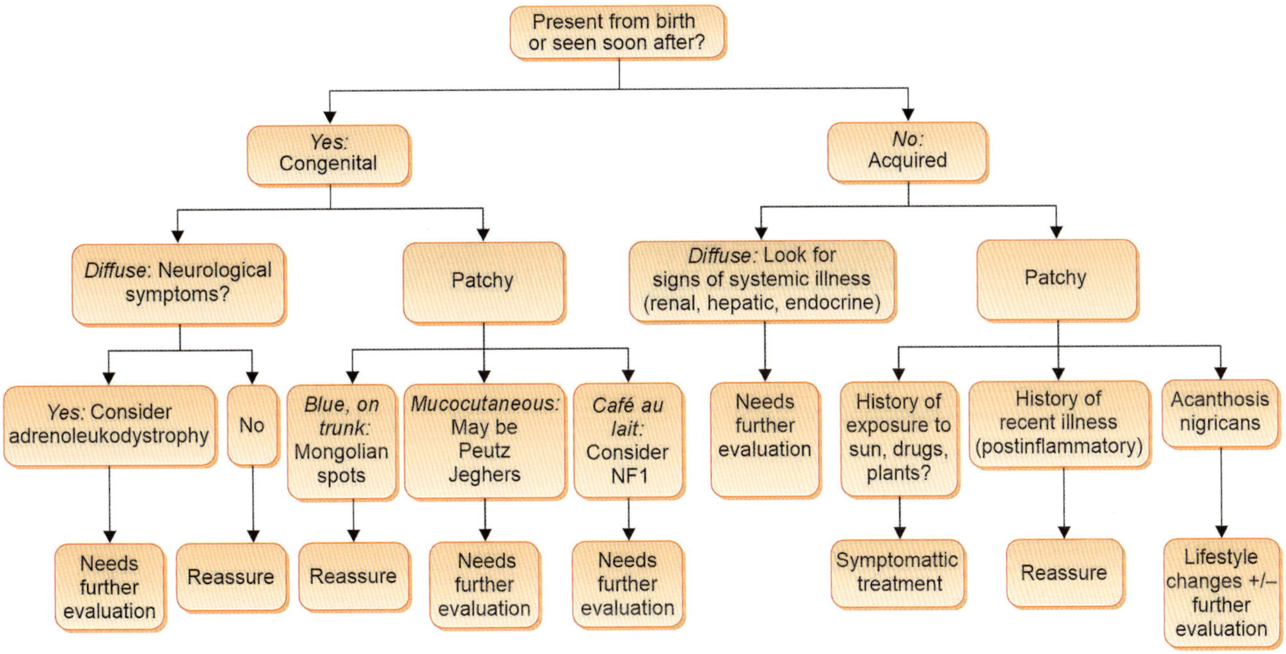

Suggested Reading

- Gulati R, Balaji J, Rathod R. (2022). IAP Standard Treatment Guidelines 2022. Hyperpigmented Lesions in Children. [online]. Available from https://iapindia.org/pdf/Ch-122-Hyperpigmented-Lesions-in-Children.pdf [Last accessed August, 2024].
- Pride HB, Yan AC, Zaenglein AL (Eds). Pediatric Dermatology: Requisites in Dermatology. Philadelphia: Saunders, Elsevier; 2008.
- Sori T, Jaisankar TJ, Thappa DM, Nath AK. Hyperpigmentary disorders in children: A hospital-based study in a tertiary care center. Indian Dermatol Online J. 2013;4(2):148-52.
- Weinberg S, Prose NS, Kristal L (Eds). Weinberg's Color Atlas of Pediatric Dermatology, 4th edition. New York, NY: McGraw Hill; 2007. pp. 267-84.

Scrotal Swelling

140

Section Editor: **Gnanamurthy Narasimha**
Section Co-Editor: **Nagalatha Chidananda**
Authors: **Soundharya S, Ramesh Santhana Krishnan**

Inguinal Hernia

- *Etiology:* Failure of closure of processus vaginalis with persistent communication between abdomen and scrotum causing herniation of bowel and other contents
- *Incidence:* 0.8–4.4%; Higher incidence in premature infants (16–25%)
- *Age:* Most commonly presents during the 1st year of life, but can be seen at any age
- *Sex:* Higher incidence in males than females
- *Laterality:* Right more common than left; bilateral hernias are seen in 10% of cases

Clinical Presentation

- Bulge in the inguinal region and/or scrotum and labia
- *Intermittent:* Increases with increased abdominal pressure like crying and straining and decreases on rest

Examination

- Swelling in inguinal/inguinoscrotal region
- Cry impulse or cough impulse present
- Reducible
- *Silk glove sign:* Finger is rubbed over the cord from side to side at the site of pubic tubercle. Positive sign is the feeling of rubbing two pieces of silk together. This sign is subjective and may not be accurate.
- Sometimes, hernia may not be demonstrable on examination, but parents have photographic evidence of hernia, which is accepted by most surgeons.

Complications

- *Incarcerated hernia:* It is the entrapment of bowel or other organs within the hernia sac. Child presents with an irreducible swelling in the inguinoscrotal region with pain and irritability, which progresses to symptoms of intestinal obstruction like abdominal distension, and vomiting.
- *Strangulated hernia:* Incarcerated hernia when not reduced can lead to loss of vascularity of trapped contents and gangrene of bowel. There may be features of peritonitis.

Investigations

- *Ultrasonography (USG):* Some studies have shown accuracy up to 97%; hence, it is a fairly reliable investigation, especially in equivocal cases.

Management

- Inguinal hernia will not resolve spontaneously.
- Surgery is the treatment of choice—inguinal herniotomy.
- *Approaches for surgery:* it can be done by open repair or laparoscopic repair depending on the age of the patient and the expertise of the surgeon.
- *Timing of surgery:* Surgery is recommended soon after diagnosis to prevent complications. For premature infants, surgery is recommended before discharge, after the baby has reached a weight of 2 kg.
- Surgery is performed as a daycare procedure for older children and advised overnight stay for neonates and infants.
- *Incarcerated hernia:* Manual reduction of hernia can be attempted after making the child calm or by using sedation. If reduced, surgery is performed after 24–48 hours to allow time for reduction of edema.
- Incarcerated hernia that has failed attempts of manual reduction and strangulated hernia require emergency surgery.

Congenital Hydrocele

Etiology: Collection of fluid around the testis between the layers of tunica.

Types

- *Communicating hydrocele:* Has a patent processus vaginalis with free flow of fluid between peritoneum and scrotum.
- *Noncommunicating hydrocele (more common):* Collection of fluid around the testis with obliteration of processus vaginalis proximal to it.

Clinical Features

- Scrotal swelling, painless.
- If communicating, there is a history of scrotal swelling that varies in size. Size increases during the day in an upright position and decreases at night in the supine position.

Examination

- Scrotal swelling, nontender, and transillumination positive.

Investigations

- USG can be used for radiological confirmation of hydrocele, if required.

Management

- Noncommunicating hydrocele usually resolves by 2 years of age, so initial management is to wait and watch.
- Communicating hydrocele or hydroceles that persist beyond 2 years of age require surgery (inguinal herniotomy).

Clinical Algorithm

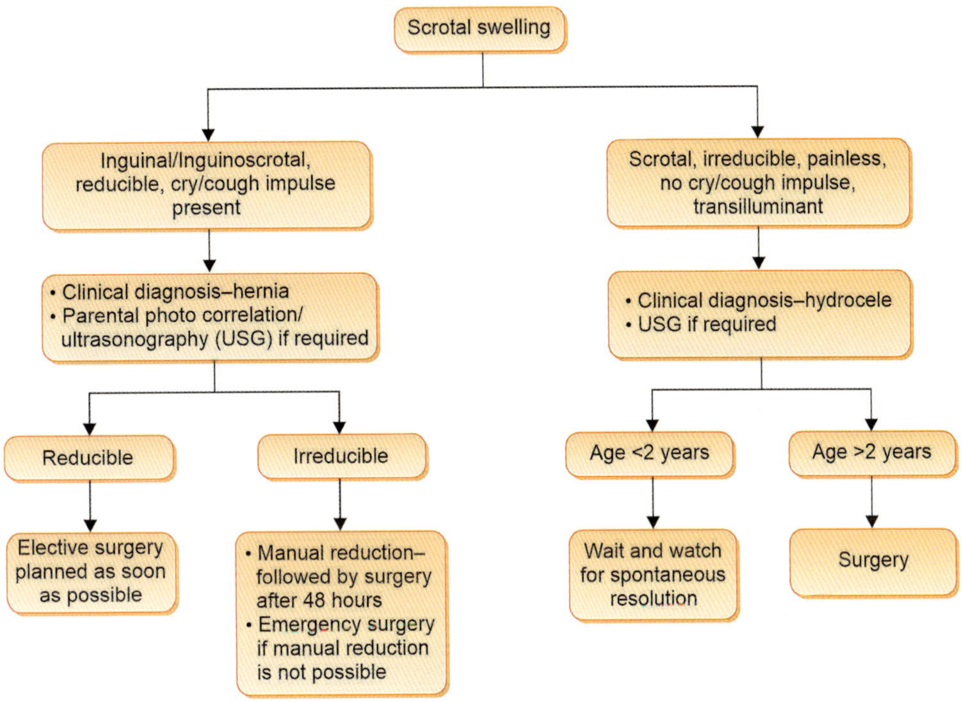

Suggested Reading

- Esposito C, Escolino M, Turrà F, Roberti A, Cerulo M, Farina A, et al. Current concepts in the management of inguinal hernia and hydrocele in pediatric patients in laparoscopic era. Semin Pediatr Surg. 2016;25(4): 232-40.
- Glick PL, Boulanger SC. Inguinal hernias and hydroceles. In: Coran AG, Caldamone A, Adzick NS, Krummel TM, Laberge JM, Shamberger R (Eds.). Pediatric Surgery, 7th edition. Philadelphia: Elsevier Saunders; 2012. pp. 985-1001.
- Lau ST, Lee YH, Caty MG. Current management of hernias and hydroceles. Semin Pediatr Surg. 2007;16(1):50-7.

Annexure

Congenital Orthopedic Malformation

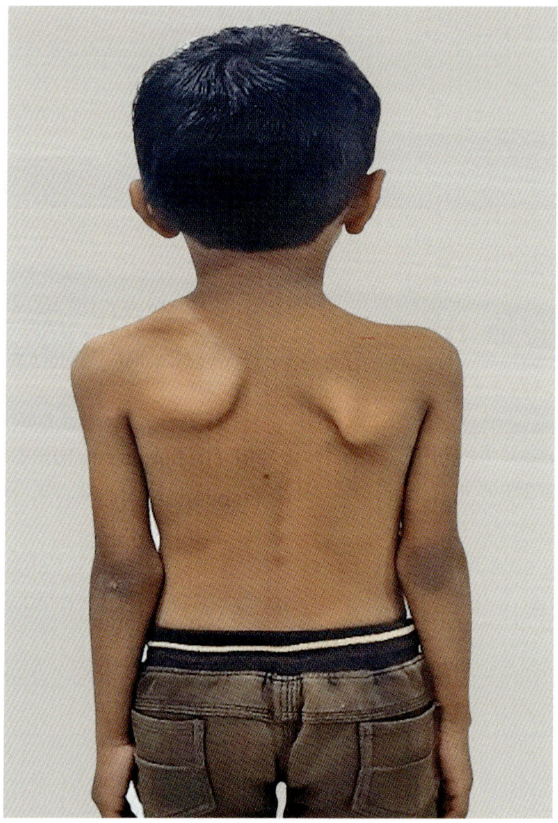

FIG. 1: Left Sprengel's shoulder with elevated scapula.

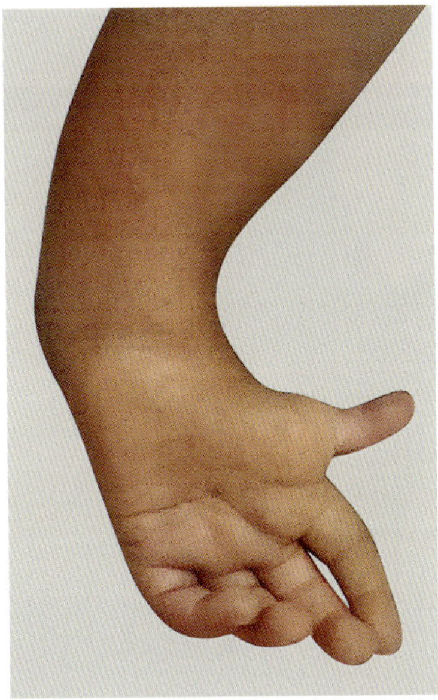

FIG. 2: Radial club hand with deformity at wrist.

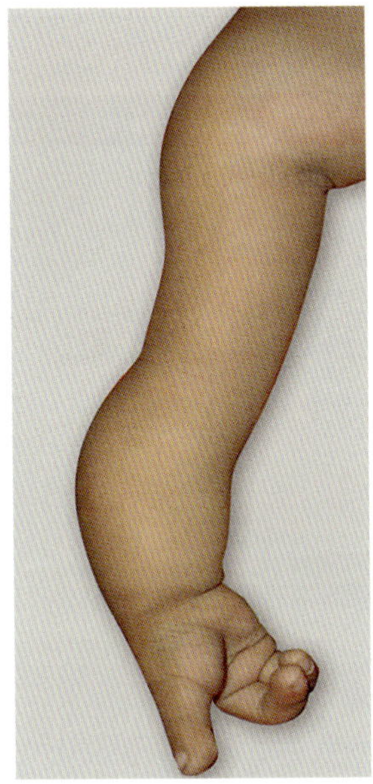

FIG. 3: Ulnar club hand with absent medial fingers.

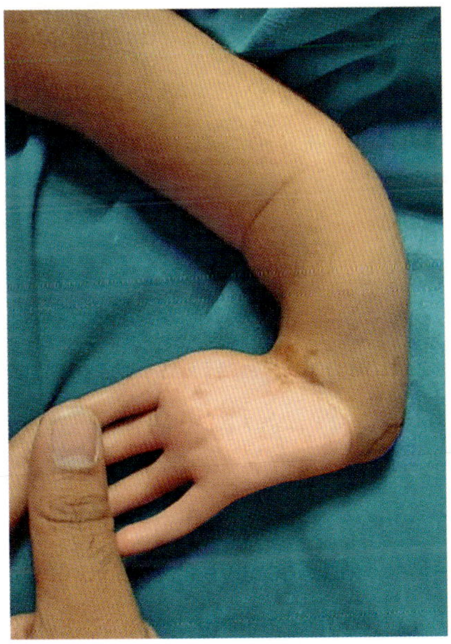

FIG. 4: *Absent thumb:* Hypoplastic/absent thumb (could be part of radial club hand).

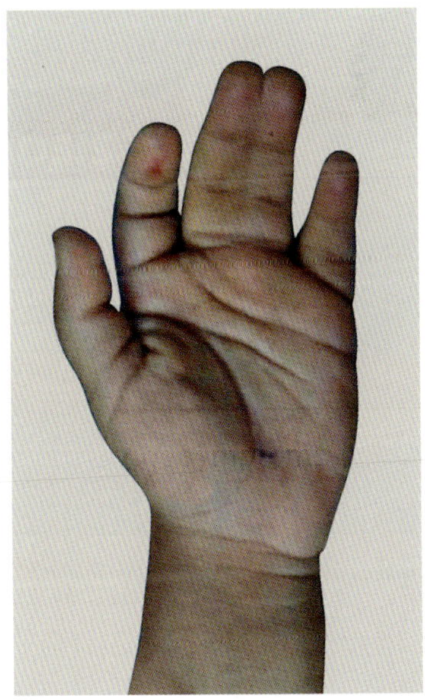

FIG. 5: Syndactyly: Fused 3rd–4th fingers.

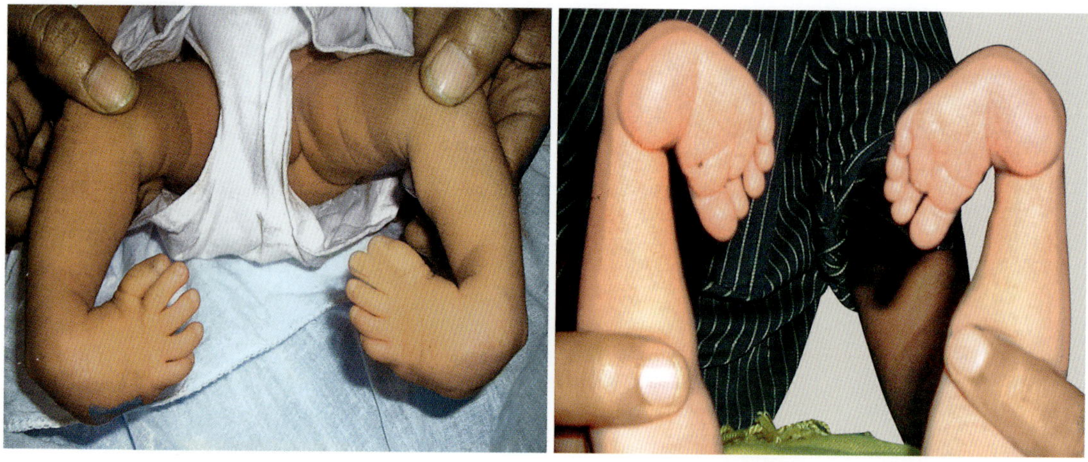

FIG. 6: Bilateral congenital talipes equinovarus (CTEV)/clubfeet.

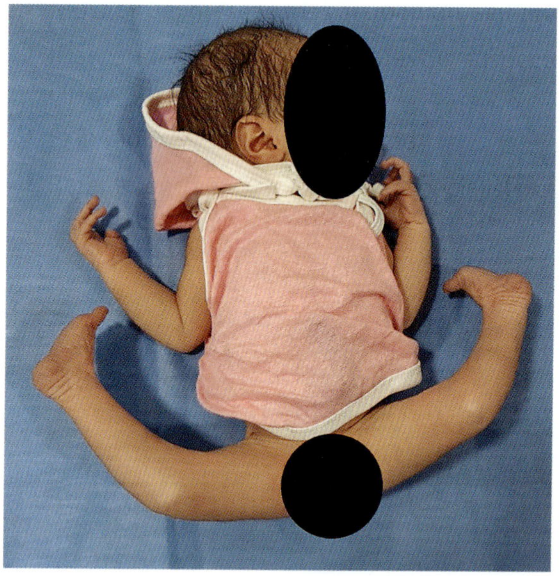

FIG. 7: Bilateral congenital dislocation of knee.

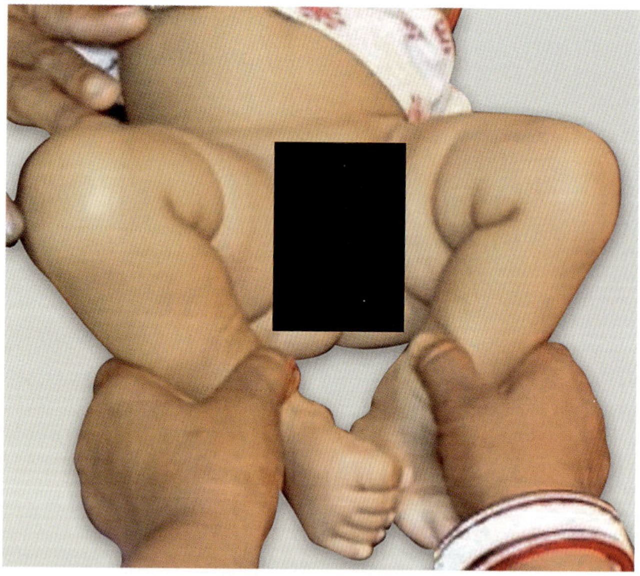

FIG. 8: Right developmental dysplasia of the hip (DDH) with short thigh segment and decreased hip abduction.

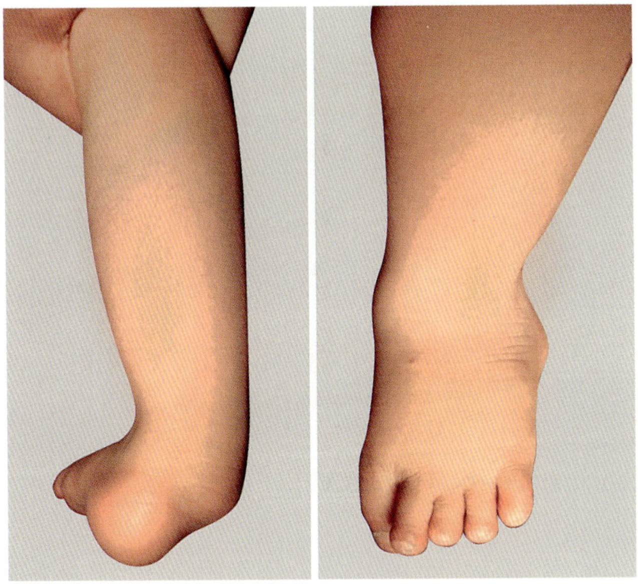

FIG. 9: Right fibular hemimelia.

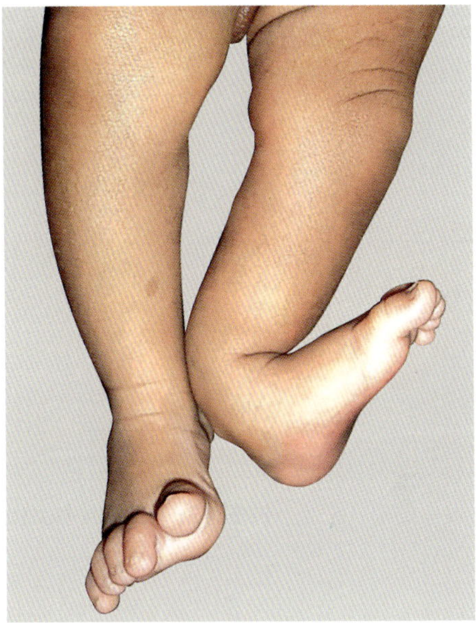

FIG. 10: Posteromedial bowing of leg.

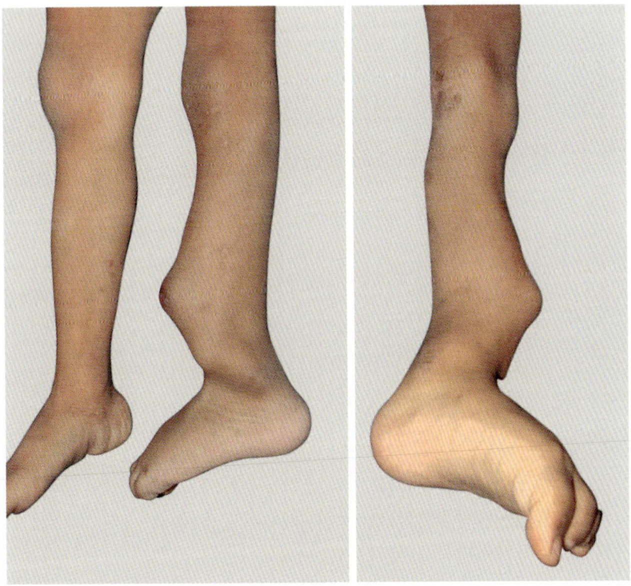

FIG. 11: Anterolateral bowing of leg.

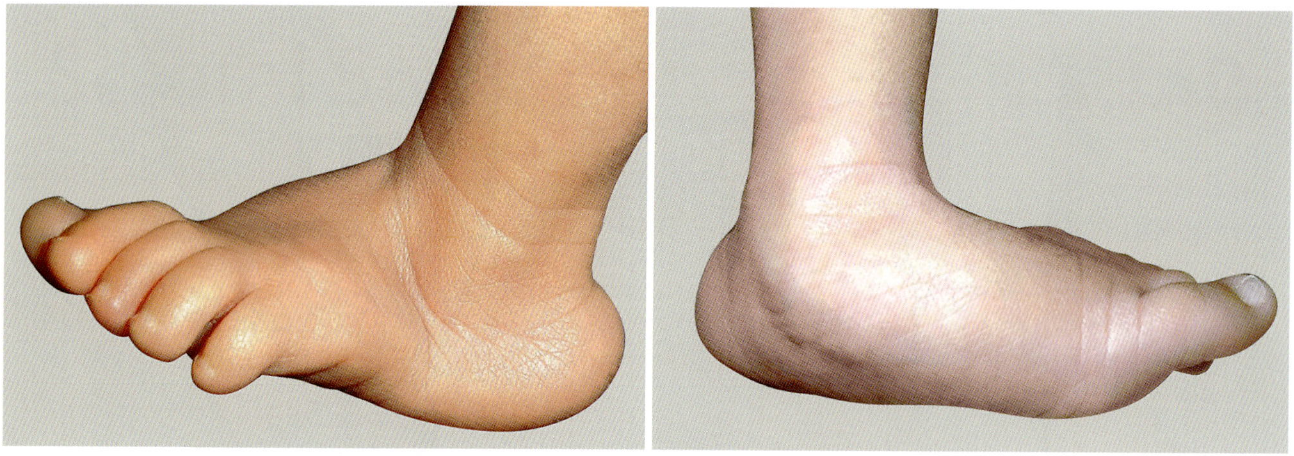

FIG. 12: Rocker-bottom foot of congenital vertical talus (CVT).

Note: All the clinical pictures are original and prior written consent has been obtained from parents.

Index

Page numbers followed by *b* refer to box, *f* refer to figure, *fc* refer to flowchart, and *t* refer to table.

A

B

D

E

F

I

J

K

L

M

P

R

S

V

W

X

Y

Z